AF753380

Thieme

# Mammography Casebook

## 100 Studies in Breast Imaging

Uwe Fischer, M.D.
Professor
Women's Health Care Center
Goettingen, Germany

Friedemann Baum, M.D.
Women's Health Care Center
Goettingen, Germany

With contributions by
Laszlo Fuezesi and Dorit von Heyden

1715 illustrations
168 tables

Thieme
Stuttgart · New York

The bookmark included with this book lists the most important parameters in breast diagnosis (description of lesions, xray, MR mammography and sonography criteria, BI-RADS categorization, MRI score etc.). Please note that this data is also repeated on page 1.

*Library of Congress Cataloging-in-Publication Data*
Fischer, Uwe, 1949–
[Trainer mammadiagnostik. English]
Mammography casebook / Uwe Fischer, Friedemann Baum.
p. ; cm.
Authorized translation of: Trainer mammadiagnostik, 2005.
ISBN 3-13-140351-9 (alk. paper) –
ISBN 1-58890-350-8 (alk. paper)
1. Breast–Radiography–Case studies.
2. Breast–Imaging–Case studies.
3. Breast–Diseases–Diagnosis–Case studies.
4. Breast–Cancer–Diagnosis–Case studies.

[DNLM: 1. Breast Neoplasms–diagnosis–Case Reports. 2. Diagnosis, Differential–Case Reports. 3. Mammography–methods–Case Reports. WP 870 F536t 2006a] I. Baum, Friedemann. II. Title.

RG493.5.R33F5713 2006
618.1'907572–dc22

2005028398

This book is an authorized translation of the German edition published and copyrighted 2005 by Georg Thieme Verlag, Stuttgart, Germany. Title of the German edition: Trainer Mammadiagnostik. Fallsammlung – 100 kommentierte Kasuistiken.

Illustrator: Barbara Gay, Stuttgart

**Important note:** Medicine is an ever-changing science undergoing continual development. Research and clinical experience are continually expanding our knowledge, in particular our knowledge of proper treatment and drug therapy. Insofar as this book mentions any dosage or application, readers may rest assured that the authors, editors, and publishers have made every effort to ensure that such references are in accordance with **the state of knowledge at the time of production of the book.**

Nevertheless, this does not involve, imply, or express any guarantee or responsibility on the part of the publishers in respect to any dosage instructions and forms of applications stated in the book. **Every user is requested to examine carefully** the manufacturers' leaflets accompanying each drug and to check, if necessary in consultation with a physician or specialist, whether the dosage schedules mentioned therein or the contraindications stated by the manufacturers differ from the statements made in the present book. Such examination is particularly important with drugs that are either rarely used or have been newly released on the market. Every dosage schedule or every form of application used is entirely at the user's own risk and responsibility. The authors and publishers request every user to report to the publishers any discrepancies or inaccuracies noticed. If errors in this work are found after publication, errata will be posted at www.thieme.com on the product description page.

© 2006 Georg Thieme Verlag
Rüdigerstraße 14
70469 Stuttgart
Germany
http://www.thieme.de
Thieme New York
333 Seventh Avenue
New York, NY 10 001 USA
http://www.thieme.com

Cover photo background: Photo Alto, Paris
Typesetting by Ziegler und Müller, Kirchentellinsfurt
Printed in Germany by Karl Grammlich GmbH, Pliezhausen

ISBN 3-13-140351-9 (GTV)
ISBN 1-58890-350-8 (TNY)

1 2 3 4 5

Some of the product names, patents, and registered designs referred to in this book are in fact registered trademarks or proprietary names even though specific reference to this fact is not always made in the text. Therefore, the appearance of a name without designation as proprietary is not to be construed as a representation by the publisher that it is in the public domain.

This book, including all parts thereof, is legally protected by copyright. Any use, exploitation, or commercialization outside the narrow limits set by copyright legislation, without the publisher's consent, is illegal and liable to prosecution. This applies in particular to photostat reproduction, copying, mimeographing, preparation of microfilms, and electronic data processing and storage.

# Preface

Breast cancer is one of the most common malignant tumors among women in many parts of the world today. In addition, it is also one of the leading causes of cancer death. In contrast to the situation for many other malignant tumors, modern imaging modalities allow the early diagnosis of breast cancers, most often in asymptomatic women. Generally, the earlier a cancerous lesion is detected, the better the prognosis. The early detection of a suspicious lesion is not only, however, the conclusion of the diagnostic work-up. In many situations it is important to further clarify the nature of the lesion by performing additional imaging and/or percutaneous biopsy. Furthermore, in the case of malignancy, it is necessary to rule out or verify the presence of additional cancerous manifestations. A complete diagnostic work-up is the prerequisite for achieving the best possible individual outcome on the one hand, and for reducing the number of unnecessary open biopsies on the other.

Terminology and strategic proceedings in breast diagnostics have changed to a greater extent than in other diagnostic imaging areas over the last years. The limitations of certain imaging techniques can often be compensated for by the performance of additional procedures. To attain the maximum of relevant diagnostic information, it is important to be aware and informed about the strengths and weaknesses of the physical examination, x-ray mammography, ultrasonography, and MR mammography. Numerous studies have evaluated the efficiency and limitations of each of these components of breast diagnostics. X-ray mammography remains the primary technique in the early diagnosis of breast cancer. It allows the detection of breast carcinoma in its earliest stages, when prognosis is best, through the visualization of minimal tumor induced changes. In addition, when mammography is performed in asymptomatic women, it allows the detection of occult carcinomas. For these reasons, mammography continues to be indispensable. Screening programs in European countries and the USA, however, have shown the performance of x-ray mammography alone to have major limitations. Its sensitivity in women with dense breast tissue, a relevant number, is significantly reduced.

The complementary performance of breast ultrasonography in women with dense breast tissue can often compensate for the limitations of mammography in these cases. Especially in the hands of an experienced examiner, ultrasonography allows the visualization of mammographically inaccessible areas of the breast due to dense tissue. Furthermore, ultrasound has no known health risks and is the standard imaging method used for examining younger women, and is also obligatory in the work-up of a patient with an indeterminate palpable lesion. In contrast to mammography and ultrasound, MR mammography not only provides information on the morphology of breast lesions, but also investigates vascularization as a metabolic-dependant characteristic. As with x-ray mammography, however, MR mammography is a widely standardized procedure which allows the acquisition of comparable image sets over time. Specialized image post-processing accentuates suspicious findings for the viewer.

In addition to the importance of the appropriate application of the various examination modalities in the diagnostic work-up of breast lesions, examination techniques, image analysis, assessment, and the ensuing therapeutic consequences should be in agreement with national and international standards. The image quality of mammography, for example, has been categorized according to the PGMI-criteria of the British national health service breast screening program (NHSBSP). The basis for terminology and lesion assessment used in mammographic image analysis was presented in the BI-RADS ™ lexicon by the American College of Radiology (ACR), and has since been firmly established in the German speaking countries of Europe. An analogous US-BIRADS lexicon serving as the basis for breast ultrasound image analysis was presented by the breast sonography work group of the "Deutsche Gesellschaft für Ultraschall in der Medizin" (DEGUM, German Society for Medical Ultrasound Applications). For the interpretation and assessment of MR mammograms there is the so-called "Goettinger Score" and its derivative, the MRM-BIRADS-categorization. New aspects considered in MR mammographic interpretation pertain to the degree of contrast enhancement seen in the normal parenchyma (MRM-Density-Type 1 – 4), and the extent of motion artifacts in the subtraction image (MRM-Artifact-Score 1 – 4). Both parameters represent a measure of the diagnostic sensitivity of the examination. Pictorial representations of the relevant classifications are included in this book in tabular form as a removable appendix.

The detection of a suspicious lesion in the breast usually requires the performance of further diagnostic procedures. In the presented clinical cases we show examples where the interventional diagnostic work-up usually conforms with the well-established guidelines and standards. In some cases, however, deviations from the standard course of action are shown to illustrate alternative procedures when the individual case demands it, or to allow for patients' wishes.

This book offers the reader the opportunity to make deliberations and decisions on 100 example cases in breast diagnostics. Each case includes information about patient complaints, personal history, risk profile, and clinical findings. The reader is able to view the relevant image material at his/her leisure and come to his/her own conclusions. He/She is able to practice analyzing and describing the images, as well as making an assessment after taking the possible differential diagnoses into account. On the pages following each case, an explicit commentary explains which diagnostic procedures were performed and the actual, often histologically verified diagnosis is revealed. In this way the interested reader is able to achieve a maximal training effect.

Because most of the presented images in this book are digital, the printed images are of high quality without loss of image information. This provides the reader with image material that allows a realistic evaluation. There are only a few exceptions when patients presented in our clinic with recently performed conventional mammograms. When not otherwise indicated as examinations not performed by the authors, all breast sonograms were performed with a Logic 5 (General Electric MS). The digital mammograms were performed using the full field digital mammography system Senograph 2000D (General Electric MS). MR mammography and MR interventions were performed using the Echospeed system (General Electric MS; MRI Device). Stereotactic interventions were performed on the Lorad-Premium intervention table (Medicor). The Vacora System (Bard) was used for stereotactic vacuum biopsies.

Our special thanks for helping make this book possible go to the team at the Diagnostisches Brustzentrum Goettingen: Anja El Hajab, Doris Hermes, Gudrun Meyer, Jutta Rüschoff, and Christina Vujecic.

Uwe Fischer
Friedemann Baum

# Contents

Numbers in **bold** type refer to case numbers, normal type refers to page numbers.

# Abbreviations

| | |
|---|---|
| **ACR** | American College of Radiology |
| **ADH** | atypical ductal hyperplasia |
| **BCT** | breast conservation therapy |
| **BIRADS** | Breast Imaging Reporting and Data System (ACR) |
| **C1-5** | cytology classification of malignancy 1 – 5 |
| **CC** | craniocaudal (view) |
| **LCIS** | lobular carcinoma in situ |
| **CM** | contrast medium |
| **DC** | ductal carcinoma |
| **DCIS** | ductal carcinoma in situ |
| **EIC** | extensive intraductal component |
| **FNAP** | Fine needle aspiration punction |
| **G1–4** | tumor cell grade 1 – 4 |
| **G** | good (PGMI) |
| **I** | intermediate (PGMI) |
| **IDC** | invasive ductal carcinoma |
| **ILC** | invasive lobular carcinoma |
| **IR** | inversion recovery |
| **LH** | lobular hyperplasia |
| **LM** | lateromedial (view) |
| **M** | moderately good (PGMI) |
| **M 0–1** | hematomatous metastases |
| **MIP** | maximum intensity projection |
| **ML** | mediolateral (view) |
| **MLO** | mediolateral oblique (view) |
| **MR** | magnetic resonance |
| **MRI** | magnetic resonance imaging |
| **MRM** | magnetic resonance mammography |
| **OPTIPACK concept** | digital dose-reduced one-view-mammography plus contrast-enhanced MR imaging of the breast |
| **P** | perfect (PGMI) |
| **PGMI** | UK system of mammogram classification: P (Perfect), G (Good), M (Moderate), I (Inadequate) |
| **pN** | lymph node status classification (histologically verified) |
| **pT** | tumor size classification (histologically verified) |
| **pTis** | histologically verified intraductal carcinoma |
| **R0–2** | residual tumor classification 0 – 2 |
| **R1** | microscopic residual tumor (incomplete tumor resection) |
| **ROI** | region of interest |
| **SN** | Sentinel node activity at axillary dissection |
| **TC** | tubular carcinoma |
| **US** | ultrasound/ultrasonography |
| **VB** | vacuum biopsy |
| **VNPI** | Van Nuys Prognostic Index |

# TNM Classification of Breast Carcinomas

Breast cancers are classified based on histopathology of the primary tumor (T stage), regional nodal status as confirmed by histopathology (N stage), and distant metastases (M stage).

In case multiple simultaneous carcinomas exist in one breast, T stage is determined by the carcinoma with the highest T stage. If carcinomas exist in both breasts, each breast is staged separately. The size of invasive carcinomas is determined based on the size of the invasive component only.

| | |
|---|---|
| TX | Primary tumor cannot be assessed (for example: no histology available) |
| T0 | No primary tumor detected (p is added if tissue was histopathologically assessed) |
| pTis | ductal carcinoma in situ (DCIS) or lobular carcinoma in situ (LCIS) or Paget's disease of the nipple without DCIS, LSIS or invasive tumor in the breast. (If invasive tumor, DCIS, or LCIS is detected in the breast, the disease is staged based on these entities.) |
| pT1 | tumor ≤ 20 mm |
| T1mic | microinvasion: The basal membrane has been exceeded in one or more foci. No focus exceeds 1 mm in size |
| pT1a | ≤ 5mm |
| pT1b | 5mm < tumor ≤ 10 mm |
| pT1c | 10mm < tumor ≤ 20 mm |
| pT2 | 20mm < tumor ≤ 50 mm |
| pT3 | tumor > 50 mm |
| pT4 | tumor of any size that invades skin or chest wall* |
| pT4a | invasion of chest wall* |
| pT4b | skin edema, ulceration, or cutaneous satellite nodule** |
| pT4c | T4a + b |
| pT4d | inflammatory carcinoma (inflammatory carcinoma without proof of in-breast tumor and with negative skin biopsy is classified as pTX) |
| N | concerns histopathologic staging of the regional lymph nodes (lymph node groups, see Appendix 2). So far this included at least sampling of ≥ six lymph nodes of level 1. |
| NX | regional lymph nodes cannot be assessed (for example: had been removed before or were not sampled) |
| pN0 | no regional lymph-node metastases |
| pN1 | mobile metastatic lymph node(s) of the ipsilateral axilla |
| pN1a | only micrometastases (≤ 2 mm) |
| pN1b | at least one metastasis > 2 mm |
| i | one ore more metastases in 1 – 3 lymph nodes all < 20 mm |
| ii | ≥ 4 lymph nodes with all foci < 20 mm |
| iii | metastatic involvement exceeds lymph-node capsule, but all foci < 20 mm |
| iv | metastatic focus or foci ≥ 20 mm |
| pN2 | metastatic lymph nodes located in the ipsilateral axilla and fixed to one another or to surrounding structures |
| pN3 | metastatic involvement of internal mammary lymph nodes |
| M1 | involvement of supraclavicular, cervical, or contralateral lymph nodes<br>distant metastases |

**References**

Heywang-Köbrunner et al. Diagnostic Breast Imaging. Stuttgart, New York: Thieme; 2001.

* The chest wall includes ribs and intercostal muscles, but not the pectoral muscles.

** Skin retraction alone does not lead to a T4 classification.

## Lesions (all modalities)

**Shape**

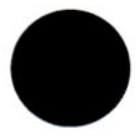
round

oval

lobulated

irregular

**Border**

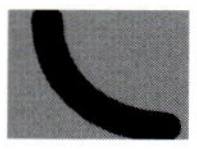
well-defined

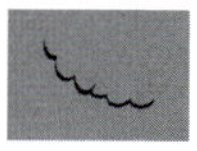
microlobulated

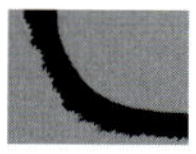
ill-defined

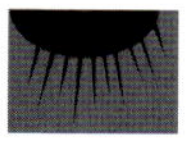
spiculated

## Mammography

### PGMI image classification

| | |
|---|---|
| P | perfect |
| G | good |
| M | moderately good |
| I | inadequate (imaging should be repeated) |

### Parenchymal Density Type

| | |
|---|---|
| ACR 1 | predominantly lipomatous tissue |
| ACR 2 | fibroglandular tissue |
| ACR 3 | inhomogeneously dense tissue |
| ACR 4 | extremely dense tissue |

### Lesion density

| | | | |
|---|---|---|---|
| equivalent to fat | hypodense (but not lipomatous) | isodense (with parenchyma) | hyperdense (denser than parenchyma) |

### Microcalcifications/Distribution

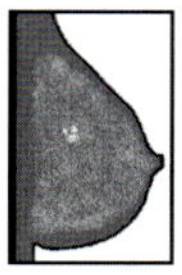
clustered

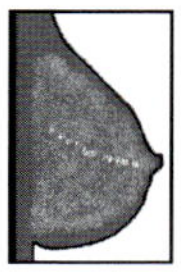
linear

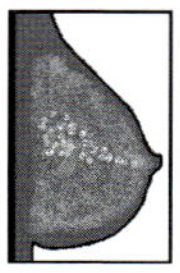
segmental

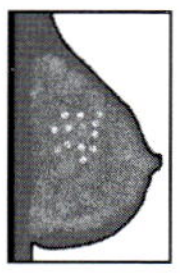
regional

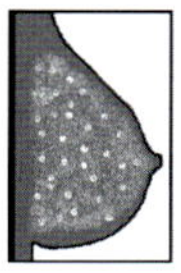
diffuse

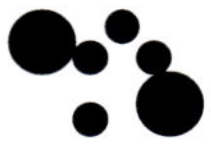
monomorphous

amorphous

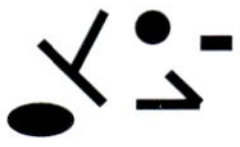
polymorphous/ pleomorphous

### Architectural distortion

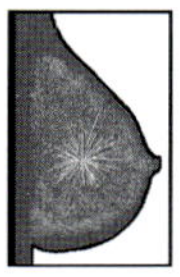

☐ yes ☐ no

## BI-RADS Categorizations (all modalities)

| | | |
|---|---|---|
| BI-RADS 1 | no findings | (risk of cancer 0%) |
| BI-RADS 2 | benign findings | (risk of cancer 0%) |
| BI-RADS 3 | probably benign findings | (risk of cancer < 2%) |
| BI-RADS 4 | probably malignant findings | (risk of cancer ~ 30%) |
| BI-RADS 5 | highly suspect findings | (risk of cancer ~ 95%) |
| BI-RADS 6 | histologically verified cancer | |

## Ultrasound of the Breast

### Lesions

**Echo pattern comparison**

| | |
|---|---|
| Surroundings | anechoic – hypoechoic – isoechoic – hyperechoic |
| Acoustic transmission | diminished – indeterminate – increased – mixed |
| Compressibility | good – low – absent |
| Internal structure | homogeneous – inhomogeneous |
| Lesion axis | horizontal – vertical – indeterminate |
| Surrounding structures | intact – displaced – disrupted |
| Mobility | good – low – immobile |
| Calcifications | macrocalcifications – microcalcifications |
| Perfusion | increased – slightly increased – not increased |

## MR Mammography

### MRI Artifact Category

| | |
|---|---|
| MRI Artifact Category 1 | no motion/subtraction artifacts |
| MRI Artifact Category 2 | minor motion/subtraction artifacts |
| MRI Artifact Category 3 | distinct motion/subtraction artifacts |
| MRI Artifact Category 4 | unacceptable motion/subtraction artifacts |

### Density Type

| | |
|---|---|
| MRI Density Type 1 | no enhancement of the parenchyma |
| MRI Density Type 2 | patchy enhancement of the parenchyma |
| MRI Density Type 3 | widespread patchy enhancement of the parenchyma |
| MRI Density Type 4 | strong enhancement of the parenchyma |

### MRI scoring system (Göttingen score)

| **Points** | **0** | **1** | **2** |
|---|---|---|---|
| **Shape** | round, oval | irregular, dendritic | – |
| **Margins** | well-defined | ill-defined | – |
| **Contrast uptake** | homogeneous | inhomogeneous | ring enhancement |
| **Initial SI increase (for 2D)** | < 50% | 50% – 100% | > 100% |
| **Post-initial SI** | increase | plateau | wash-out |

### MRI BI-RADS

| | |
|---|---|
| 0 Points | MRI BI-RADS 1 |
| 1–2 Points | MRI BI-RADS 2 |
| 3 Points | MRI BI-RADS 3 |
| 4–5 Points | MRI BI-RADS 4 |
| 6–8 Points | MRI BI-RADS 5 |

**Indication:** Palpable mass in the left breast, upper outer quadrant, discovered 8 weeks prior to examination.
**History:** Unremarkable.
**Risk profile:** No increased risk.
**Age:** 78 years.

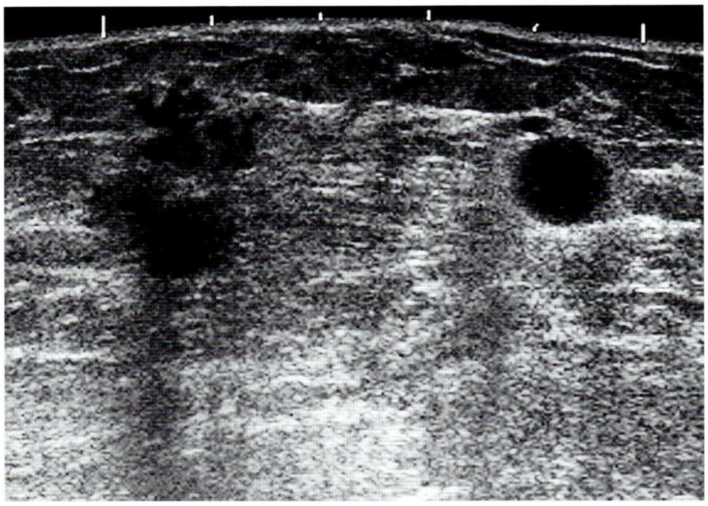

Fig. 1.**1** Sonography of the left breast. Panoramic view.

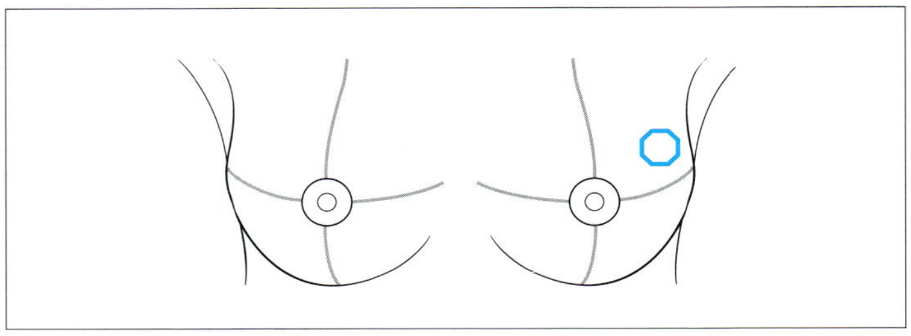

## Clinical Findings

Dense, mobile mass of diameter 2 cm in the upper outer quadrant of the left breast. Ptosis of the left breast.

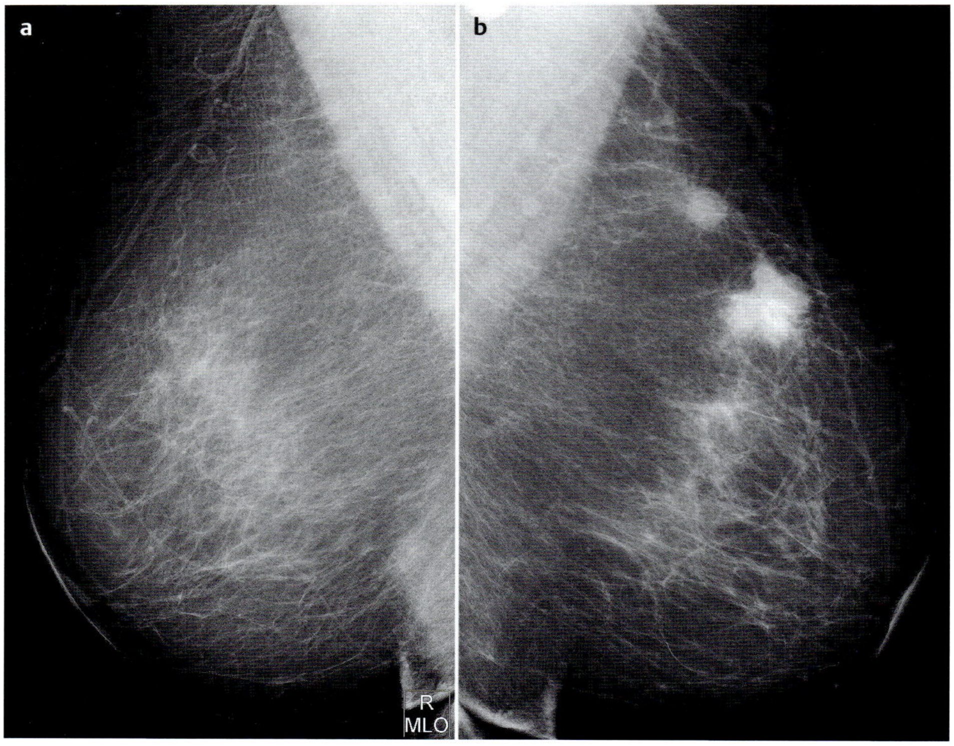


Fig. 1.**2 a, b** Digital mammography, MLO view.

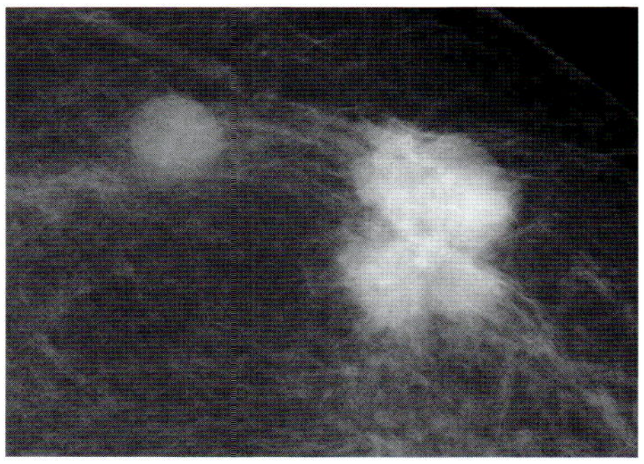

Fig. 1.**3** Magnification view of the upper outer quadrant of the left breast, CC view.

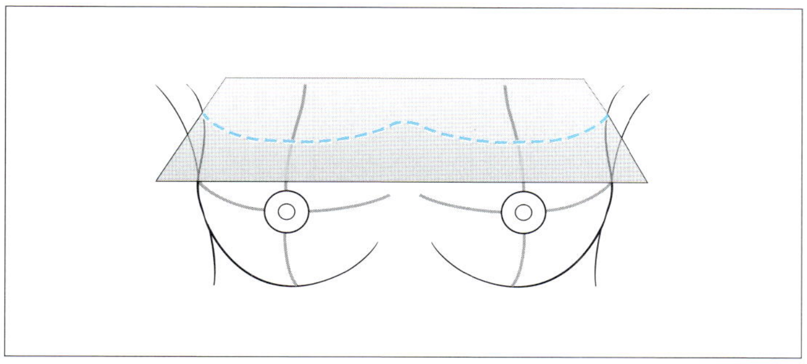

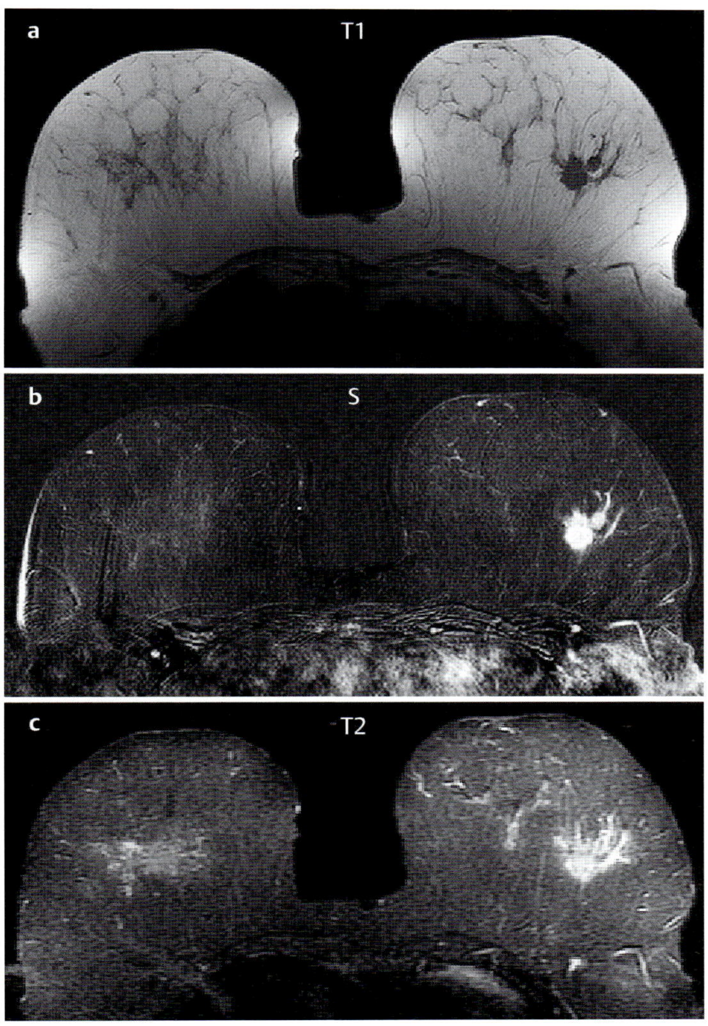


Fig. 1.4 **a–c** Contrast-enhanced MRI of the breasts.

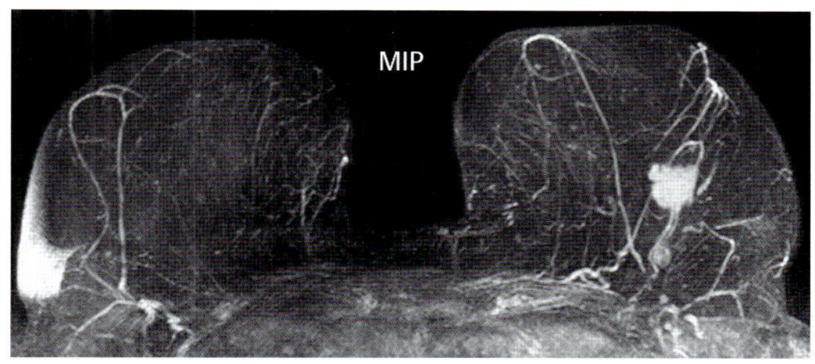


Fig. 1.**5** Contrast-enhanced MR mammography. Maximum intensity projection.

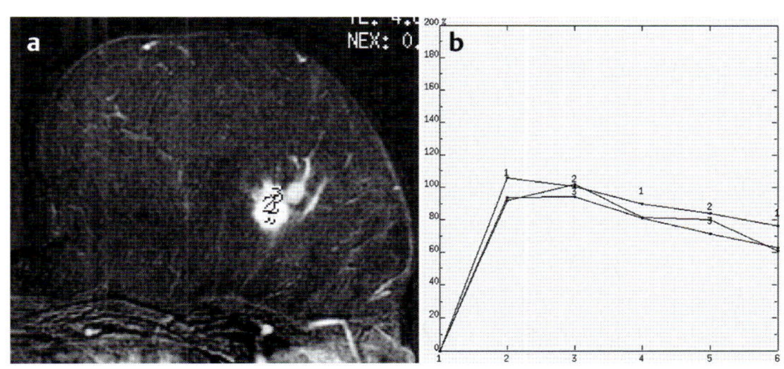


Fig. 1.**6 a, b** Signal-to-time curve.

Please characterize the ultrasound, mammography and MRI findings.
What is your preliminary diagnosis?
What are your next steps?

This case describes the imaging findings in an older symptomatic woman. Clinical findings strongly suggest the diagnosis of invasive breast cancer in the left breast.

### Ultrasound

Corresponding to the palpable mass, ultrasound demonstrates a suspect lobulated lesion with predominantly ill-defined borders and a hyperechoic marginal area. This lesion disturbs ligaments and leads to retraction of the surrounding parenchyma. Close to this lesion, ultrasound shows a pathologically enlarged lymph node. Assessment: US BI-RADS left 5.

### Mammography

Mammography shows symmetric lipomatous breast tissue of ACR type 1. There are no pathological findings in the right breast. In the upper outer quadrant of the left breast, there is a lobulated mass (2 cm diameter) with ill-defined borders. A bridge of dense tissue is seen between the lesion and a prepectoral lymph node about 2 cm away. There is a further partially visible, enlarged lymph node in the left upper axilla. No microcalcifications are detectable (BI-RADS right 1/left 5). PGMI: G (the inframammary fold was not clearly discernible).

### MR Mammography

MRI shows a mass 2 cm in diameter in the upper outer quadrant of the left breast. There is a second small nodule nearby. After administration of contrast the tumor shows marked initial enhancement, followed by washout. There is ductal enhancement extending from the primary tumor to the lateral parts of the left breast (Fig. 1.**7**; arrow). MIP demonstrates pathological enhancement of the prepectoral lymph node as well as the bridgelike connection between tumor and lymph node.

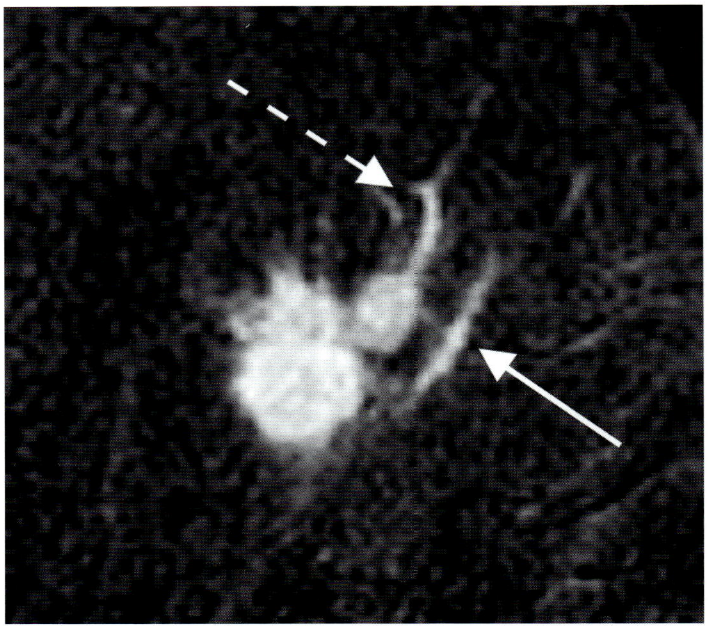

Fig. 1.**7** Contrast-enhanced MR mammography. Magnification view of the left breast, upper outer quadrant.

**Caution:** Other linear structures with increased vascularization correlate with contrast-enhanced veins (broken arrow).

**MRI Artifact Category:** 2
**MRI Density Type:** 1

| MRM score | Finding | Points |
|---|---|---|
| **Shape** | lobulated | 0 |
| **Border** | ill-defined | 1 |
| **CM Distribution** | inhomogeneous | 1 |
| **Initial Signal Intensity Increase** | strong | 2 |
| **Post-initial Signal Intensity Character** | wash-out | 2 |
| **MRI score (points)** | | **6** |
| **MRI BI-RADS** | | **5** |

### → Preliminary Diagnosis

Invasive breast cancer of the left breast with lymph node metastases, stage T2. No differential diagnosis.

| BIRADS Categorization | | |
|---|---|---|
| Clinical Findings | right 1 | left 5 |
| Ultrasound | right 1 | left 5 |
| Mammography | right 1 | left 5 |
| MR Mammography | right 1 | left 5 |
| **BI-RADS Total** | **right 1** | **left 5** |

**Next step according to guidelines**

US-guided core biopsy of the palpable mass in the left breast.

**Performed step (departing from guidelines)**

Due to the age of the patient and the clear findings in all imaging modalities, and in response to the patient's own request, a US-guided core biopsy for preoperative histopathological diagnosis was not performed. The tumor was examined histopathologically following mastectomy.

## Histology

Medullary carcinoma of the left breast.

MC pT2 (2.5 cm), pN1a (2/18), G2.

## Treatment

Mastectomy (subsequent radiation therapy was declined by the patient).

This case shows a typical breast cancer in all imaging modalities.
But beware: The following cases are trickier!

**Indication:** Screening.
**History:** Hodgkin disease 20 years ago. Supradiaphragmal irradiation therapy. No relapse.
**Risk profile:** Irradiation therapy of the chest. No increased familial risk.
**Age:** 42 years.

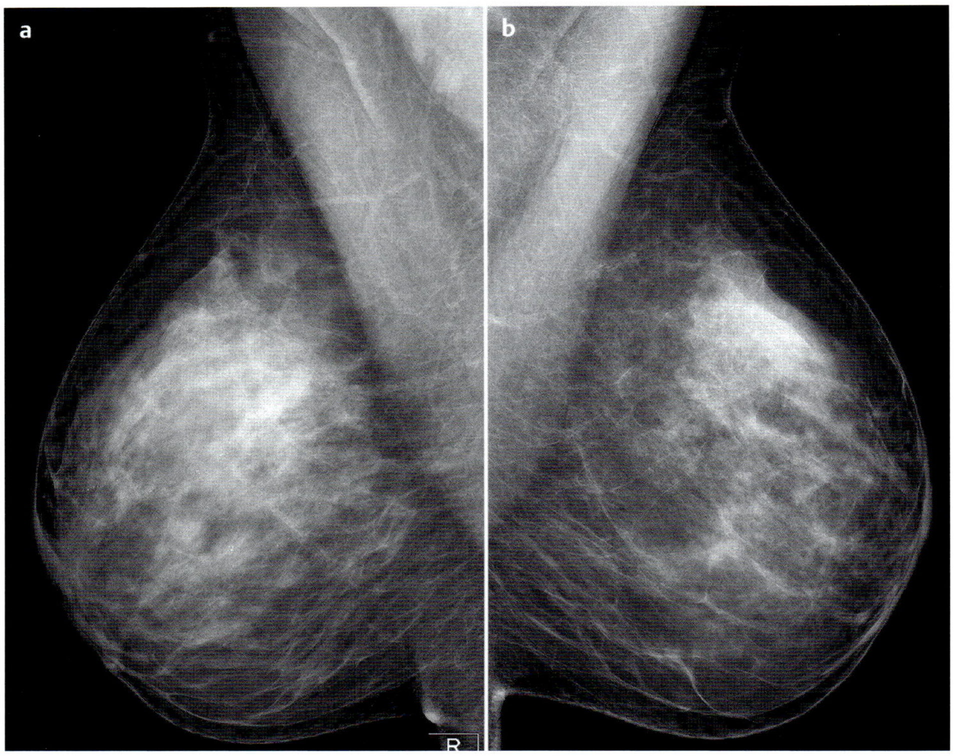

Fig. 2.**1 a, b** Digital mammography, MLO view.

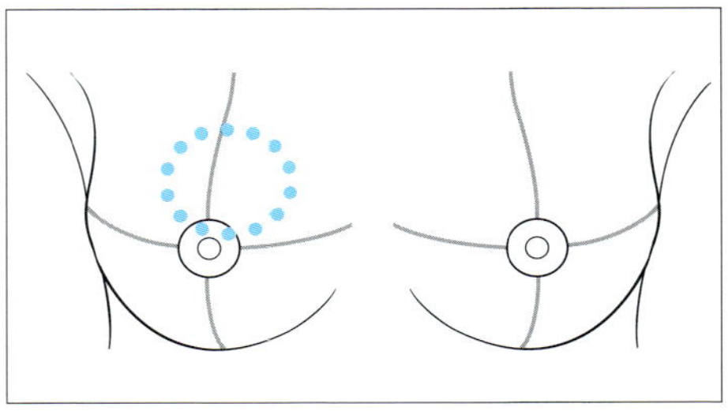

### Clinical Findings

Slightly increased parenchymal resistance in the upper quadrants of the right breast, compared to left. No palpable mass.

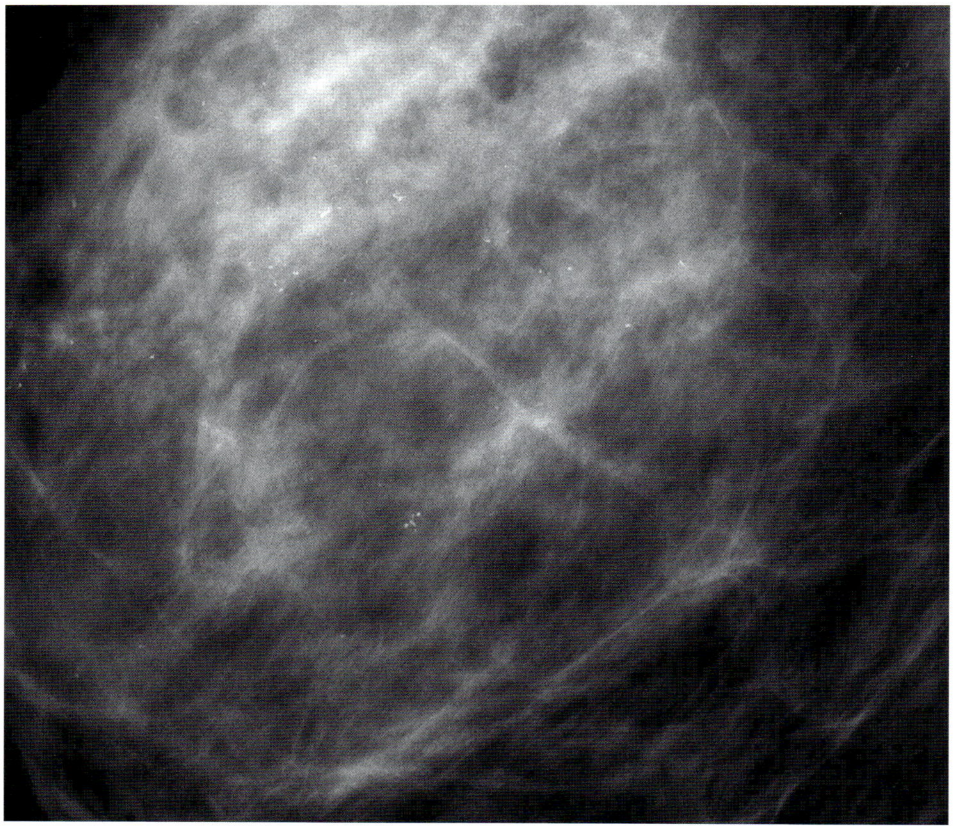

Fig. 2.**2** Magnification view of the central region of the right breast.

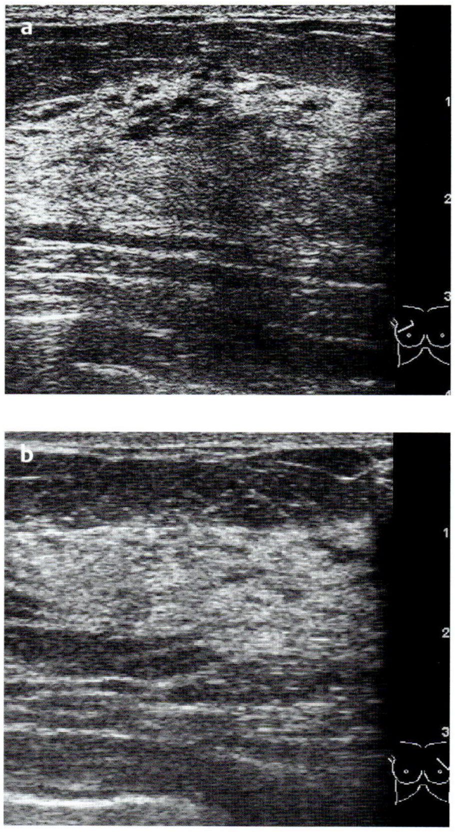

Fig. 2.**3 a, b** Sonography (comparison of upper outer quadrants bilaterally).

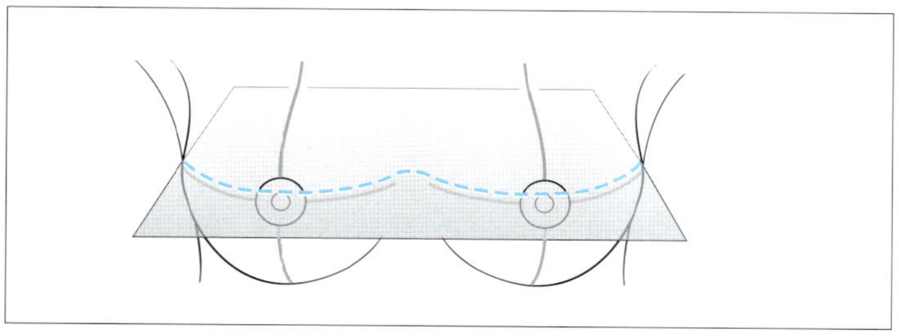

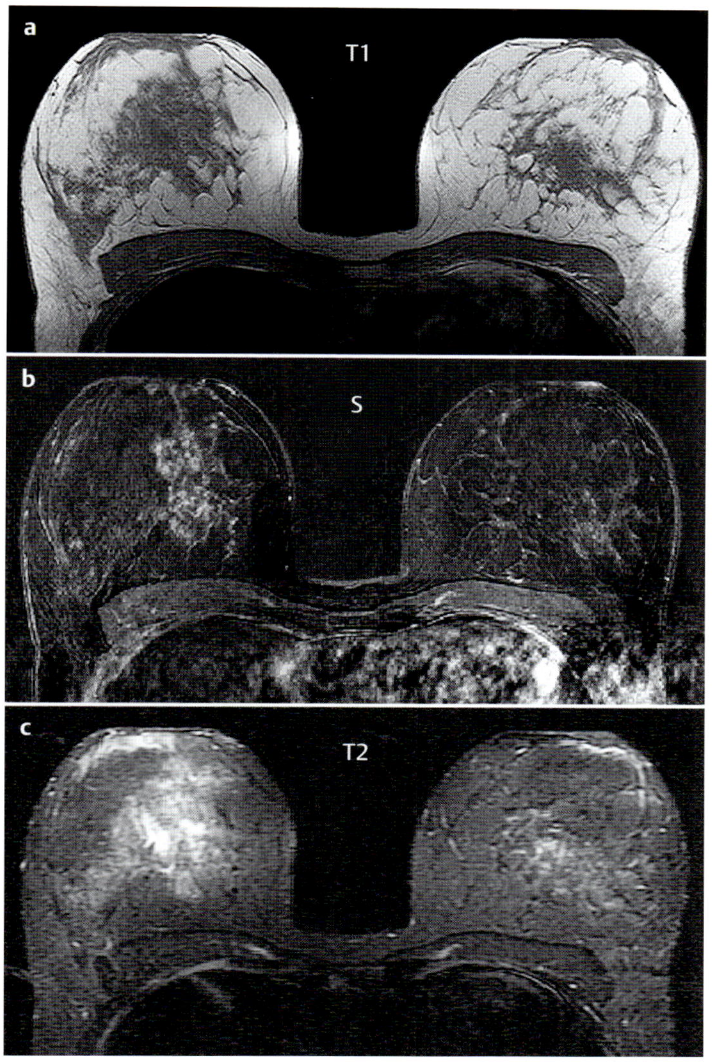


Fig. 2.**4 a – c** Contrast-enhanced MRI of the breasts.

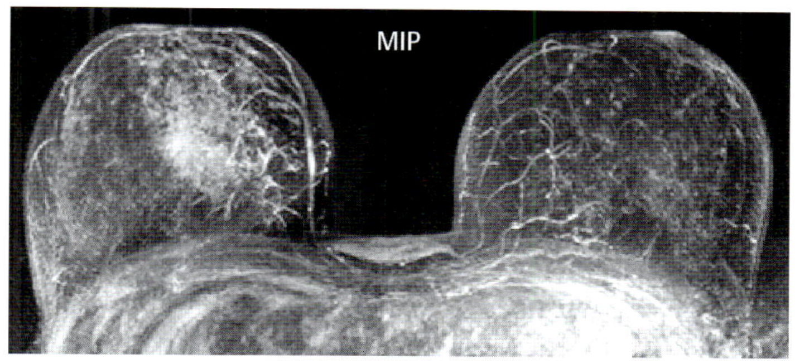


Fig. 2.**5** Contrast-enhanced MR mammography. Maximum intensity projection.

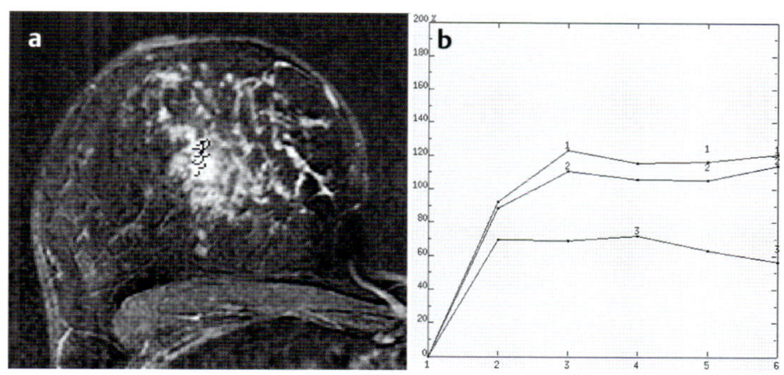


Fig. 2.**6 a, b** Signal-to-time curves.

**?**
Please characterize ultrasound, mammography, and MRI findings.
What is your preliminary diagnosis?
What are your next steps?

Presented here are all the imaging studies of a younger woman who presented for screening and has a markedly increased risk of breast cancer due to radiation therapy to the mantle field 20 years previously.

**Ultrasound**

There is a marked difference in the calibers of the milk ducts (right > left), a sign of possible duct ectasia in the right breast. No circumscribed lesion. US BI-RADS right 3/left 1.

**Mammography**

Asymmetric inhomogeneous dense parenchyma of ACR type 4. No opacities. Polymorphous (round, linear, v-shaped) microcalcifications within the dense parenchyma of the right breast visible in the enlarged view. BI-RADS right 5/left 1). PGMI: P.

**MR Mammography**

MRI shows no suspect findings on T1-weighted images and on water-sensitive IR sequence. There is a suspicious segmental dendritic signal enhancement in the upper quadrants of the right breast after administration of contrast medium. Signal–time curve is unspecific. However, in cases with a dendritic enhancement pattern, the placement of an adequate region-of-interest (ROI) is difficult or impossible. MRI shows no circumscribed enhancing masses. MRI of the left breast is normal.

**MRI Artifact Category:** 2
**MRI Density Type:** 1

| MRM score | Finding | Points |
|---|---|---|
| Shape | irregular | 1 |
| Border | ill-defined | 1 |
| CM Distribution | dendritic | 1 |
| Initial Signal Intensity Increase | strong | 2 |
| Post-initial Signal Intensity Character | plateau | 1 |
| **MRI score (points)** | | **6** |
| **MRI BI-RADS** | | **5** |

## → Preliminary Diagnosis

Extensive intraductal, possibly partially microinvasive tumor of the right breast.

## Differential Diagnosis

Segmental adenosis, inflammation (both very unlikely).

| BI-RADS Categorization | | |
|---|---|---|
| Clinical Findings | right 3 | left 1 |
| Ultrasound | right 3 | left 1 |
| Mammography | right 5 | left 1 |
| MR Mammography | right 5 | left 1 |
| **BI-RADS Total** | **right 5** | **left 1** |

**Procedure**

Stereotactic vacuum core biopsy of the right breast to obtain histological confirmation of preliminary diagnosis.

Compression with the probe of one of the tissue samples retrieved in the area of a calcification, visible here, produced "blackhead"-like emissions from the core. This is evidence of the presence of intraductal tumor.

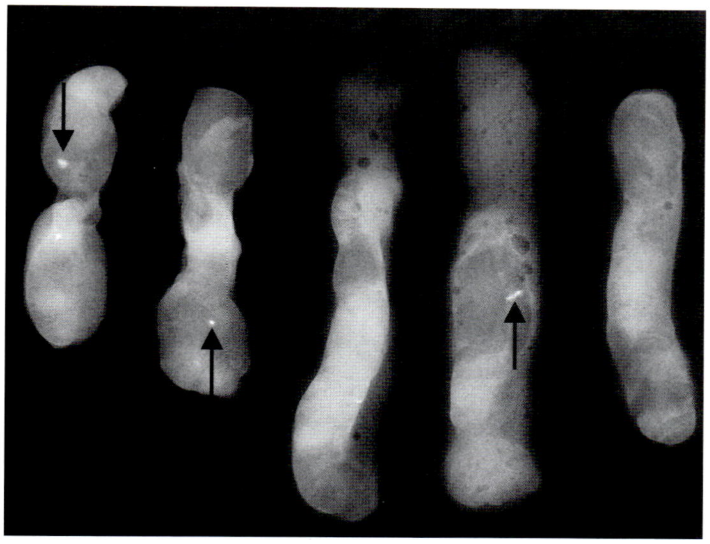

Fig. 2.**7** Specimen radiography of some of the core biopsies with positive findings of microcalcifications (arrows).

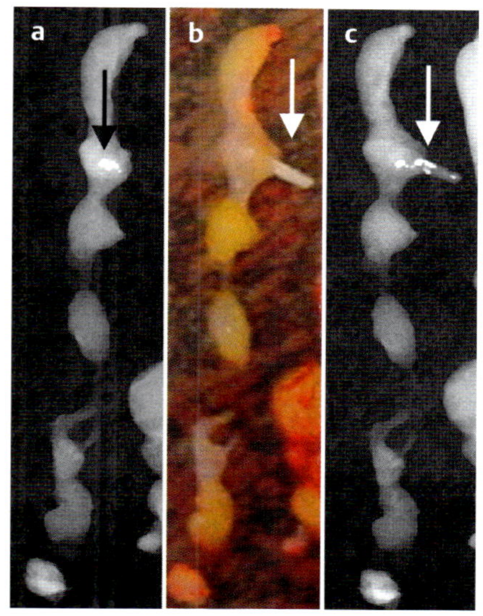


Fig. 2.**8 a–c** Specimen of a single core biopsy before and after compression of the tissue including the microcalcification. Photography of the necrotic comedo tissue (arrow) after compression.

### Histology of the specimen

Comedo-type DCIS, Grade 2.

### Histology of the right breast

Tricentric intraductal breast carcinoma in the central part of the right breast including the nipple (see the linear enhancement in MRI reaching the nipple region).

pTis (Paget disease), pN0 (sentinel Node 0/2), G2, R1 (upper inner quadrant), VNPI 10 points.

### Treatment

Mastectomy of the right breast with subsequent resection in the upper inner quadrant (primary R1 resection).

Earlier radiation therapy near the area of the breasts carries an increased risk of breast cancer developing up to 15–25 years later.

**Indication:** Screening.
**History:** Unremarkable.
**Risk profile:** Postmenopausal breast cancer in mother, premenopausal in an aunt, postmenopausal in a second cousin.
**Age:** 40 years.

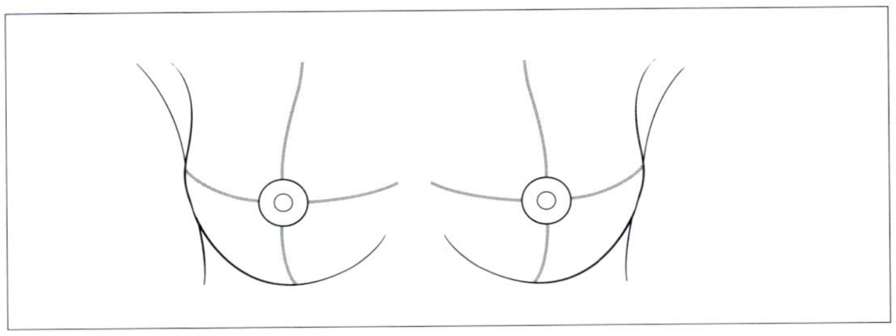

### Clinical Findings

No findings.

### Sonography

No findings (not shown).

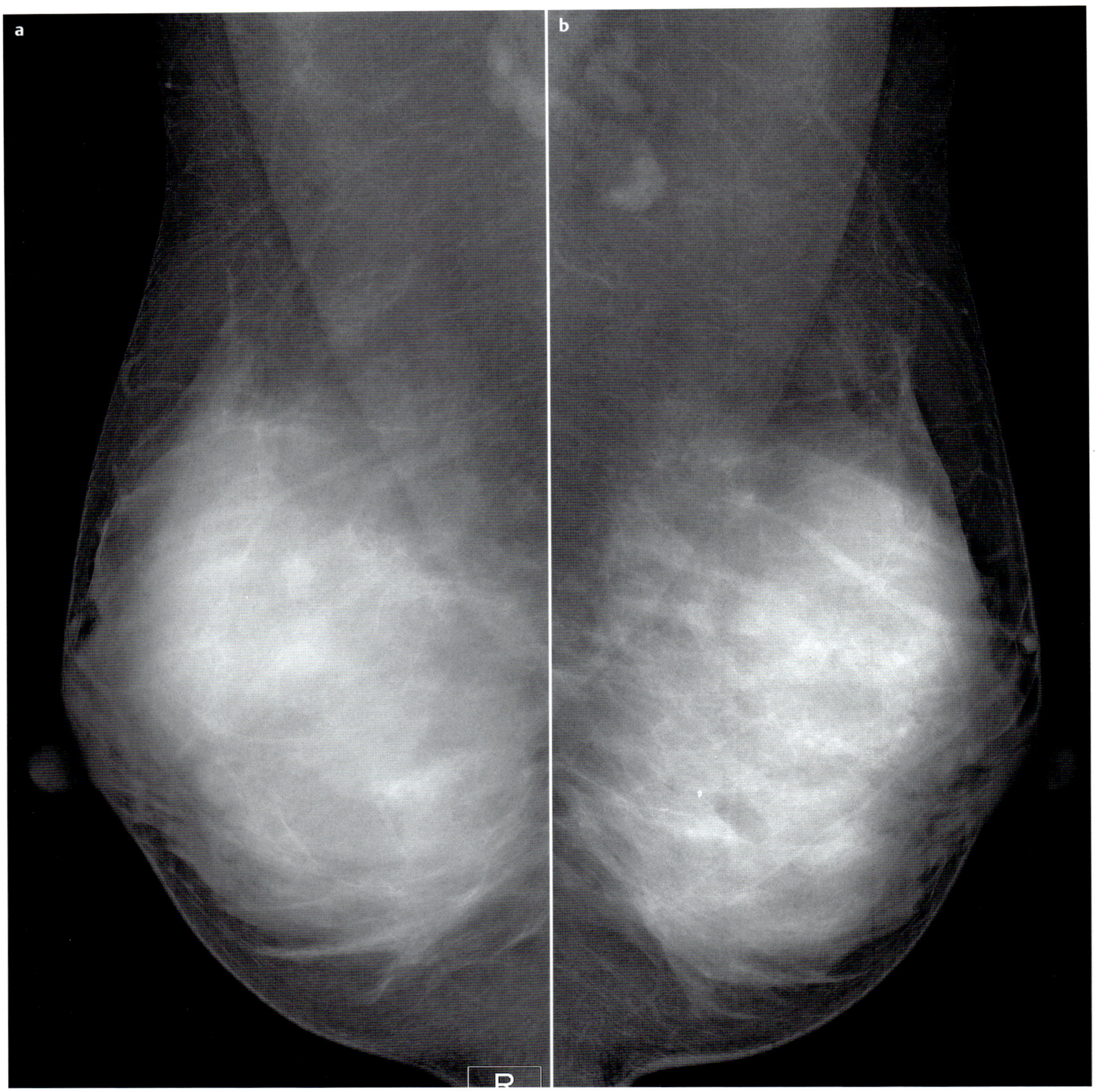

Fig. 3.1 **a, b** Digital mammography of both breasts, MLO view.

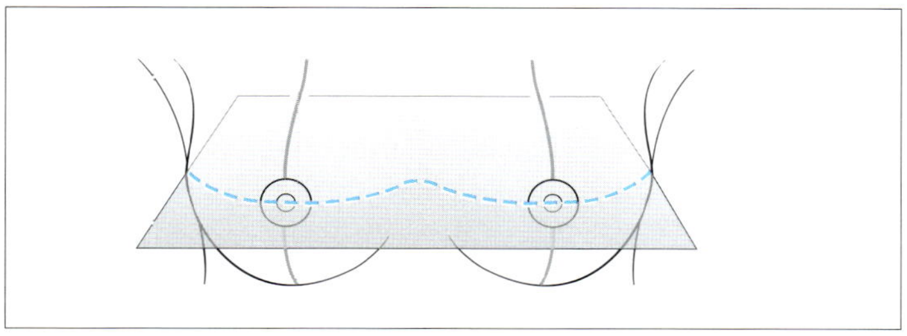

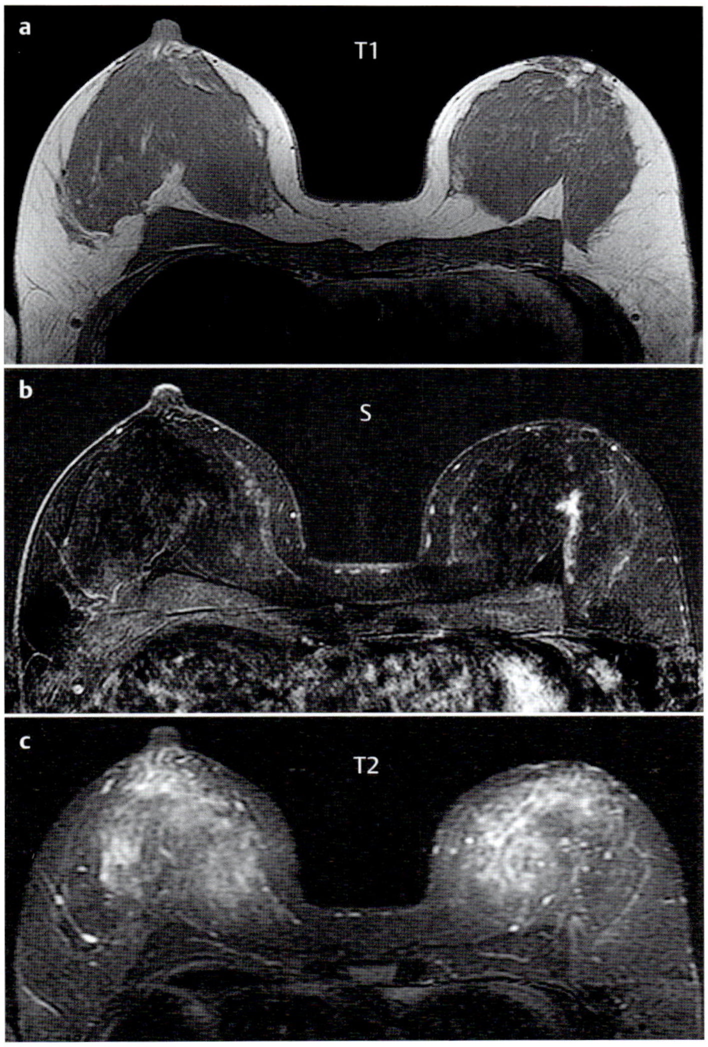


Fig. 3.**2 a–c** Contrast-enhanced MRI of the breasts.

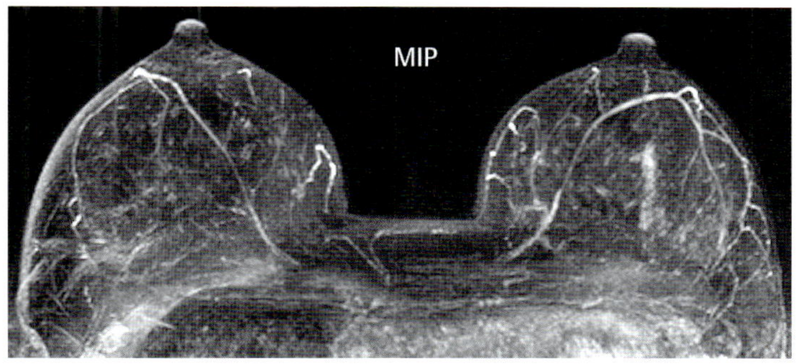


Fig. 3.**3** Contrast-enhanced MR mammography. Maximum intensity projection.

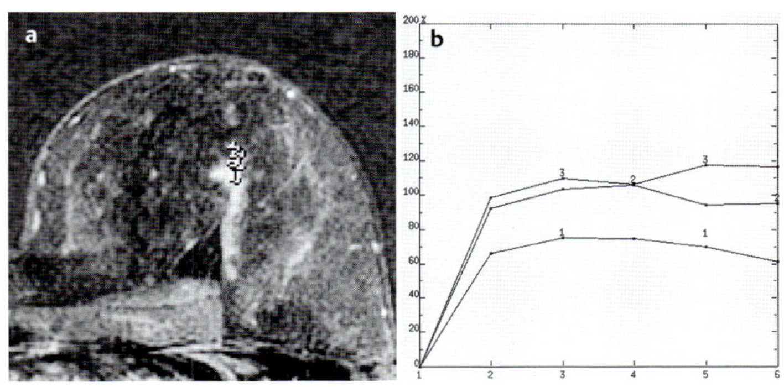


Fig. 3.**4 a, b** Signal-to-time curves.

Please characterize mammography and MRI findings.
What is your preliminary diagnosis?
What are your next steps?

These are the imaging studies of a younger woman presenting for screening with a high risk profile due to three relatives having breast cancer.

### Ultrasound

Ultrasound showed no suspicious changes (not shown).

### Mammography

Bilaterally symmetric, extremely dense parenchymal pattern, ACR type 4. Within the limitations of these conditions, there were no abnormal findings in the left breast central area–where MRI findings are significant–or anywhere else. There is no hyperdensity, no mass, no architectural distortion. No microcalcifications corresponding to the linear enhancement observed in MRI (BI-RADS right 1/left 1). PGMI: MLO view P.

### MR Mammography

There is linear and partially dendritic enhancement, likely representing a milk duct, visible in the central sections of the left breast. Signal–time curves are nonspecific. No further observations.

**MRI Artifact Category:** 1
**MRI Density Type:** 1

| MRM score | Finding | Points |
|---|---|---|
| **Shape** | linear | 1 |
| **Border** | ill-defined | 1 |
| **CM Distribution** | homogeneous | 0 |
| **Initial Signal Intensity Increase** | strong | 2 |
| **Post-initial Signal Intensity Character** | plateau | 1 |
| **MRI score (points)** | | **5** |
| **MRI BI-RADS** | | **4** |

### → Preliminary Diagnosis

DCIS.

### Differential Diagnosis

Segmental papillomatosis, inflammation of the milk ducts.

| BI-RADS Categorization | | |
|---|---|---|
| Clinical Findings | right 1 | left 1 |
| Ultrasound | right 1 | left 1 |
| Mammography | right 1 | left 1 |
| MR Mammography | right 1 | left 4 |
| **BI-RADS Total** | **right 1** | **left 4** |

### Procedure

Histological verification of the suspicious findings in MRI, preferably with MR-guided percutaneous vacuum biopsy to avoid open biopsy.

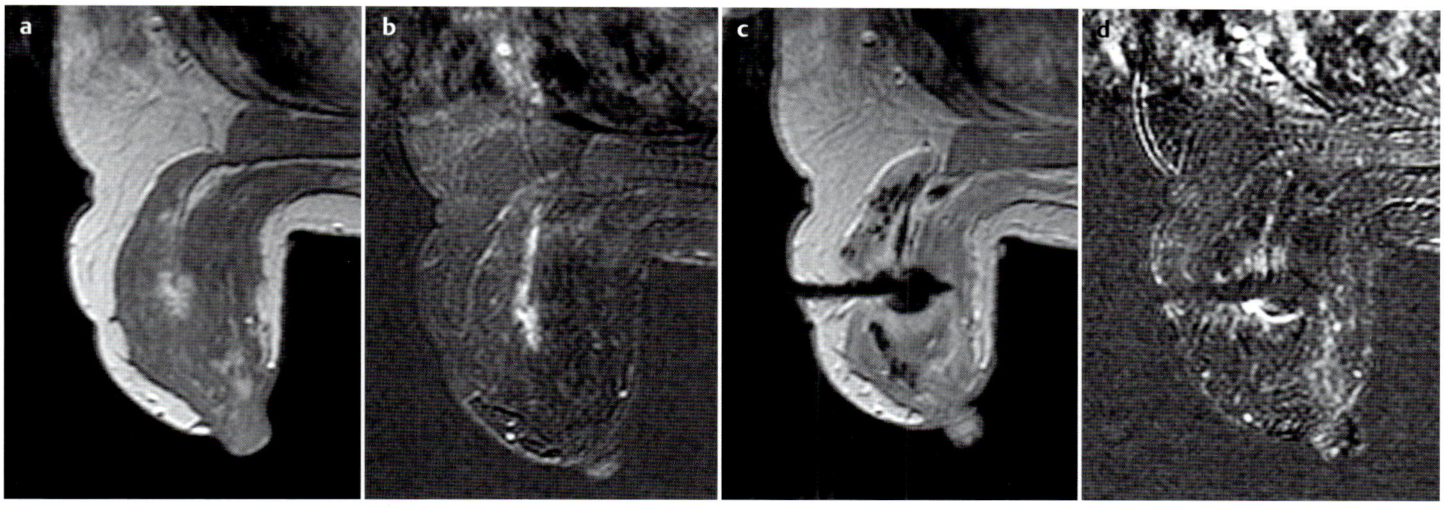


Fig. 3.5 **a–d** Documentation of the MR-guided vacuum biopsy: T1-weighted precontrast image of the left breast positioned within the stereotactic device (**a**). Precise reproducibility of the linear enhancement in subtraction image (**b**). Position of the biopsy needle after removal of 20 core biopsies (11 gauge) (**c**). Documentation of parts of the enhancing area in a second contrast-enhanced MRI sequence (subtraction image) (**d**).

### Histopathological result of the left breast

Chronic fibrocystic mastopathy with a single intraductal papilloma. Low-grade sclerosing adenosis.
No malignancy.

### Treatment

None. One follow-up MRI after 6 months.

Suspicious findings visible on MRI only can be reliably corroborated with MR-guided vacuum core biopsy.
This strategy helps avoid a large number of unnecessary open biopsies.

**Indication:** Screening.
**History:** Unremarkable.
**Risk profile:** No increased risk.
**Age:** 52 years.

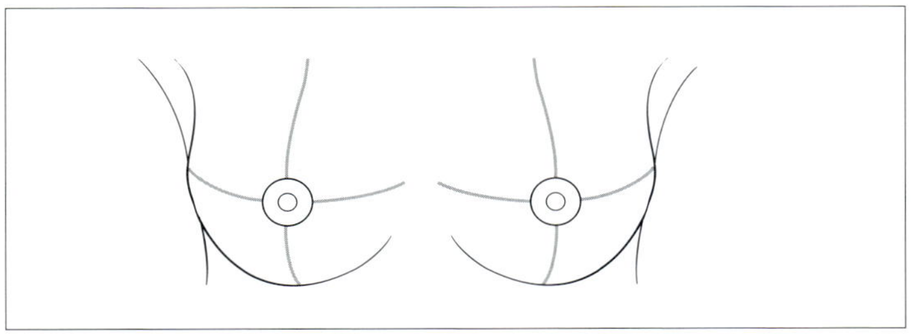

## Clinical Findings

Normal.

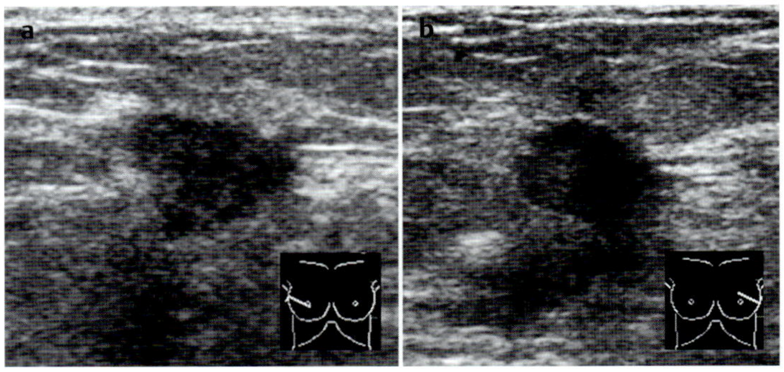

Fig. 4.**1 a, b** Sonography.

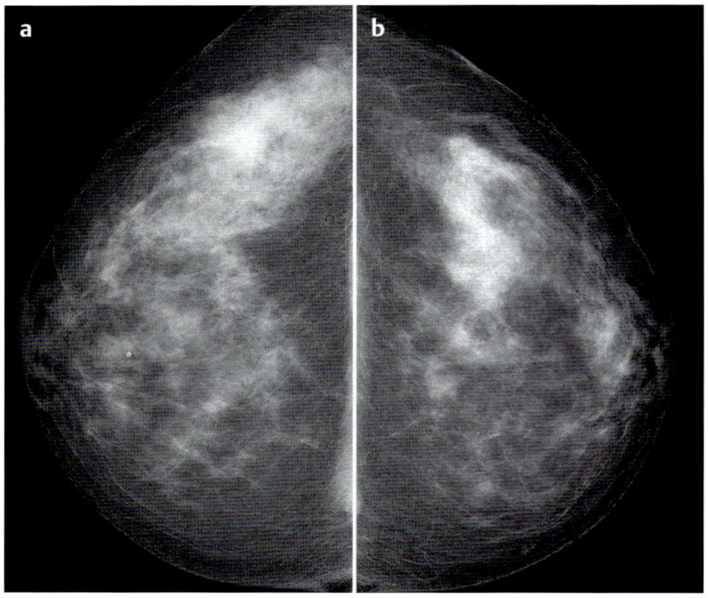

Fig. 4.**2 a, b** Digital mammography, CC view.

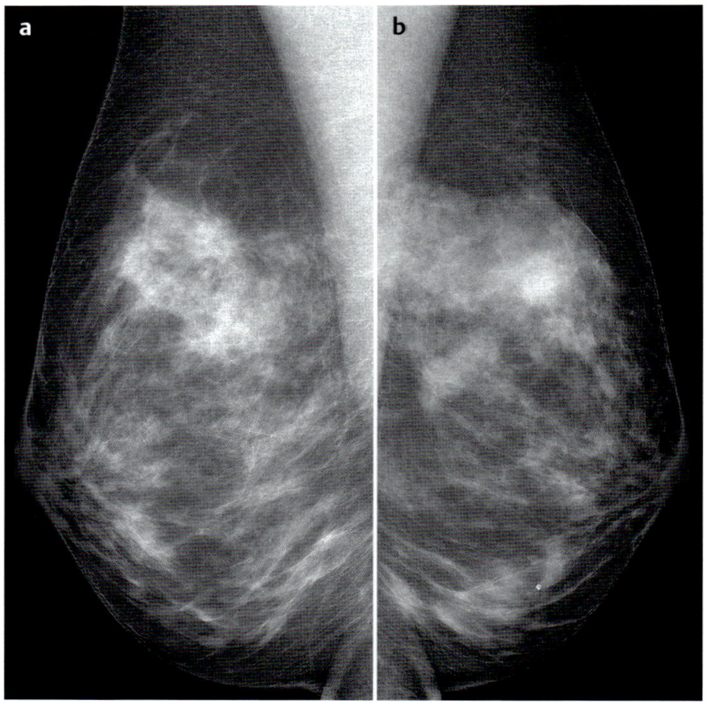

Fig. 4.**3 a, b** Digital mammography, MLO view.

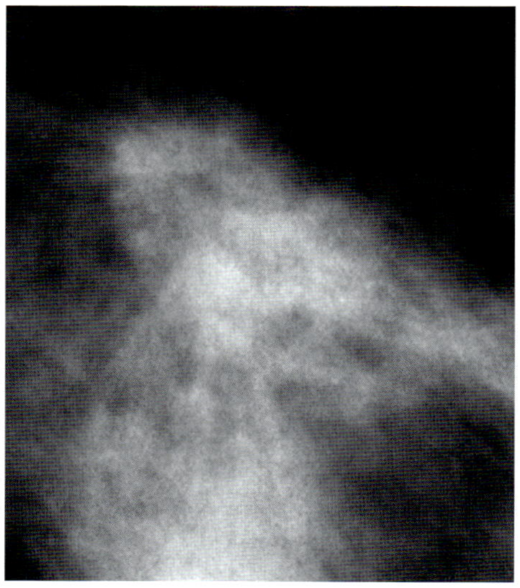

Fig. 4.**4** Zoomed view of upper outer quadrant of the left breast, CC view.

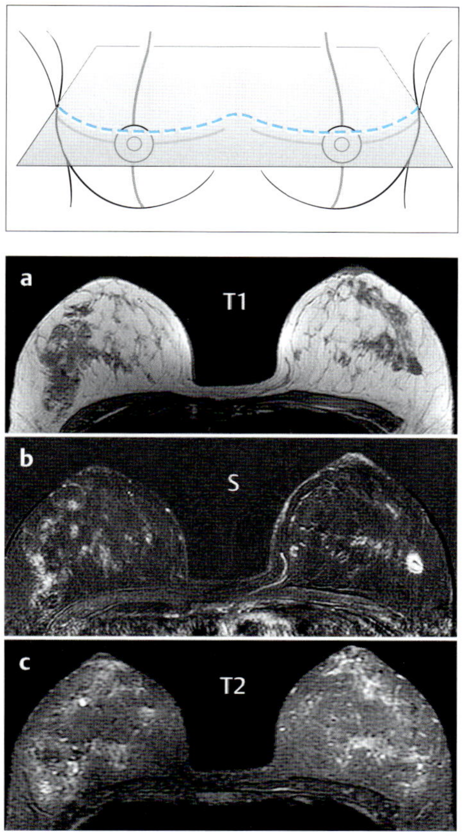


Fig. 4.5 **a – c**

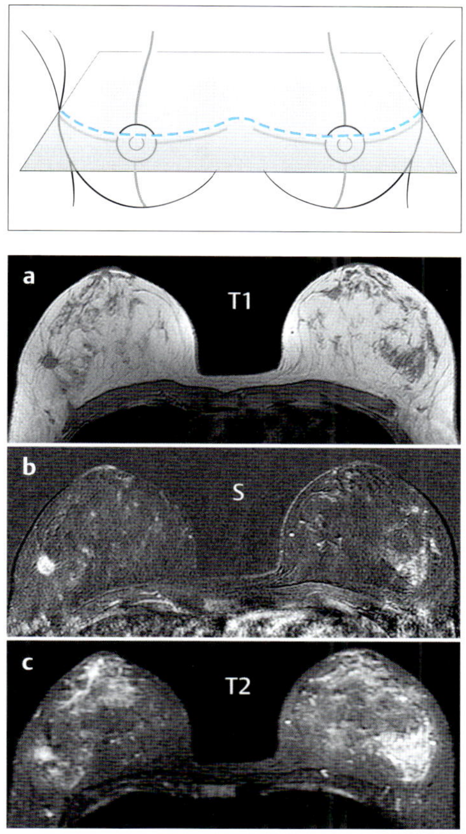


Fig. 4.6 **a – c**

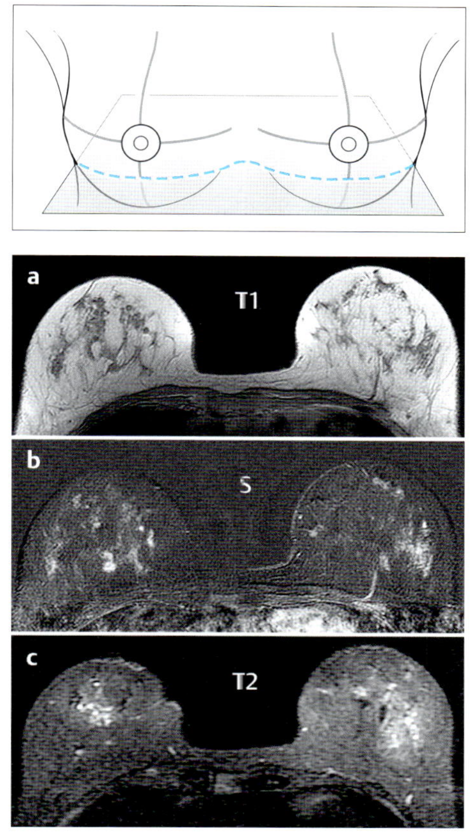


Fig. 4.7 **a – c**

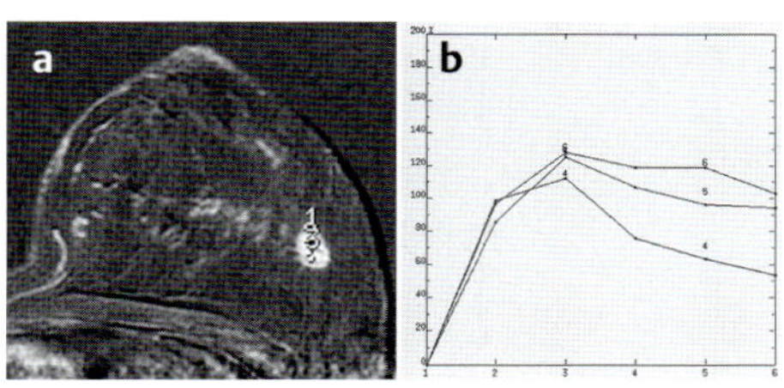


Fig. 4.8 **a, b** Signal-to-time curves.

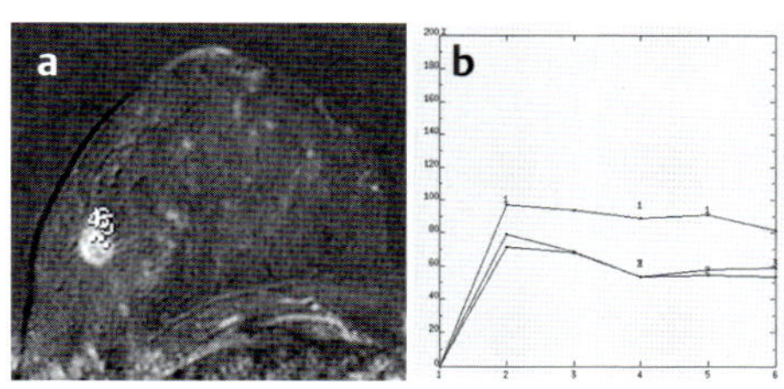


Fig. 4.9 **a, b** Signal-to-time curves.

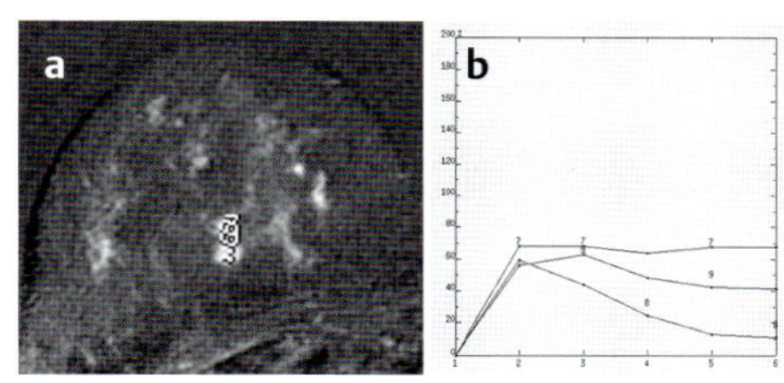


Fig. 4.10 **a, b** Signal-to-time curves.

Fig. 4.5 – 4.10 Contrast-enhanced MR mammography.

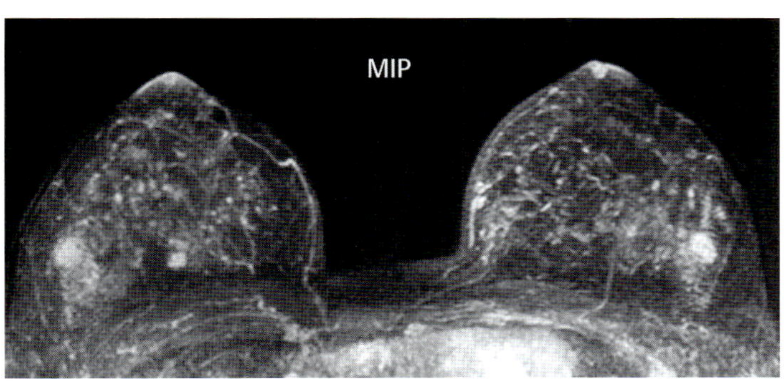


Fig. 4.11 Contrast-enhanced MR mammography. Maximum intensity projection.

?

Please characterize ultrasound, mammography, and MRI findings.
What is your preliminary diagnosis?
What are your next steps?

This asymptomatic woman presented for screening mammography. There was no increased familial risk.

## Ultrasound

There is a lobulated hypoechoic lesion with microlobulated borders and partially peripheral hyperechogenicity as well as a disruption of a ligament structure in the upper outer quadrant of the right breast. Moreover, there is a round hypoechoic lesion with partially ill-defined borders and disruption of the continuity of a ligament in the outer upper quadrant of the left breast. Neither lesion shows any pathological distal echo alteration. US BI-RADS right 5/left 4.

## Mammography

Both breasts show inhomogeneous dense tissue, ACR type 3. There is a hyperdense round lesion 1 cm in diameter with spiculated borders within the dense parenchyma in the upper outer quadrant of the right breast. There are no associated microcalcifications. In the upper outer quadrant of the left breast, there is also a hyperdense round lesion (1 cm) with spiculated borders. There are microcalcifications in the region of this lesion (BI-RADS right 5/left 5). PGMI: CC view P; MLO view M (inframammary fold, pectoral angle < 20°).

## MR Mammography

Corresponding to ultrasound and digital mammography findings, there is a round hypervascularized tumor of 1 cm diameter in the upper outer quadrant of each breast. Additionally, MRI shows another small hypervascularized tumor in the caudal area of the right breast (in line with the nipple) with a stronger contrast uptake in the early subtraction phase compared to the surrounding tissue. All lesions showed intermediate signal intensity in water-sensitive IR sequence.

**MRI Artifact Category:** 2
**MRI Density Type:** 2

| MRM score | Left breast, upper outer quadrant | Points | Right breast, upper outer quadrant | Points | Right breast, caudal lesion | Points |
|---|---|---|---|---|---|---|
| **Shape** | oval | 0 | oval | 0 | round | 0 |
| **Border** | spiculated | 1 | ill-defined | 1 | ill-defined | 1 |
| **CM Distribution** | rim sign | 2 | rim sign | 2 | rim sign | 2 |
| **Initial Signal Intensity Increase** | strong | 2 | moderate | 1 | moderate | 1 |
| **Post-initial Signal Intensity Character** | wash-out | 2 | wash-out | 2 | wash-out | 2 |
| **MRI score (points)** | | **7** | | **6** | | **6** |
| **MRI BI-RADS** | | **5** | | **5** | | **5** |

## → Preliminary Diagnosis

Multicentric invasive breast cancer of the right breast. Invasive breast cancer of the left breast, probably with an extensive intraductal component (EIC, see microcalcifications).

| BI-RADS Categorization | | |
|---|---|---|
| Clinical Findings | right 1 | left 1 |
| Ultrasound | right 5 | left 4 |
| Mammography | right 5 | left 5 |
| MR Mammography | right 5 (suspected MCC) | left 5 |
| **BI-RADS Total** | **right 5 (suspected MCC)** | **left 5** |

### Procedure

Histological verification of the suspect lesion in the upper outer quadrants of both breasts with US-guided core biopsy. Additionally, histology of the suspect lesion in the caudal area of the right breast with MR-guided vacuum biopsy.

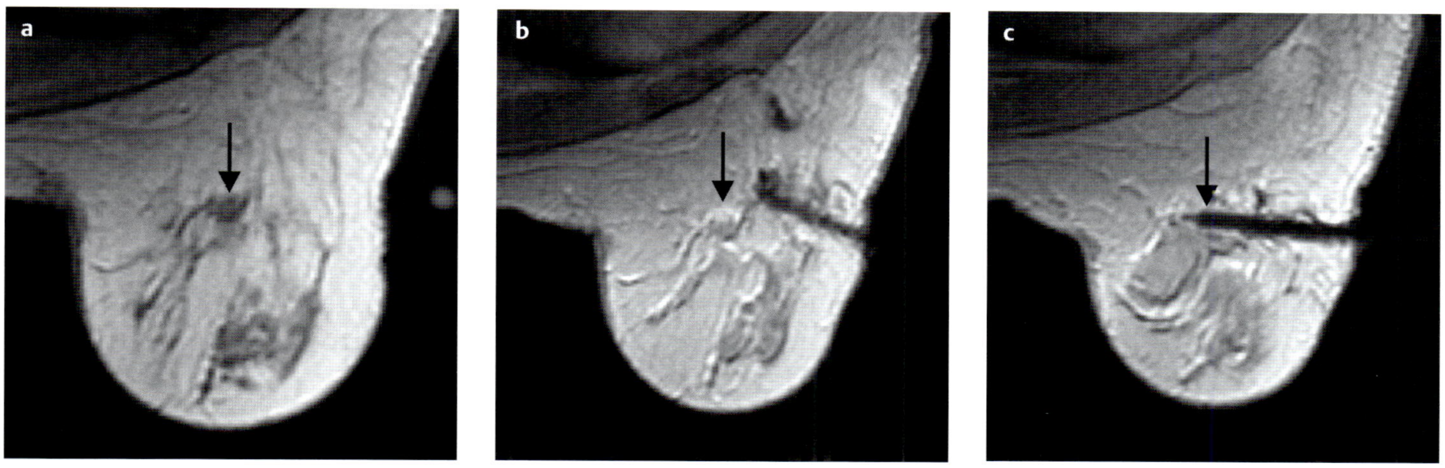


Fig. 4.**12 a – c** MR-guided vacuum biopsy of the right breast (caudal lesion). Reproducibility of the lesion (arrow) (**a**). Misplacement of the coaxial needle with deviation toward the thoracic wall (**b**). Repositioning of the coaxial needle and documentation of its correct position after excision of the tissue specimen. (**c**).

## Histology

Histology of US-guided core biopsy, upper outer quadrant, right breast: IDC.
Histology of US-guided core biopsy upper outer quadrant, left breast: IDC.
Histology of MR-guided vacuum biopsy right caudal lesion: ILC.

## Histology

| | |
|---|---|
| Right breast: | IDC and ILC pT1c (multicentric: 12 mm + 7 mm), pN0 (0/11)*, G1 + G2. |
| Left breast: | IDC pT1b (8 mm) + pTis (EIC 4 mm + 5 mm), pN0 (0/5 sn), G1. |

* Sentinel node resection is not recommended in cases with multicentricity.

## Treatment

Right breast: Mastectomy, plastic breast reconstruction.
Left breast: Wide segmental resection, cosmetic quadrantectomy.

In cases with microcalcifications surrounding a primary tumor, the radiologist should consider the possibility of an additional extensive intraductal component (EIC).

**Indication:** Screening.
**History:** Unremarkable.
**Risk profile:** No increased risk.
**Age:** 39 years.

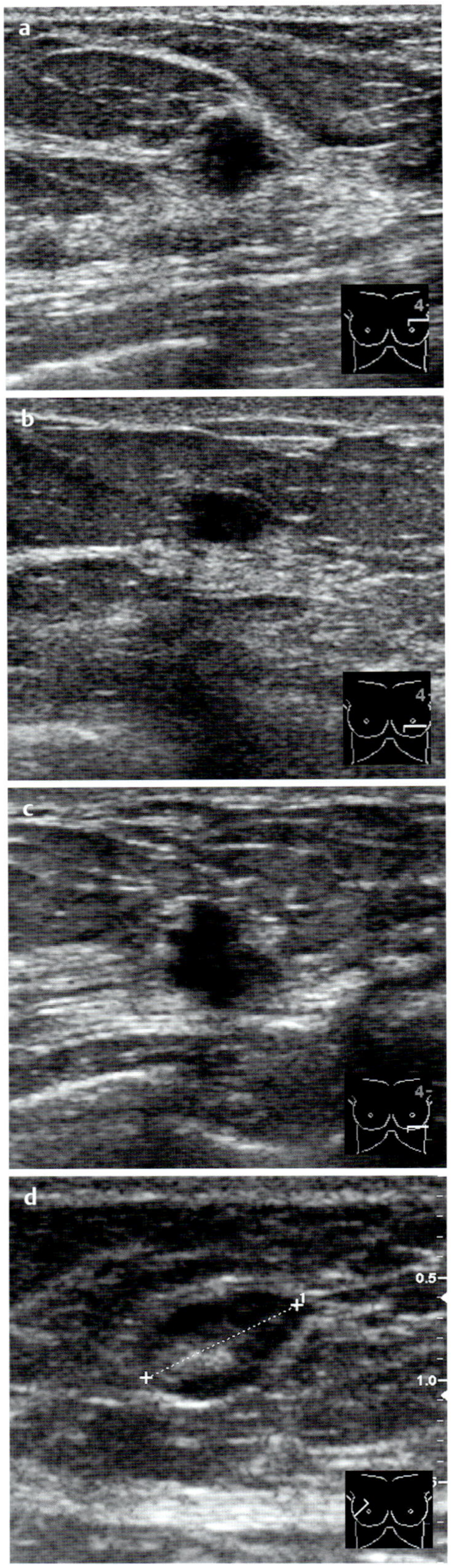


Fig. 5.**1 a–d** Sonography.

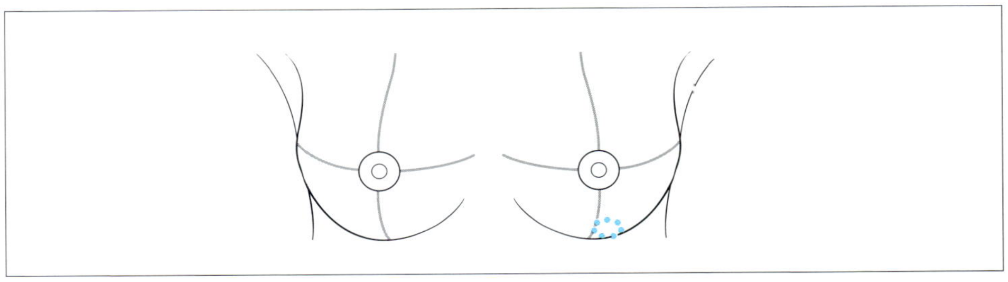

## Clinical Findings

Circumscribed resistance in the area of the inframammary fold of the left breast.

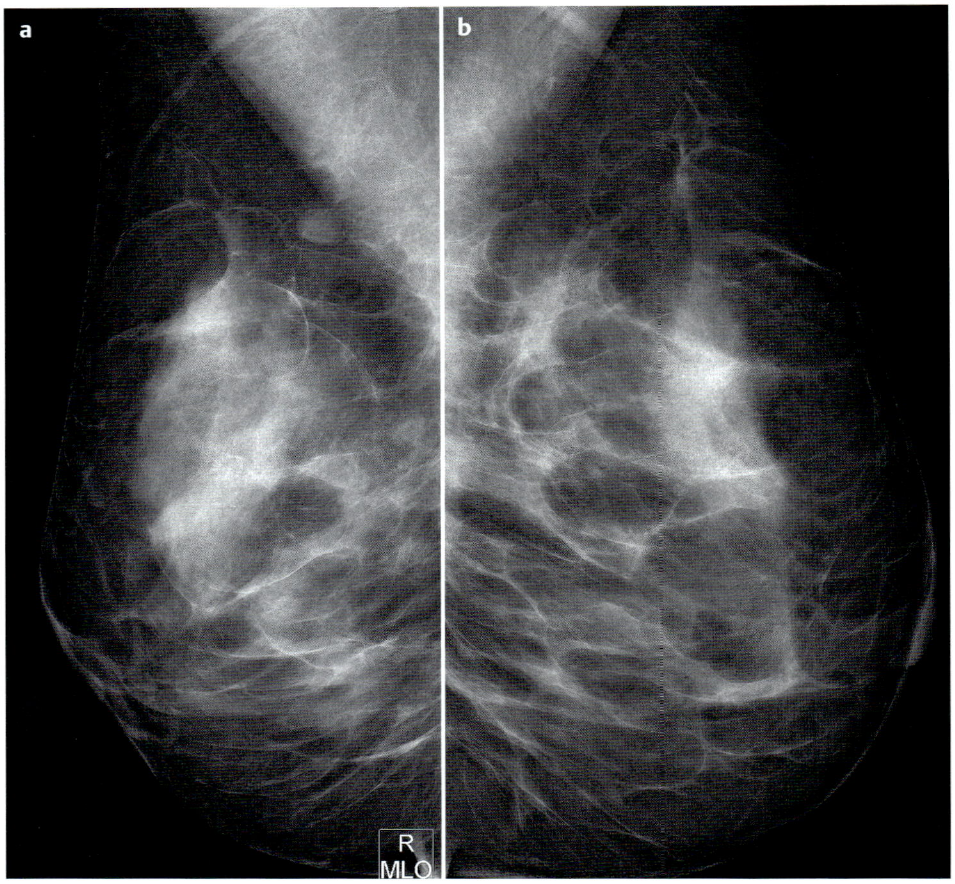


Fig. 5.**2 a, b** Digital mammography, MLO view.

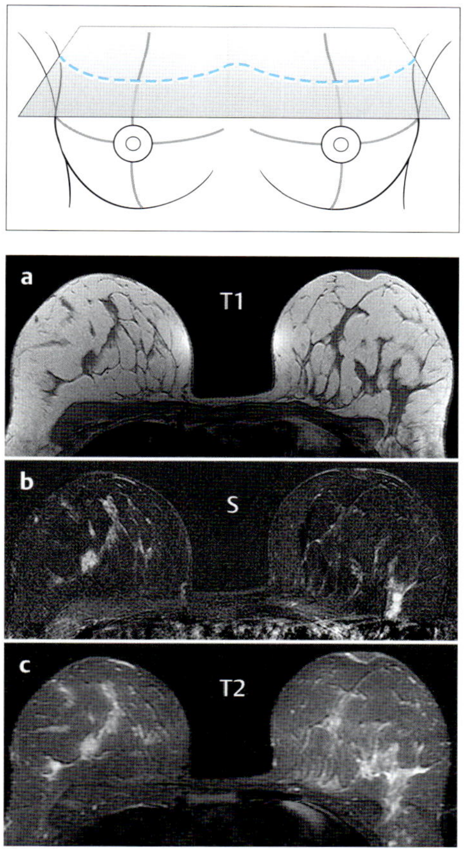


Fig. 5.**3 a – c**

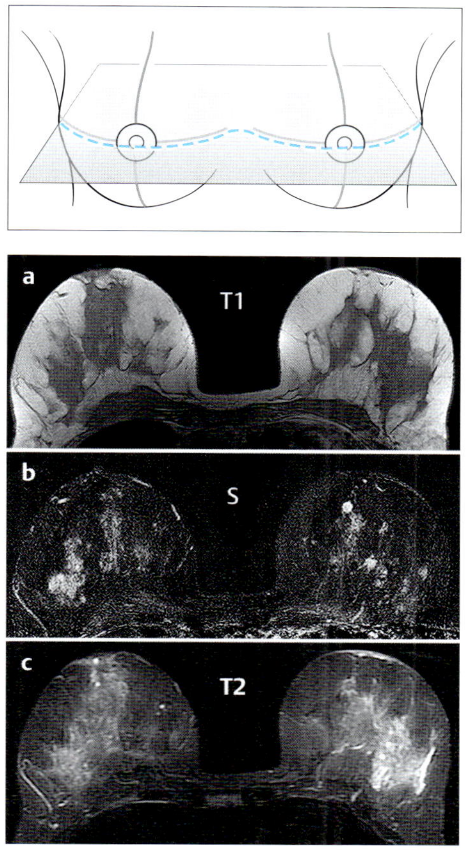


Fig. 5.**4 a – c**

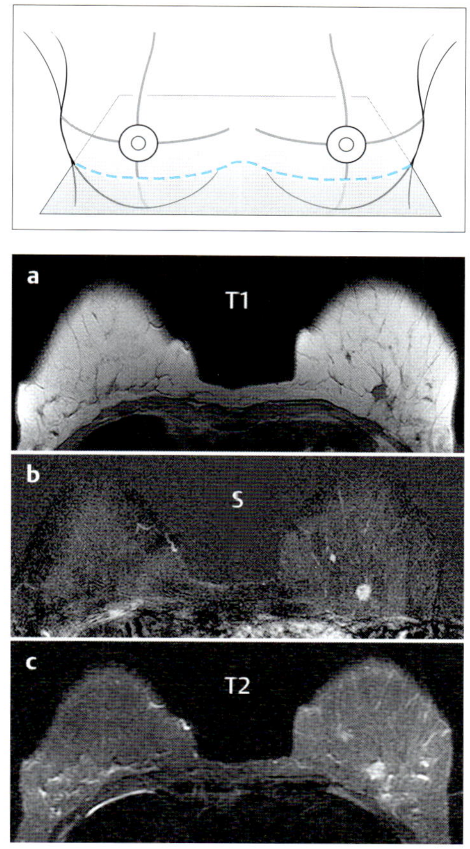


Fig. 5.**5 a – c**

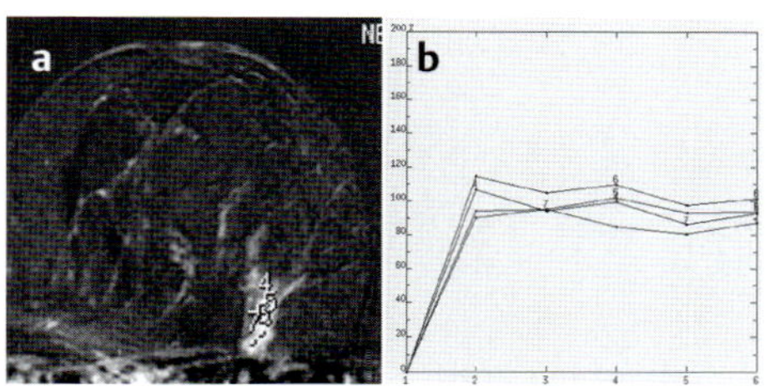


Fig. 5.**6 a, b** Signal-to-time curves.

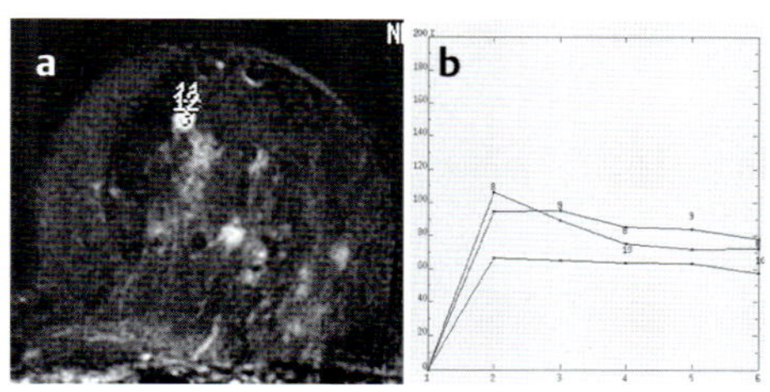


Fig. 5.**7 a, b** Signal-to-time curves.

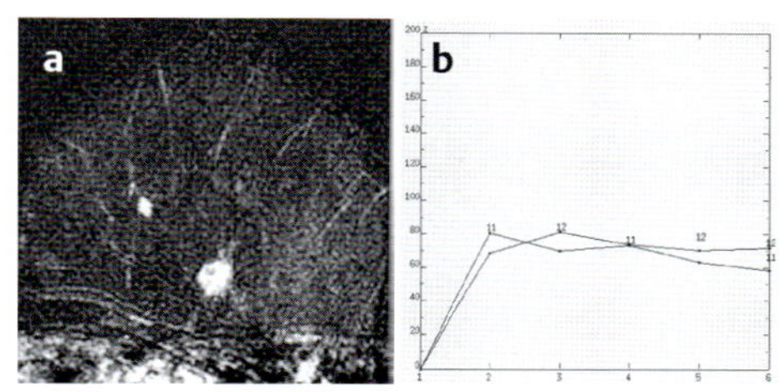


Fig. 5.**8 a, b** Signal-to-time curves.

Fig. 5.**3** – 5.**8** Contrast-enhanced MR mammography.

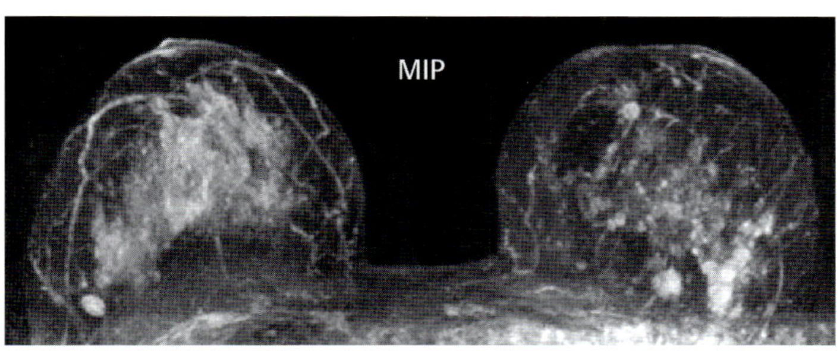


Fig. 5.**9** Contrast-enhanced MR mammography. Maximum intensity projection.

**?**

Please characterize ultrasound, mammography, and MRI findings.
What is your preliminary diagnosis?
What are your next steps?

This is the imaging study of an asymptomatic woman without any increased familial risk.

### Ultrasound

Ultrasound shows a round hypoechoic lesion with well-defined margins and a markedly hyperechoic wall in the upper outer quadrant of the left breast. This lesions disrupts ligamental structures. Directly inferior to the nipple of the left breast, there is another hypoechoic lesion with a hyperechoic wall. In the region of the caudal inframammary fold, there is a third hypoechoic lesion with hyperechoic wall, distortion of the surrounding tissue, and possibly infiltration of deeper structures. None of the lesions show distal shadowing. In the right breast there was a normal prepectoral lymph node with a central fatty hilum. US BI-RADS right 1/left 5 (MCC).

### Mammography

Both breasts demonstrated inhomogeneous dense breast tissue ACR type 3. In the upper parts of the left breast (near the edge of the MLO view image) is a mild architectural distortion of the parenchyma, corresponding to the cranial and central ultrasound finding. Right mammogram demonstrates a normal lymph node. There are no pathological calcifications in either breast (BI-RADS right 1/left 4. PGMI: MLO view G (inframammary fold).

### MR Mammography

MRI depicted a chainlike grouping of hypervascularized lesions in the upper outer quadrant of the left breast, each lesion being nearly 1 cm in diameter. A second lesion of approx. 1 cm diameter is seen directly caudal of the left nipple. The third hypervascularized lesion, with ring enhancement, is located in the area of the caudal inframammary fold. The signal curves are indicative of malignancy.

**MRI Artifact Category:** 1
**MRI Density Type:** 3

| MRM score | Left breast, upper outer quadrant | Points | Left breast, central lesion | Points | Left breast, caudal lesion | Points |
|---|---|---|---|---|---|---|
| **Shape** | round | 0 | round | 0 | round | 0 |
| **Border** | well-defined | 0 | ill-defined | 1 | ill-defined | 1 |
| **CM Distribution** | rim sign | 2 | rim sign | 2 | rim sign | 2 |
| **Initial Signal Intensity Increase** | strong | 2 | strong | 2 | moderate | 1 |
| **Post-initial Signal Intensity Character** | wash-out | 2 | wash-out | 2 | plateau | 1 |
| **MRI score (points)** | | **6** | | **7** | | **5** |
| **MRI BI-RADS** | | **5** | | **5** | | **4** |

### → Preliminary Diagnosis

Multicentric invasive carcinoma of the left breast.

| BI-RADS Categorization | | |
|---|---|---|
| Clinical Findings | right 1 | left 4 |
| Ultrasound | right 1 | left 5 |
| Mammography | right 1 | left 4 |
| MR Mammography | right 1 | left 5 |
| **BI-RADS Total** | **right 1** | **left 5** |

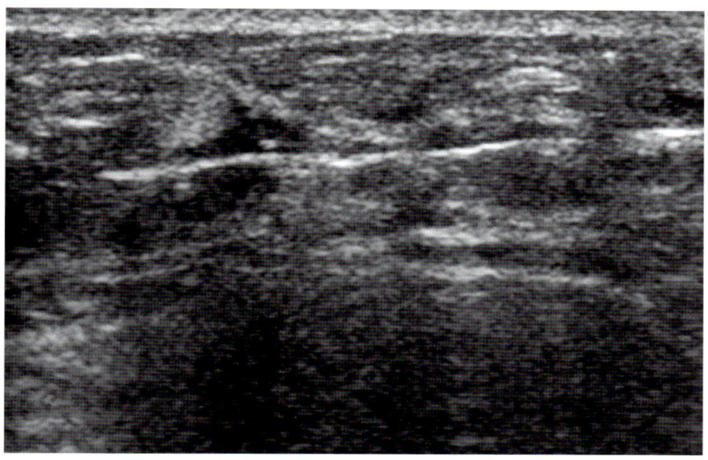

Fig. 5.**10** US-guided core biopsy (14-gauge) of the caudal lesion in the left breast. Post-fire documentation.

**Procedure**

US-guided core biopsy of at least two of the three lesions in the left breast to obtain histological data and to verify (or exclude) multicentricity.

The lesion visible in mammography in the prepectoral region of the right breast can be seen in the ultrasound imaging to have all the criteria of a benign lymph node. Therefore, no additional assessment is necessary.

### Histology

Histology left breast upper outer quadrant: IDC, grade 2.
Histology left breast caudal: IDC, grade 2.

### Histology

IDC pT2 (multicentric), pN3a (20/38), G2.

### Treatment

Mastectomy.

Carcinoma multicentricity is generally a contraindication for breast conservation therapy.

**Indication:** Screening.
**History:** Unremarkable.
**Risk profile:** Breast cancer of mother (premenopausal) and sister (perimenopausal).
**Age:** 59 years.

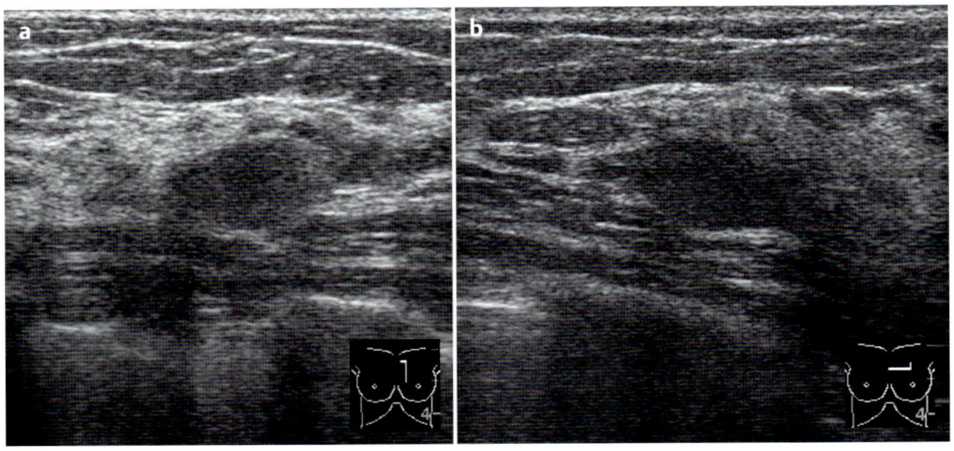

Fig. 6.**1 a, b** Sonography.

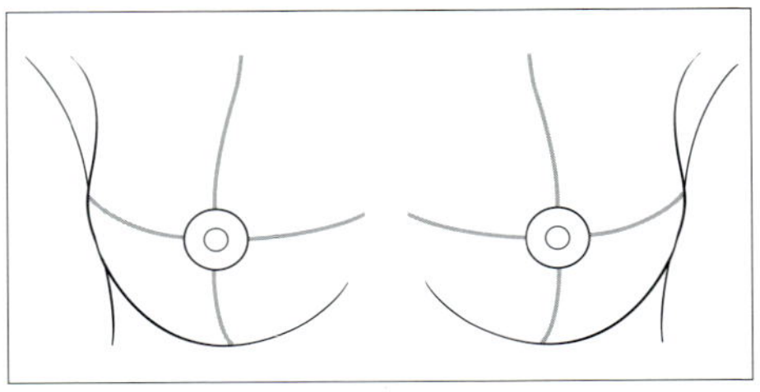

**Clinical Findings**

Normal.

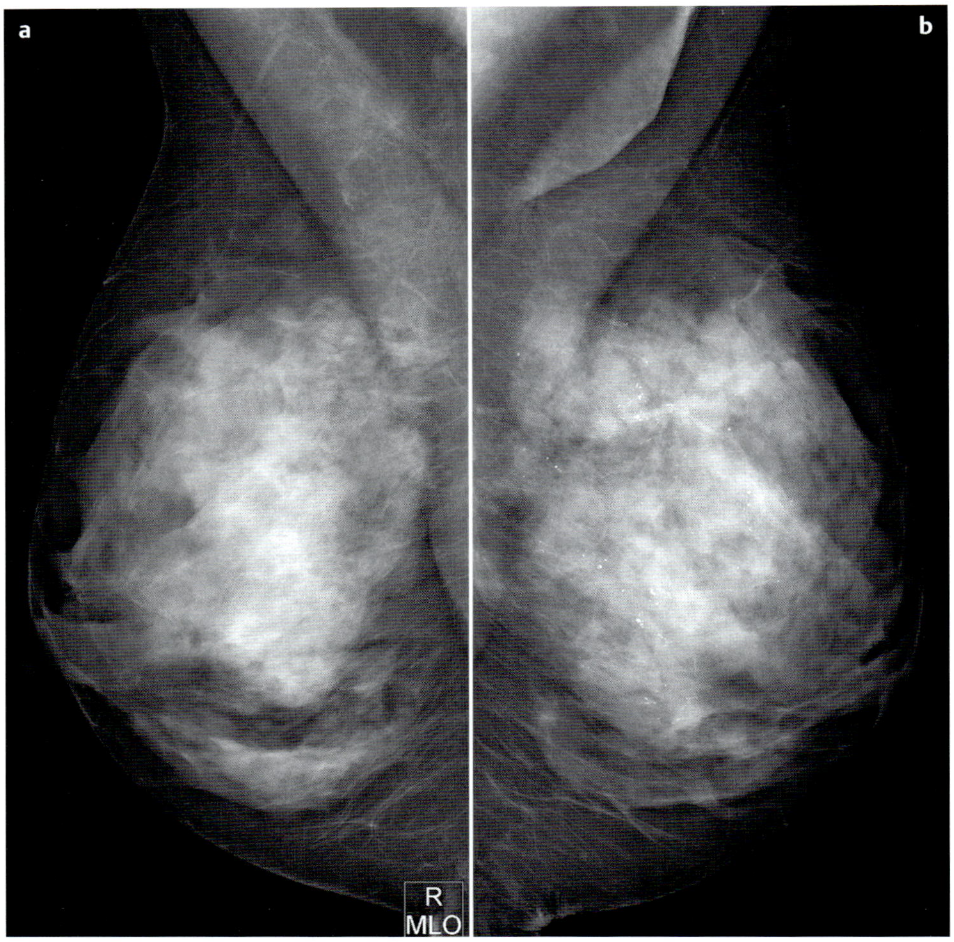


Fig. 6.**2 a, b** Digital mammography, MLO view.

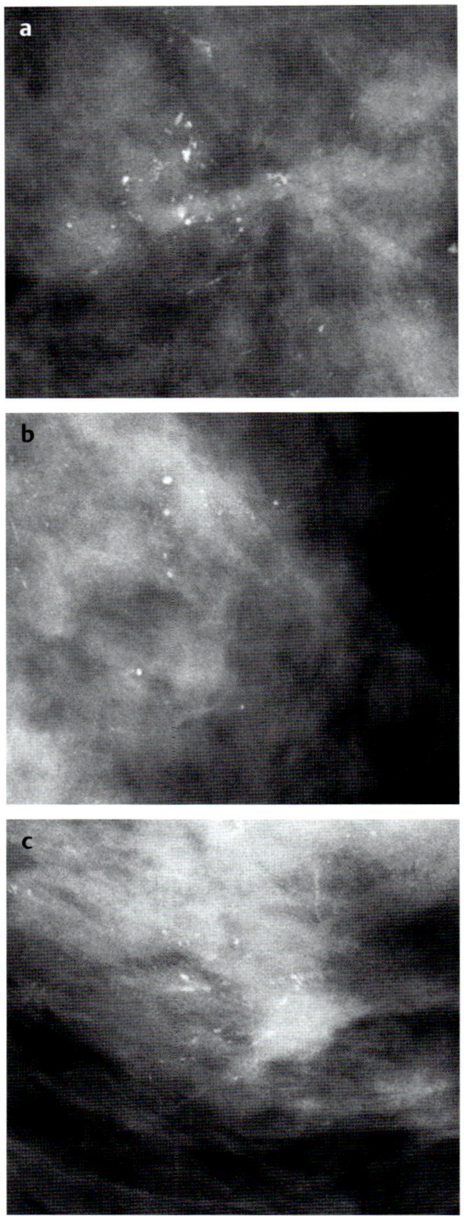

Fig. 6.**3 a – c** Magnification view of the left breast cranial (**a**), central (**b**) and caudal (**c**).

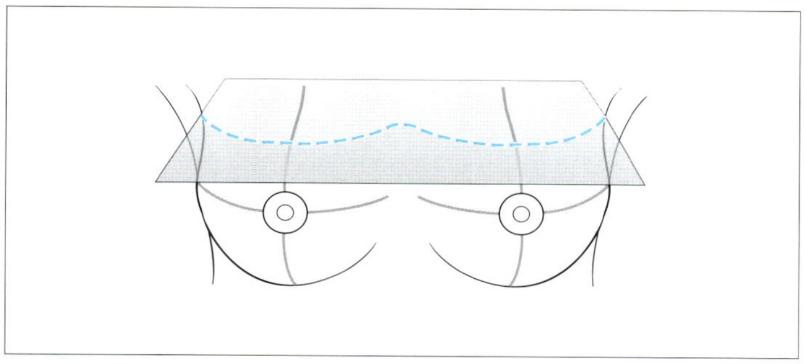

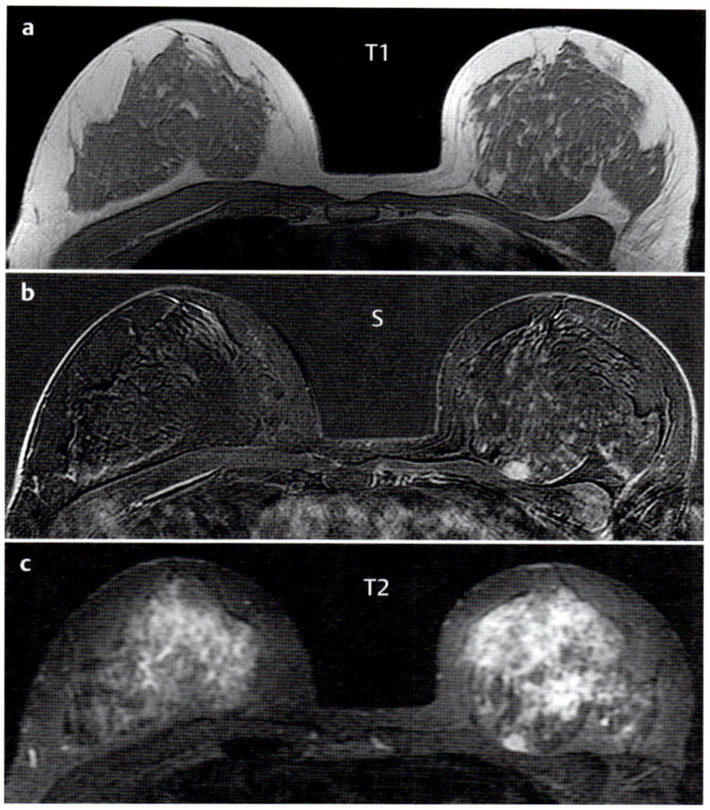

Fig. 6.4 **a – c** Contrast-enhanced MRI of the breasts.

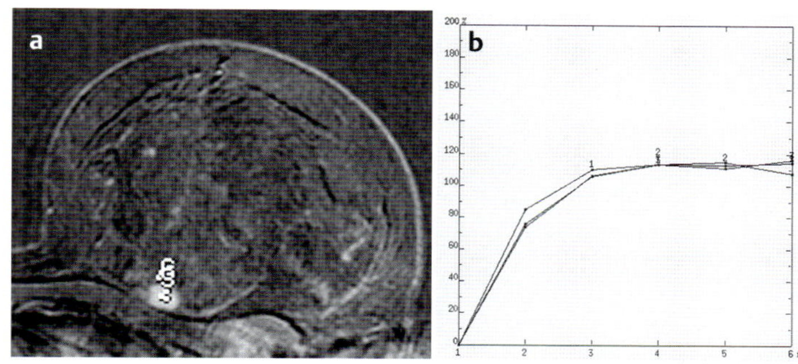

Fig. 6.5 **a, b** Signal-to-time curves.

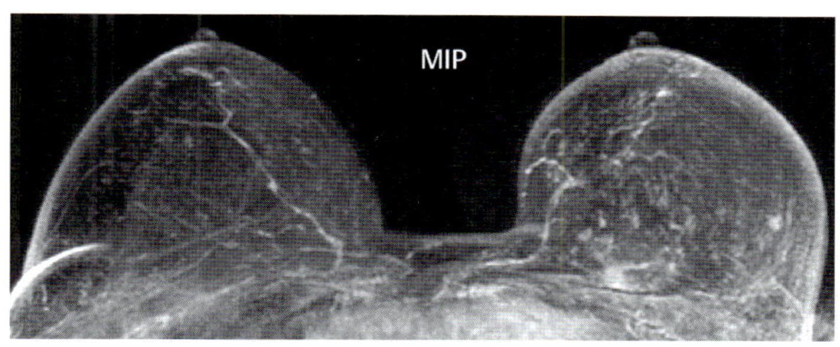

Fig. 6.**6** Contrast-enhanced MR mammography. Maximum intensity projection.

?

Please characterize ultrasound, mammography, and MRI findings.
What is your preliminary diagnosis?
What are your next steps?

This asymptomatic woman underwent screening imaging because of her increased familial risk.

### Ultrasound

Round lesion with smooth borders in the upper inner quadrant of the left breast close to the pectoral muscle. Homogeneous internal echo pattern. Long axis parallel to skin. Slight distal acoustic enhancement. No definitive criteria of malignancy. US BI-RADS 3.

### Mammography

Bilaterally symmetric extremely dense parenchymal pattern, ACR type 4. Within the limitations of these conditions, no mass was detected. No architectural distortion. Diffuse microcalcifications in the left breast, with varying characteristics:

Cranial: regionally polymorphous (BI-RADS 4)
Central: regionally monomorphous (round) (BI-RADS 2)
Caudal: segmentally polymorphous (BI-RADS 5)

Did you note the microcalcifications in the axillary region of the right breast (Fig. 6.**7**)? How do you interpret these?

**Categorization of mammography findings:** BI-RADS right 3/left 5. PGMI: MLO view P (despite axillary fold visible left).

### MR Mammography

There is a round hypervascularized lesion 1 cm in diameter in the upper inner quadrant of the left breast, obviously corresponding to the lesion seen in ultrasound. This lesion has high signal intensity (water content) in the inversion recovery sequence and a nonspecific signal–time curve with maximum 110% initial increase and subsequent plateau.

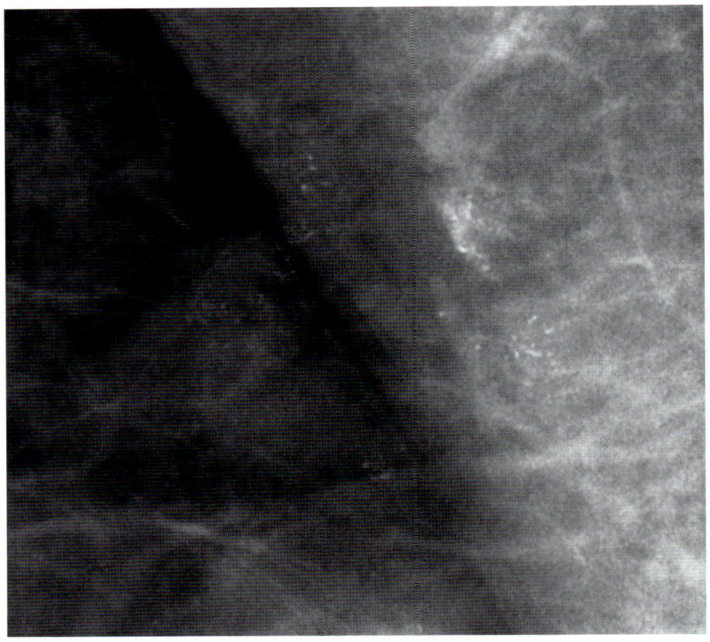

Fig. 6.**7** Mammography, magnification view of the upper outer quadrant of the right breast.

**MRI Artifact Category:** 2
**MRI Density Type:** 1

### → Differential Diagnosis

| | |
|---|---|
| Left breast, upper inner quadrant: | Fibroadenoma, papilloma, phyllodes tumor, carcinoma (mucinous, medullary?) |
| Left breast, cranial and caudal regions: | DCIS, IDC |
| Left breast, central region: | adenosis, DCIS |
| Right axillary region: | adenosis, DCIS |

| MRM score | Finding | Points |
|---|---|---|
| **Shape** | round | 0 |
| **Border** | well-defined | 0 |
| **CM Distribution** | homogeneous | 0 |
| **Initial Signal Intensity Increase** | strong | 2 |
| **Post-initial Signal Intensity Character** | plateau | 1 |
| **MRI score (points)** | | **3** |
| **MRI BI-RADS** | | **3** |

| BI-RADS Categorization | | |
|---|---|---|
| Clinical Findings | right 1 | left 1 |
| Ultrasound | right 1 | left 3 |
| Mammography | right 3 | left 5 |
| MR Mammography | right 1 | left 3 |
| **BI-RADS Total** | **right 3** | **left 5** |

### Procedure

MR-guided vacuum core biopsy of the lesion in the left breast close to the chest wall. Alternatively, US-guided core biopsy, it being likely although not certain that this lesion corresponds with the US findings. Stereotactic vacuum core biopsy of the cranially or caudally located microcalcifications. Excisional biopsy for diagnostic purposes of the calcifications of the right axillary region after preoperative marking.

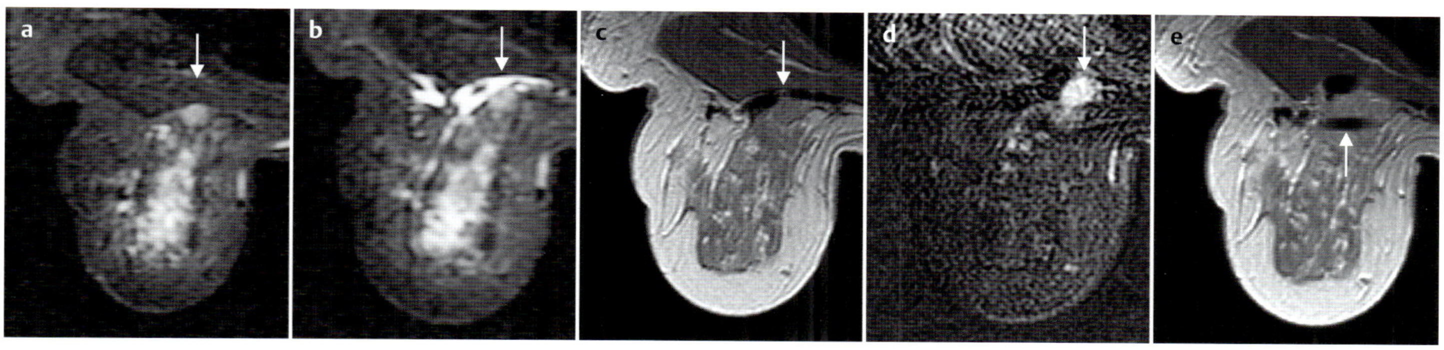


Fig. 6.**8 a – e** MR-guided vacuum biopsy of the hypervascularized lesion in the left breast. Documentation of the lesion (arrow) in water-sensitive IR-sequence before (**a**) and after local anaesthesia (**b**). T1-weighted image (**c**), subtraction image (**d**) and documentation of the positioned coaxial canula (arrow) after removal of specimen (**e**).

### Histology of the lesion close to the chest wall, left breast

Mucinous carcinoma.

### Histology of the microcalcifications, left breast cranial region:

Intraductal carcinoma.

### Histology

Left breast: Invasive mucinous carcinoma pT1c (11 mm) + extensive DCIS pN0 (0/14 sn), G3 (DCIS)
Right breast: Adenofibrous dysplasia. No malignancy.

### Treatment

Mastectomy of the left breast. Segmental biopsy of the right breast.

Where diffuse microcalcifications are present, all affected parts of the breast must be carefully evaluated. Both benign and malignant calcifications can occur in the same breast.

**Indication:** Screening.
**History:** Unremarkable.
**Risk profile:** Bilateral breast cancer in mother at 45 and 65 years.
**Age:** 41 years.

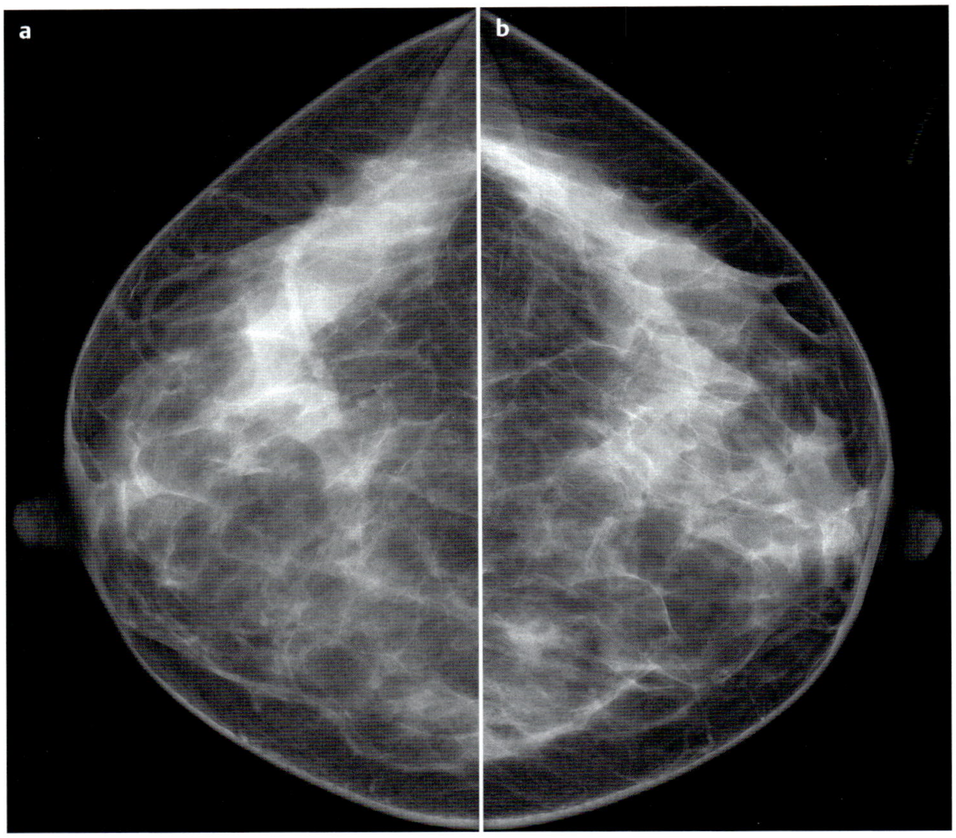


Fig. 7.1 **a, b** Digital mammography, CC view.

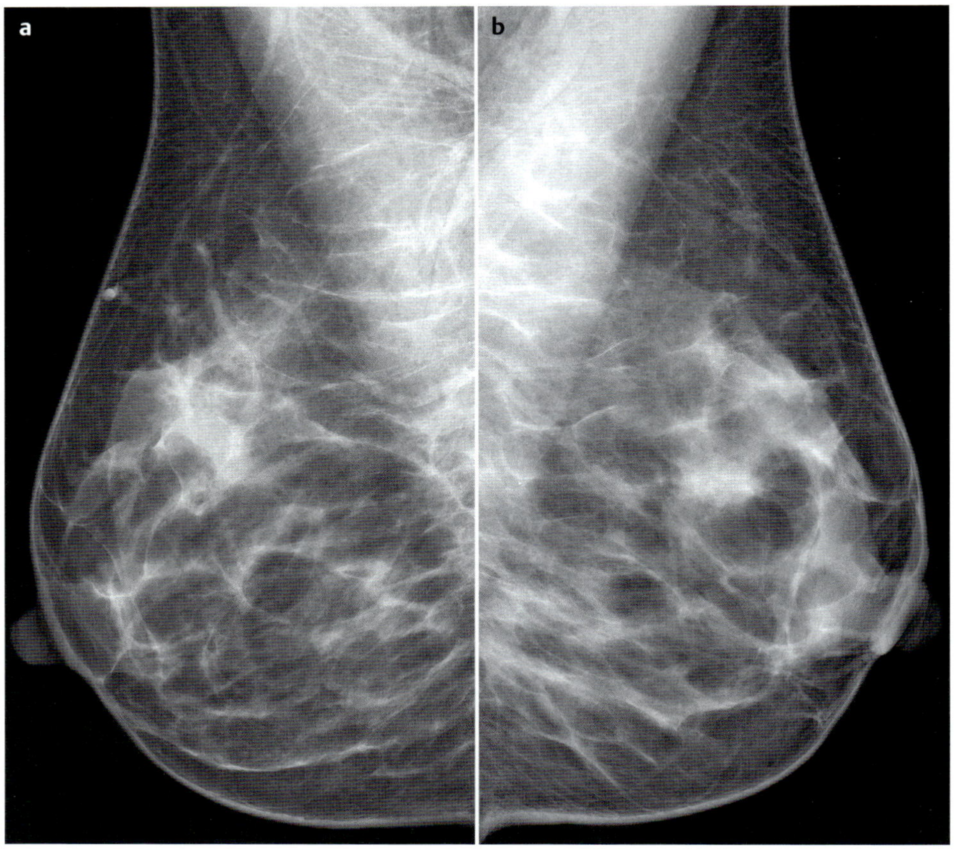


Fig. 7.2 **a, b** Digital mammography, MLO view.

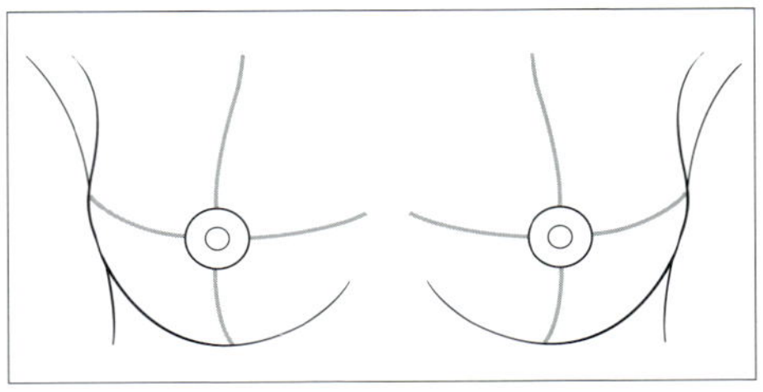

## Clinical Findings

No pathological findings on inspection or palpation.

## Ultrasound

No pathological findings.

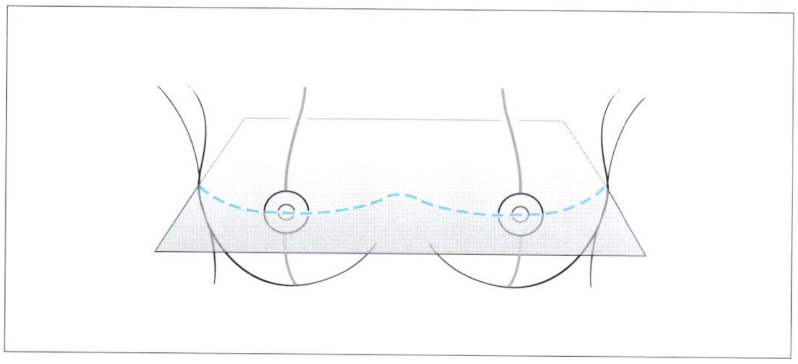

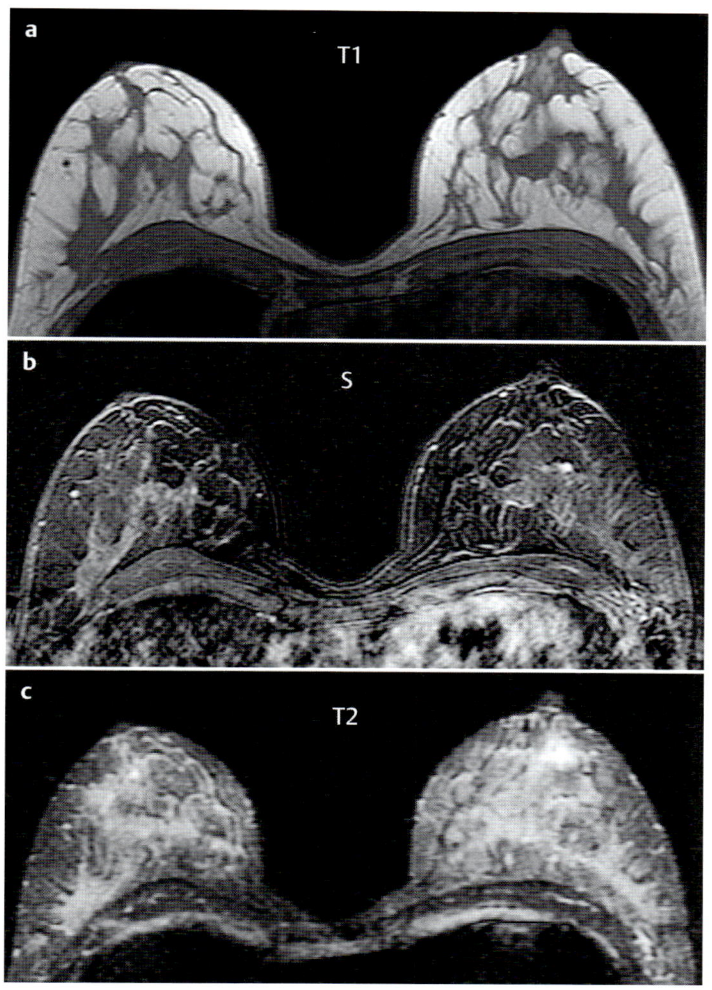


Fig. 7.3 **a – c** Contrast-enhanced MRI of the breasts.

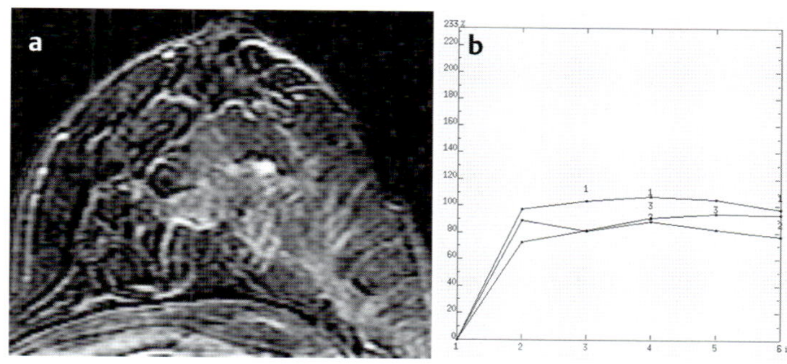


Fig. 7.4 **a, b** Signal-to-time curves.

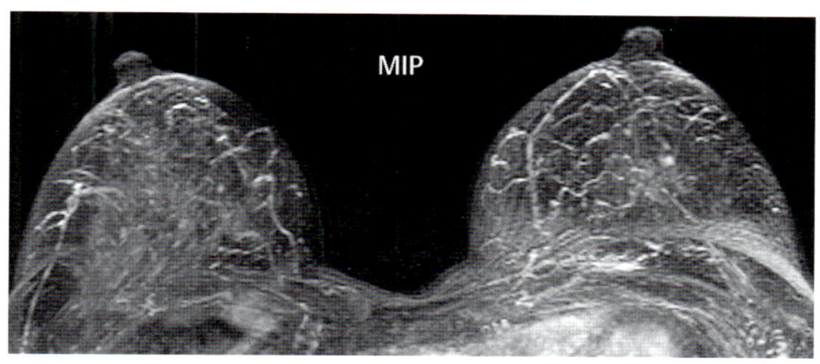


Fig. 7.**5** Contrast-enhanced MR mammography. Maximum intensity projection.

?

Please characterize mammography and MRI findings.
What is your preliminary diagnosis?
What are your next steps?

These examinations were performed in a screening situation in a woman with an increased familial risk.

### Ultrasound

Ultrasound showed no pathological findings. In particular, there was no circumscribed lesion corresponding to the enhancing area in the left breast seen in MRI.

### Mammography

Digital mammograms demonstrated bilaterally symmetric, extremely dense parenchymal structures, ACR type 4. Under these limiting conditions, no lesions or masses were visible. No calcifications (BI-RADS right 1/left 1). PGMI: CC view P; MLO view P.

### MR Mammography

MRI depicted a 5 mm mass in the central part of the left breast with increased vascularization. No other findings.

**MRI Artifact Category:** 3
**MRI Density Type:** 2

| MRM score | Finding | Points |
|---|---|---|
| **Shape** | round | 0 |
| **Border** | well-defined | 0 |
| **CM Distribution** | inhomogeneous | 1 |
| **Initial Signal Intensity Increase** | moderate | 1 |
| **Post-initial Signal Intensity Character** | plateau | 1 |
| **MRI score (points)** | | **3** |
| **MRI BI-RADS** | | **3** |

### → Differential Diagnosis

Fibroadenoma, adenoma, papilloma, small carcinoma.

| BI-RADS Categorization | | |
|---|---|---|
| Clinical Findings | right 1 | left 1 |
| Ultrasound | right 1 | left 1 |
| Mammography | right 1 | left 1 |
| MR Mammography | right 1 | left 3 |
| **BI-RADS Total** | **right 1** | **left 3** |

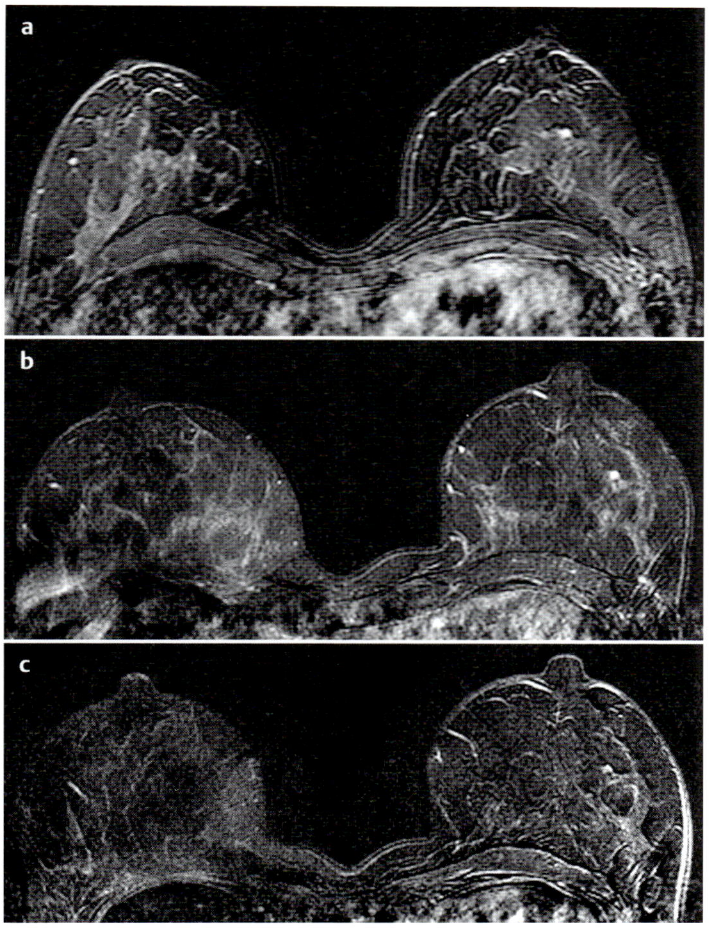

Fig. 7.6 **a – c** Monitoring of findings.
**a** First examination.
**b** Second examination 6 months after first MRI.
**c** Second examination 12 months after first MRI.

**Procedure**

Follow-up examination (MRI) in 6 months.

## Diagnosis (without histopathological verification, but MRI findings consistent over 12 months)

Benign mass in the left breast (fibroadenoma, adenoma, papilloma?)

### Treatment

None. Next complete examination (mammography, US, MRI) in 12 months.

A single enhancing mass in MRI with no corresponding findings in ultrasound or mammography, and no spiculation, washout, or rim sign findings, can simply be followed up at intervals of 6 months.

**Indication:** Screening.
**History:** Unremarkable.
**Risk profile:** No increased risk.
**Age:** 68 years.

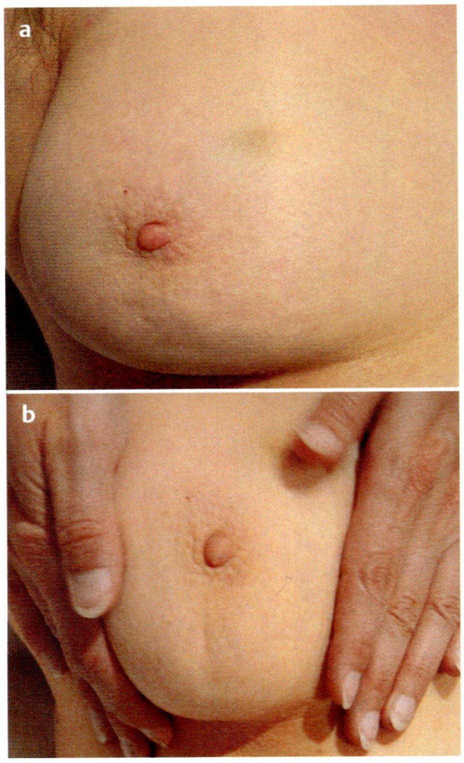

Fig. 8.1 **a, b** Clinical examination of the right breast. No palpable mass.

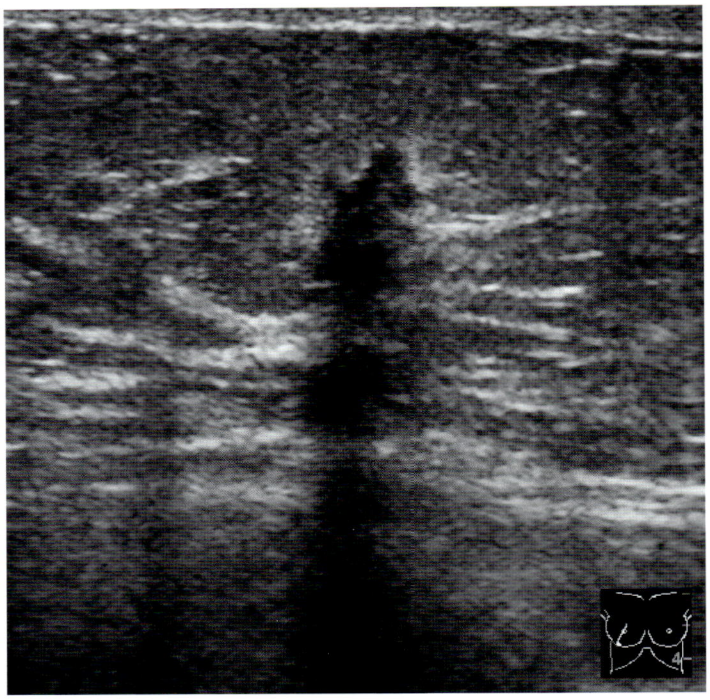

Fig. 8.**2** Sonography.

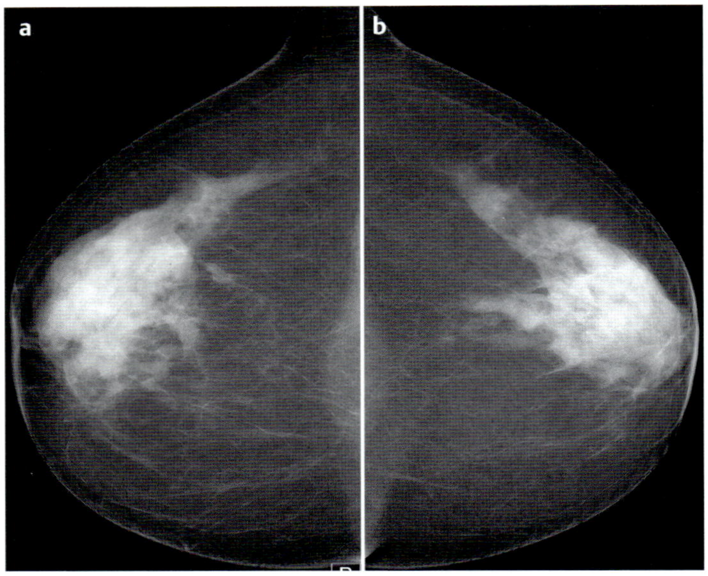

Fig. 8.**3 a, b** Digital mammography, CC view.

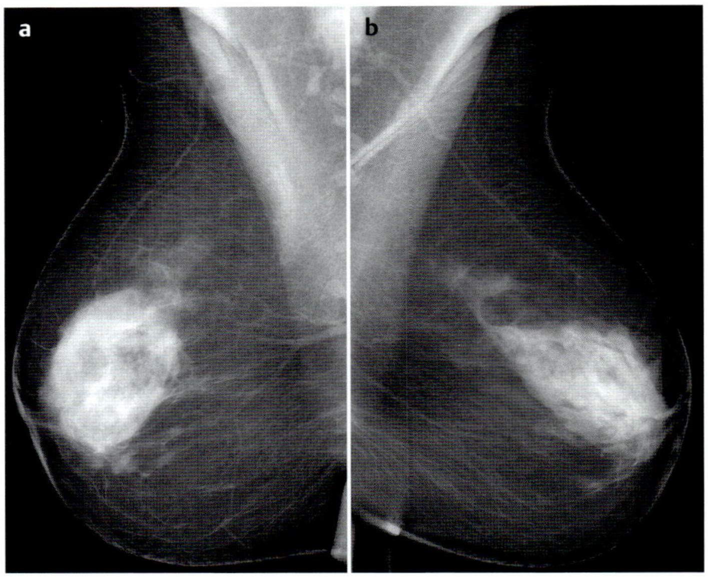

Fig. 8.**4 a, b** Digital mammography, MLO view.

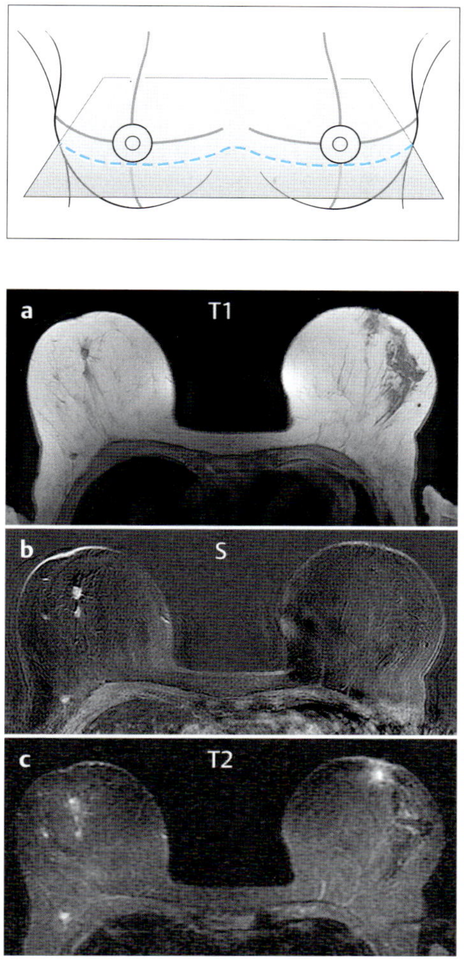


Fig. 8.**5 a – c** Contrast-enhanced MRI of the breasts.

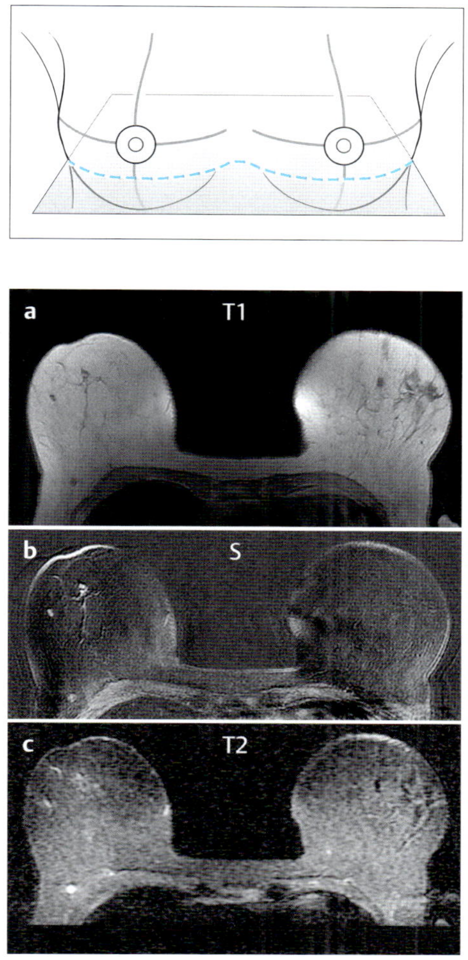


Fig. 8.**6 a – c** Contrast-enhanced MRI of the breasts.

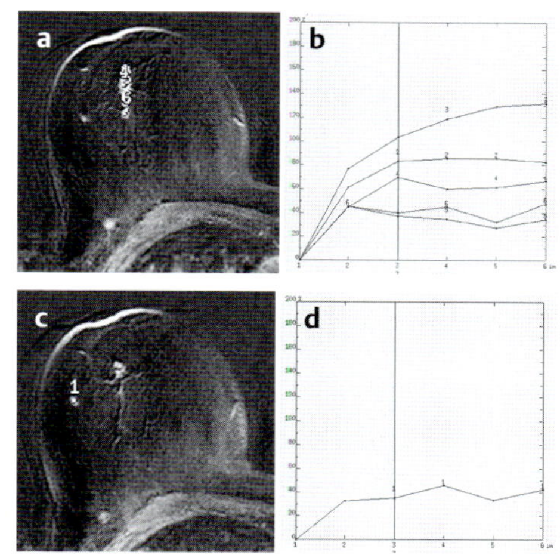


Fig. 8.**7 a – d** Signal-to-time curves.

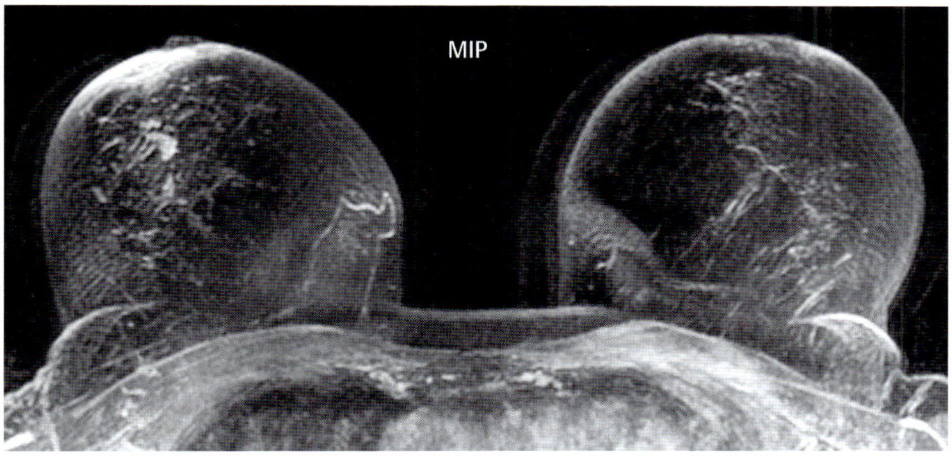


Fig. 8.**8** Contrast-enhanced MR mammography. Maximum intensity projection.

?

Please characterize ultrasound, mammography, and MRI findings.
What is your preliminary diagnosis?
What are your next steps?

Clinical symptoms were present and imaging was performed for screening purposes.

## Clinical Examination

With the patient's arms raised, and on compression of the right breast with both hands, there was a suspicious skin retraction below the nipple.

## Ultrasound

Ultrasound demonstrated a suspect 6 mm-long mass with a hyperechoic margin. The long axis of this lesion was perpendicular to the skin, disrupting the continuity of the surrounding ligaments. US BI-RADS right 5.

## Mammography

The parenchyma in both breasts was dense, ACR type 4, and bilaterally symmetric. No calcifications. The MLO view of the right breast showed a lobulated density of approx. 8 mm diameter caudal of the glandular tissue However, this finding was obscured by the parenchyma in the CC view (BI-RADS right 3/left 1). For better differentiation, spot compression of the unclear density in the right breast was performed (Fig. 8.**9**b). This view depicted the spiculated periphery of this lesion (BI-RADS including spot view: right 4). PGMI: CC view P; MLO view G (caudal inframammary fold).

## MR Mammography

Corresponding to ultrasound and mammography findings, MRI showed a hypervascularized lesion in the right breast inferior to the nipple. A second small lesion with increased vascularization was visible toward the chest wall. A third lesion was seen lateral to the primary tumor. Hypervascularized lymph nodes.

**MRI Artifact Category:** 2
**MRI Density Type:** 1

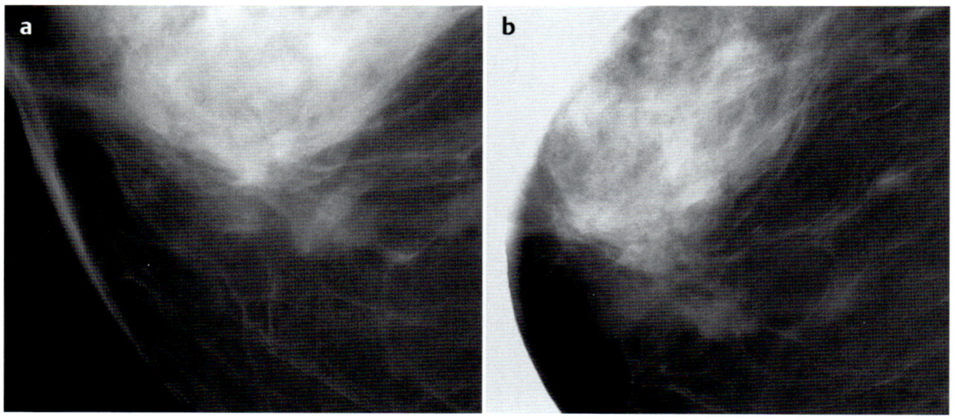


Fig. 8.**9 a, b** Magnification of the MLO view (right breast) and additional spot compression.

| MRM score | Finding | Points |
|---|---|---|
| **Shape** | oval | 0 |
| **Border** | spiculated | 1 |
| **CM Distribution** | inhomogeneous | 1 |
| **Initial Signal Intensity Increase** | moderate | 1 |
| **Post-initial Signal Intensity Character** | plateau | 1 |
| **MRI score (points)** | | **4** |
| **MRI BI-RADS** | | **4** |

## → Preliminary Diagnosis

Multifocal breast cancer. No differential diagnoses.

| BI-RADS Categorization | | |
|---|---|---|
| Clinical Findings | right 4 | left 1 |
| Ultrasound | right 5 | left 1 |
| Mammography | right 3 (4 after spot) | left 1 |
| MR Mammography | right 4 (multifocal) | left 1 |
| **BI-RADS Total** | **right 4** | **left 1** |

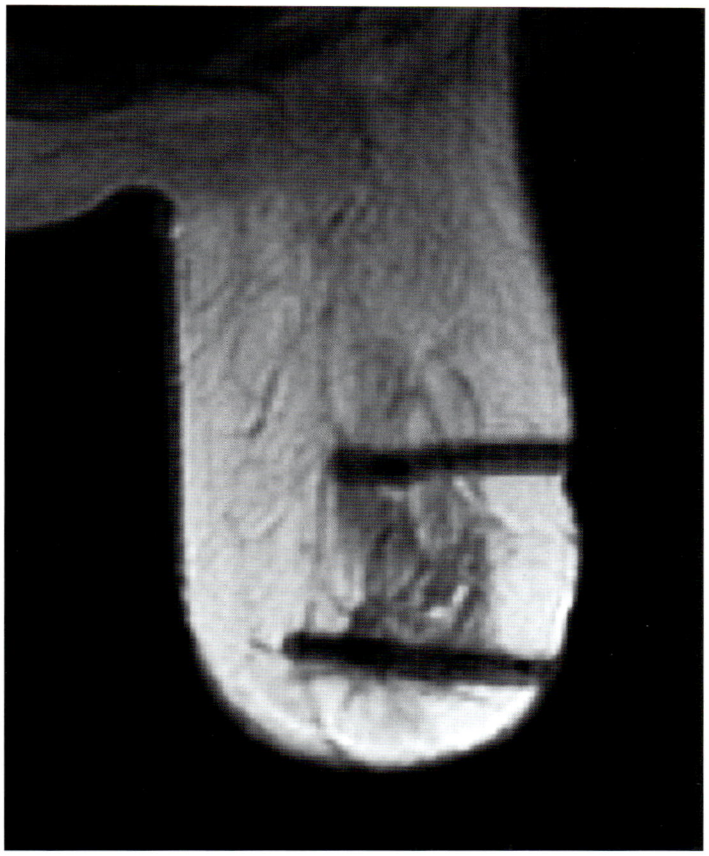

Fig. 8.**10** Preoperative MR-guided localization with two hook-wires.

**Procedure**

Histological verification of the primary tumor of the right breast by percutaneous US-guided core biopsy.

**Histopathology of the right breast after US-guided core biopsy**

Invasive ductal carcinoma.

Preoperative MR-guided localization of the multifocal nodules peripheral to the primary tumor (Fig. 8.**10**).

## Diagnosis

Bifocal invasive ductal carcinoma of the right breast (13 mm, 7 mm).

IDC pT1c (bifocal), pN1 (1/5 sn), G2

## Treatment

Segmentectomy.

Any clinical findings such as tissue resistance, a palpable mass, or skin or nipple retraction raise suspicion of malignancy. In this situation, imaging is required either to exclude the possibility of malignancy with a great degree of certainty or, as in this case, to confirm it.

**Indication:** Palpable mass between upper quadrants of the left breast.
**History:** Unremarkable.
**Risk profile:** Breast cancer in grandmother at the age of 82 years.
**Age:** 52 years.

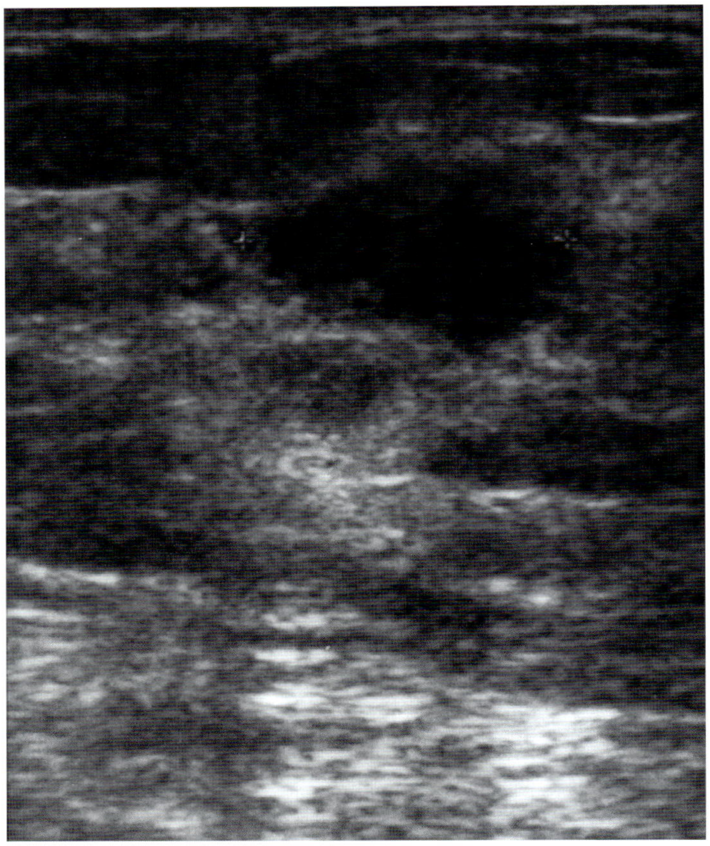

Fig. 9.**1** Ultrasound image of the palpable mass.

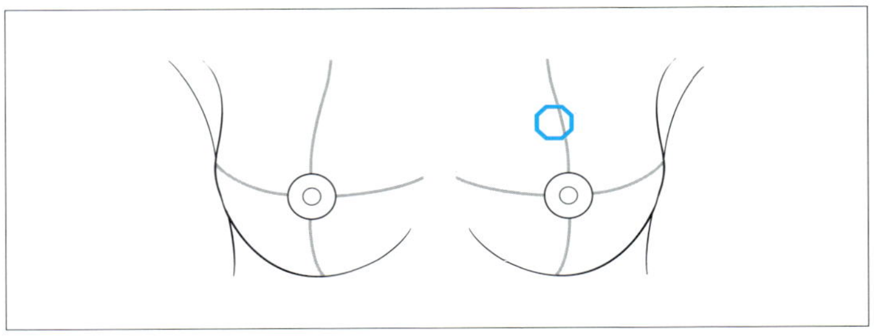

## Clinical Findings

Palpable mass of approx. 1.5 cm located in line with the nipple between the upper quadrants of the left breast. Generally lumpy parenchymal texture.

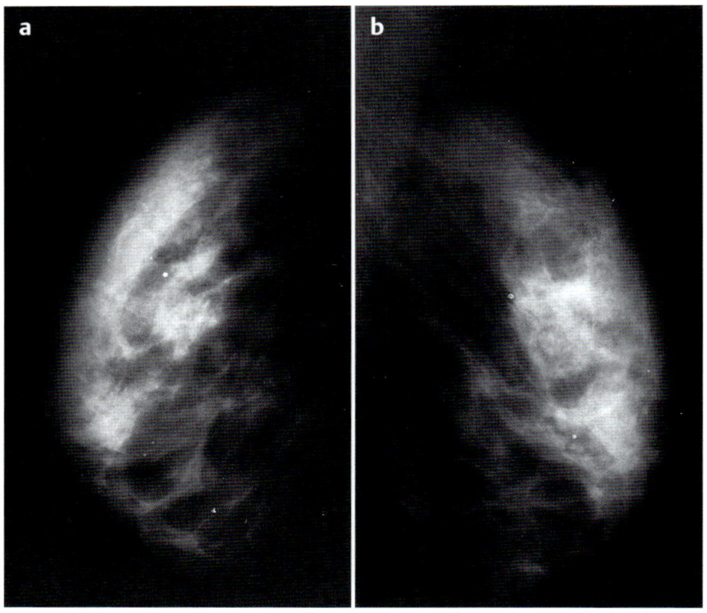


Fig. 9.**2 a, b** Conventional mammography, CC view [imaging not performed by authors].

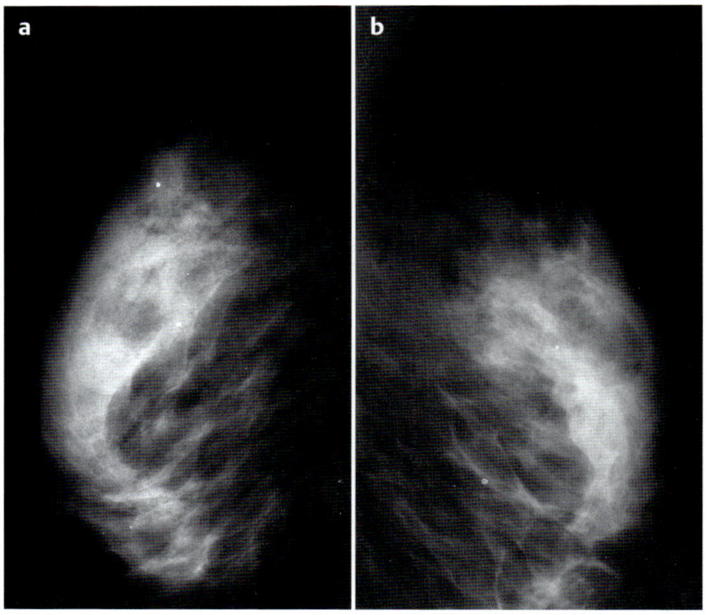


Fig. 9.**3 a, b** Conventional mammography, MLO view [imaging not performed by authors].

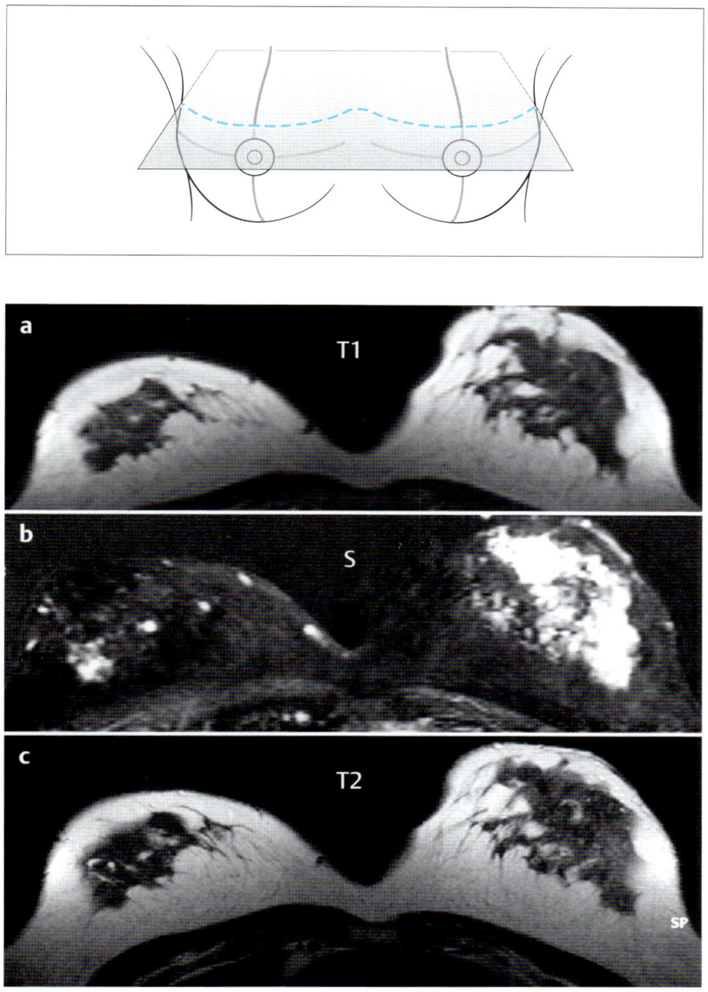


Fig. 9.**4 a–c** Contrast-enhanced MRI of the breasts, 3-D technique [imaging not performed by authors].

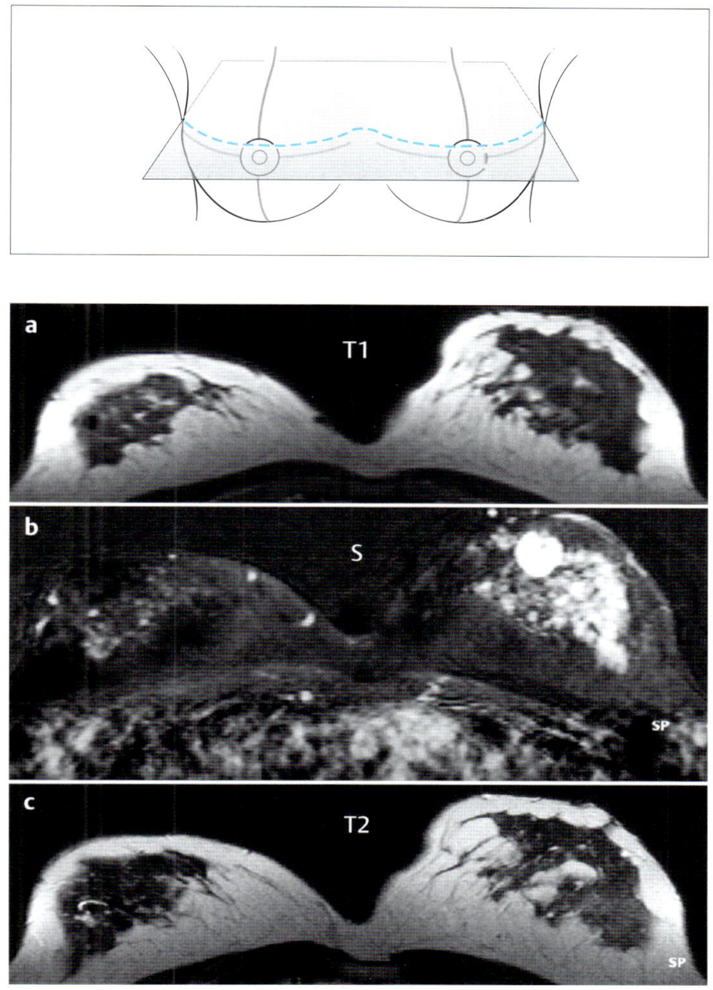


Fig. 9.**5 a–c** Contrast-enhanced MRI of the breasts, 3-D technique [imaging not performed by authors].

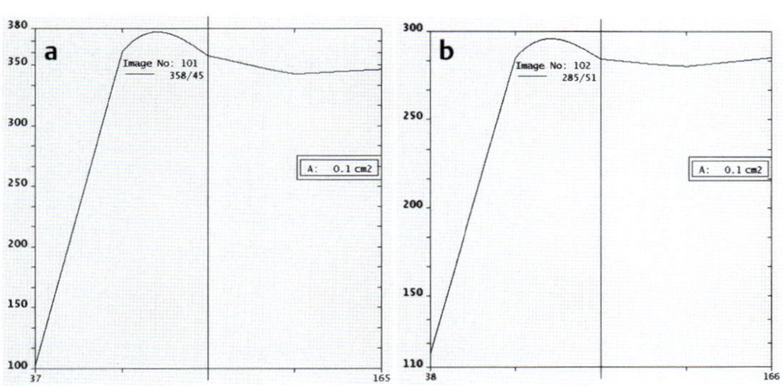


Fig. 9.**6 a, b** Signal-to-time curve [data not prepared by authors].

?

Please characterize ultrasound, mammography, and MRI findings.
What is your preliminary diagnosis?
What are your next steps?

This case demonstrates the imaging of a symptomatic woman presenting with a palpable mass between the upper quadrants of the left breast. The breast cancer of her grandmother at 82 years does not represent an increased risk.

### Ultrasound

Corresponding to the palpable resistance there is an irregular hypoechogenic lesion with partially echogenic borders and indeterminate distal echo characteristics in the left breast. US BI-RADS left 4.

### Mammography

Mammography showed bilaterally symmetric inhomogeneous dense parenchyma (ACR type 3). There was a hyperdense lesion with a diameter of 1 cm accompanied by architectural distortion in the center of the left breast (Fig. 9.**7**). Imaging showed no suspicious microcalcifications. BI-RADS right 1/left 4. PGMI: MLO view I (incomplete presentation of the parenchyma; minimal presentation of the pectoral muscle); CC view I (exposure, nipples projected into breast tissue).

### MR Mammography

Corresponding to the clinical and ultrasound findings, MRI demonstrated a round, hypervascularized, partially spiculated lesion 1.3 cm in diameter in the left breast. Initial signal increase of more than 280% (NB: 3-D technique!) and postinitial plateau. There was evident asymmetry of the parenchymal perfusion (left > right).

**MRI Artifact Category:** 2
**MRI Density Type:** 3*

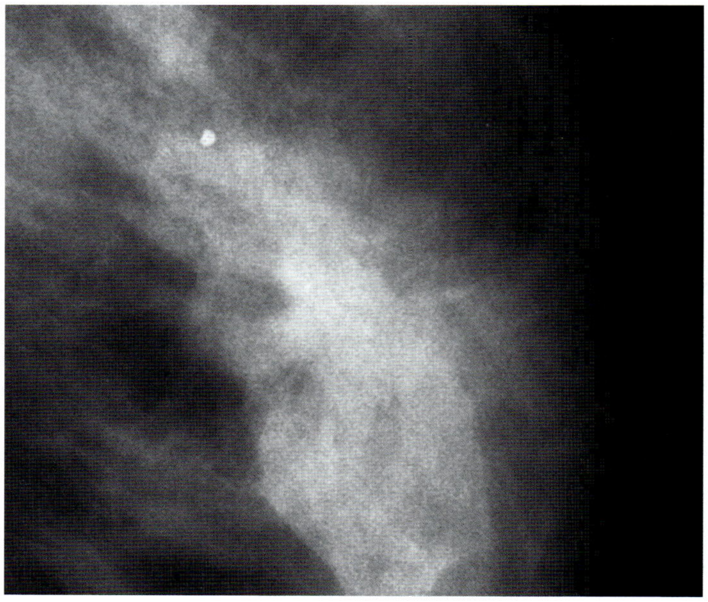

Fig. 9.**7** Magnification of the MLO view, left breast.

| MRM score | Finding | Points |
|---|---|---|
| **Shape** | round | 1 |
| **Border** | ill-defined | 1 |
| **CM Distribution** | ring (?)* | 2 |
| **Initial Signal Intensity Increase#** | strong | 2 |
| **Post-initial Signal Intensity Character** | plateau | 1 |
| **MRI score (points)** | | **7** |
| **MRI BI-RADS** | | **5** |

* Contrast in MR images too high.
\# note: 3-D technique

### → Preliminary Diagnosis

Breast cancer. Considerably less likely: fibroadenoma.

| BI-RADS Categorization | | |
|---|---|---|
| Clinical Findings | right 1 | left 4 |
| Ultrasound | right 1 | left 4 |
| Mammography | right 1 | left 4 |
| MR Mammography | right 1 | left 5 |
| **BI-RADS Total** | **right 1** | **left 5** |

**Procedure recommended elsewhere (departing from guidelines)**

Open biopsy of the left breast for histological analysis of the lesion.

**Procedure according to guidelines**

Ultrasound guided core biopsy.

### Histology

Fibrocystic mastopathy including an intraductal papilloma (2 mm) and a fibroadenoma (3 mm).

Papilloma and fibroadenoma

### Treatment

Excisional biopsy for diagnostic purposes. No consequences.

Mammographic images classed "level I" (inadequate) in PGMI must be repeated, with the exception of cases where specific anatomical conditions prevent the acquisition of better imaging.

Are you completely satisfied with the analysis and follow-up in this case?
Are the histopathology and imaging findings really compatible?
Part 2 of this case (Case 10) is required reading!

**Indication:** Status 2 years after excisional biopsy (benign) for suspected cancer. New lump near scar.
**History:** Unremarkable.
**Risk profile:** Breast cancer in grandmother at the age of 82 years.
**Age:** 54 years.

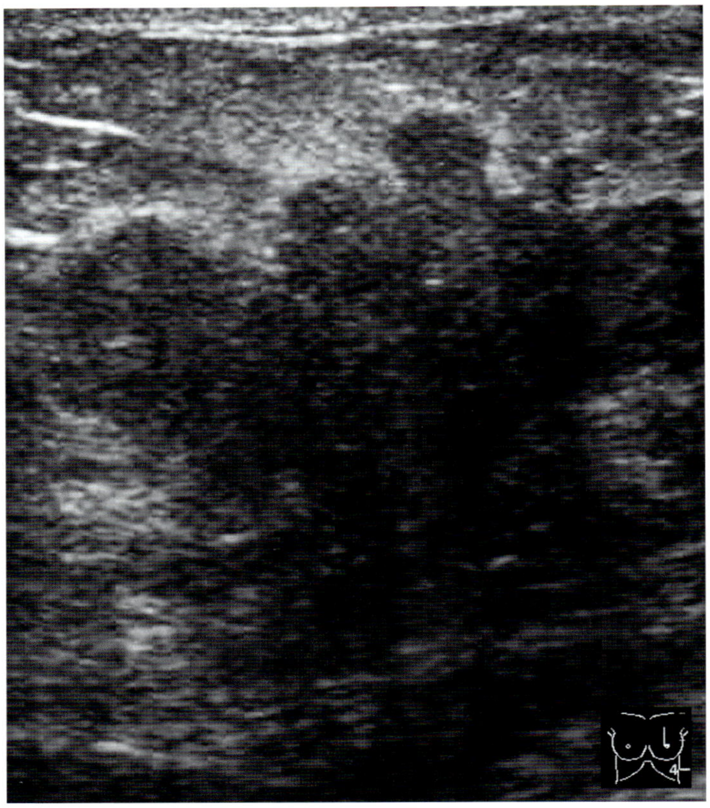

Fig. 10.**1** Ultrasound image from the area of the palpable mass.

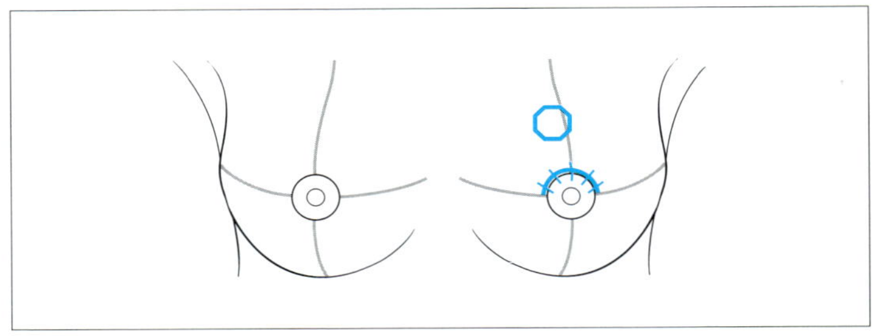

## Clinical Findings

2 cm resistance in the upper inner quadrant of the left breast in the region of the previous open biopsy. Uncomplicated scar.

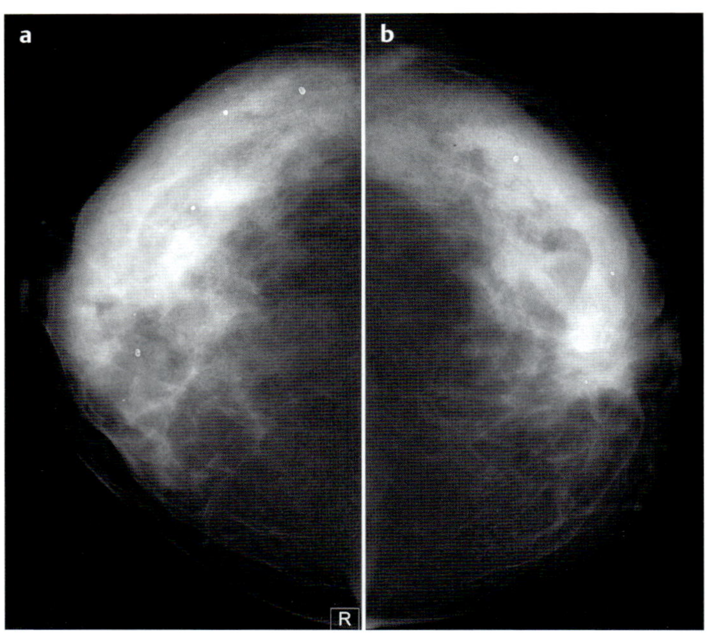


Fig. 10.**2 a, b** Digital mammography, CC view.

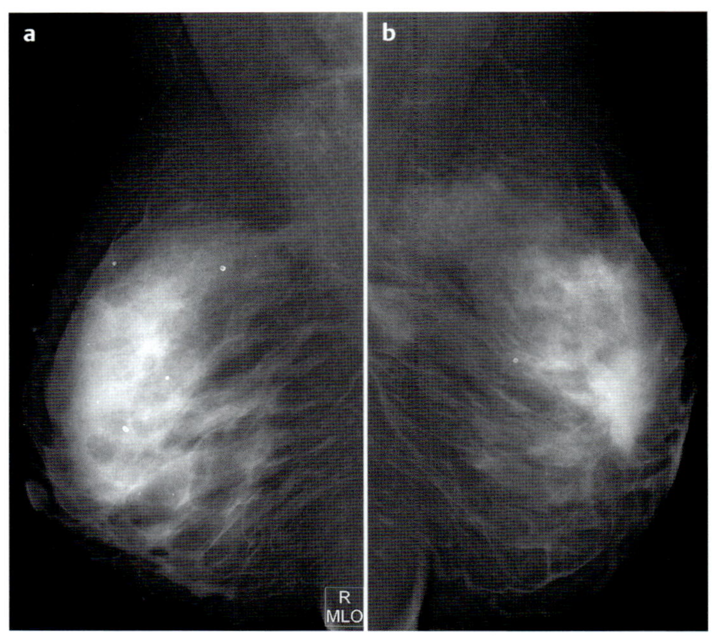


Fig. 10.**3 a, b** Digital mammography, MLO view.

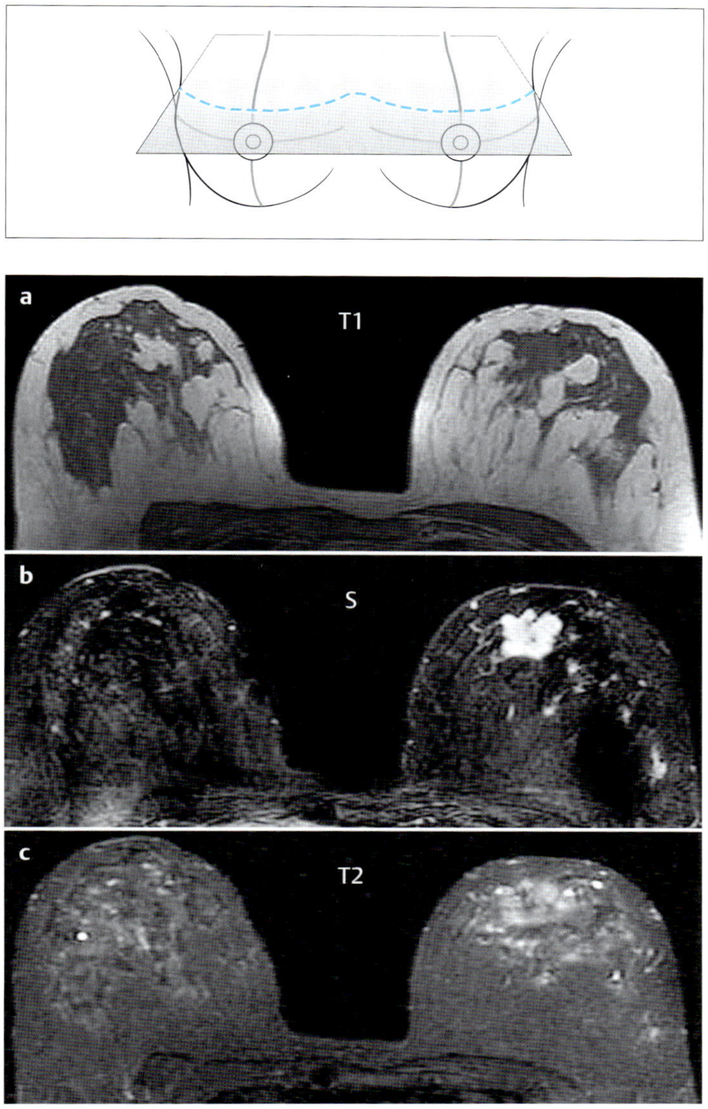


Fig. 10.**4 a – c** Contrast-enhanced MR mammography.

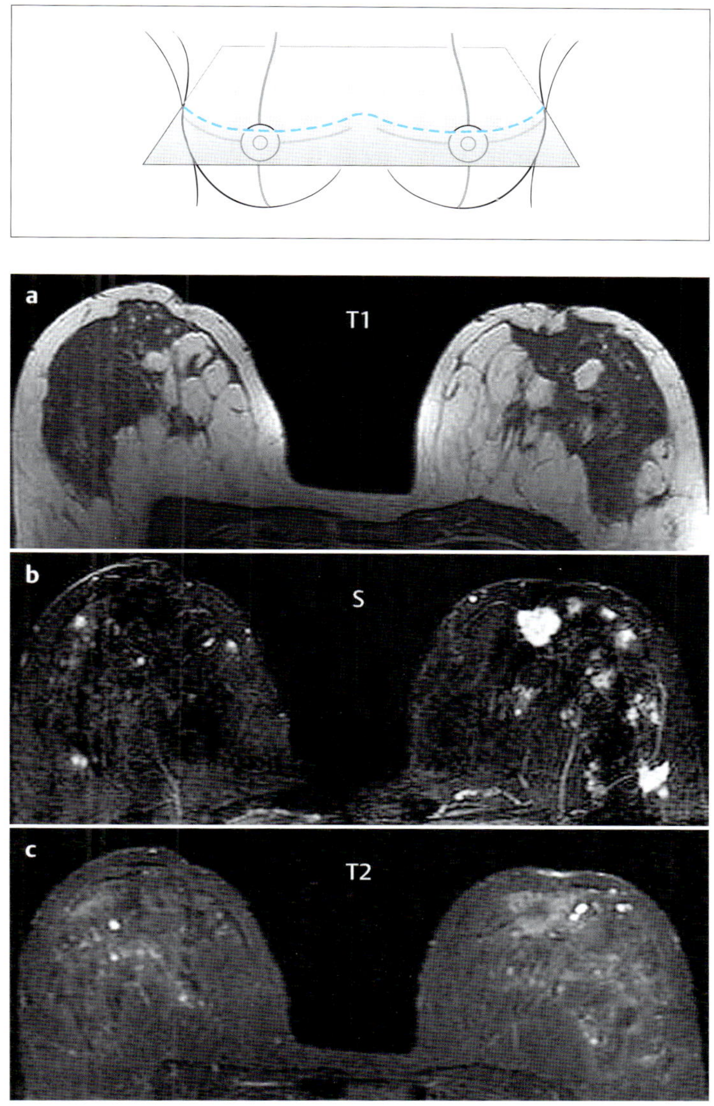


Fig. 10.**5 a – c** Contrast-enhanced MR mammcgraphy.

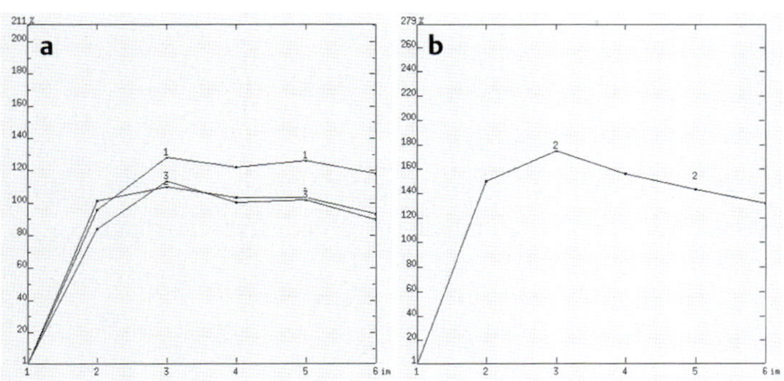


Fig. 10.**6 a, b** Signal-to-time curves of the lesion in the left breast.

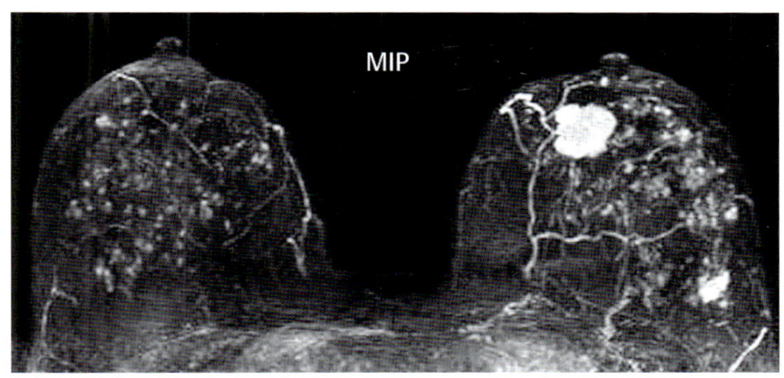


Fig. 10.**7** Contrast-enhanced MR mammography. Maximum intensity projection.

Please characterize ultrasound, mammography, and MRI findings.
What is your preliminary diagnosis?
What are your next steps?

This is the first screening examination after an open biopsy of a benign lesion 2 years previously (see Case 9). The patient noted postoperative resistance in the region of the left breast, which had been operated on, and interpreted this as scar tissue.

### Ultrasound

Within the previously operated region there was a lobulated, hypoechogenic mass, now of 3 cm diameter, with echogenic borders, distortion of the parenchymal architecture, and indeterminate distal echo characteristics (US BI-RADS left 5).

### Mammography

Mammograms showed a bilaterally symmetric, very dense parenchyma ACR type 4. Between the upper quadrants of the left breast there was visible a lobulated, hyperdense, partially superimposed mass with a diameter of 2.5 cm accompanied by architectural distortion. There were no suspicious microcalcifications. BI-RADS right 1/left 4. PGMI: MLO view P; CC view P.

### MR Mammography

Corresponding to the clinical, mammographic, and ultrasound findings, MRI demonstrated a lobulated, partially ill-defined hypervascularized mass 3 cm in diameter. After administration of contrast medium, this lesion showed a pathological perfusion pattern (ring enhancement, washout) and intermediate signal intensity in T2 imaging. There was another partially ill-defined, spiculated mass of 2 cm diameter in the upper outer quadrant of the left breast. This also demonstrated inhomogeneous contrast uptake, washout, and an intermediate signal in the T2 sequence.

**MRI Artifact Category:** 1
**MRI Density Type:** 2

| MRM score | Left breast, upper outer quadrant | Points | Left breast, between upper quadrants | Points |
|---|---|---|---|---|
| **Shape** | lobulated | 1 | lobulated | 1 |
| **Border** | ill-defined | 1 | ill-defined | 1 |
| **CM Distribution** | ring | 2 | inhomogeneous | 1 |
| **Initial Signal Intensity Increase** | strong | 2 | strong | 2 |
| **Post-initial Signal Intensity Character** | wash-out | 2 | wash-out | 2 |
| **MRI score (points)** | | **8** | | **7** |
| **MRI BI-RADS** | | **5** | | **5** |

### → Preliminary Diagnosis

Breast cancer (previous biopsy having failed to excise the original mass). Indications of multicentricity. No differential diagnosis.

| BI-RADS Categorization | | |
|---|---|---|
| Clinical Findings | right 1 | left 4 |
| Ultrasound | right 1 | left 5 |
| Mammography | right 1 | left 4 |
| MR Mammography | right 1 | left 5 (multicentric) |
| **BI-RADS Total** | **right 1** | **left 5** |

**Procedure Step 1**

Histopathological examination of the primary tumor (between the upper quadrants of the left breast) after US-guided core biopsy.

**Histopathology**

Invasive ductal carcinoma.

**Procedure Step 2**

Open biopsy of the primary tumor between the upper quadrants of the left breast as well as the mass in the upper outer quadrant after preoperative MR-guided hook-wire localization of this lesion (Fig. 10.**8**).

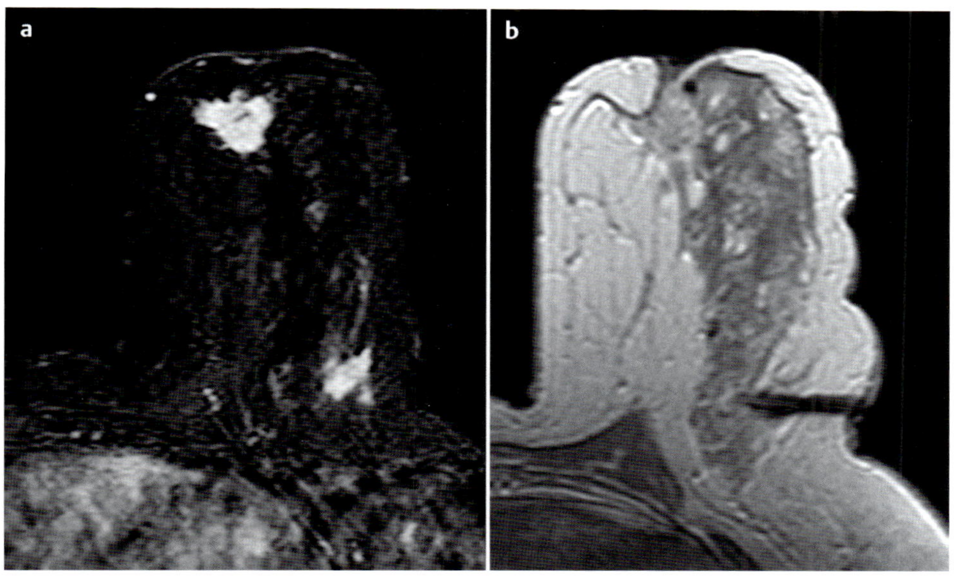


Fig. 10.**8** Preoperative MR-guided hook-wire localization of the second tumor.

## Histology

Bifocal invasive ductal carcinoma (diameters 2.9 cm and 1.7 cm).

IDC pT2 (bifocal), pN1bi (1/13), G2

## Treatment

Mastectomy.

Correspondence between imaging and histopathology must be carefully verified in all cases after open biopsy (see Case 9). The results of the open biopsy 2 years previously did not match the imaging findings. Such discrepancies should be discussed in interdisciplinary conferences and taken into account when deciding the course of action (for example, repetition of imaging or operation).

**Indication:** Ultrasound examination performed elsewhere raised suspicion of breast cancer.
**History:** Unremarkable.
**Risk profile:** No increased risk.
**Age:** 45 years.

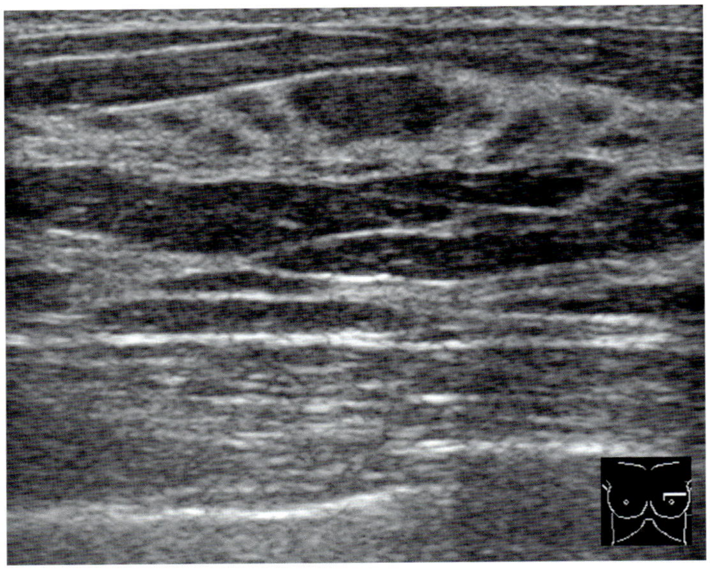

Fig. 11.**1** Sonography.

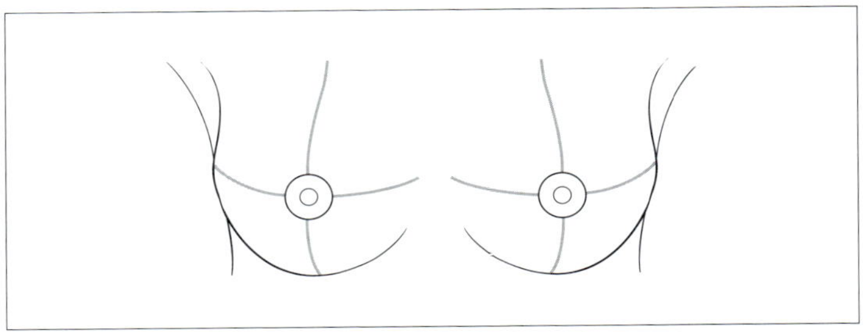

## Clinical Findings

No findings.

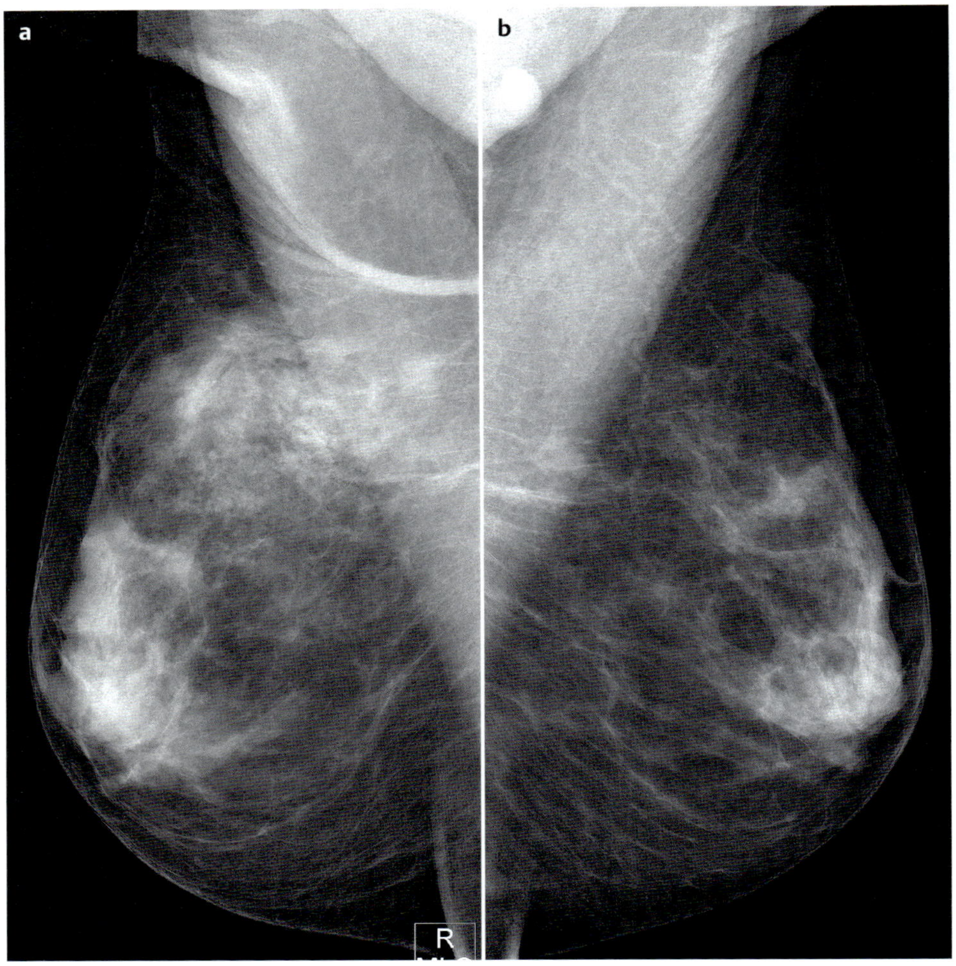


Fig. 11.**2 a, b** Digital mammography, MLO view.

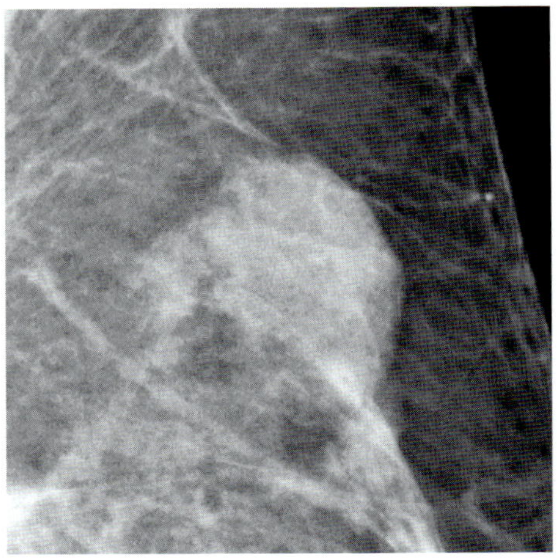

Fig. 11.**3** Magnification view of the left breast, upper outer quadrant (MLO).

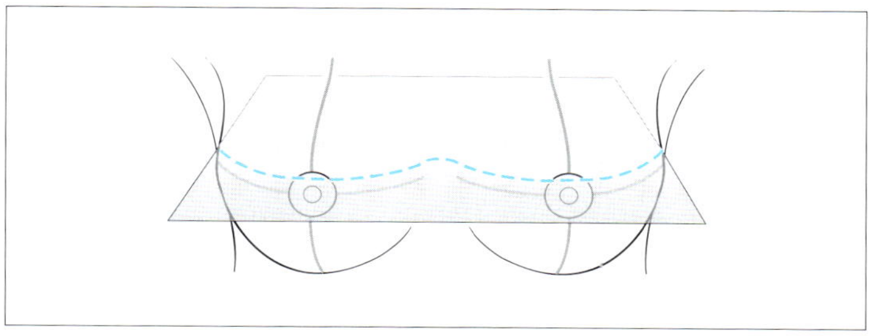

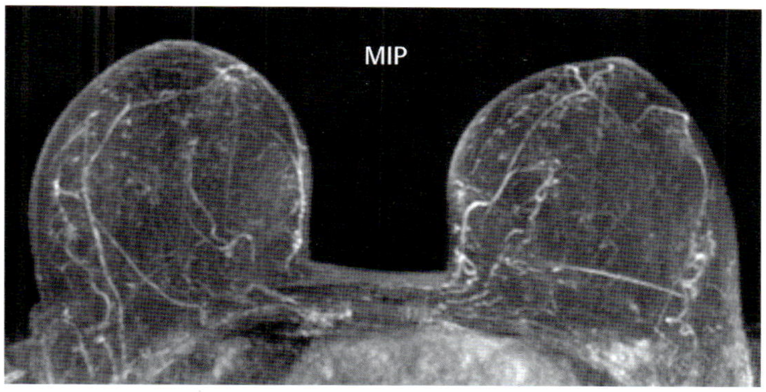


Fig. 11.5 Contrast-enhanced MR mammography. Maximum intensity projection.

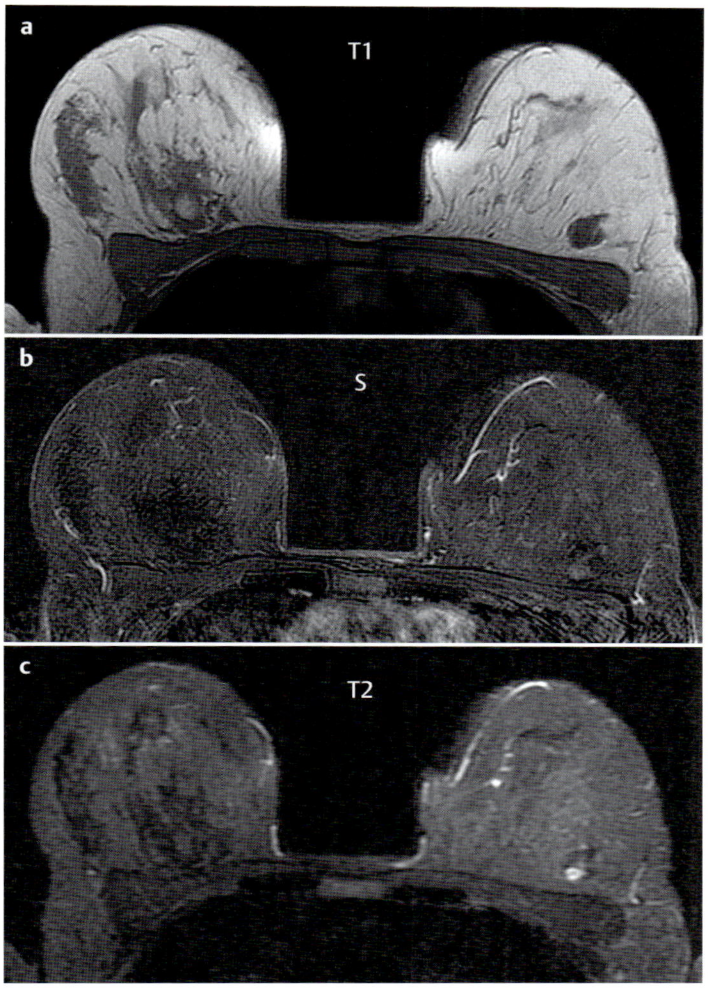


Fig. 11.4 a – c Contrast-enhanced MR mammography.

Please characterize ultrasound, mammography, and MRI findings.
What is your preliminary diagnosis?
What are your next steps?

Further imaging studies were performed following suspicious findings in an initial ultrasound examination.

### Ultrasound

There was an oval, mostly well-defined mass with a maximum diameter of 8 mm in the upper outer quadrant of the left breast. The long axis of this lesion was parallel to the skin. Homogeneous internal structure. There were no unusual echo patterns in surrounding tissue. US BI-RADS left 3.

### Mammography

Digital mammography showed bilaterally symmetric, extremely dense parenchyma, especially in the retromamillary regions (ACR type 4). There were no pathological findings in the right breast. There was an oval mass with largely well-defined borders and a hypodense internal pattern in the upper outer quadrant of the left breast. Mammograms showed no calcifications and no architectural distortion. BI-RADS right 1/left 3. PGMI: G (inframammary and axillary folds visible).

### MR Mammography

MRI demonstrated an oval mass in the upper outer quadrant of the left breast, consistent with ultrasound and mammographic findings. This mass showed a well-defined margin and no enhancement after administration of contrast medium. In the water-sensitive inversion recovery sequence, this lesion showed a moderate signal increase.

**MRI Artifact Category:** 1
**MRI Density Type:** 1

| MRM score | Finding | Points |
|---|---|---|
| **Shape** | – | 0 |
| **Border** | – | 0 |
| **CM Distribution** | – | 0 |
| **Initial Signal Intensity Increase** | – | 0 |
| **Post-initial Signal Intensity Character** | – | 0 |
| **MRI score (points)** | | **0** |
| **MRI BI-RADS** | | **1** |

### → Preliminary Diagnosis

Predominantly fibrotic fibroadenoma. No evidence of malignancy.

| BI-RADS Categorization | | |
|---|---|---|
| Clinical Findings | right 1 | left 1 |
| Ultrasound | right 1 | left 3 |
| Mammography | right 1 | left 3 |
| MR Mammography | right 1 | left 1 |
| **BI-RADS Total** | **right 1** | **left 3** |

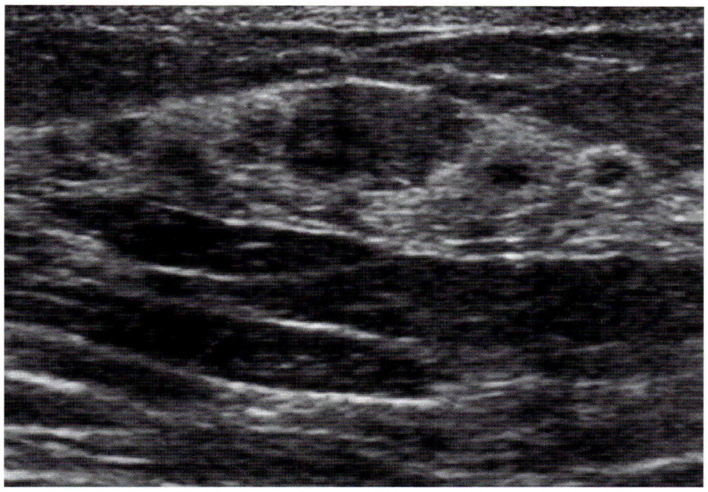

Fig. 11.**6** The follow-up ultrasound 6 months later (using light compression with the transducer) showed no changes in the findings.

**Procedure**

No biopsy required. Follow-up ultrasound in 6 months.

## Diagnosis (without histopathological verification)

Fibroadenoma. Adenoma.

## Treatment

None.

A mass with no enhancement on MRI excludes malignancy with high reliability.

**Indication:** Screening.
**History:** Unremarkable.
**Risk profile:** No increased risk.
**Age:** 48 years.

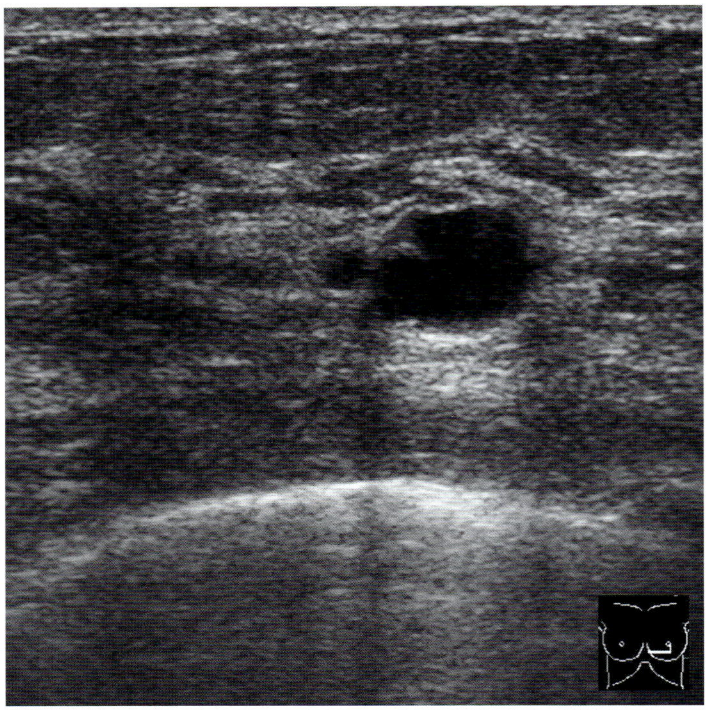

Fig. 12.**1** Sonography.

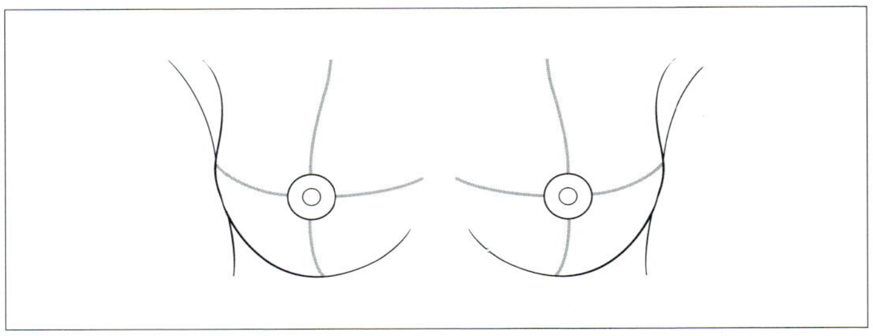

### Clinical Findings

Normal.

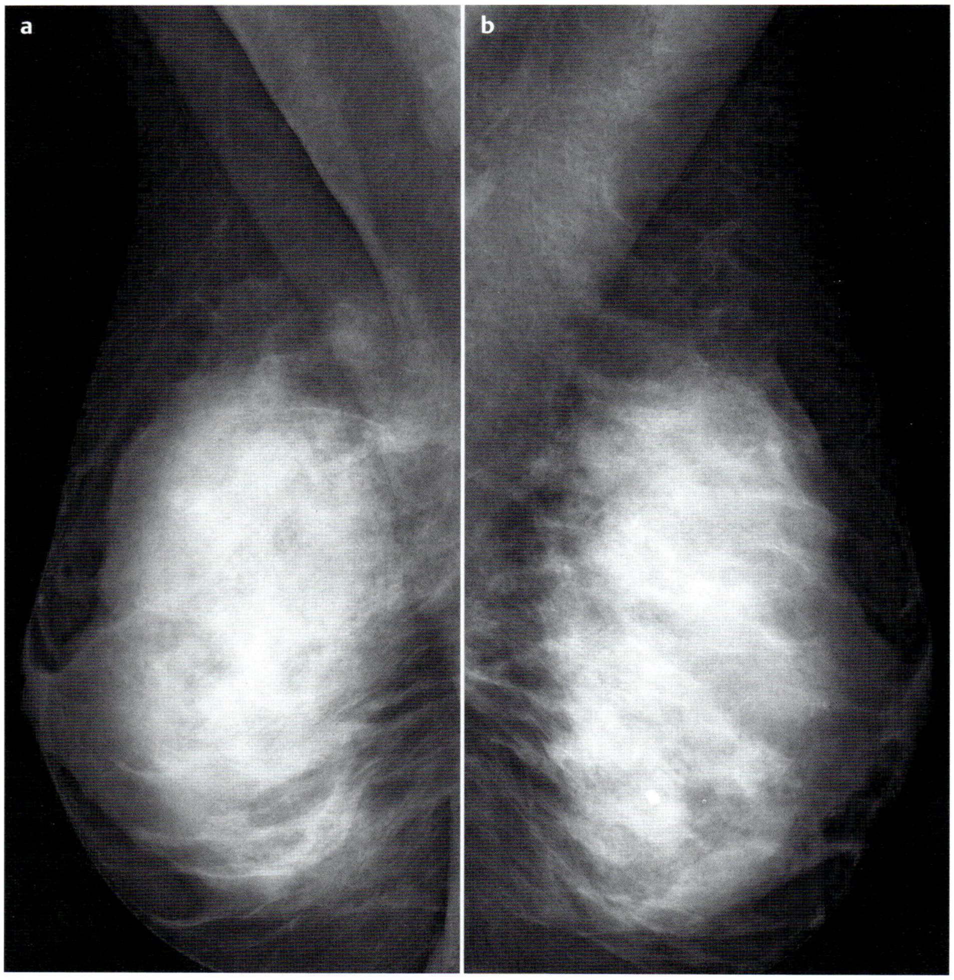

Fig. 12.**2 a, b** Digital mammography, MLO view.

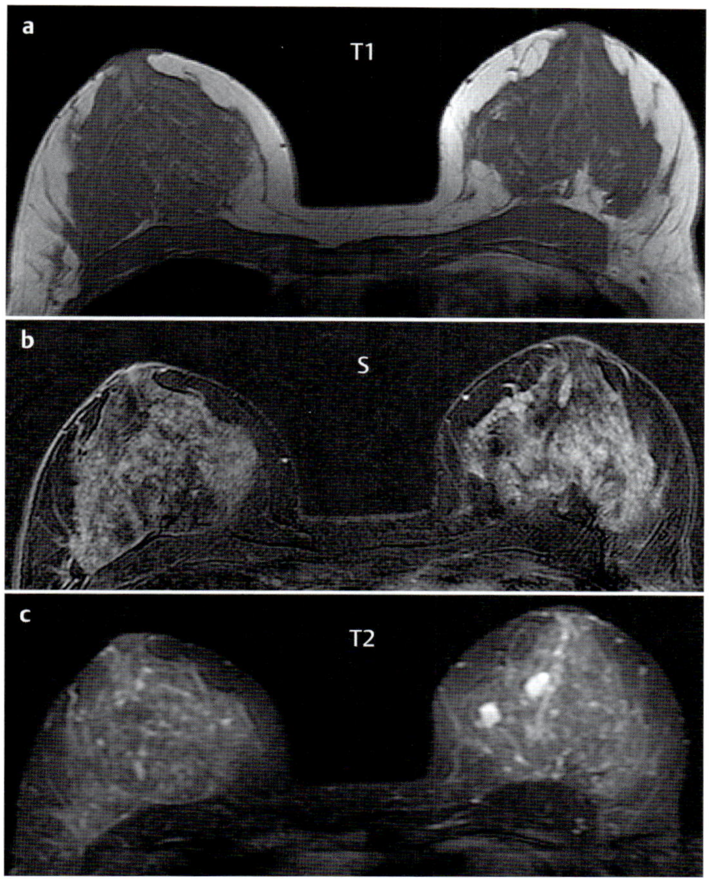


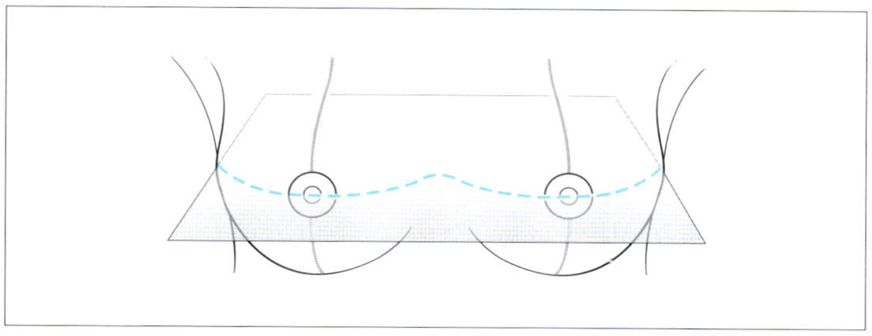

Fig. 12.3 **a – c** Contrast-enhanced MR mammography.

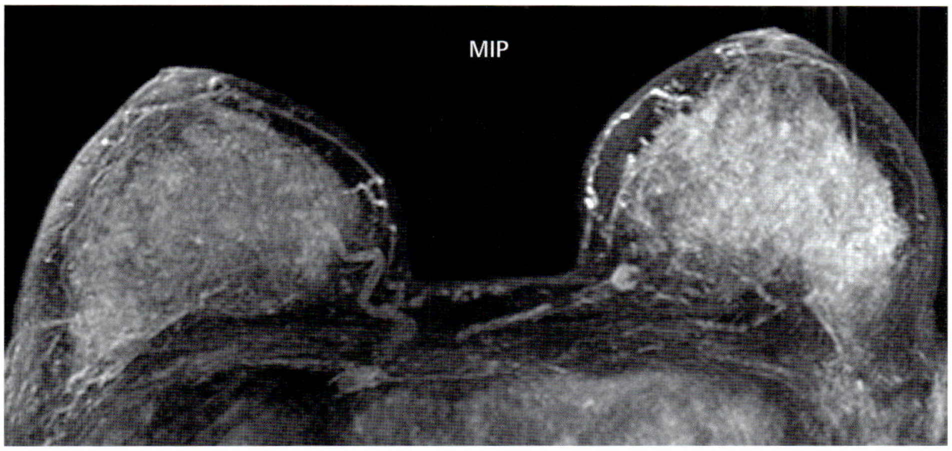


Fig. 12.4 Contrast-enhanced MR mammography. Maximum intensity projection.

?

Please characterize ultrasound, mammography, and MRI findings.
What is your preliminary diagnosis?
What are your next steps?

Because of the density of the parenchyma, mammography was performed in one view only (MLO) and supplemented by contrast-enhanced MR mammography (so-called optipack-concept).

#### Ultrasound

The US image is of the lower inner quadrant of the left breast. It demonstrates a cyst compatible with the information provided by T2-weighted MRI. US BI-RADS left 2.

#### Mammography

The mammogram shows extremely dense parenchyma of both breasts, ACR type 4. Under these limiting conditions, no abnormalities were detectable. The macrocalcifications in the center of the left breast can be considered harmless and irrelevant. (BI-RADS right 1/left 1). PGMI: MLO view G (inframammary fold not clearly depicted).

#### MR Mammography

Subtraction images were obtained by subtracting the precontrast image from images derived from the second measurement after administration of contrast (approx. 3 minutes after introduction of contrast into peripheral veins). These early subtraction images show strong enhancement of all glandular tissue, meaning that no further differentiation of circumscribed lesions was possible. However, a round enhancing area was observed in the inner region of the left breast (not shown on the slices reproduced here).

**MRI Artifact Category:** 2
**MRI Density Type:** 4

| MRM score | Finding | Points |
|---|---|---|
| **Shape** | – | 0 |
| **Border** | – | 0 |
| **CM Distribution** | – | 0 |
| **Initial Signal Intensity Increase** | – | 0 |
| **Post-initial Signal Intensity Character** | – | 0 |
| **MRI score (points)** | | **0** |
| **MRI BI-RADS** | | **1** |

### → Preliminary Diagnosis

No remarkable findings from imaging.
Caution: It must be remembered that the sensitivity of x-ray mammography and MRI is limited by the circumstances of very dense parenchymal patterns (here ACR type 4, MRM density type 4).

| BI-RADS Categorization | | |
|---|---|---|
| Clinical Findings | right 1 | left 1 |
| Ultrasound | right 1 | left 2 |
| Mammography | right 1 | left 1 |
| MR Mammography | right 1 | left 1 |
| **BI-RADS Total** | **right 1** | **left 2** |

## Diagnosis (without histological verification)

No pathological findings. No evidence of malignancy.

However–you should *not* be satisfied with this diagnosis! Note the following comment.

In the present case, given the strongly enhancing characteristics of the parenchyma, besides the standard early subtraction (images of second measurement after contrast administration minus precontrast images), a subtraction of the **earliest** data (images from first measurement after contrast, minus precontrast images) should also have been performed to increase the sensitivity of the MRI studies. See part 2 of this case on the following pages (Case 13).

**Indication:** Screening.
**History:** Unremarkable.
**Risk profile:** Not increased.
**Age:** 48 years.

In addition to the conventional MR mammography imaging seen in Case 12, a **very** early subtraction (images of first measurement after contrast minus precontrast images) was performed.

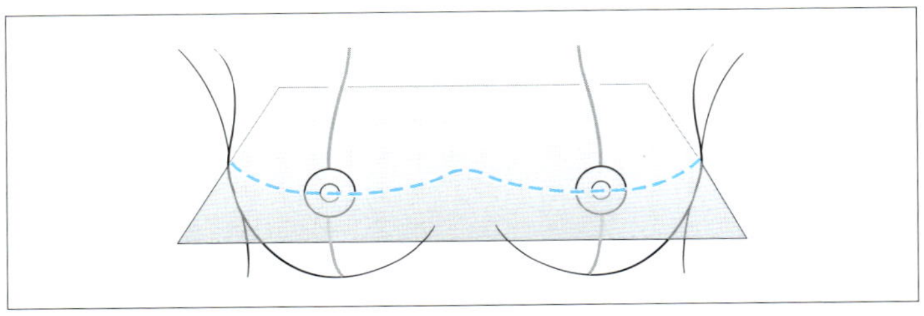

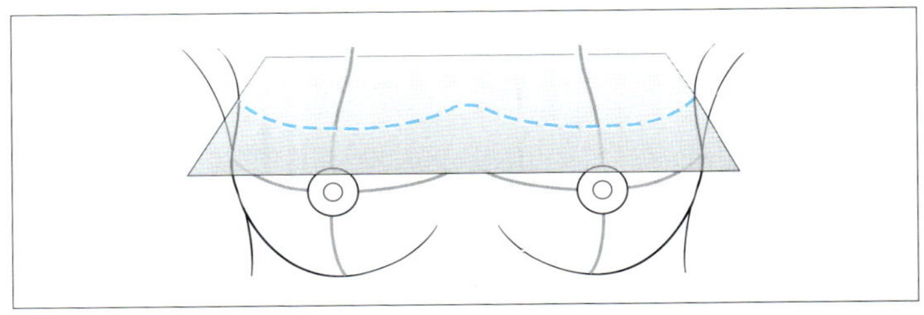

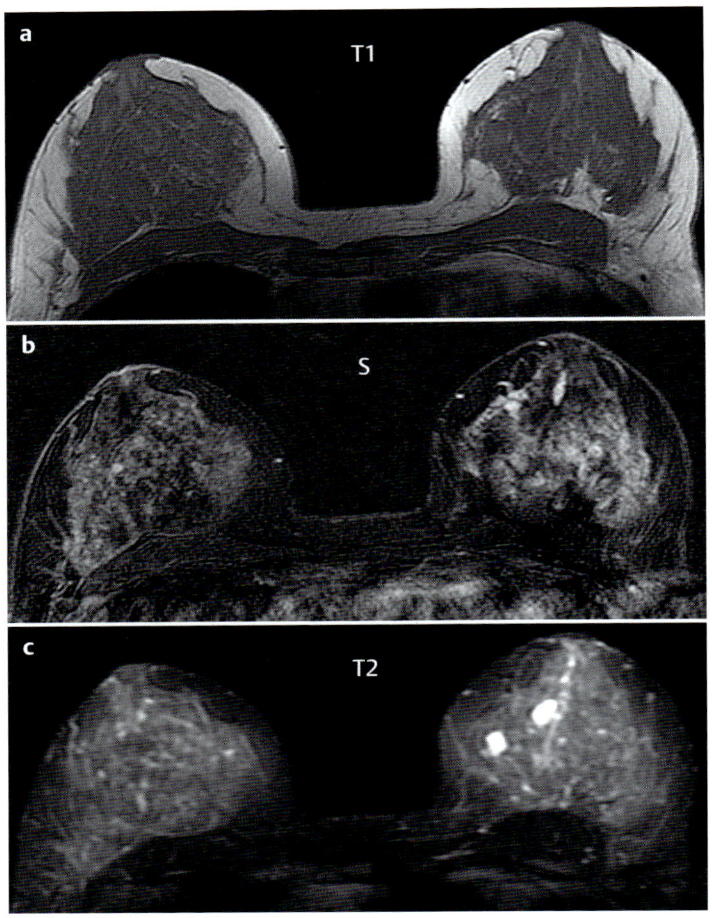


Fig. 13.**1 a–c** MR mammography (*earliest* subtraction).

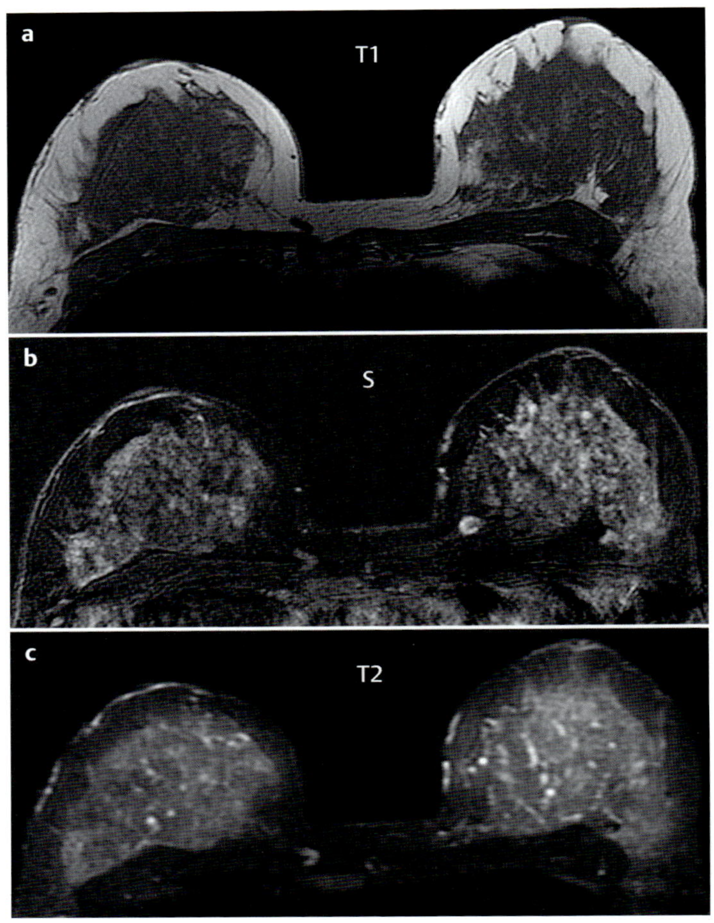


Fig. 13.**2 a–c** MR mammography (*earliest* subtraction).

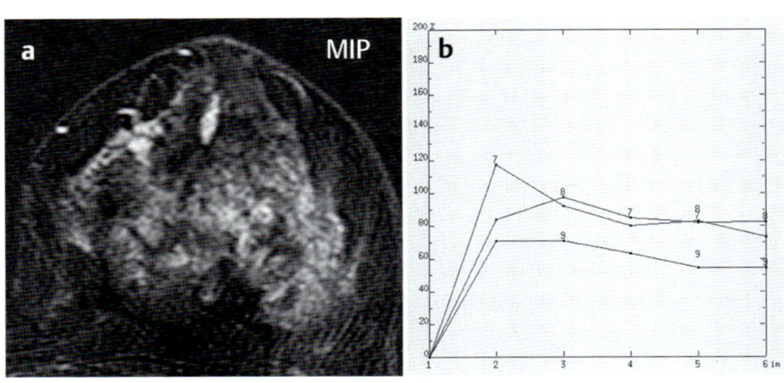


Fig. 13.**3 a, b** Signal-to-time curves of the linear enhancement.

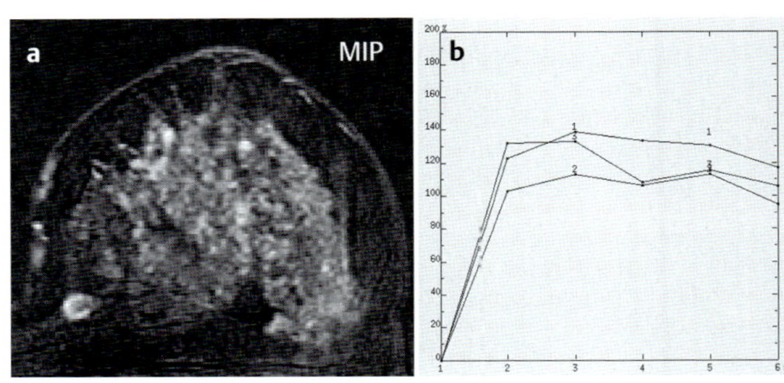


Fig. 13.**4 a, b** Signal-to-time curves of the round enhancement.

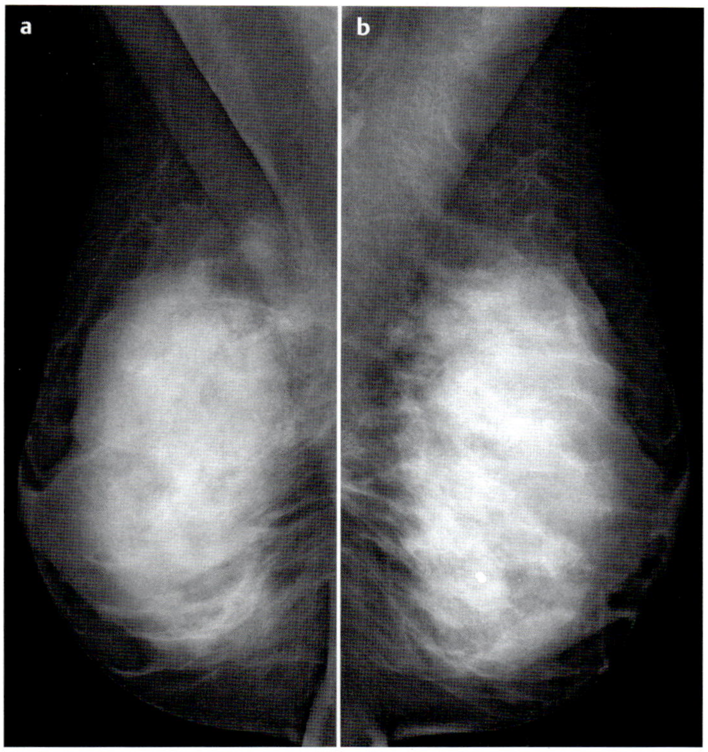


Fig. 13.5 a, b Digital mammography, MLO view.

## Clinical Findings

Normal.

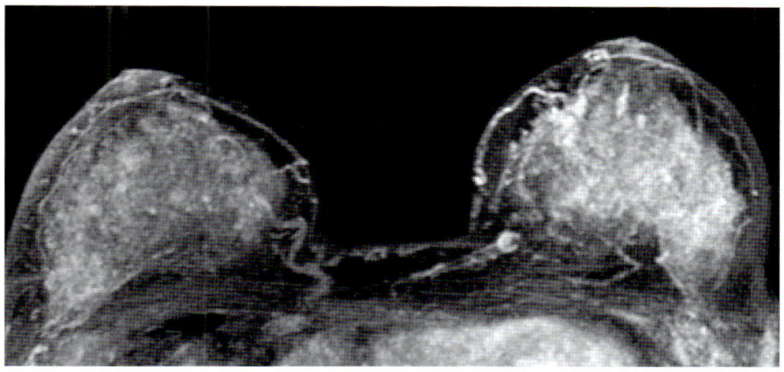

Fig. 13.6 Contrast-enhanced MR mammography. Maximum intensity projection.

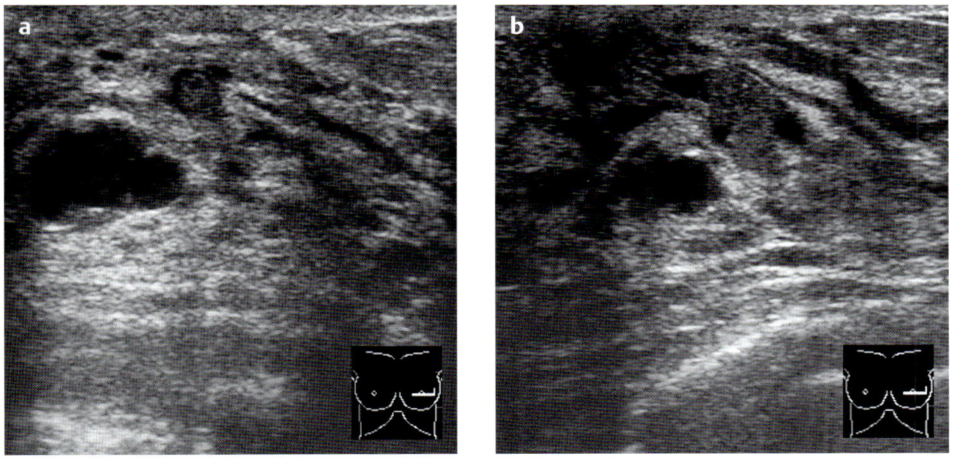


Fig. 13.7 a, b Targeted sonography in region of MRI findings, behind the left nipple.

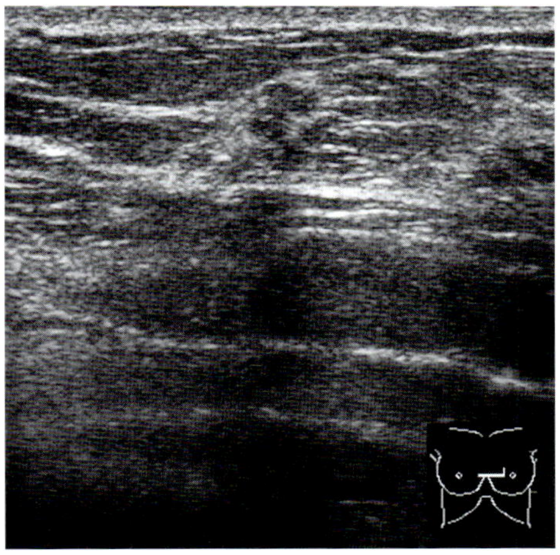

Fig. 13.8 Targeted sonography in region of MRI findings, left upper inner quadrant.

?

Please characterize ultrasound, mammography, and MRI findings.
What is your preliminary diagnosis?
What are your next steps?

It is clear that performing an additional *earliest* image subtraction can indeed be worthwhile.

### MR Mammography

The very early subtraction (i.e., images from first measurement after CM administration, 1 minute after contrast, minus precontrast imaging) enabled much better differentiation between the extremely high contrast uptake of specific structures and the early enhancement of the surrounding breast tissue. Behind the nipple of the left breast there was a spindle-shaped linear enhancing area with early signal peak followed by washout (Fig. 13.**9a**, arrow). In the upper inner quadrant of the left breast there was an additional round hypervascularized lesion with nonspecific signal curve (Fig. 13.**9b**, double arrow).

### Mammography

Due to the high density of the parenchyma (ACR type 4), no additional information is provided by conventional mammograms (BI-RADS right 1/left 1).

### Ultrasound

Ultrasound images were obtained directly behind the nipple of the left breast and in the upper inner quadrant of the left breast. In the immediate area of the cyst shown in Case 12 (Fig. 12.**1**) at least one ectatic duct showed a solid intraductal mass (Fig. 13.**10a**, arrow) (US BI-RADS left 3). In the upper inner quadrant of the left breast, US demonstrated a hypoechoic lesion with a hyperechoic marginal pattern (US BI-RADS 4).

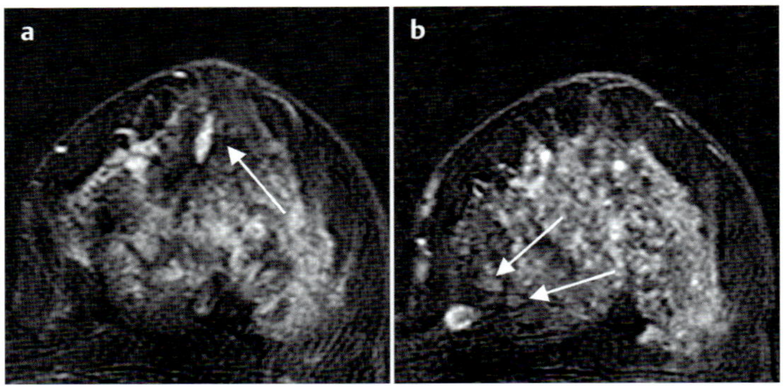


Fig. 13.**9a, b** *Earliest* subtraction findings.

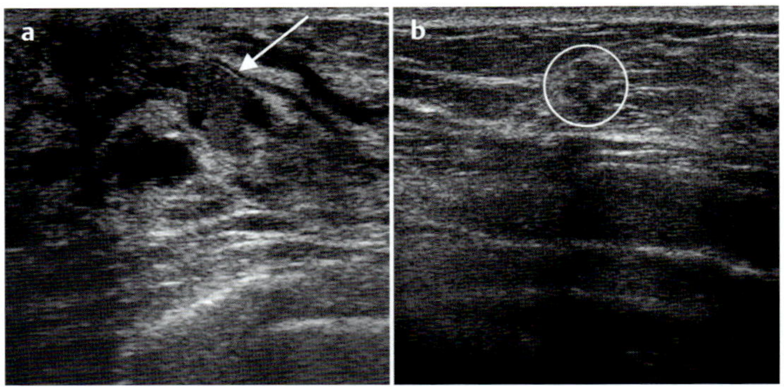


Fig. 13.**10a, b** Targeted ultrasound findings.

| MRM score | Left breast, below the nipple | Points | Left breast, upper inner quadrant | Points |
|---|---|---|---|---|
| **Shape** | linear | 1 | round | 0 |
| **Border** | well-defined | 0 | well-defined | 0 |
| **CM Distribution** | homogeneous | 0 | inhomogeneous | 1 |
| **Initial Signal Intensity Increase** | strong | 2 | strong | 2 |
| **Post-initial Signal Intensity Character** | wash-out | 2 | plateau | 1 |
| **MRI score (points)** | | **5** | | **4** |
| **MRI BI-RADS** | | **4** | | **4** |

| BI-RADS Categorization | | |
|---|---|---|
| Clinical Findings | right 1 | left 1 |
| Ultrasound | right 1 | left 4 |
| Mammography | right 1 | left 1 |
| MR Mammography | right 1 | left 4 |
| **BI-RADS Total** | **right 1** | **left 4** |

**Interpretation of findings and procedure**

The findings in the left breast (lesions behind the nipple and in the upper inner quadrant) provided reason for further investigation (BI-RADS 4). Due to the questionable correlation between US and MRI findings, an MR-guided vacuum core biopsy of the dendritic enhancement behind the left nipple was performed (Fig. 13.**11**).

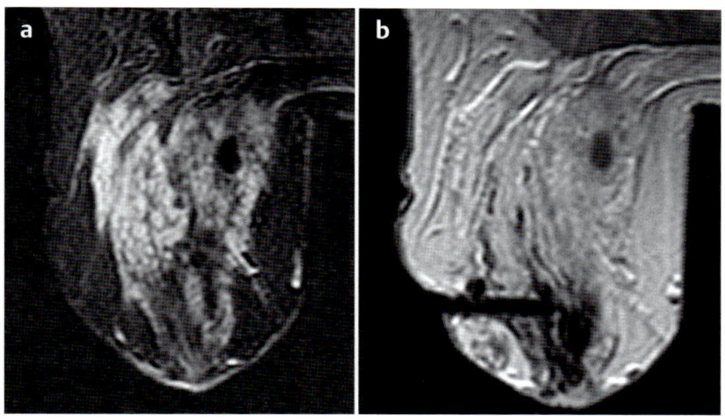


Fig. 13.**11 a, b** MR-guided vacuum biopsy.
**a** Subtraction image.
**b** Position of coaxial needle (pre-fire).

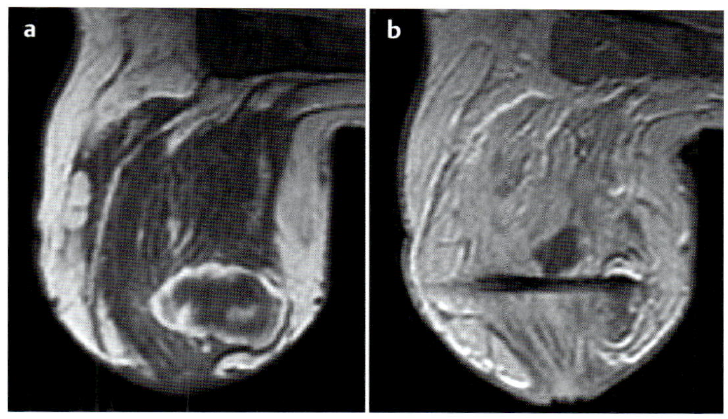


Fig. 13.**12** MR-guided preoperative localization.
**a** Hematoma after vacuum biopsy.
**b** Hook-wire in position.

## Histology of vacuum biopsy from the left breast

Ductal carcinoma in situ, grade 2. No invasive tumor components.

Open biopsy was performed on the affected duct behind the left nipple, after MR-guided marker wire localization, and on the hypervascularized lesion in the upper inner quadrant after US-guided localization and external marking.

## Final diagnosis

Left central: High-grade DCIS, VNPI 8, G2
Left upper inner quadrant: ILC, pT1b, 8 mm, G2, pN0

## Treatment

Mastectomy of the left breast.

In patients with very marked early enhancement of the breast tissue in MRI, subtraction of very early images (so-called **earliest** subtraction) is recommended for better differentiation between benign tissue and malignant lesions.

**Indication:** Screening.
**History:** Unremarkable.
**Risk profile:** No increased risk.
**Age:** 57 years.

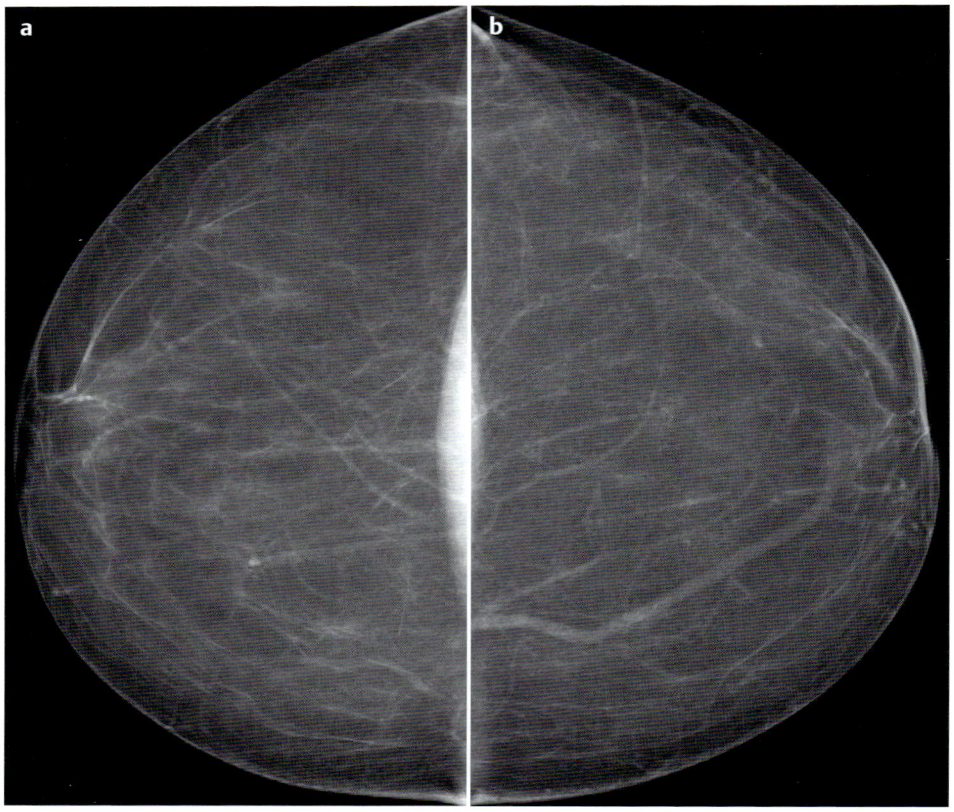


Fig. 14.**1 a, b** Digital mammography, CC view [imaging not performed by authors].

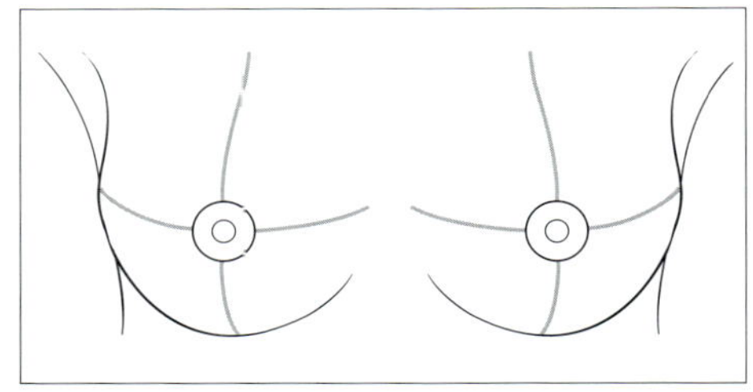

### Clinical Findings

Normal.

### Ultrasound

No suspicious findings (not shown).

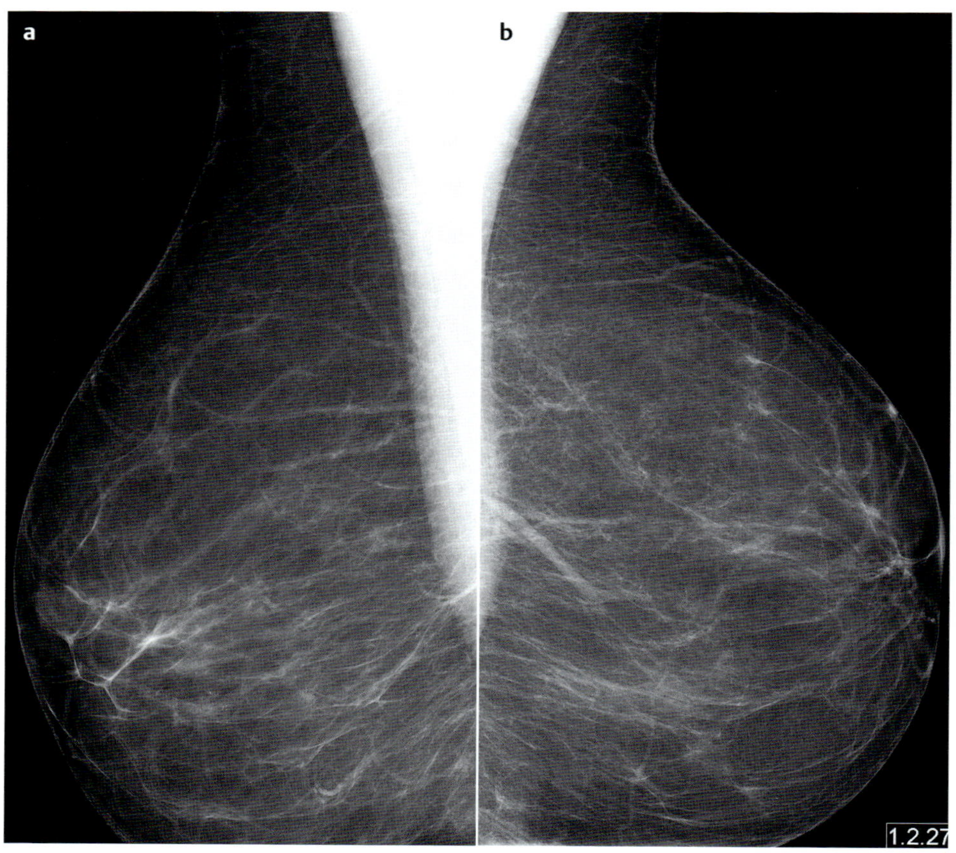


Fig. 14.**2 a, b** Digital mammography, MLO view [imaging not performed by authors].

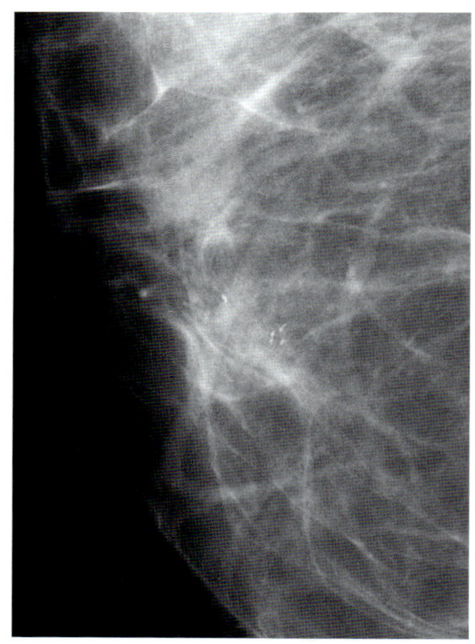

Fig. 14.**3** Magnification view of the right breast, behind the nipple.

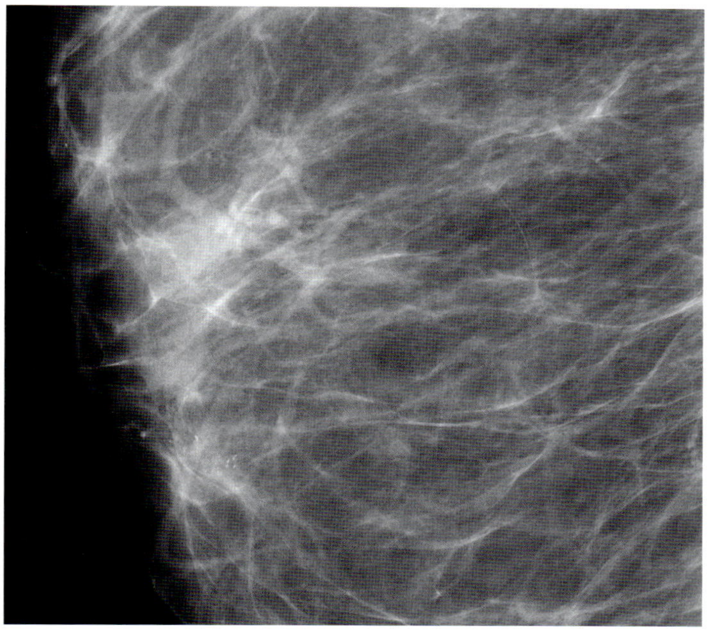

Fig. 14.**4** Magnification view at first examination.

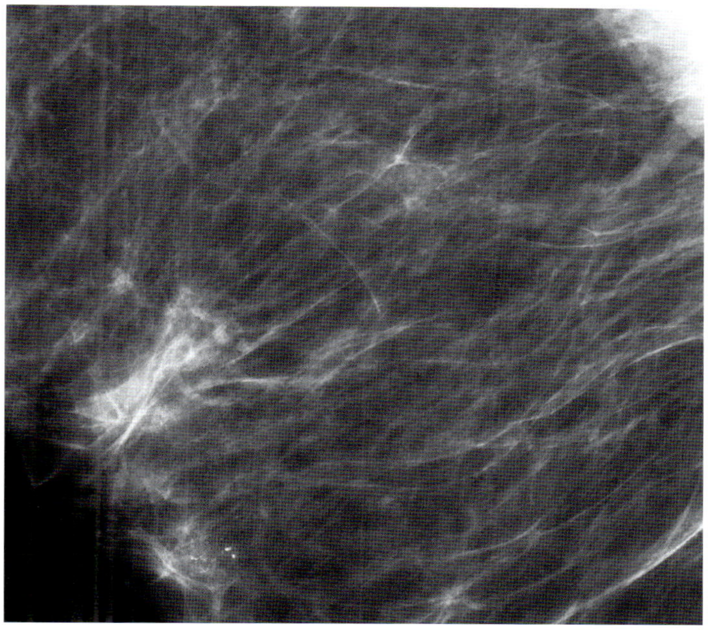

Fig. 14.**5** Magnification view at follow-up 7 months later.

?

Please characterize the calcifications on the mammograms.
What is your preliminary diagnosis?
What are your next steps?

### Mammography

Mammography showed predominantly lipomatous tissue in both breasts, ACR type 1. There were no lesions or masses. There is, however, a cluster of polymorphous microcalcifications in the region behind the nipple of the right breast (Fig. 14.**4**). These calcifications were categorized as BI-RADS 3. (BI-RADS right 3/left 1).

Follow-up mammography of the right breast in 6 months was recommended.

The follow-up mammography 7 months later (Fig. 14.**5**), showed no changes and the findings were again categorized as BI-RADS 3. Another follow-up mammography was recommended in a further 6 months.

Unfortunately, the patient did not attend for the follow-up mammography 6 months later, but rather 24 months after the original examination (Fig. 14.**6**).

### Mammography (Fig. 14.6)

There was a round lesion containing microcalcifications behind the nipple of the right breast–i.e., exactly where calcifications had been identified 2 years previously (1). There was a further cluster of polymorphous microcalcifications in the central part of the right breast (2). Retrospectively, this second cluster was not visible in the earlier images.

### MR Mammography

MRI demonstrated a hypervascularized mass behind the right nipple, corresponding to the lesion with calcifications (1) as seen in mammography (Fig. 14.**6**). There was no increased vascularization corresponding to the second cluster of microcalcifications (2) in the center of the right breast.

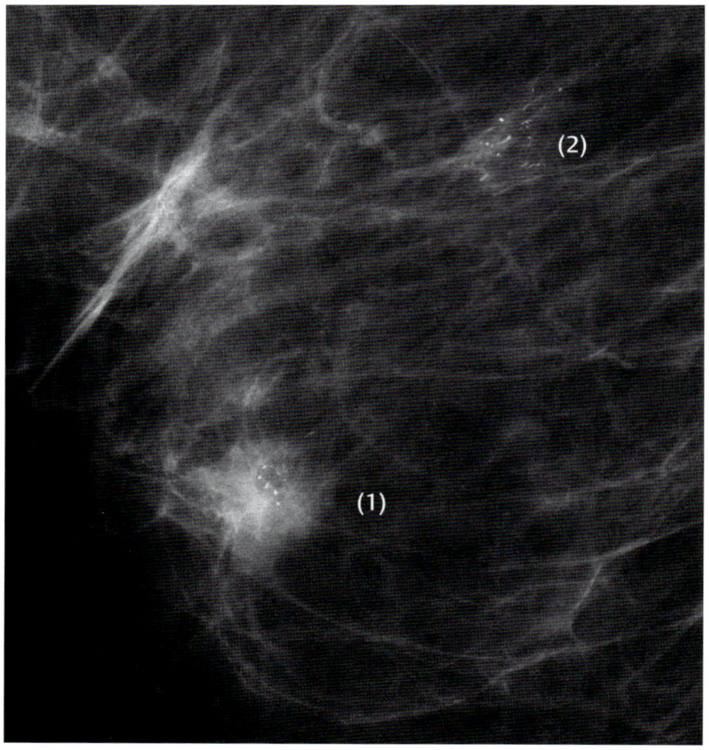


Fig. 14.**6** Mammography 24 months after first examination.

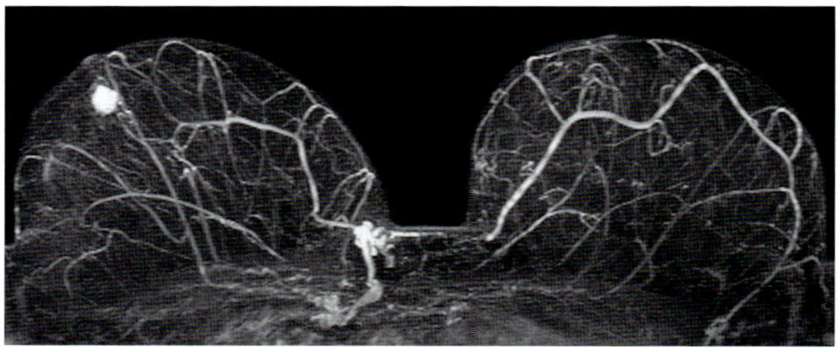

Fig. 14.**7** MR imaging performed at the same time as the mammogram seen in Fig. 14.**6**.

| BI-RADS Categorization (First examination and follow-up after 7 months) | | |
|---|---|---|
| Clinical Findings | right 1 | left 1 |
| Ultrasound | right 1 | left 1 |
| Mammography | right 3 | left 1 |
| MR Mammography | – | – |
| **BI-RADS Total** | **right 3** | **left 1** |

| BI-RADS Categorization (Follow-up examination after 2 years) | | |
|---|---|---|
| Clinical Findings | right 1 | left 1 |
| Ultrasound | right 1 | left 1 |
| Mammography | right 5 (bifocal) | left 1 |
| MR Mammography | right 5 | left 1 |
| **BI-RADS Total** | **right 5** | **left 1** |

## → Preliminary Diagnosis

Bifocal breast cancer of the right breast (presumed invasive in the region behind the nipple, presumed intraductal in the central region).

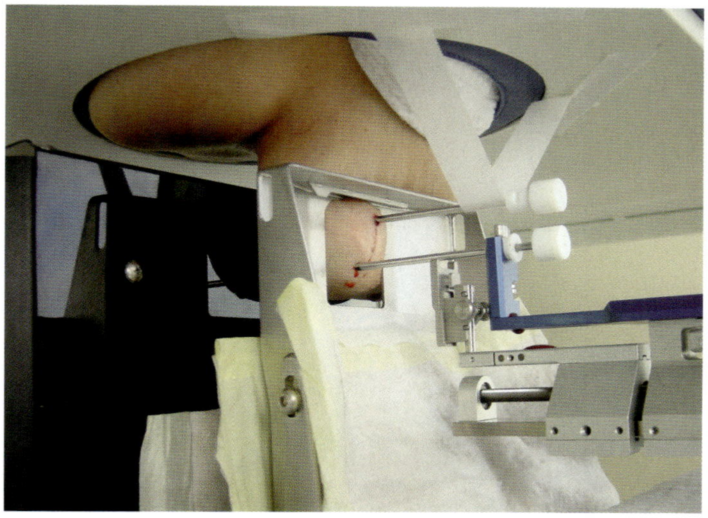

Fig. 14.**8** Simultaneous stereotactic vacuum biopsy of both findings.

## Procedure

Stereotactic vacuum biopsy.

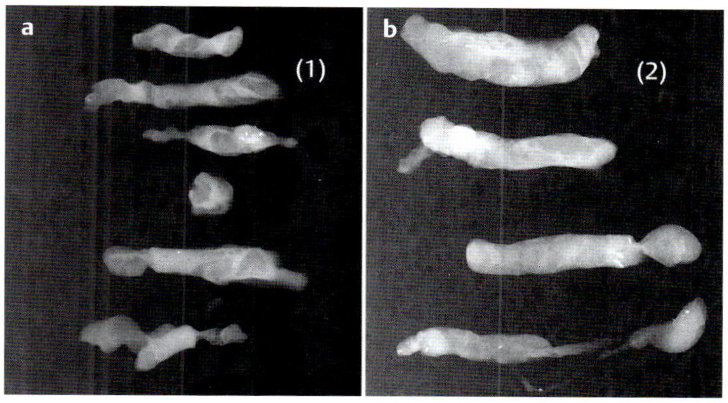


Fig. 14.**9** Specimen radiograms.
**a** Specimen from the lesion behind the nipple (marked [1] in Fig. 14.**6**).
**b** Specimen from the central clustered calcifications (marked [2] in Fig. 14.**6**).

## Diagnosis

Right breast behind nipple: IDC pT1b (5 mm), pN0 (0/15), R0, G2
Right breast central: DCIS (no residual tumor in excised specimens)

## Treatment

Mastectomy of the right breast.

Microcalcifications categorized as BI-RADS 3 that show no changes after 6 months should be checked a second time after a further 6 months.

**Indication:** Resistance in upper outer quadrant of the right breast.
**History:** No abnormalities.
**Risk profile:** No increased risk.
**Age:** 51 years.

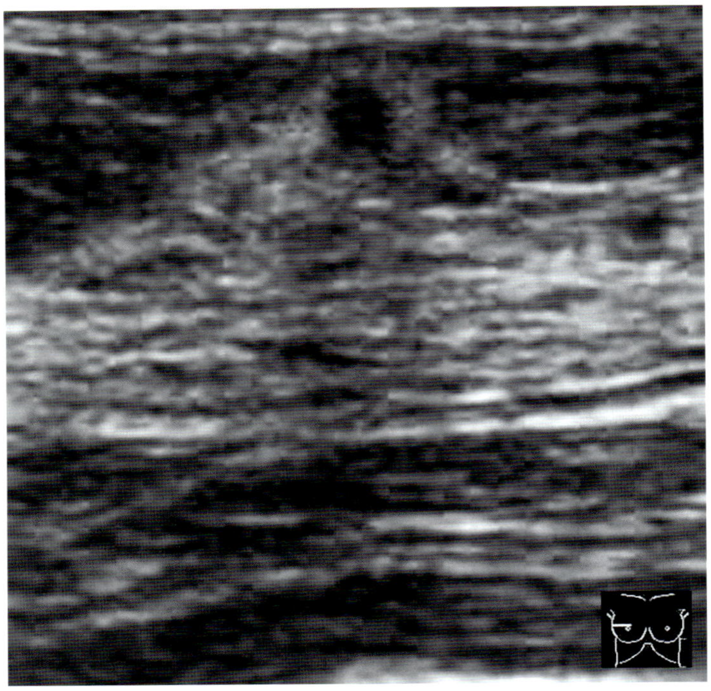

Fig. 15.**1** Ultrasound image from the area of the palpable mass.

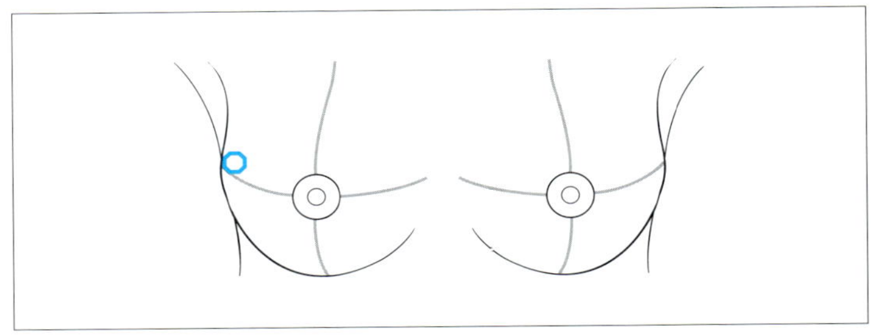

### Clinical Findings

Well-defined resistance of approximately 3 mm diameter in the upper outer quadrant of the right breast. Generally lumpy parenchymal structure.

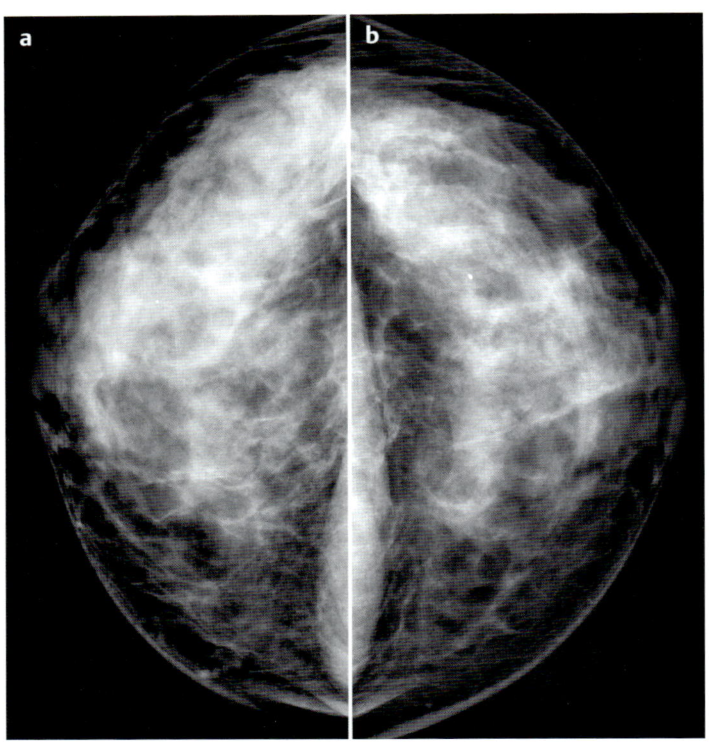


Fig. 15.**2 a, b** Digital mammography, CC view.

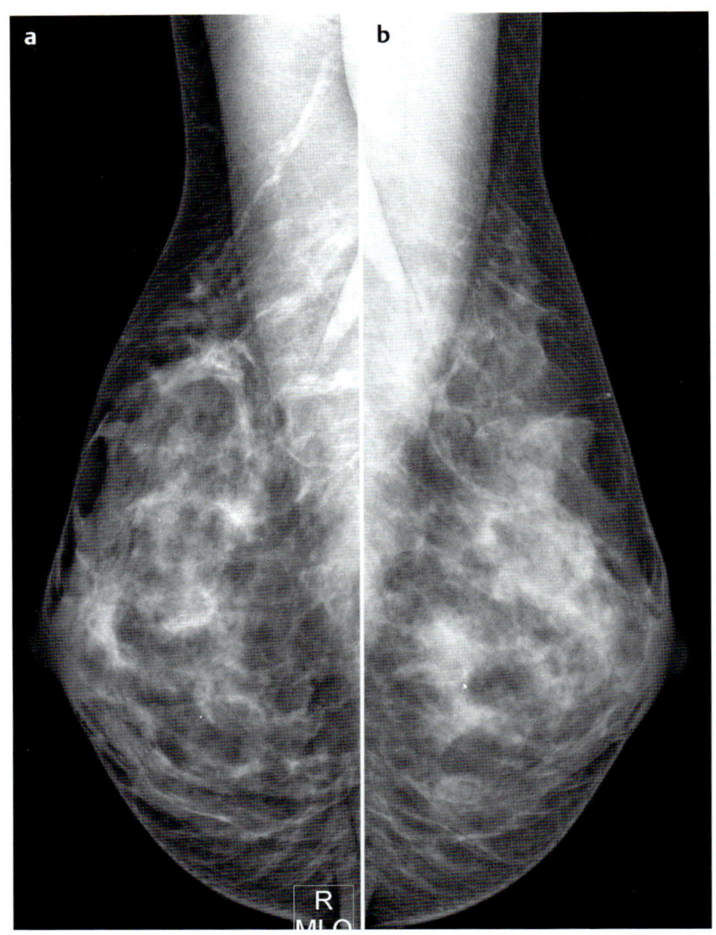


Fig. 15.**3 a, b** Digital mammography, MLO view.

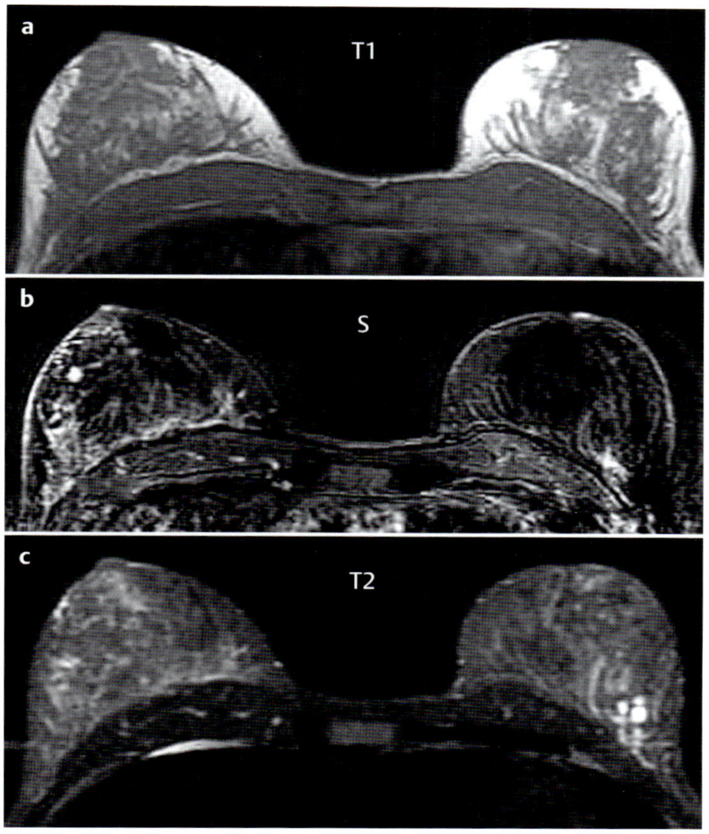


Fig. 15.**4 a – c** Contrast-enhanced MR mammography.

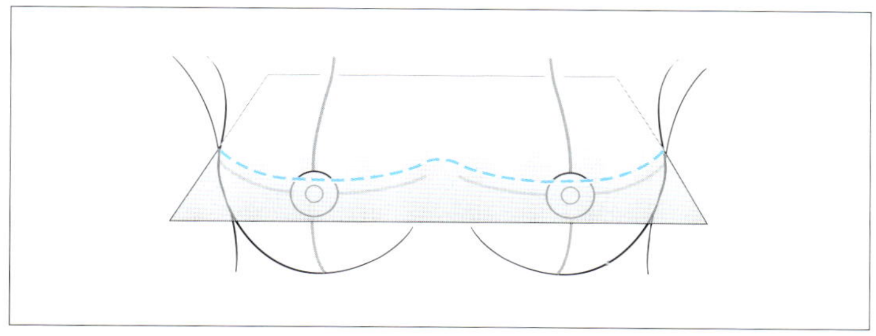

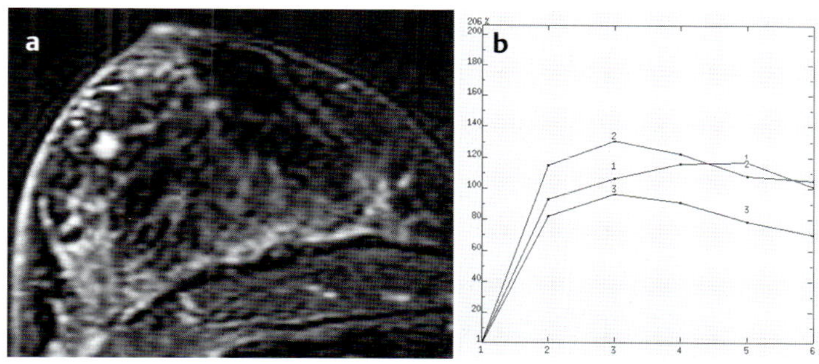


Fig. 15.**5 a, b** Signal-to-time curves.

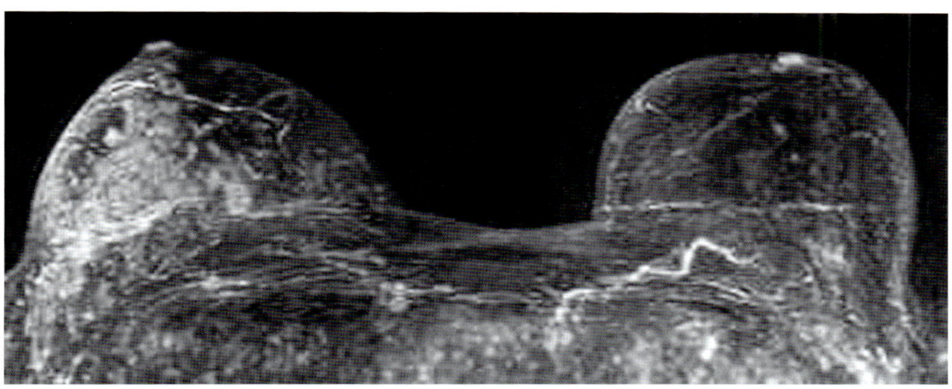

Fig. 15.**6** Contrast-enhanced MR mammography. Maximum intensity projection.

?

Please characterize ultrasound, mammography, and MRI findings.
What is your preliminary diagnosis?
What are your next steps?

This is the imaging study of a symptomatic woman. The resistance in the right upper outer quadrant had the characteristics of a harmless nodular gland. Nevertheless, this was the reason the patient presented for mammography. The risk profile was not increased.

### Ultrasound

Corresponding to the location of the resistance in the right breast, there is a well-defined, lobulated mass of 2 mm diameter with markedly hyperechogenic borders. The architectural structure is distorted in this area. US BI-RADS right 5.

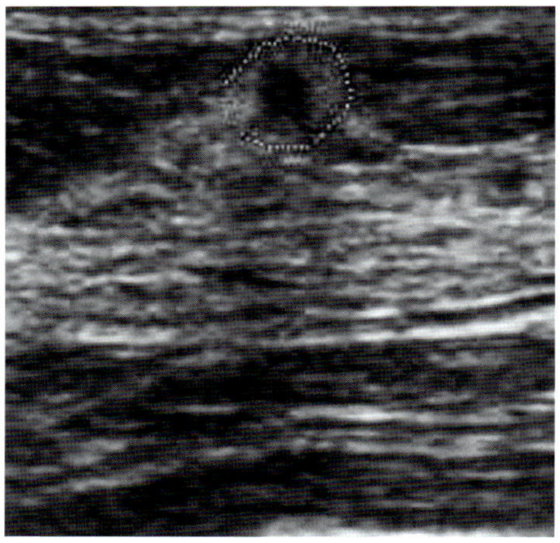

Fig. 15.**7** Lesion in ultrasound.

### Mammography

The parenchyma was bilaterally symmetric and extremely dense, ACR type 4. Under these limiting conditions, mammography showed no specific findings in the area of the clinically observed mass or elsewhere. There were no visible masses, densities, calcifications, or architectural distortion (BI-RADS right 1/left 1). PGMI: CC view P; MLO view P.

### MR Mammography

Corresponding to the clinical and ultrasound findings, MRI shows a hypervascularized, round, partially ill-defined mass of approx. 1 cm diameter, lateral to the right nipple. This lesion showed an intermediate signal on T2-weighted images.

**MRI Artifact Category:** 2
**MRI Density Type:** 2

| MRM score | Finding | Points |
|---|---|---|
| **Shape** | round | 0 |
| **Border** | ill-defined | 1 |
| **CM Distribution** | homogeneous | 0 |
| **Initial Signal Intensity Increase** | strong | 2 |
| **Post-initial Signal Intensity Character** | wash-out | 2 |
| **MRI score (points)** | | **5** |
| **MRI BI-RADS** | | **4** |

### → Preliminary Diagnosis

Carcinoma, fibroadenoma

| BI-RADS Categorization | | |
|---|---|---|
| Clinical Findings | right 3 | left 1 |
| Ultrasound | right 5 | left 1 |
| Mammography | right 1 | left 1 |
| MR Mammography | right 4 | left 1 |
| **BI-RADS Total** | **right 5** | **left 1** |

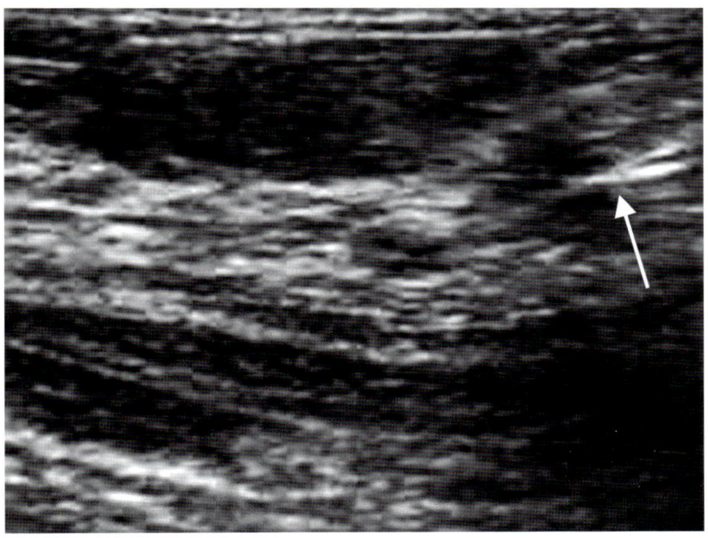

Fig. 15.**8** US-guided FNAP with needle visible in lesion (arrow).

**Procedure**

Normally: histopathological evaluation of the palpable mass following US-guided core biopsy.

**Procedure followed here (departing from guidelines)**

US-guided fine-needle aspiration cytology (FNAP), because of the small size of the lesion.

**Cytology**

Prolific cancer cells. Category C5.

## Histology

Invasive lobular carcinoma 6 mm in diameter. Axillary lymph node status normal.

ILC pT1b, pN0, M0, G2.

## Treatment

Breast conservation therapy.

Hyperechoic margins of lesions as seen in ultrasound are an extremely important criterion for malignancy.

**Indication:** Screening.
**History:** No abnormalities.
**Risk profile:** No increased risk.
**Age:** 45 years.

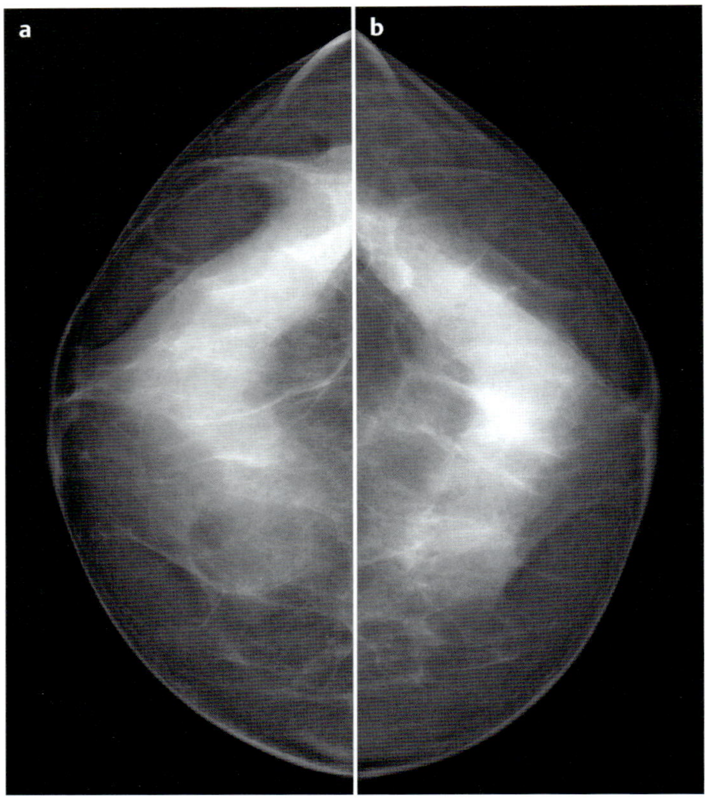


Fig. 16.**1 a, b** Digital mammography, CC view.

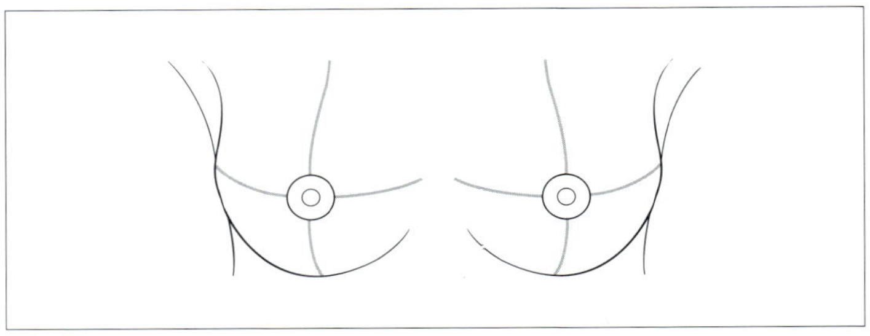

### Clinical Findings

Lumpy parenchymal texture. No resistance.

### Ultrasound

No findings.

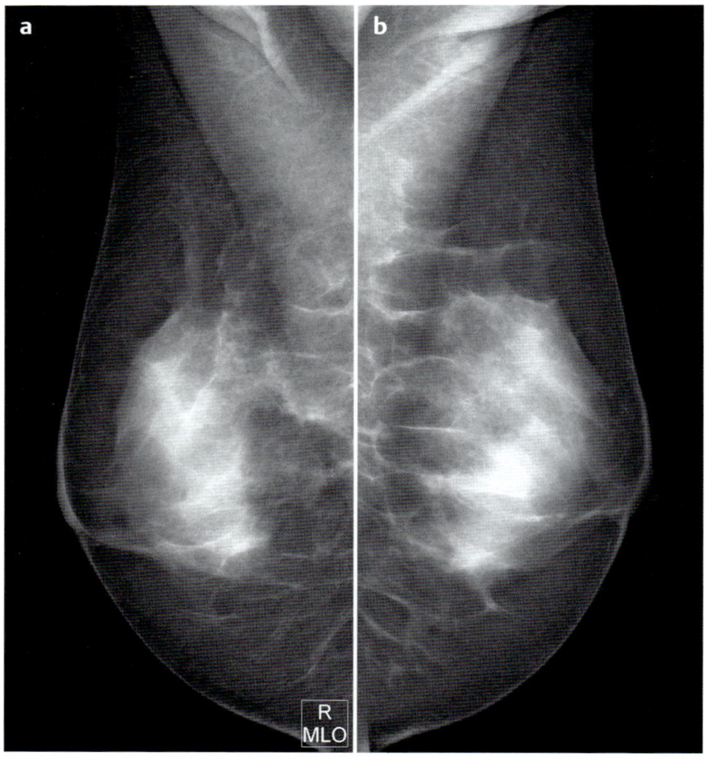


Fig. 16.**2 a, b** Digital mammography, MLO view.

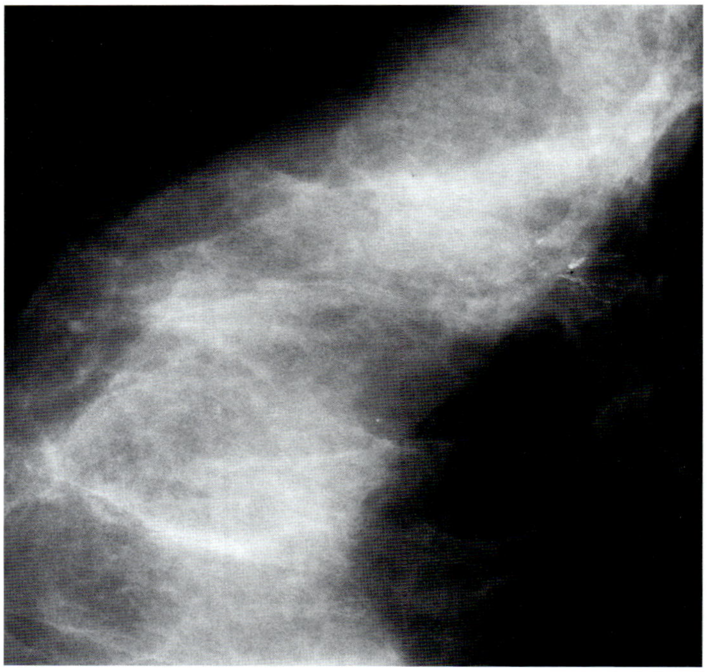

Fig. 16.**3** Magnification view of the right breast (CC).

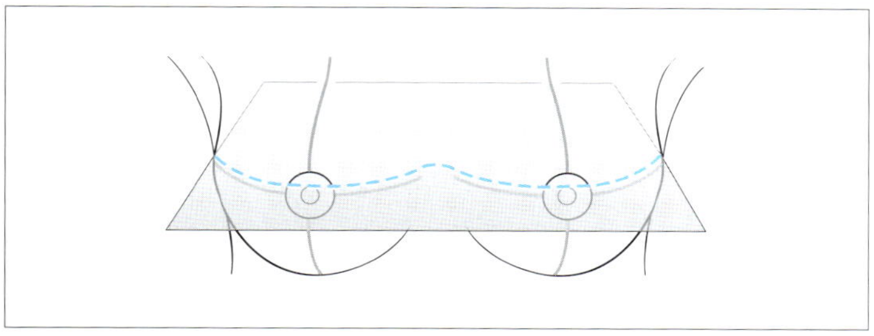

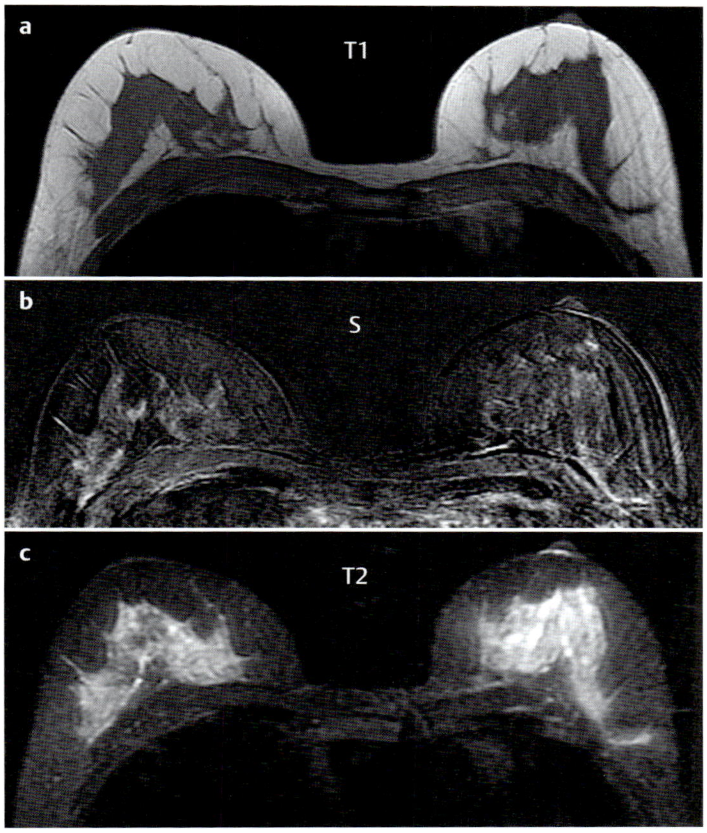


Fig. 16.**4 a – c** Contrast-enhanced MR mammography.

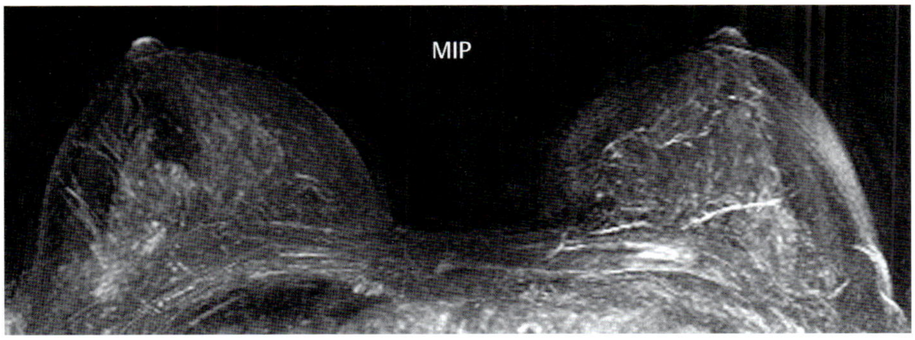


Fig. 16.**5** Contrast-enhanced MR mammography. Maximum intensity projection.

?

Please characterize mammography and MRI.
What is your preliminary diagnosis?
What are your next steps?

This case investigated microcalcifications that were discovered in screening mammography.

## Ultrasound

Ultrasound showed no abnormalities in either breast. Even with the mammography data as a guide, no echo alteration was detected in the upper outer quadrant of the right breast.

## Mammography

Mammography demonstrated bilaterally symmetric, extremely dense parenchyma, ACR type 4. In the upper outer quadrant of the right breast a cluster of polymorphous microcalcifications was visible in a segmental orientation. Magnification mammography depicted the polymorphous character in more detail (linear and Y-shaped calcifications). No hyperdensities or architectural distortion. BI-RADS right 4/left 1. PGMI: CC view P; MLO view P.

## MR Mammography

There were no pathological findings in MR mammography. In the right upper outer ROI, strong contrast uptake throughout the parenchyma meant that no focal, linear or dendritic enhancements were detected.

**MRI Artifact Category:** right 2/left 3
**MRI Density Type:** 2

| MRM score | Finding | Points |
|---|---|---|
| **Shape** | – | 0 |
| **Border** | – | 0 |
| **CM Distribution** | – | 0 |
| **Initial Signal Intensity Increase** | – | 0 |
| **Post-initial Signal Intensity Character** | – | 0 |
| **MRI score (points)** | | **0** |
| **MRI BI-RADS** | | **1** |

## → Preliminary Diagnosis

Intraductal carcinoma (occult on US and MRI), probably minimally invasive.

| BI-RADS Categorization | | |
|---|---|---|
| Clinical Findings | right 1 | left 1 |
| Ultrasound | right 1 | left 1 |
| Mammography | right 4 | left 1 |
| MR Mammography | right 1 | left 1 |
| **BI-RADS Total** | **right 4** | **left 1** |

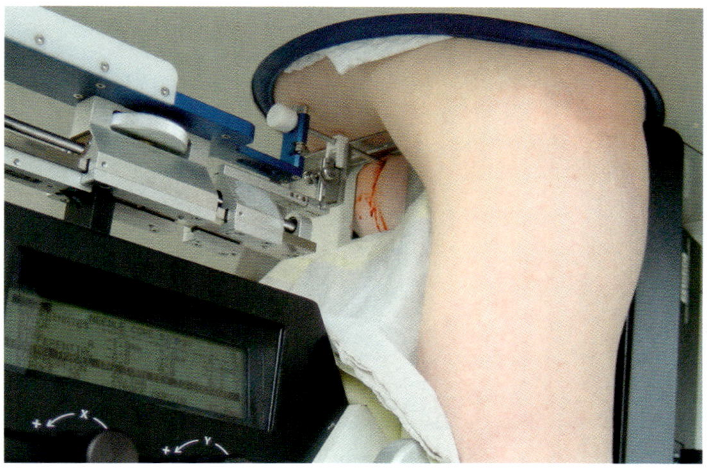

Fig. 16.**6** Vacuum biopsy using a Lorad table. An atypical positioning of the arm was adopted because the calcifications were very close to the chest wall.

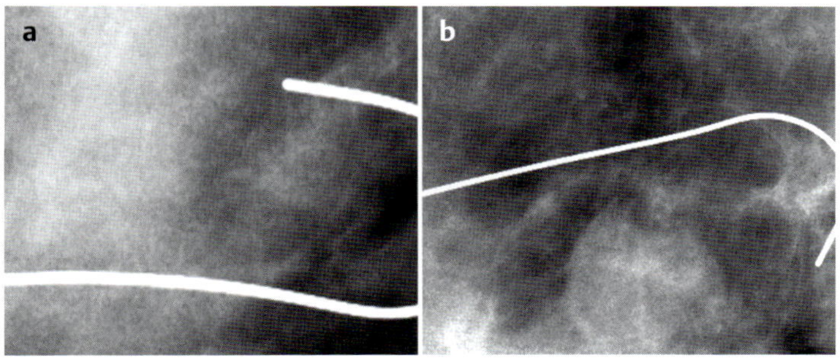

Fig. 16.**7 a, b** Preoperative hook-wire localization, CC and MLO magnifications.

**Procedure**

Histopathological evaluation of the microcalcifications in the upper outer quadrant of the right breast by stereotactic vacuum biopsy (Fig. 16.**6**).

**Histopathology of the core biopsy specimen:** Invasive lobular carcinoma.

**Further procedure:** Preoperative hook-wire localization of the calcification cluster (Fig. 16.**7a, b**).

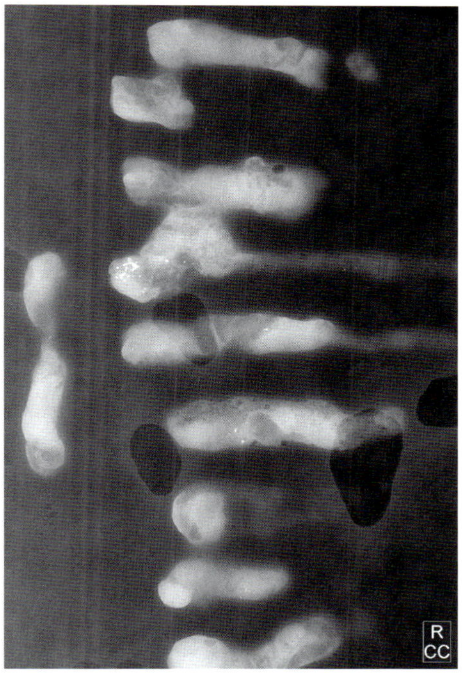


Fig. 16.**8** Specimen radiography.

## Histology

Invasive lobular carcinoma 12 mm in maximum diameter. Axillary lymph node status normal.

ILC* pT1b, pN0, M0, Estrogen receptor (+), Gestagen receptor (+).

* The microcalcifications suggested the likelihood of a ductal carcinoma.

## Treatment

Breast conservation therapy.

Mammography is the method of choice for the very early detection of breast cancer because it reliably depicts microcalcifications.

**Indication:** Screening mammography.
**History:** Unremarkable.
**Risk profile:** No increased risk.
**Age:** 47 years.

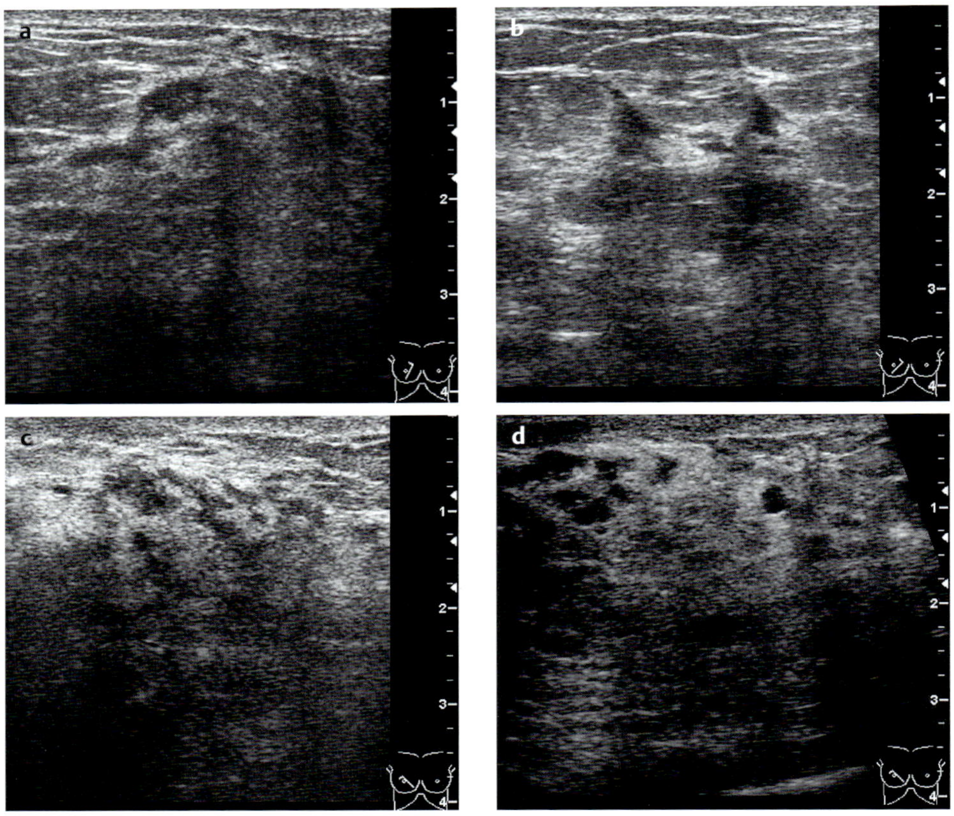

Fig. 17.**1 a – d** Ultrasound of the right breast, inner quadrants.

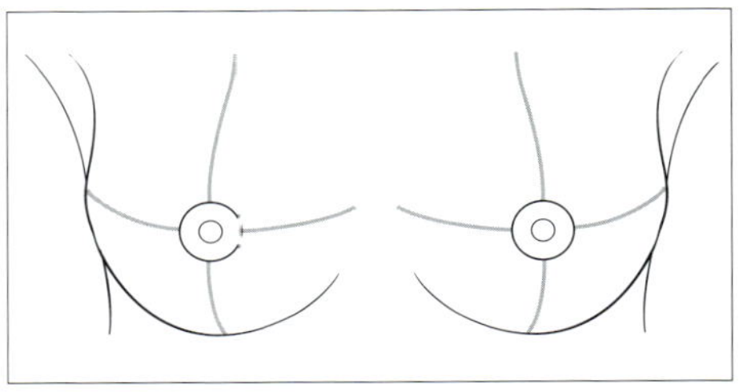

## Clinical Findings

Lumpy parenchymal texture, no suspect findings.

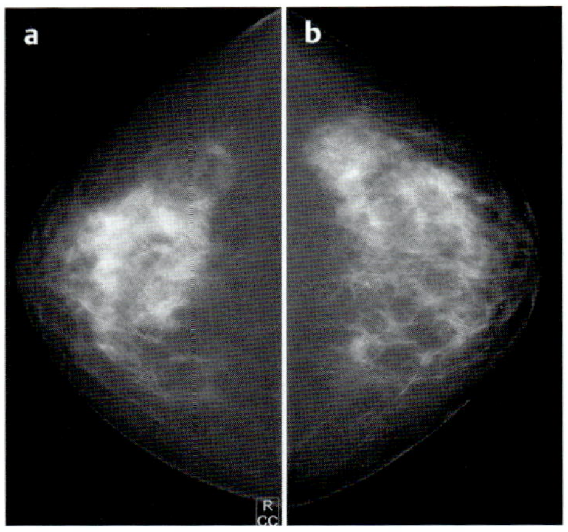

Fig. 17.**2 a, b** Digital mammography, CC view.

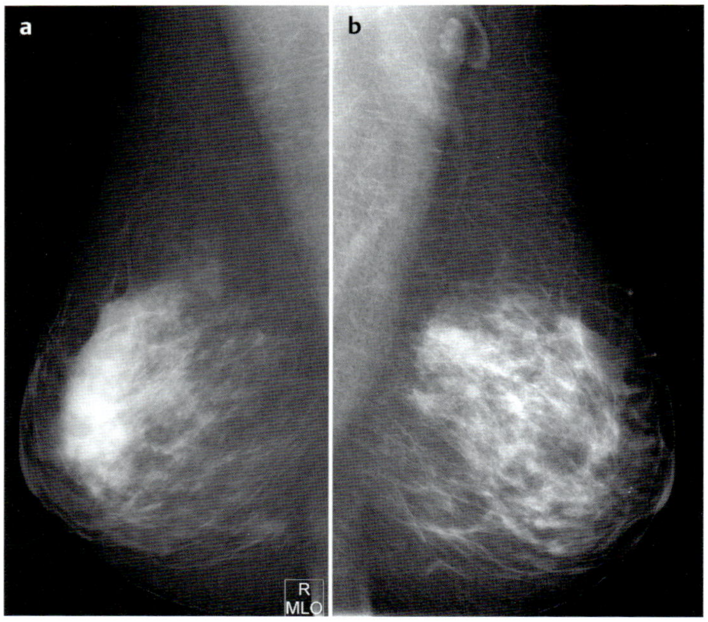

Fig. 17.**3 a, b** Digital mammography, MLO view.

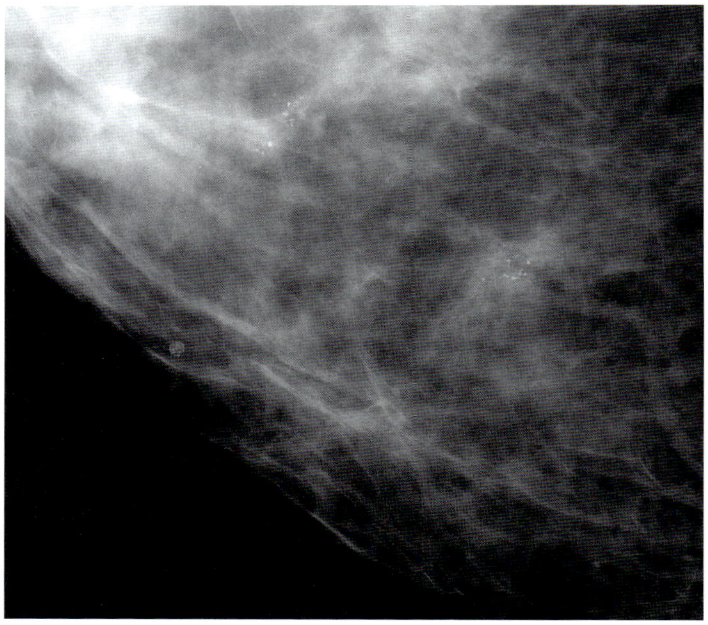

Fig. 17.**4** Magnification view of the right breast (CC).

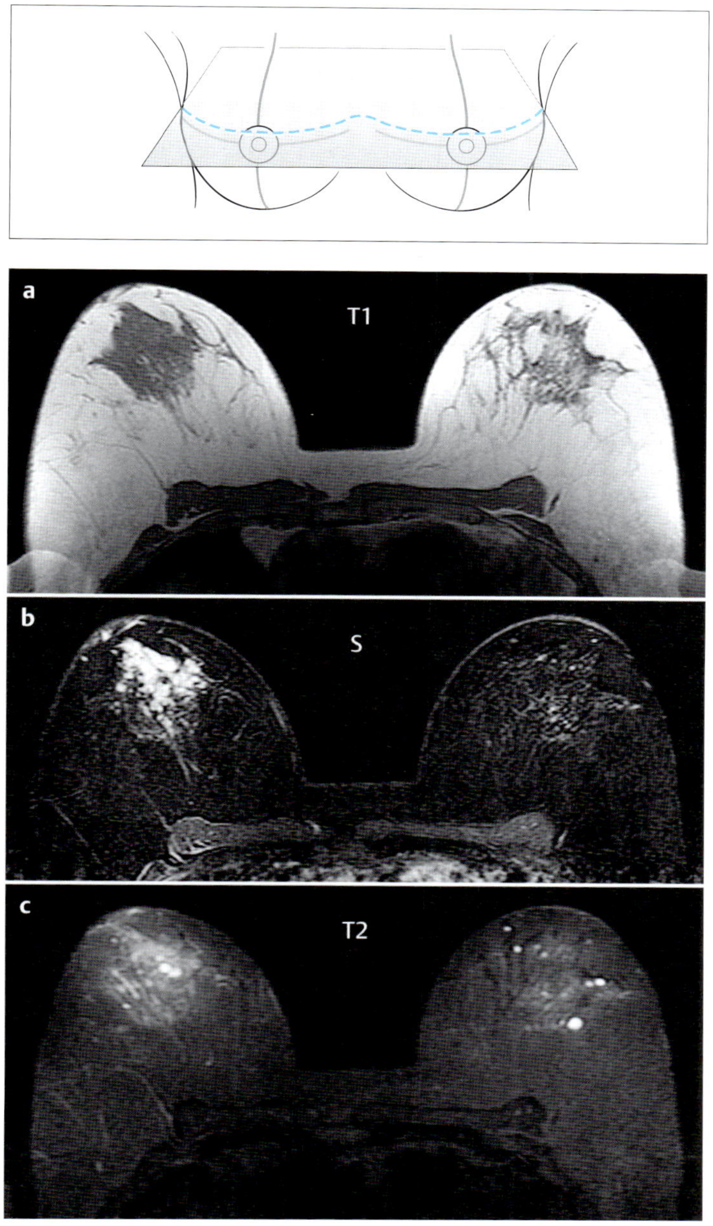


Fig. 17.**5 a – c** Contrast-enhanced MR mammography.

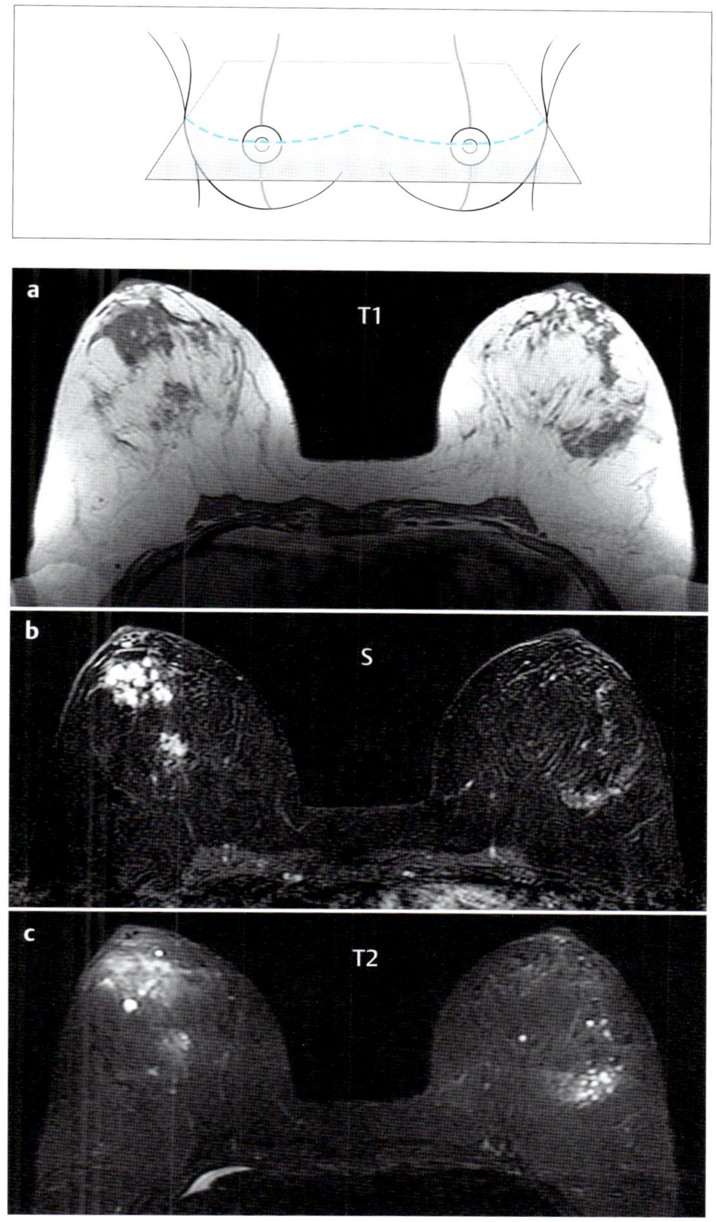


Fig. 17.**6 a – c** Contrast-enhanced MR mammography.

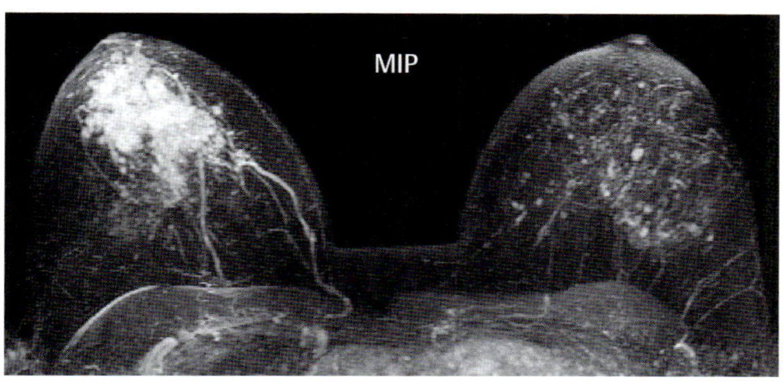


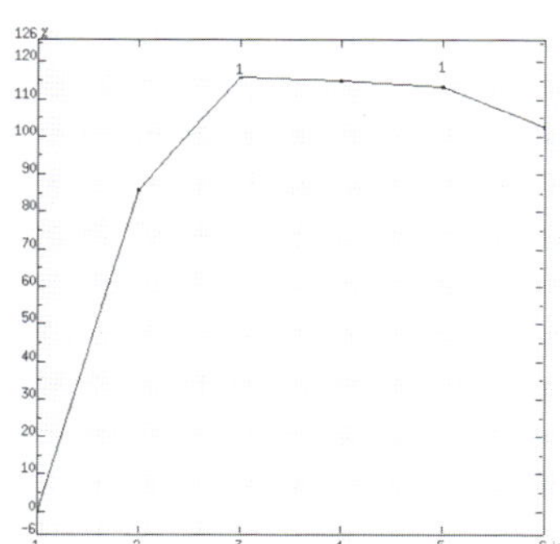

Fig. 17.**7** Contrast-enhanced MR mammography. Maximum intensity projection.

Fig. 17.**8** Signal-to-time curve (right breast, central region).

Please characterize ultrasound, mammography and MRI.
What is your preliminary diagnosis?
What are your next steps?

This case shows the imaging studies of an asymptomatic woman. In screening mammography, suspect microcalcification clusters were noted in the inner quadrants of the right breast.

### Ultrasound

Corresponding to the microcalcifications seen in mammography and the localized enhancement in MRI, the inner quadrants of the right breast showed inhomogeneous echogenicity. Multiple hypoechoic lesions 6–8 mm in diameter with nonechogenic borders and no distal shadowing. No definitively suspect findings. US BI-RADS right 3.

### Mammography

Mammograms demonstrated bilaterally symmetric inhomogeneous dense parenchyma, ACR type 3. Imaging showed two clusters of polymorphous microcalcifications between the inner quadrants of the right breast and in the central part of the right breast. There were no masses, densities, or architectural distortions. BI-RADS right 4/left 1. PGMI: CC view P; MLO view G (inframammary fold not clearly imaged).

### MR Mammography

A dendritic, partially ill-defined and inhomogeneous enhancement was seen in the upper inner quadrant of the right breast, with a strong initial signal increase (> 100%) and postinitial plateau. This enhancing focus showed low signal intensity in T2-weighted images. No findings in the left breast.

**MRI Artifact Category:** 2
**MRI Density Type:** 2

| MRM score | Finding | Points |
|---|---|---|
| **Shape** | dendritic | 1 |
| **Border** | ill-defined | 1 |
| **CM Distribution** | inhomogeneous | 1 |
| **Initial Signal Intensity Increase** | strong | 2 |
| **Post-initial Signal Intensity Character** | plateau | 1 |
| **MRI score (points)** | | **6** |
| **MRI BI-RADS** | | **5** |

### → Preliminary Diagnosis

DCIS, minimally invasive carcinoma, invasive carcinoma.

| BI-RADS Categorization | | |
|---|---|---|
| Clinical Findings | right 1 | left 1 |
| Ultrasound | right 3 | left 1 |
| Mammography | right 4 | left 1 |
| MR Mammography | right 5 | left 1 |
| **BI-RADS Total** | **right 5** | **left 1** |

### Procedure

Histopathological evaluation after US-guided core biopsy of the right upper inner quadrant.

### Histopathology

Ductal carcinoma in situ.

### Further procedure

Preoperative hook-wire localization.

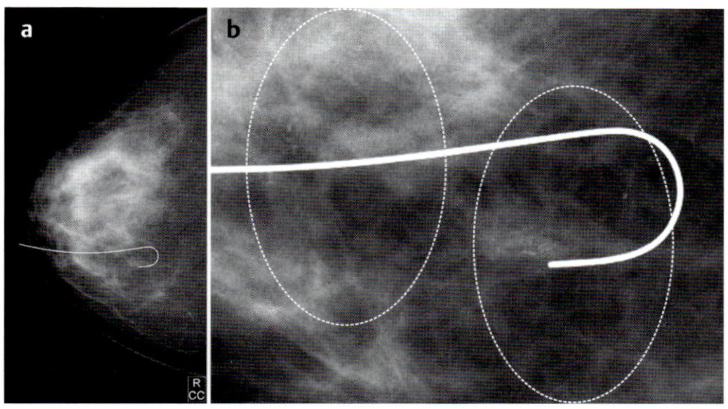


Fig. 17.**9 a, b** Preoperative localization and magnification view (CC).

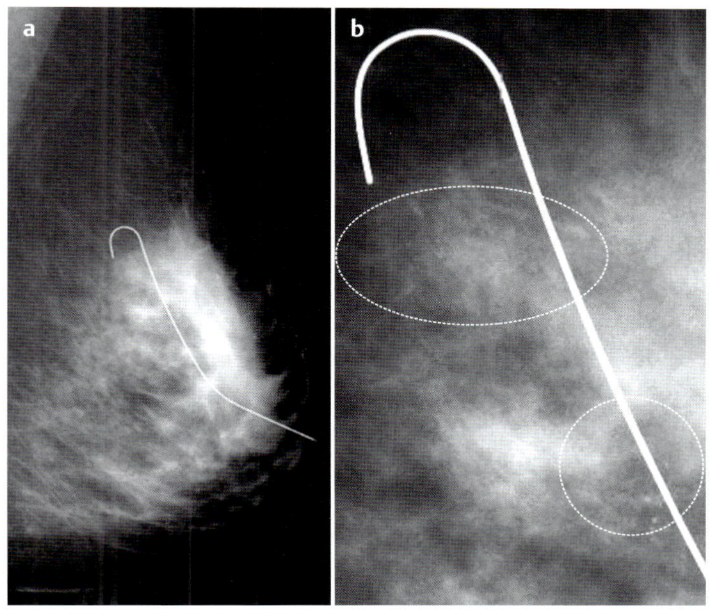


Fig. 17.**10** a, b Preoperative localization and magnification view (MLO). Both calcification groups are marked with a Homer wire.

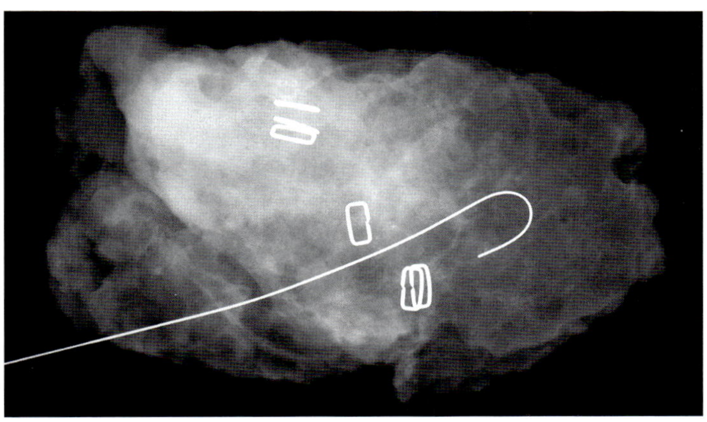

Fig. 17.**11** Specimen radiography.

### Histology

Extended ductal carcinoma in situ. As expected, no infiltration of the axillary lymph nodes.

DCIS, pN0, G2

### Treatment

Mastectomy, extent of DCIS being > 4 cm

Even intraductal carcinomas (DCIS) can show enhancement in MRI (in theory as a result of tumor-induced increase in vascular permeability).

**Indication:** Pain in right breast.
**History:** Unremarkable.
**Risk profile:** No increased risk.
**Age:** 55 years.

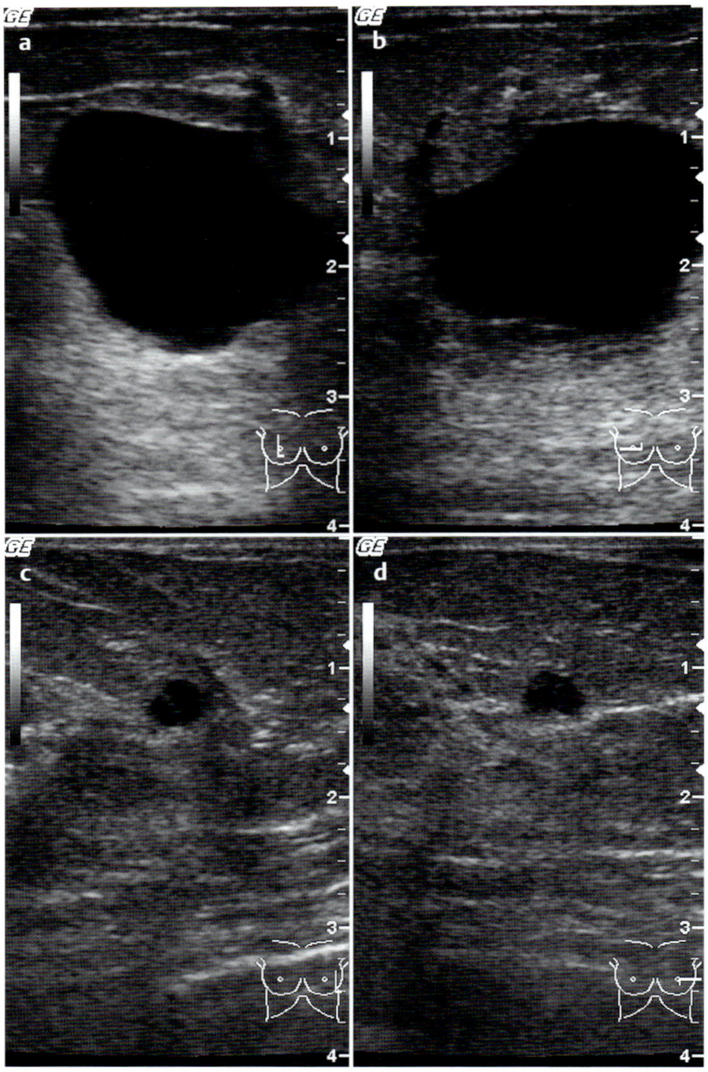

Fig. 18.**1 a – d** Ultrasound.

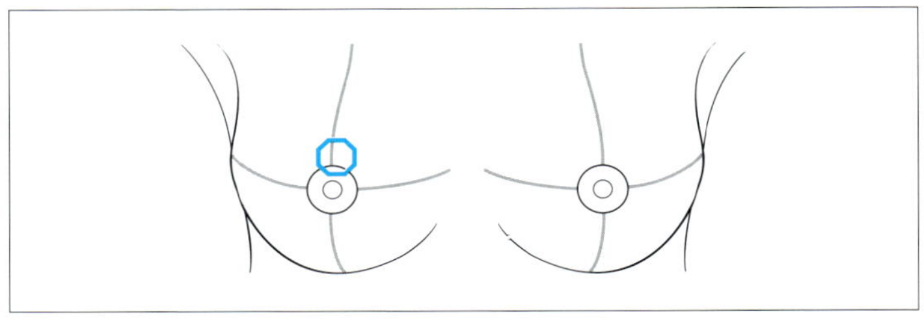

## Clinical Findings

Resistance of 2 cm diameter in the right breast, above the areola.

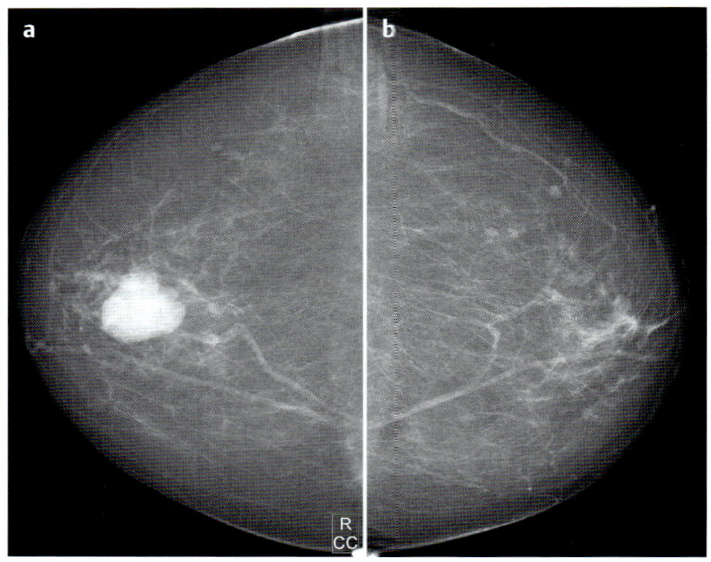

Fig. 18.**2 a, b** Digital mammography, CC view.

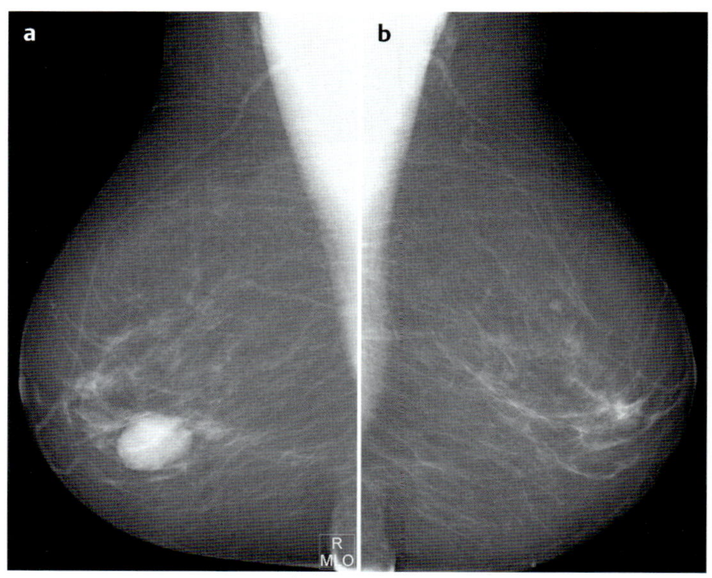

Fig. 18.**3 a, b** Digital mammography, MLO view.

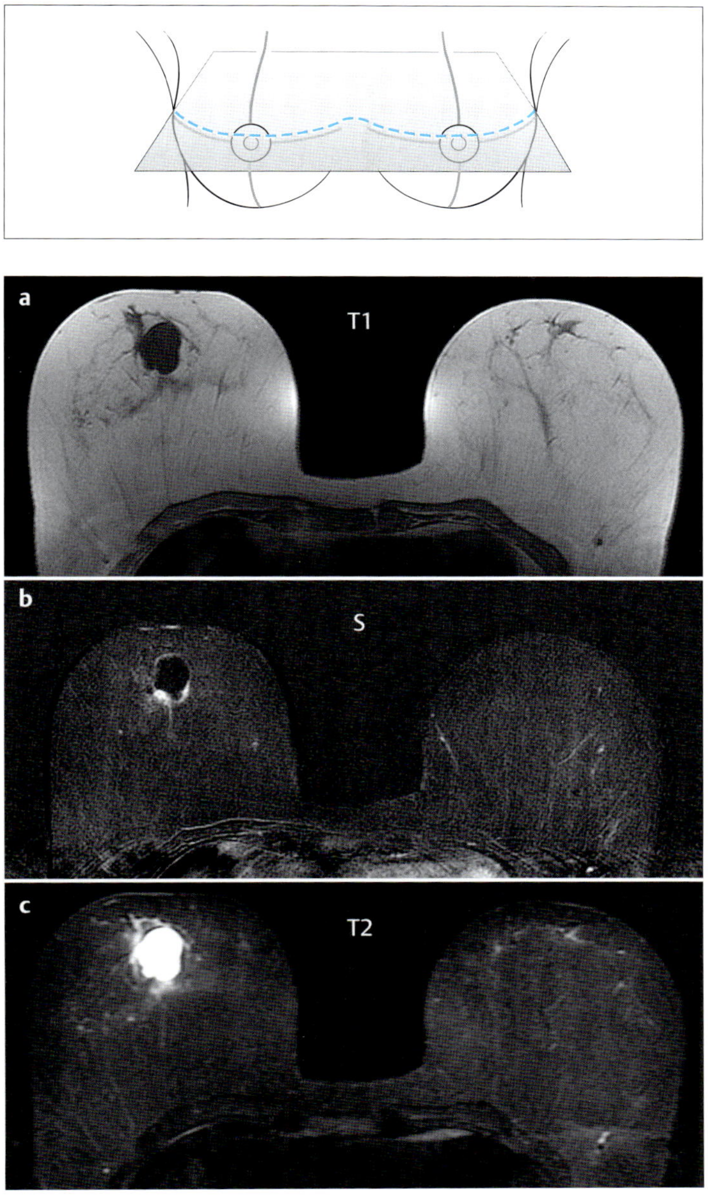


Fig. 18.4 a–c Contrast-enhanced MR mammography.

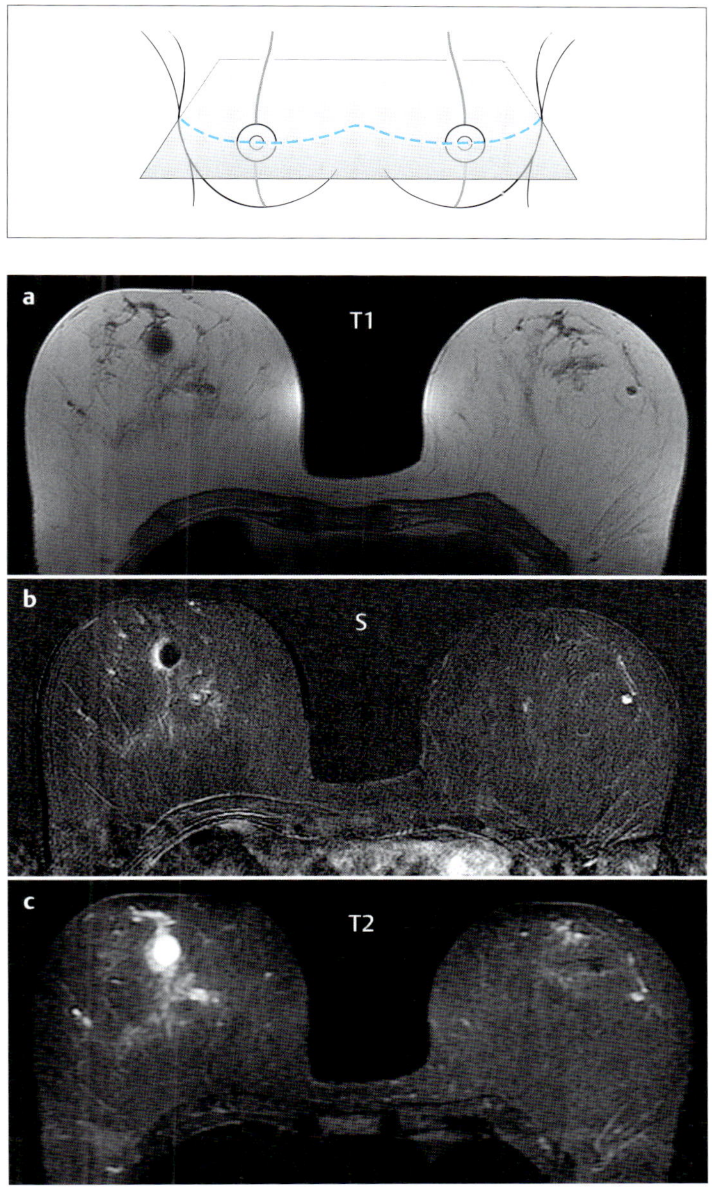


Fig. 18.5 a–c Contrast-enhanced MR mammography.

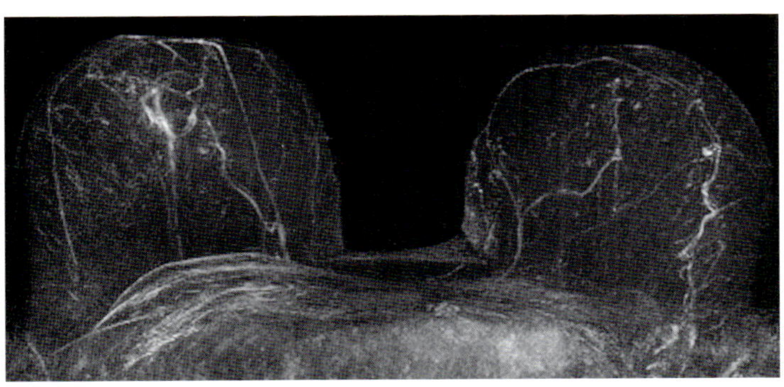

Fig. 18.6 Contrast-enhanced MR mammography. Maximum intensity projection.

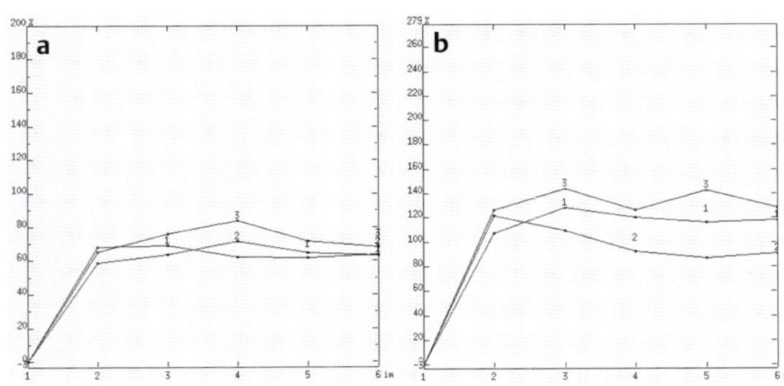


Fig. 18.7 a, b Signal-to-time curves of the cyst wall, right breast (a) and of the lesion in the left breast (b).

Please characterize ultrasound, mammography and MRI.
What is your preliminary diagnosis?
What are your next steps?

This case shows the imaging of a symptomatic woman presenting with a resistance between the upper quadrants of the right breast.

### Ultrasound

In the area of the painful resistance, ultrasound demonstrated a lobulated, anechoic lesion of 2 cm diameter with hypoechoic border components and characteristics of a complicated cyst. Additionally, ultrasound showed a lobulated hypoechoic lesion of 5 mm with indeterminate distal echo pattern between the lateral quadrants of the left breast (DD: cyst, fibroadenoma). US BI-RADS right 4/left 3.

### Mammography

Both breasts showed predominantly lipomatous tissue, ACR type 1. Mammography showed a well-defined, hyperdense, lobulated mass of 2 cm diameter in the central part of the right breast. There was a further well-defined lobulated hyperdensity of 0.5 cm in the upper outer quadrant of the left breast. Mammography depicted no architectural distortion or microcalcifications. BI-RADS right 2/left 2. PGMI: CC view P; MLO view M (pectoralis angle < 20°, inframammary fold incorrectly positioned).

### MR Mammography

Corresponding to ultrasound and mammography, MRI demonstrated a well-defined, lobulated, 2 cm lesion in the middle of the right breast with marginal contrast uptake. There was also a well-defined, lobulated, enhancing mass between the outer quadrants of the left breast with initial signal increase of 70% and increasing postinitial signal behavior. This lesion showed increased signal in T2-weighted imaging.

**MRI Artifact Category:** 1
**MRI Density Type:** 1

| MRM score | Finding right | Points | Finding left | Points |
|---|---|---|---|---|
| **Shape** | round | 0 | round | 0 |
| **Border** | well-defined | 0 | well-defined | 0 |
| **CM Distribution** | homogeneous | 0 | homogeneous | 0 |
| **Initial Signal Intensity Increase** | moderate | 1 | strong | 2 |
| **Post-initial Signal Intensity Character** | plateau | 1 | plateau | 1 |
| **MRI score (points)** | | **2** | | **3** |
| **MRI BI-RADS** | | **2** | | **3** |

### → Preliminary Diagnosis

Right: Cyst, complicated cyst, intracystic tumor.

Left: Adenoma, fibroadenoma, papilloma, carcinoma (medullary? mucinous?).

| **BI-RADS Categorization** | | |
|---|---|---|
| Clinical Findings | right 3 | left 1 |
| Ultrasound | right 4 | left 3 |
| Mammography | right 2 | left 2 |
| MR Mammography | right 2 | left 3 |
| **BI-RADS Total** | **right 4** | **left 3** |

**Procedure (as recommended by guidelines)**

US-guided core biopsy of the solid cyst wall components (right breast).

**Procedure followed here**

Since the proposed intervention was declined by the patient, follow-up ultrasound imaging was carried out after 6 months.

**Follow-up ultrasound findings after 6 months**: No findings. Complete resorption of the cyst in the right breast (not shown).

MR mammography imaging was carried out after 6 months to check whether the contrast-enhancing changes would be reproduced. Findings: right–complete resorption of previously enhancing area; left–findings unchanged.

## Diagnosis (without histopathological verification)

Right breast: Complicated Cyst
Left breast: Fibroadenoma

## Treatment

None.

You may think there is nothing exceptional about this case. All the same, it represents everyday diagnostic practice in breast clinics.

**Indication:** Check-up after vacuum biopsy.
**History:** Vacuum core biopsy 6 months previously.
**Risk profile:** No increased risk.
**Age:** 49 years.

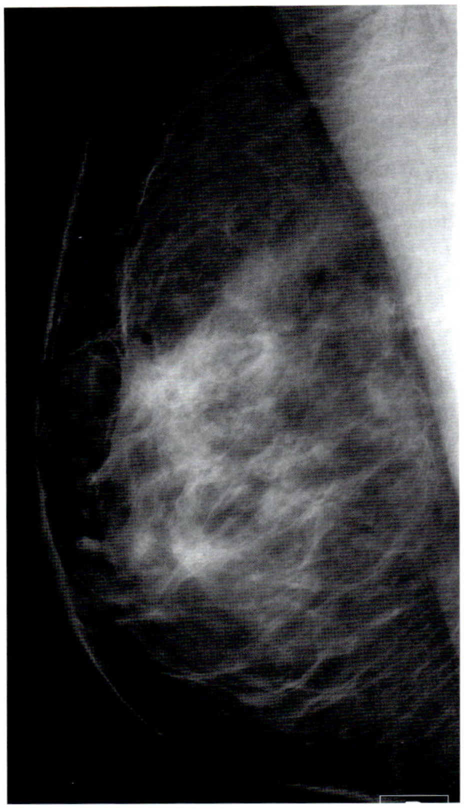

Fig. 19.1 Mammography, MLO view, before vacuum biopsy.

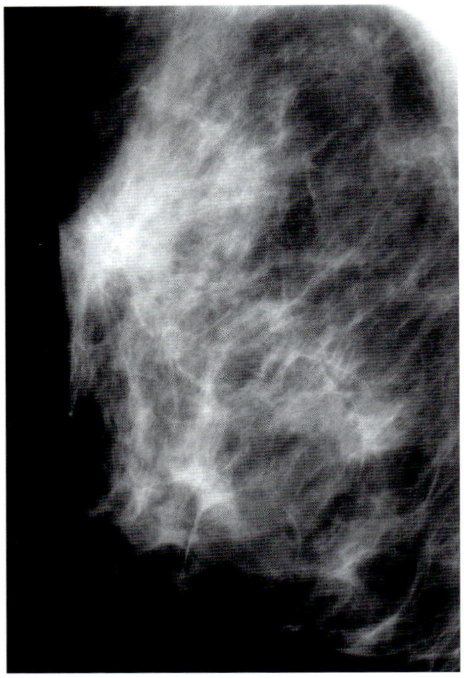

Fig. 19.2 Magnification view (MLO), before vacuum biopsy.

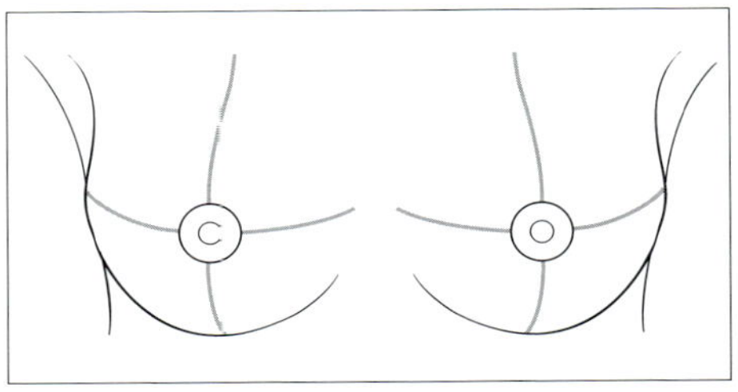

**Clinical Findings**

Normal.

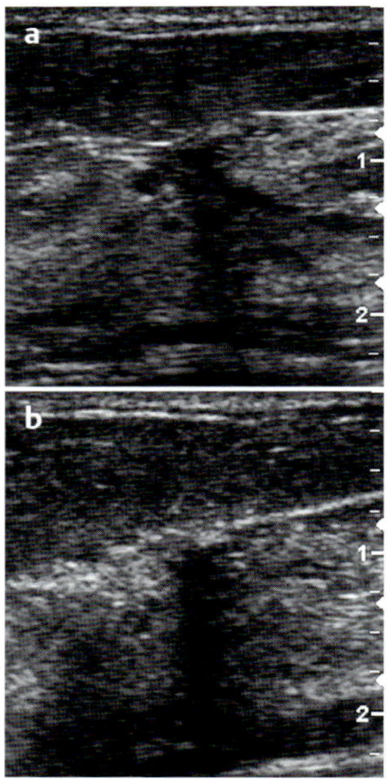


Fig. 19.3 Ultrasound of the previous biopsy region.

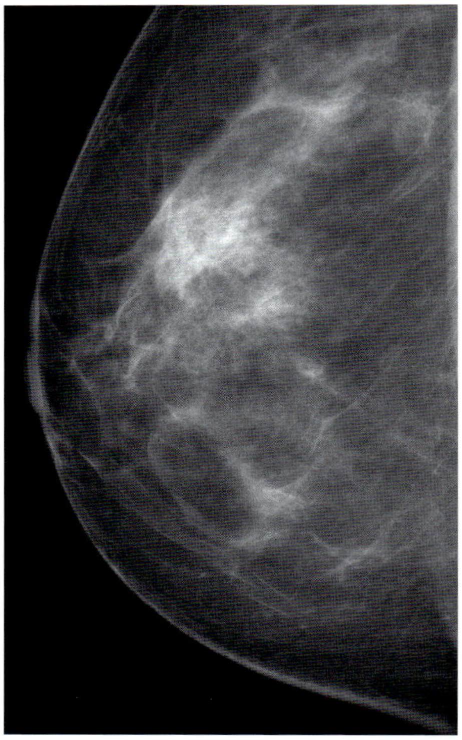

Fig. 19.4 Digital mammography, CC view, six months after biopsy.

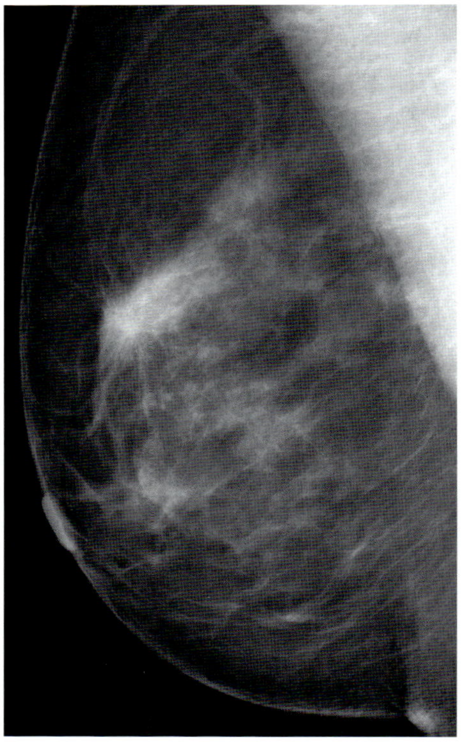

Fig. 19.5 Digital mammography, MLO view, six months after biopsy.

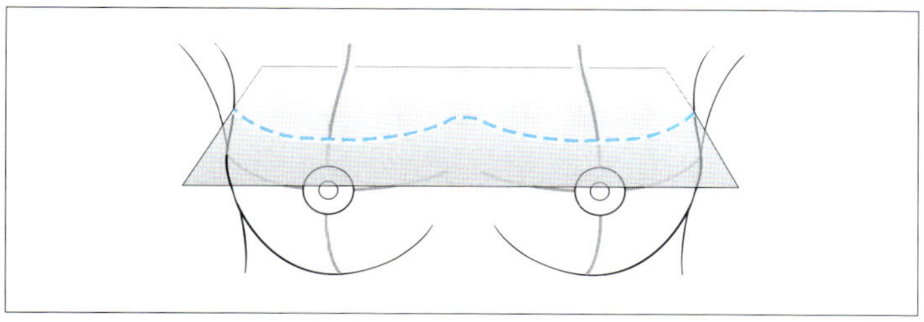

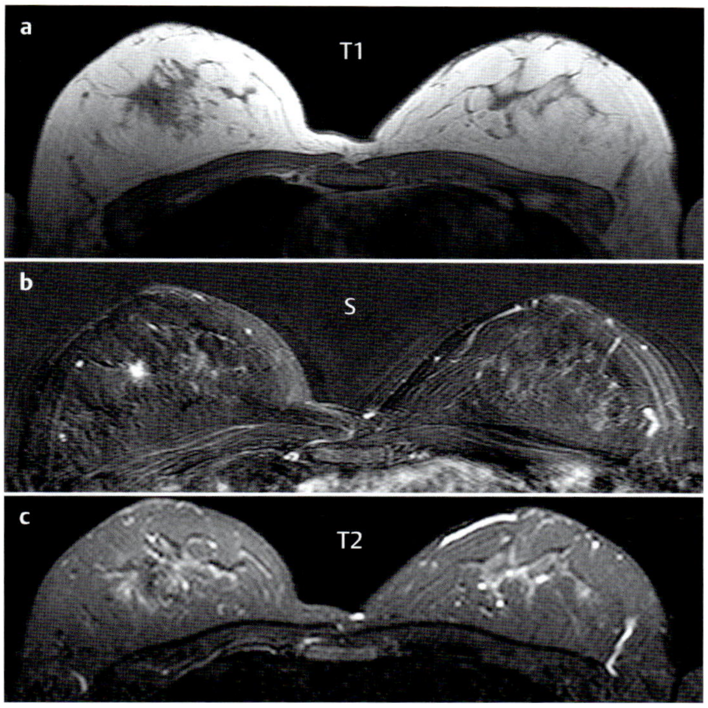


Fig. 19.**6 a – c** Contrast-enhanced MR mammography six months after biopsy.

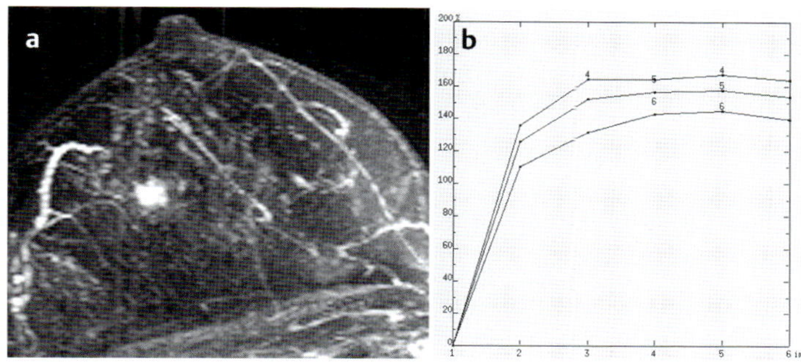


Fig. 19.**8 a, b** Signal-to-time curves.

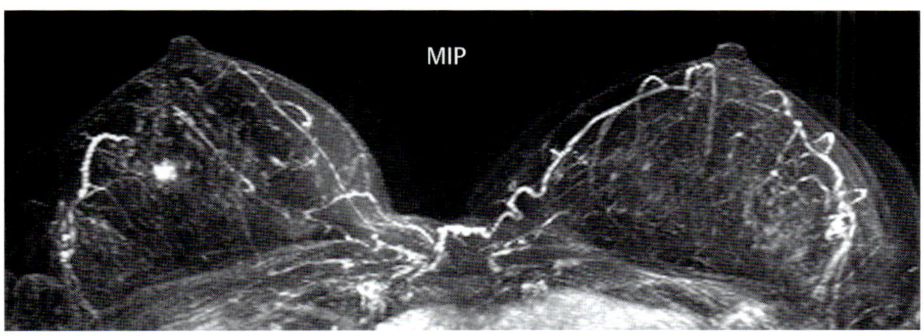


Fig. 19.**7** Contrast-enhanced MR mammography. Maximum intensity projection.

?

Please characterize ultrasound, mammography and MRI.
What is your preliminary diagnosis?
What are your next steps?

This case demonstrates imaging of an asymptomatic woman. In screening mammography 6 months previously, suspect microcalcifications were found between the upper quadrants of the right breast. Vacuum biopsy (VB) was carried out and histopathology indicated a diagnosis of sclerosing adenosis.

**Ultrasound (6 months after VB)**

Ultrasound demonstrated an ill-defined hypoechoic lesion 5 mm in diameter between the upper quadrants of the right breast, with an indeterminate distal echo pattern. US BI-RADS right 3.

**Mammography (6 months after VB,** Figs. 19.**4** and 19.**5**)

Mammograms showed fibroglandular parenchyma, ACR type 2. In comparison with the pre-biopsy imaging (Fig. 19.**1**), an ill-defined hyperdensity in the upper outer quadrant of the right breast showed an increase in diameter. No microcalcifications were visualized. BI-RADS right 4. PGMI not defined for one-sided mammography.

**MR Mammography (6 months after VB)**

MRI showed an ill-defined, spiculated, homogeneously enhancing lesion (diameter 1 cm) between the upper quadrants of the right breast, with initial signal increase of 125% and a postinitial plateau. There was a decreased signal in T2-weighted imaging. No findings in the left breast.

**MRI Artifact Category:** 2
**MRI Density Type:** 2

| MRM score | Finding | Points |
|---|---|---|
| **Shape** | spiculated | 1 |
| **Border** | ill-defined | 1 |
| **CM Distribution** | inhomogeneous | 0 |
| **Initial Signal Intensity Increase** | strong | 2 |
| **Post-initial Signal Intensity Character** | plateau | 1 |
| **MRI score (points)** | | **5** |
| **MRI BI-RADS** | | **4** |

## → Preliminary Diagnosis

Carcinoma; scarring from vacuum biopsy with atypical enhancement; focal mastitis following intervention.

| BI-RADS Categorization | | |
|---|---|---|
| Clinical Findings | right 1 | left 1 |
| Ultrasound | right 3 | left 1 |
| Mammography | right 4 | left 1 |
| MR Mammography | right 4 | left 1 |
| **BI-RADS Total** | **right 4** | **left 1** |

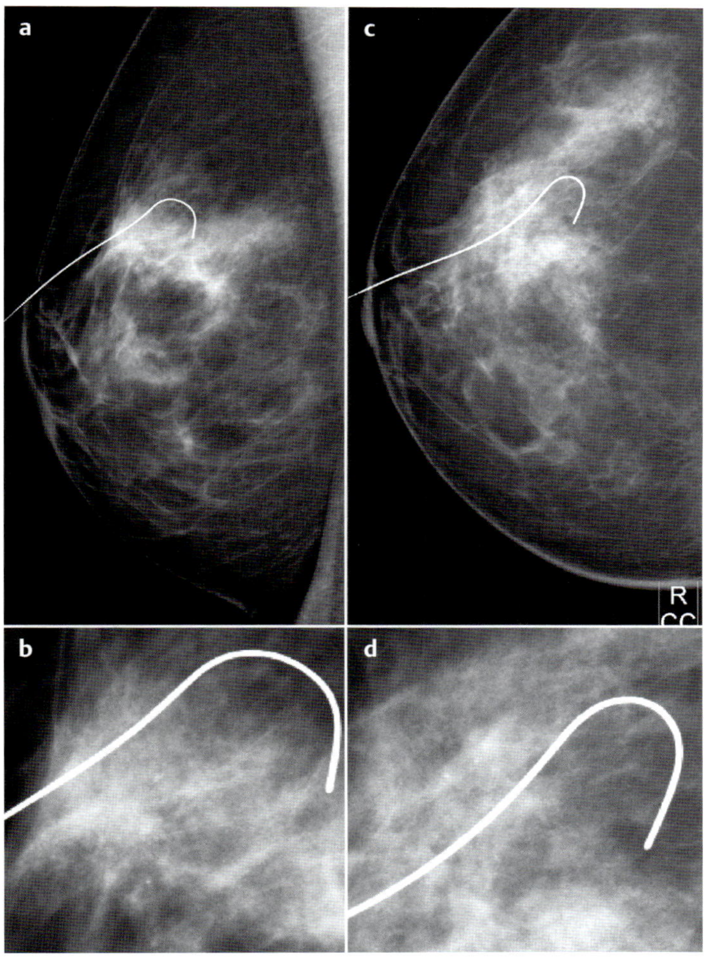


Fig. 19.**9 a – d** Localization in two planes with magnification views.

**Procedure**

Open biopsy following hook-wire localization.
Preoperative hook-wire localization and specimen radiography.

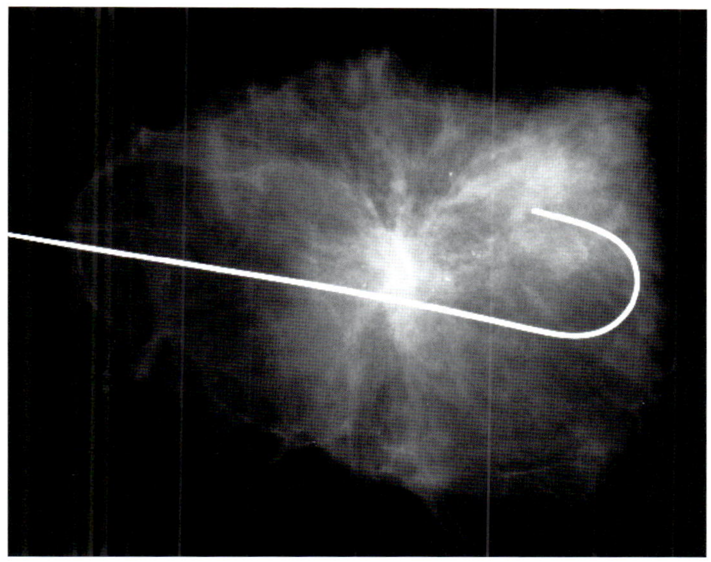

Fig. 19.**10** Specimen radiography.

## Histology

Scar tissue (from vacuum biopsy) with focal mastitis.

## Treatment

None.

Scar tissue that enhances in MRI can be a cause of false-positive findings. However, it is rare, and is usually associated with focal inflammation.

**Indication:** Lump in right breast.
**History:** Unremarkable.
**Risk profile:** No increased risk.
**Age:** 60 years.

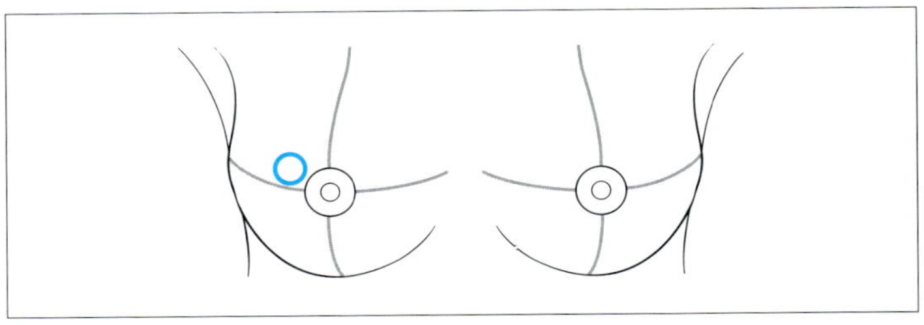

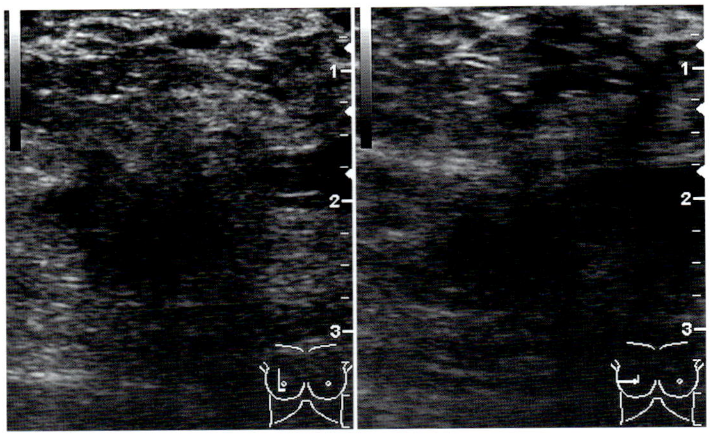

Fig. 20.1 Ultrasound, right breast.

## Clinical Findings

Palpable resistance in upper outer quadrant of the right breast. No findings in the left breast.

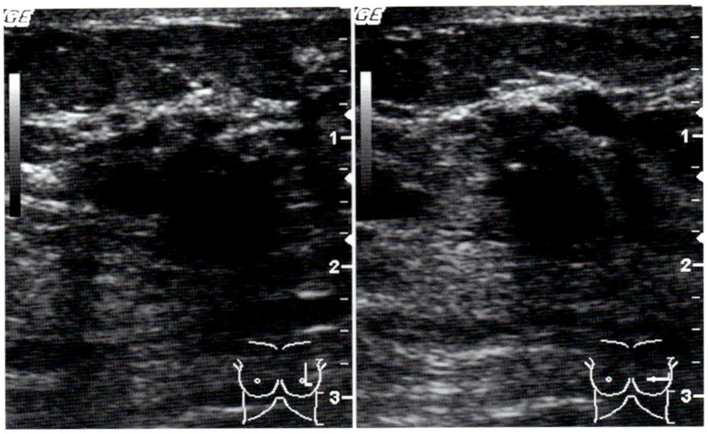

Fig. 20.2 Ultrasound, left breast.

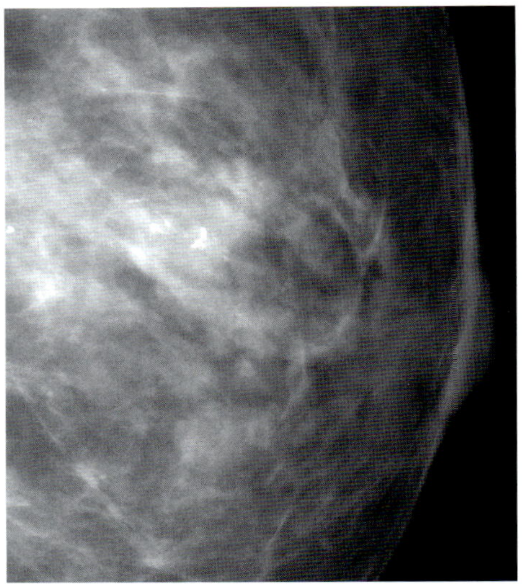

Fig. 20.3 Magnification view of the left breast (MLO).

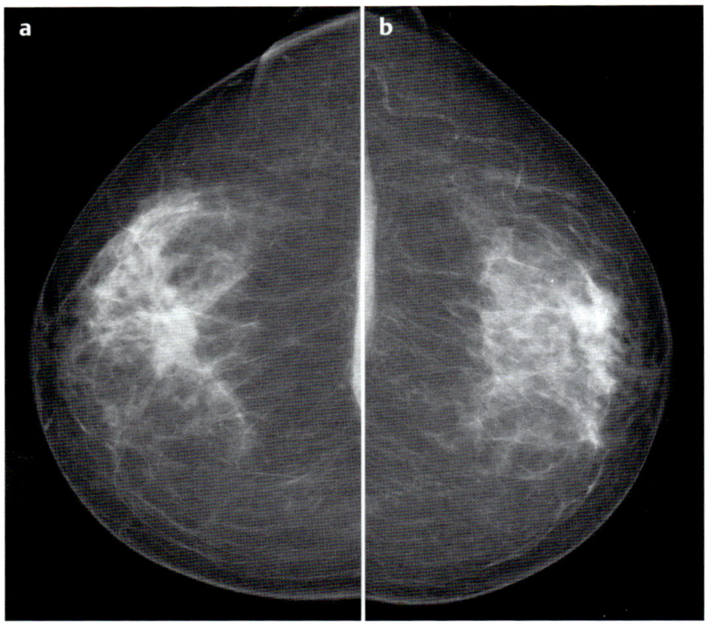

Fig. 20.4 a, b Digital mammography, CC view.

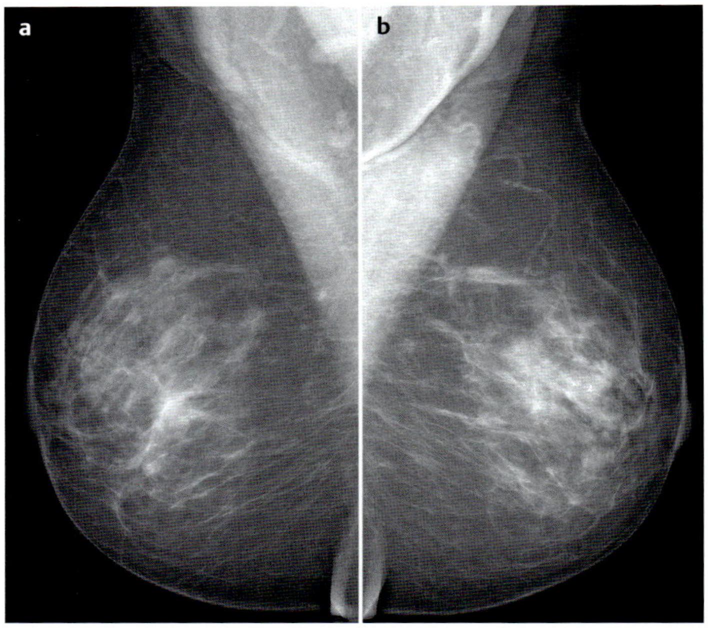

Fig. 20.5 a, b Digital mammography, MLO view.

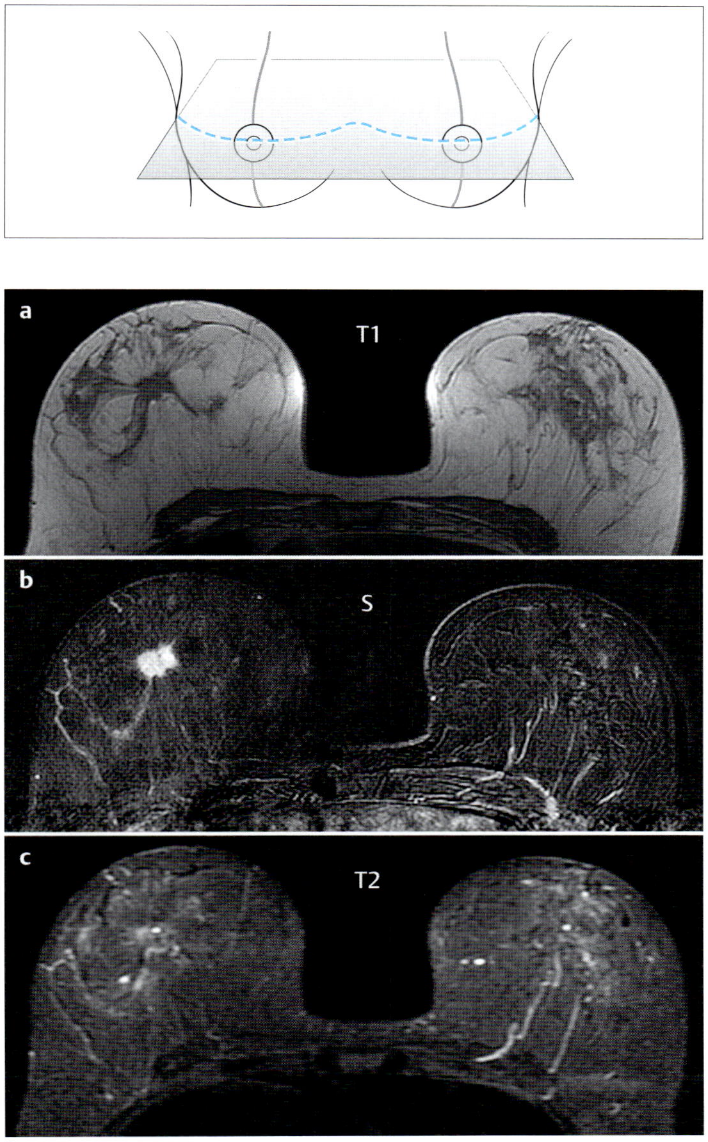


Fig. 20.6 **a – c** Contrast-enhanced MRI of the breasts.

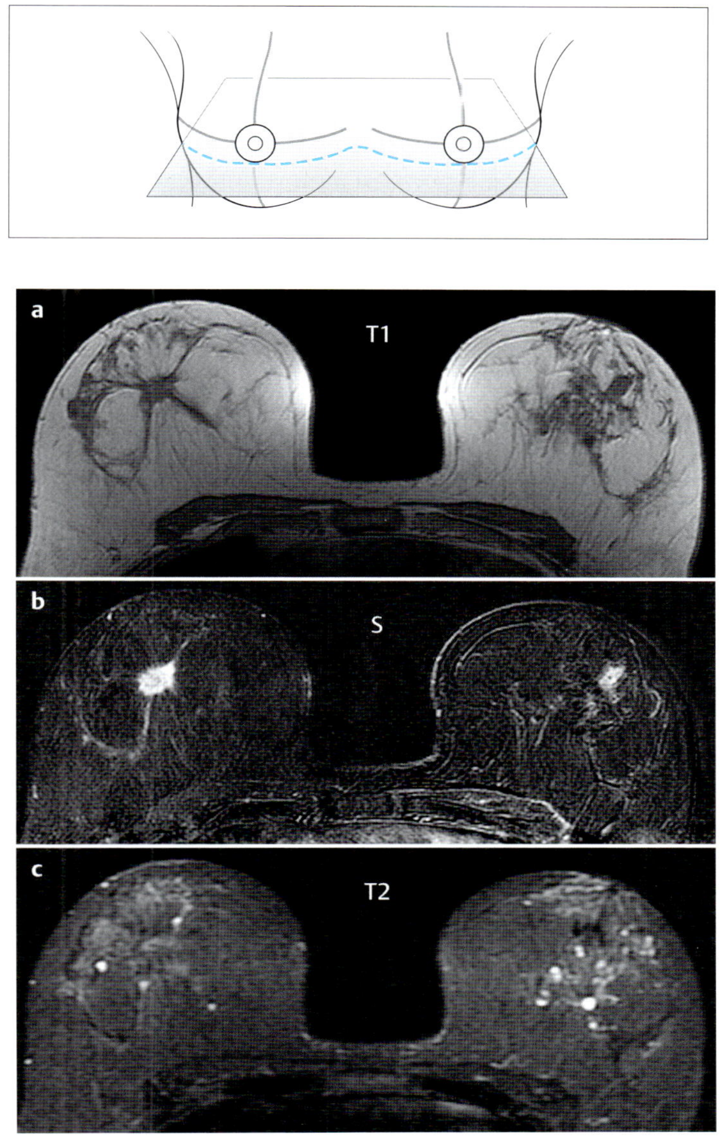


Fig. 20.7 **a – c** Contrast-enhanced MRI of the breasts.

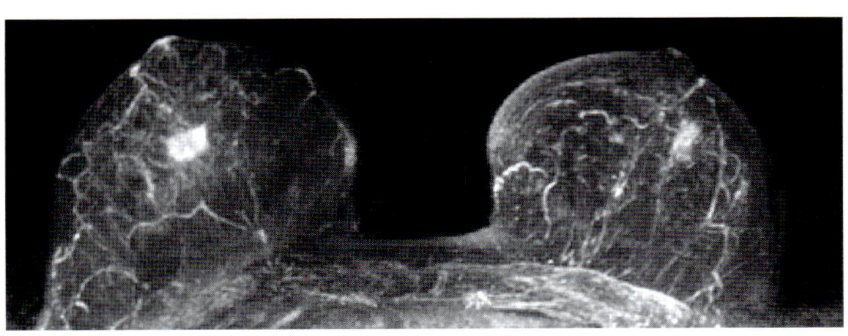

Fig. 20.**8** Contrast-enhanced MR mammography. Maximum intensity projection.

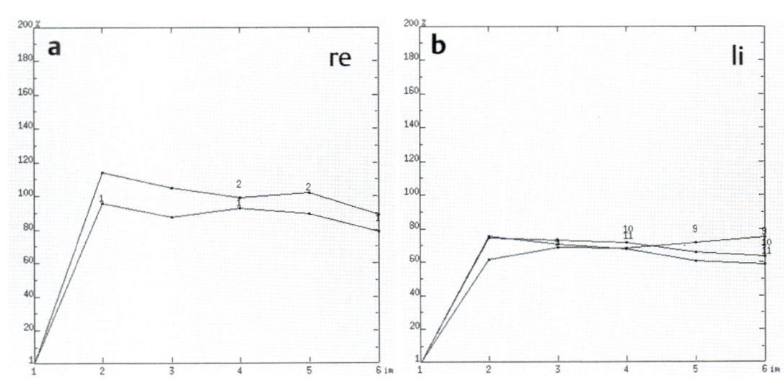


Fig. 20.**9** Signal-to-time curves of lesions in right (**a**) and left (**b**) breasts.

Please characterize ultrasound, mammography and MRI.
What is your preliminary diagnosis?
What are your next steps?

This case investigates a palpable resistance in the right breast.

### Ultrasound

Ultrasound showed a hypoechoic mass with irregular, echogenic borders and distal echo shadowing behind the nipple of the right breast (diameter 1.7 cm). This lesion caused architectural distortion. Laterally to the left nipple, ultrasound depicted a hypoechoic, lobulated lesion of 1.5 cm diameter with indeterminate distal echo behavior. No architectural distortion in the left breast. US BI-RADS right 5/left 3.

### Mammography

Imaging demonstrated bilaterally symmetric fibroglandular parenchyma, ACR type 2. Isodense, spiculated 1.8 cm mass in the central area of the right breast. Oval, isodense, partially ill-defined mass of 1.9 cm diameter with superimposition between the outer quadrants of the left breast. There were also polymorphous calcifications in this region. BI-RADS right 5/left 3. PGMI: CC view P; MLO view G (inframammary fold incorrectly positioned).

### MR Mammography

A spiculated, ill-defined lesion of 1.9 cm diameter was visible in the center of the right breast. This lesion showed ring-pattern enhancement, initial signal increase of 120%, and postinitial wash-out as well as increased signal in T2-weighted imaging. A lobulated, partially ill-defined lesion with inhomogeneous enhancement was depicted between the outer quadrants of the left breast. This tumor was 2 cm in diameter and showed an initial signal increase of 80%, postinitial plateau, and a reduced signal in T2-weighted imaging.

**MRI Artifact Category:** 2
**MRI Density Type:** 1

| MRM score | Finding right | Points | Finding left | Points |
|---|---|---|---|---|
| **Shape** | irregular | 1 | lobulated | 0 |
| **Border** | spiculated | 1 | ill-defined | 1 |
| **CM Distribution** | ring | 2 | inhomogeneous | 1 |
| **Initial Signal Intensity Increase** | strong | 2 | moderate | 1 |
| **Post-initial Signal Intensity Character** | wash-out | 2 | plateau | 1 |
| **MRI score (points)** | | **8** | | **4** |
| **MRI BI-RADS** | | **5** | | **4** |

### → Preliminary Diagnosis

Bilateral carcinoma.

### Differential Diagnosis

Left breast: Adenoma, papilloma.

| BI-RADS Categorization | | |
|---|---|---|
| Clinical Findings | right 5 | left 1 |
| Ultrasound | right 5 | left 3 |
| Mammography | right 5 | left 3 |
| MR Mammography | right 5 | left 4 |
| **BI-RADS Total** | **right 5** | **left 4** |

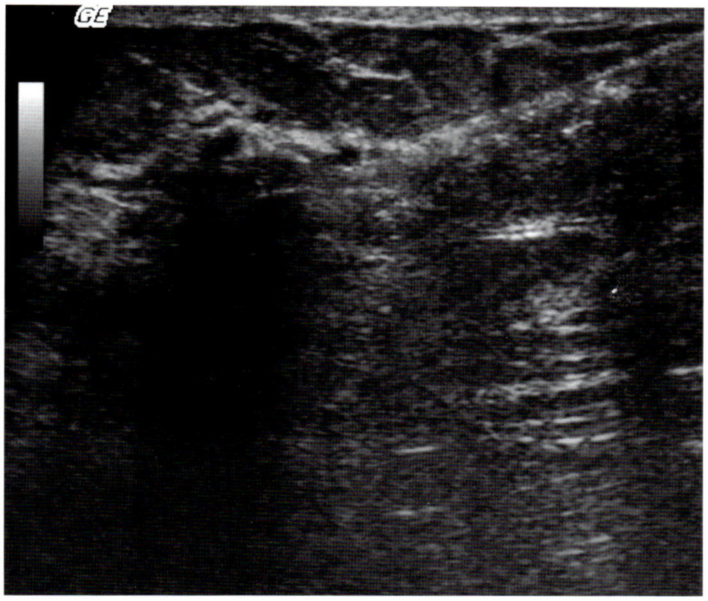


Fig. 20.**10** US-guided core biopsy of the central lesion in the right breast.

**Procedure**

Ultrasound guided investigation of the lesion in the center of the right breast.

**Histopathology of the biopsy specimen**

Invasive lobular carcinoma.

**Further procedure**

Hook-wire localization of the lesion in left breast; open biopsy of this lesion simultaneously with operation necessary on right breast.

## Histology

Right breast: invasive lobular carcinoma measuring 15 mm. Axillary lymph node status positive (1/17).
Left breast: Intraductal papilloma.

Right: ILC pT1c, pN1a (1/17), G2
Left: Papilloma

## Treatment

Breast conservation therapy of the right breast; excisional biopsy of left breast.

If tumor excision is indicated in patients with histopathologically verified carcinoma of the breast (BI-RADS 6), any further suspect lesions should also be biopsied, even though occasional false-positive findings will result.

**Indication:** Screening.
**History:** No abnormalities.
**Risk profile:** Breast cancer in sister at the age of 60 years.
**Age:** 59 years.

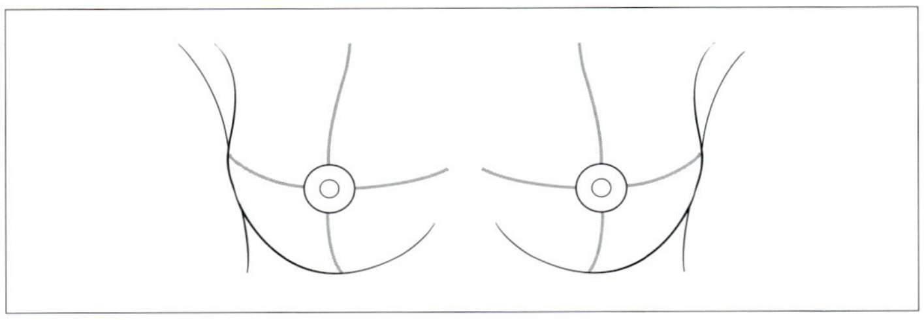

### Clinical Findings

Nodular parenchymal texture at palpation. No resistance.

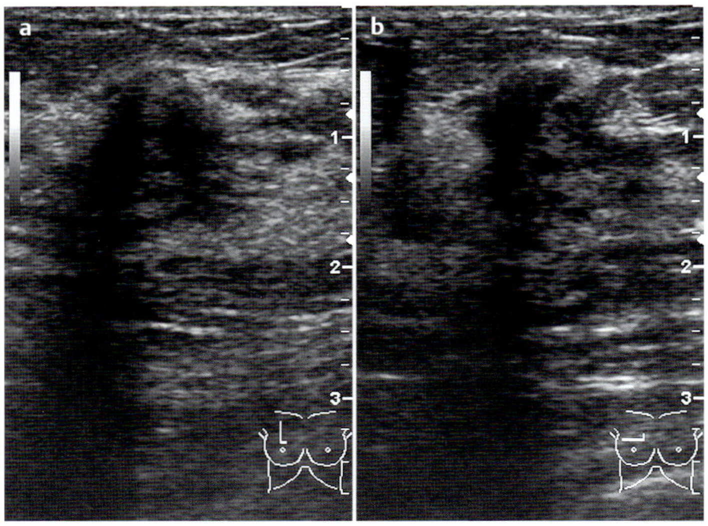

Fig. 21.**1 a, b** Ultrasound.

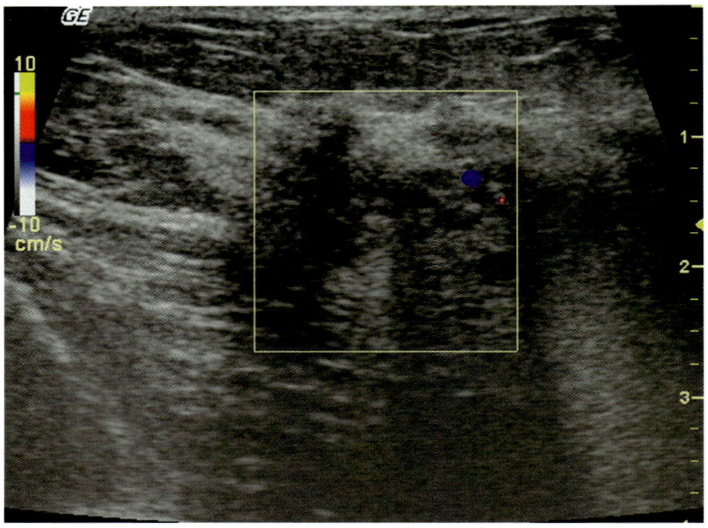

Fig. 21.**2** Color-coded Doppler sonography between the upper quadrants of the right breast.

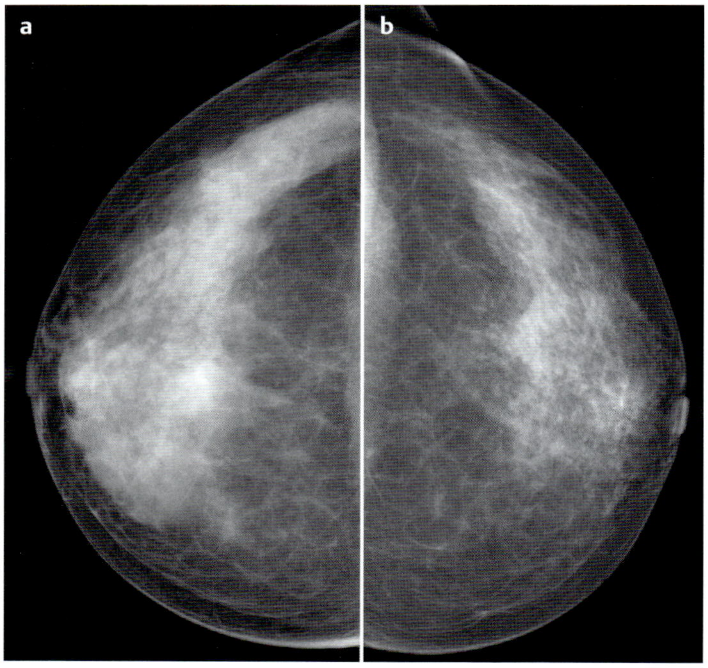

Fig. 21.**3 a, b** Digital mammography, CC view.

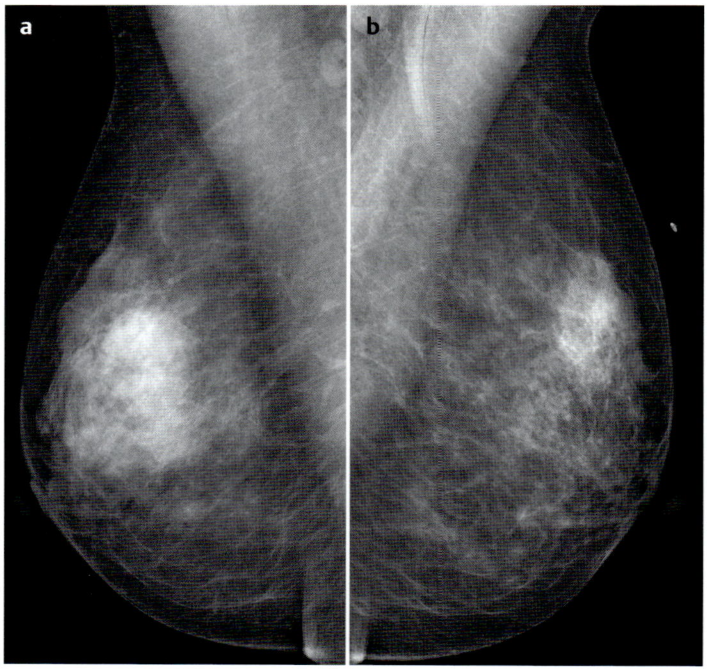

Fig. 21.**4 a, b** Digital mammography, MLO view.

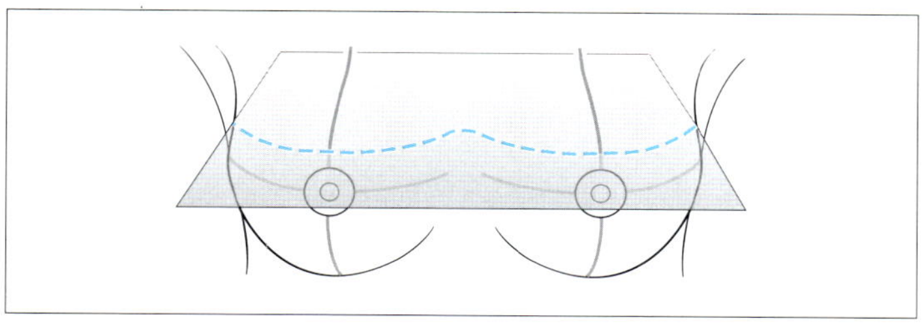

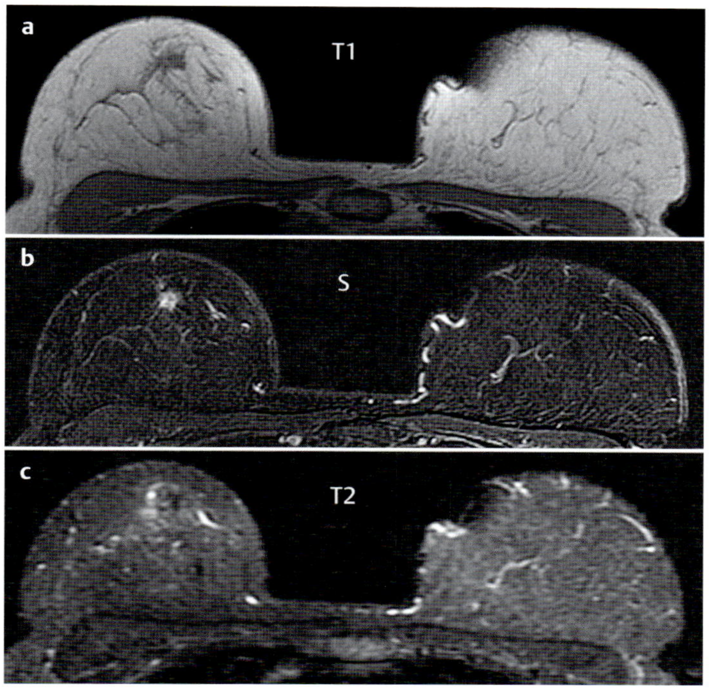


Fig. 21.5 **a–c** Contrast-enhanced MRI of the breasts.

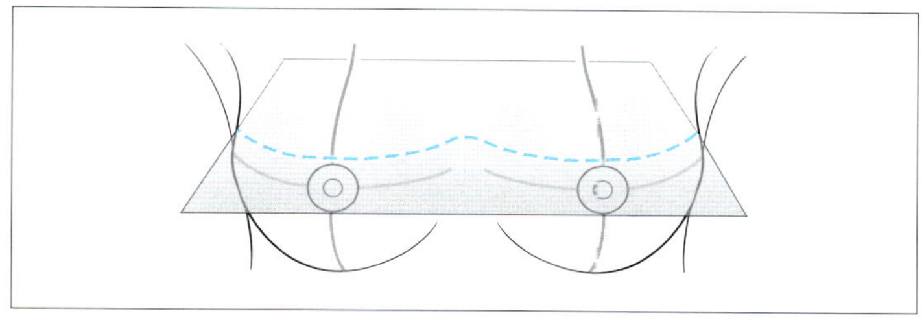

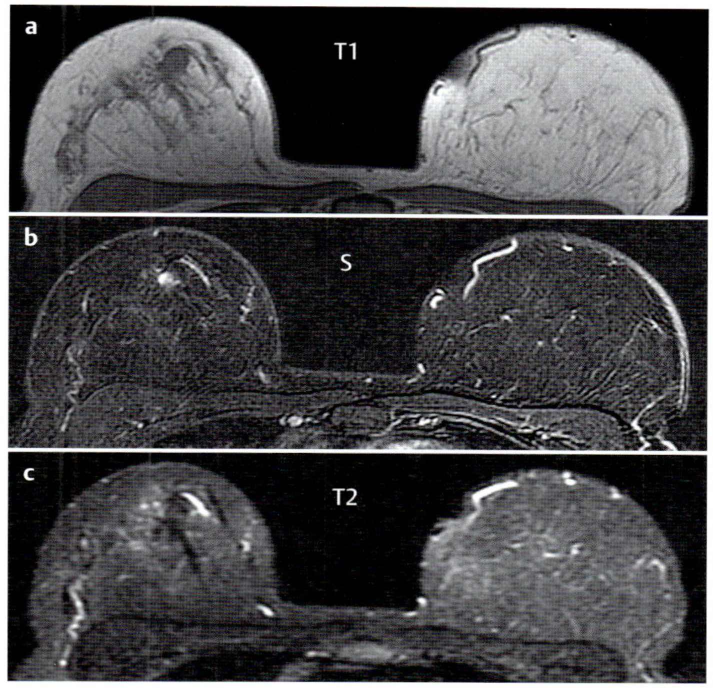


Fig. 21.6 **a–c** Contrast-enhanced MRI of the breasts.

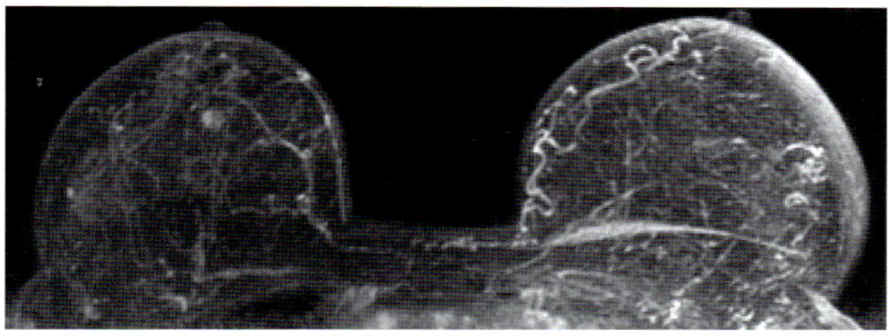

Fig. 21.7 Contrast-enhanced MR mammography. Maximum intensity projection.

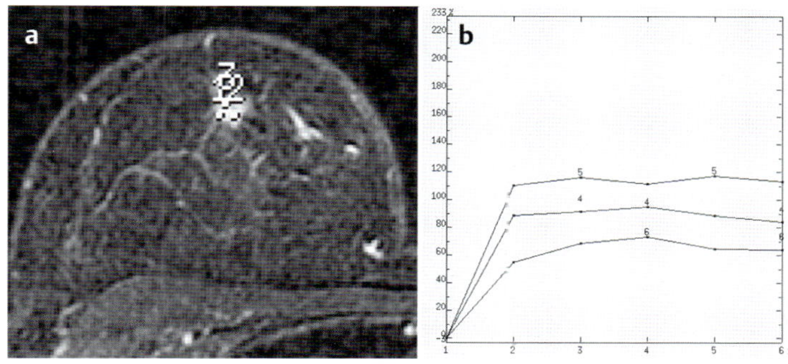


Fig. 21.8 **a, b** Signal-to-time curve.

Please characterize ultrasound, mammography, and MRI findings.
What is your preliminary diagnosis?
What are your next steps?

This case illustrates the imaging studies of an asymptomatic woman.

### Ultrasound

Ultrasound showed an inhomogeneously hypoechoic lesion with distal shadowing between the upper quadrants of the right breast. Color-coded Doppler sonography demonstrated no suspect hypervascularization. US BI-RADS right 4.

### Mammography

Mammography showed inhomogeneous dense parenchyma of both breasts (ACR type 3). There was asymmetry of the parenchyma (right > left), with focal hyperdensity in the right breast (CC view laterally, MLO view cranially). Mammograms demonstrated no architectural distortion or microcalcifications. BI-RADS right 4/left 1. PGMI: CC view G (nipple not in profile, skin folds); MLO view G (inframammary fold not correctly depicted).

### MR Mammography

MRI depicted a lobulated, partially ill-defined, hypervascularized lesion between the upper quadrants of the right breast. This lesion showed criteria of malignancy including ring enhancement, strong initial signal increase and reduced signal in T2-weighted imaging. No other suspect findings.

**MRI Artifact Category:** 1
**MRI Density Type:** 1

| MRM score | Finding | Points |
|---|---|---|
| **Shape** | irregular | 1 |
| **Border** | ill-defined | 1 |
| **CM Distribution** | ring | 2 |
| **Initial Signal Intensity Increase** | strong | 2 |
| **Post-initial Signal Intensity Character** | plateau | 1 |
| **MRI score (points)** | | **7** |
| **MRI BI-RADS** | | **5** |

## → Preliminary Diagnosis

Carcinoma (e.g., invasive lobular).

## Differential Diagnosis

Focal adenosis.

| BI-RADS Categorization | | |
|---|---|---|
| Clinical Findings | right 1 | left 1 |
| Ultrasound | right 4 | left 1 |
| Mammography | right 4 | left 1 |
| MR Mammography | right 5 | left 1 |
| **BI-RADS Total** | **right 5** | **left 1** |

### Procedure

Since a correlation was suspected between the lesion between the upper quadrants of the right breast, graded BI-RADS 4 in ultrasound, and the lesion detected in MRI, a US-guided core biopsy of the right breast was recommended to obtain histological data.

### Histopathology of core biopsy

Invasive lobular carcinoma, grade 2.

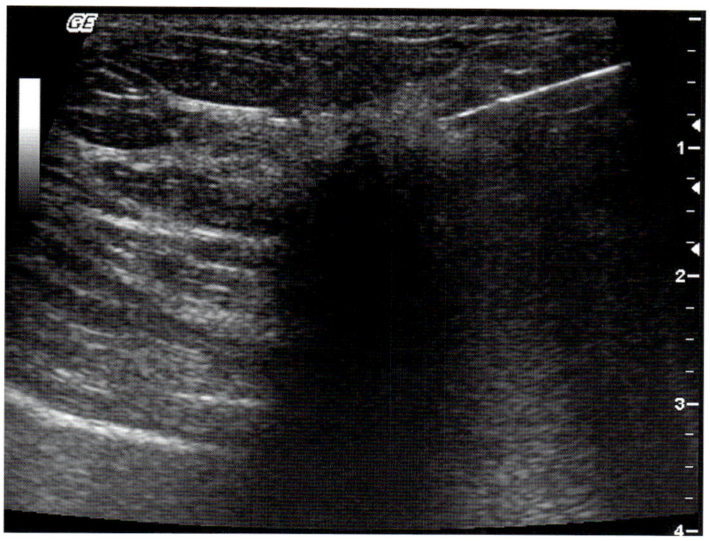

Fig. 21.**9** US-guided core biopsy. Pre-fire ultrasound image.

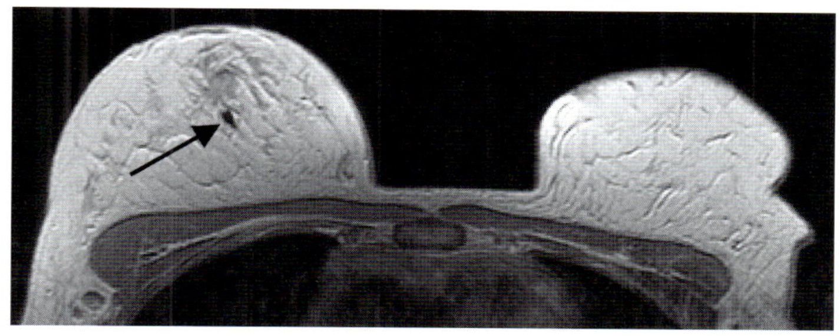

Fig. 21.**10** MR imaging was performed after US-guided biopsy to confirm the correlation between the US and MRI findings. MRI demonstrated an air bubble (arrow) resulting from the biopsy in the direct neigbourhood of the suspicious lesion in MRI.

## Histology

12 mm invasive lobular carcinoma, axillary lymph node status normal.

ILC pT1b, pN0, R0, G2.

## Treatment

BCT.

Even in the absence of palpable lesions, a focal asymmetry in mammography may be a sign of malignancy.

**Indication:** Screening.
**History:** Unremarkable.
**Risk profile:** No increased risk.
**Age:** 55 years.

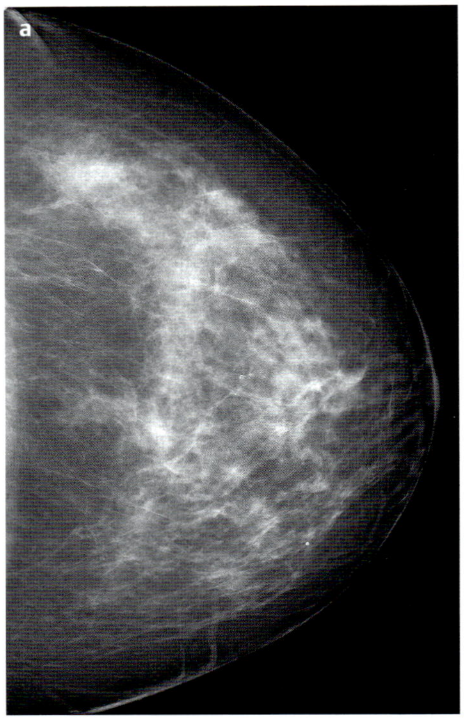

Fig. 22.1 a Digital mammography, CC view.

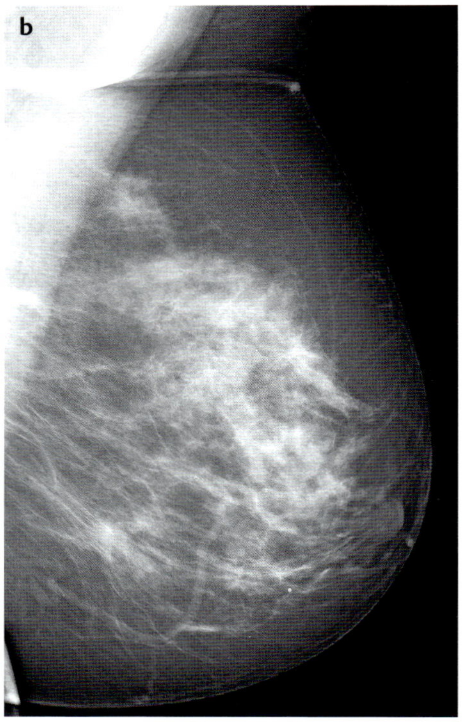

Fig. 22.1 b Digital mammography, MLO view.

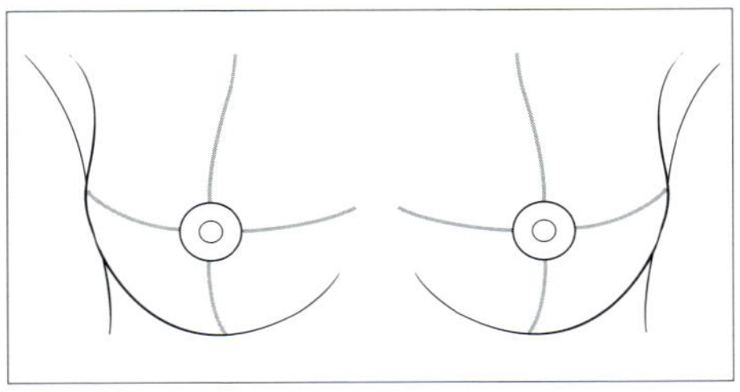

## Clinical Findings

Normal.

## Ultrasound

No pathological findings (not shown).

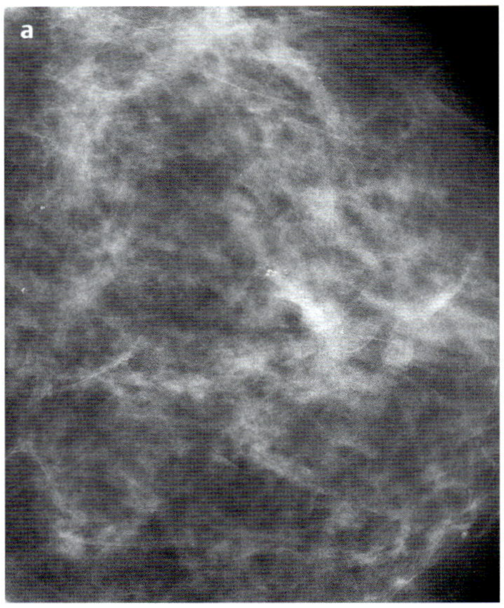

Fig. 22.2 a Magnification view (CC).

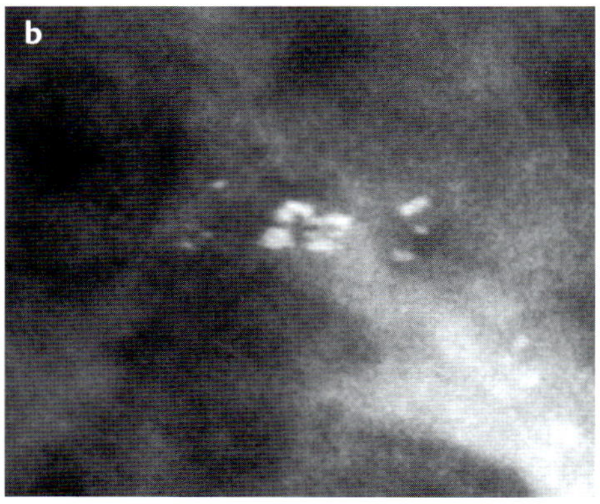

Fig. 22.2 b Zoomed view of the magnification view.

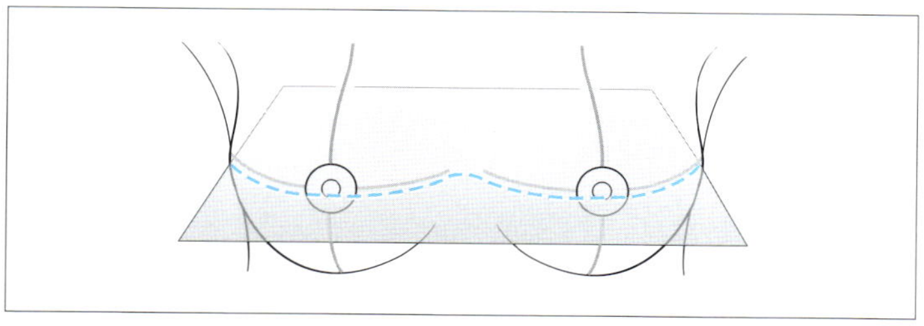

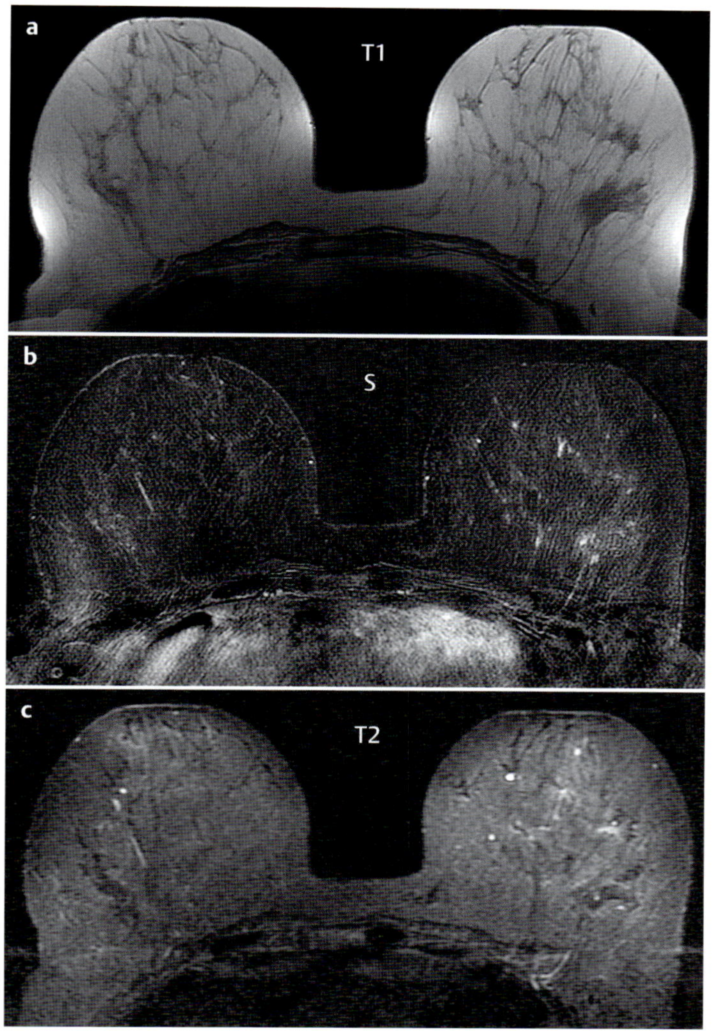


Fig. 22.3 **a – c** Contrast-enhanced MRI of the breasts.

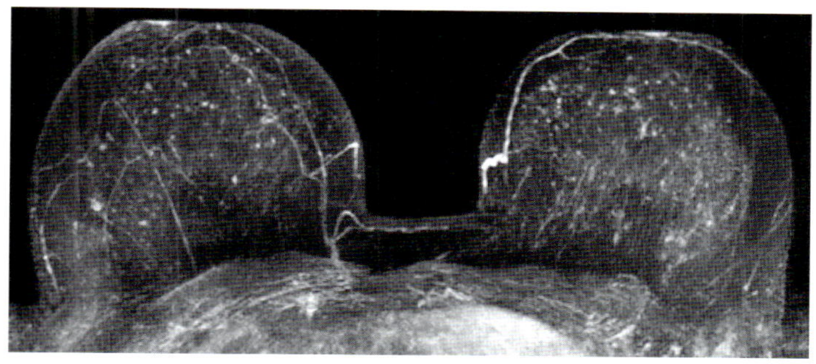

Fig. 22.**4** Contrast-enhanced MR mammography. Maximum intensity projection.

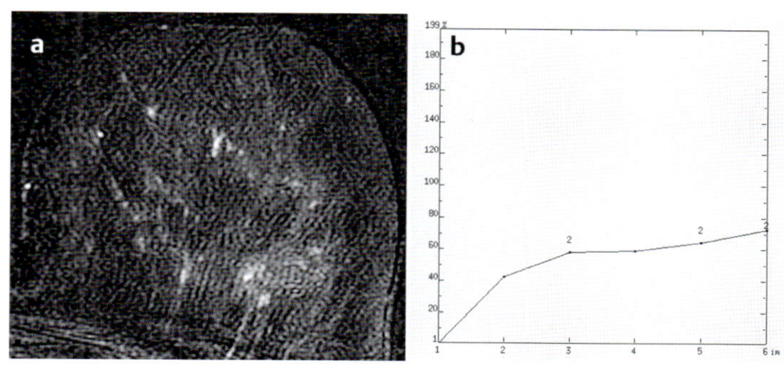


Fig. 22.**5 a, b** Signal-to-time curve of the Y-shaped enhancement.

Please characterize ultrasound, mammography, and MRI findings.
What is your preliminary diagnosis?
What are your next steps?

This case investigates a cluster of microcalcifications which was discovered in the patient's left breast during screening.

### Ultrasound

Sonography showed multiple cysts (maximum diameter 5 mm) in both breasts, and otherwise normal echo patterns. There were no suspicious findings in the central part of the left breast or elsewhere. US BI-RADS right 2/left 2.

### Mammography

Imaging showed fibroglandular parenchyma, ACR type 2. There were polymorphous microcalcifications (round and linear, no V- or Y-shaped particles) in the central part of the left breast in a linear or segmental orientation. Mammograms showed no masses or densities and no architectural distortions. BI-RADS right 1[no figure]/left 4. PGMI is defined only for bilateral mammography.

### MR Mammography

MRI depicted a Y-shaped enhancement in the center of the left breast, most likely in the same location as the microcalcifications detected in mammography (Fig. 22.**6**).

**MRI Artifact Category:** 1
**MRI Density Type:** 1

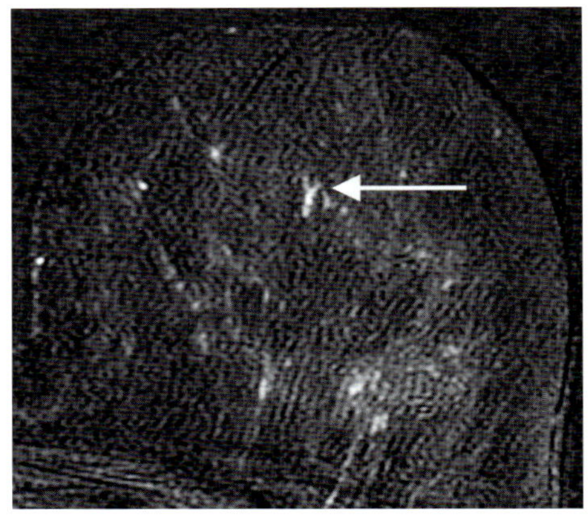

Fig. 22.**6** Y-shaped enhancement in the left breast.

| MRM score | Finding | Points |
|---|---|---|
| **Shape** | dendritic | 1 |
| **Border** | well-defined | 0 |
| **CM Distribution** | homogenous | 0 |
| **Initial Signal Intensity Increase** | moderate | 1 |
| **Post-initial Signal Intensity Character** | increasing | 0 |
| **MRI score (points)** | | **2** |
| **MRI BI-RADS** | | **2** |

## → Preliminary Diagnosis

DCIS.

## Differential Diagnosis

Papilloma, adenosis, ductal hyperplasia, focal mastitis.

| BI-RADS Categorization | | |
|---|---|---|
| Clinical Findings | right 1 | left 1 |
| Ultrasound | right 2 | left 2 |
| Mammography | right 1 | left 4 |
| MR Mammography | right 1 | left 2 |
| **BI-RADS Total** | **right 2** | **left 4** |

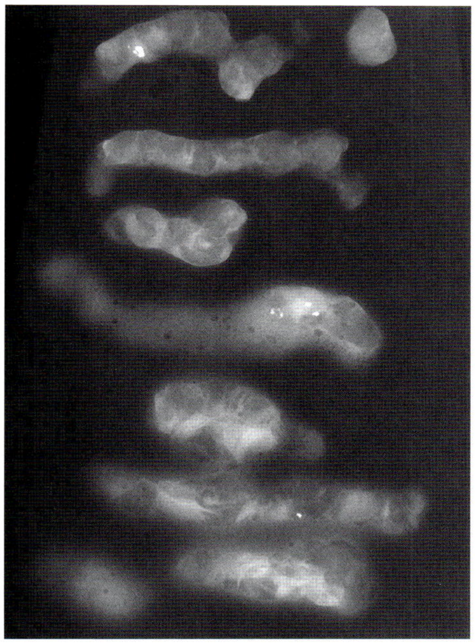

Fig. 22.**7** Radiogram of some of the specimens.

**Procedure**

Histopathological evaluation of the microcalcifications in the center of the left breast by stereotactic vacuum biopsy.

**Histopathology of the vacuum biopsy**

Multiple intraductal papillomas.

## Histology (vacuum core biopsy)

Intraductal papillomatosis.

## Treatment

None. Follow-up mammography after 6 months was indicated.

Approximately 50% of intraductal papillomas exhibit calcifications. Their linear or segmental orientation and possible polymorphous character can give rise to suspicion on mammography.
Furthermore, MR mammography shows intraductal enhancement in some cases of papilloma.

**Indication:** Screening.
**History:** Unremarkable.
**Risk profile:** No increased risk.
**Age:** 56 years.

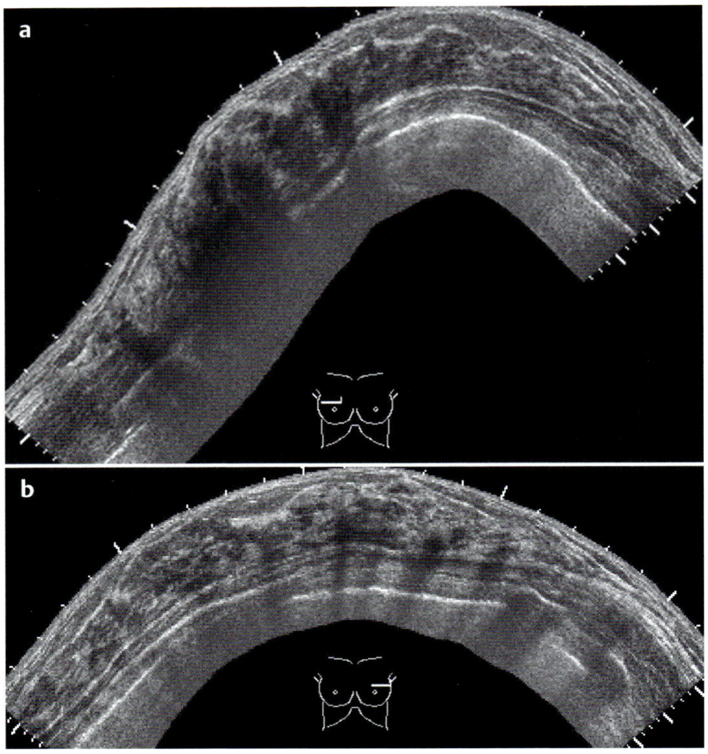


Fig. 23.**1 a, b** Sonography. Panoramic view of right and left breasts.

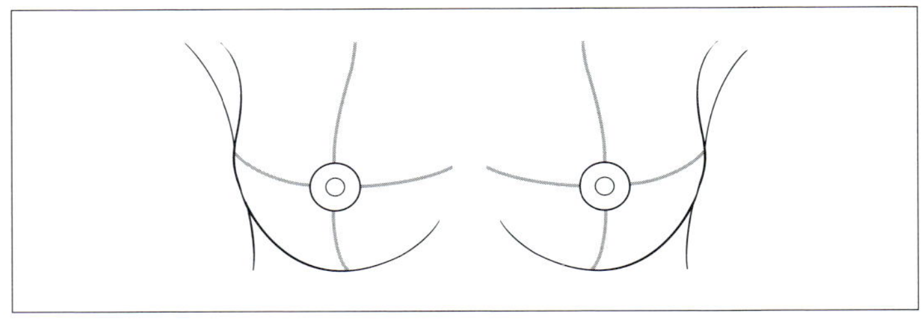

## Clinical Findings

Resistant parenchyma in the upper outer quadrants of both breasts, known and unchanged over a number of years. No circumscribed mass.

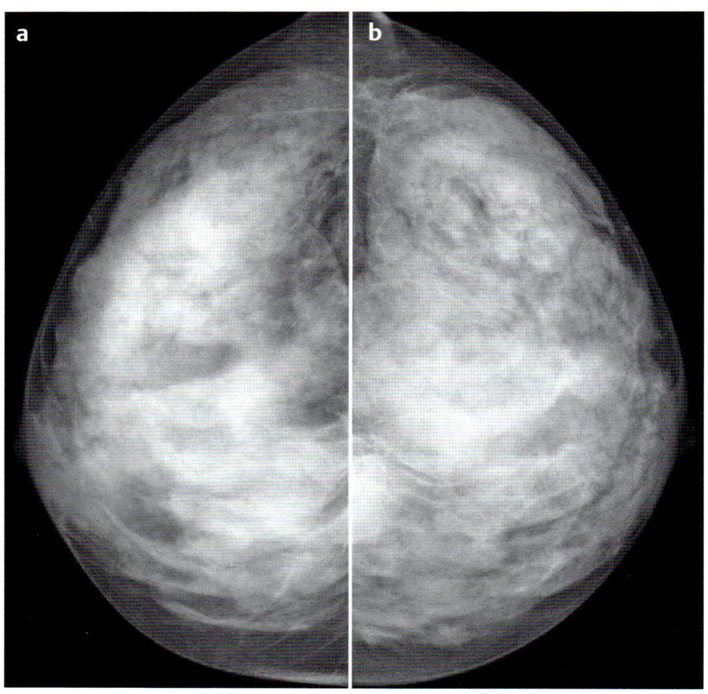


Fig. 23.**2 a, b** Digital mammography, CC view.

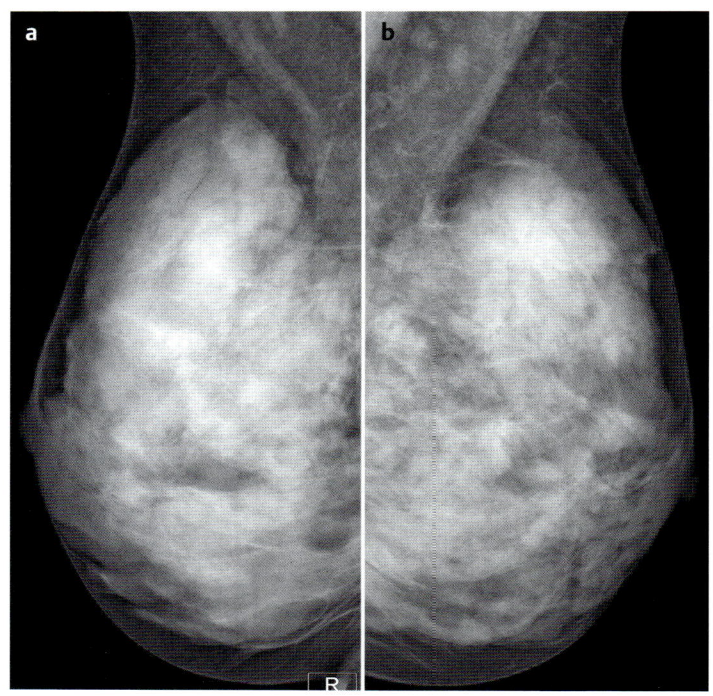


Fig. 23.**3 a, b** Digital mammography, MLO view.

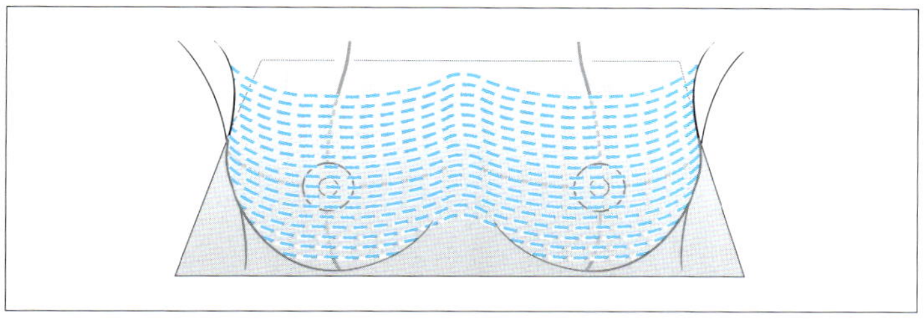

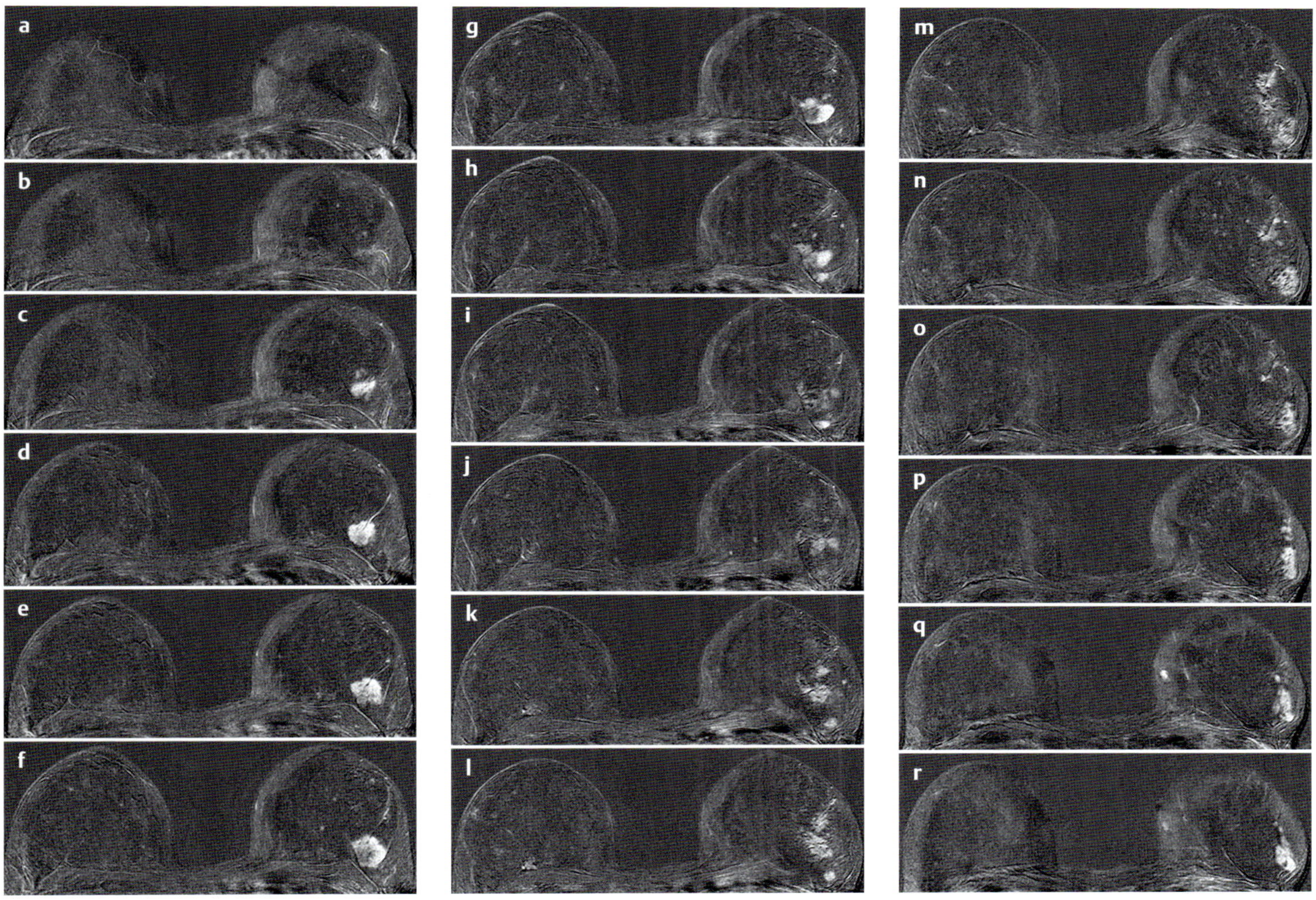


Fig. 23.**4 a – r** Contrast-enhanced MR mammography. 18 consecutive subtraction images, cranial to caudal.

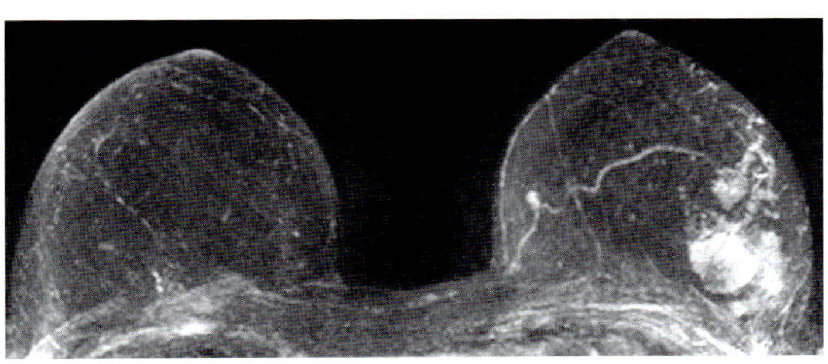

Fig. 23.**5** Contrast-enhanced MR mammography. Maximum intensity projection.

?

Please characterize ultrasound, mammography and MRI.
What is your preliminary diagnosis?
What are your next steps?

The indication for examination was a screening situation. Clinical examination did not demonstrate any difference between the right and the left breasts, even though the MRI findings suggest that this patient has a large mass, which one would expect to be palpable, in her left breast.

### Ultrasound

Panoramic views of the upper quadrants of both breasts are shown. Comparing both sides, suspect acoustic shadowing is in evidence on the right, while there are no notable ultrasound findings in the left breast. US BI-RADS right 3/left 2.

### Mammography

Imaging showed bilaterally symmetric extremely dense parenchyma, ACR type 4. Considering these limiting conditions, no masses or densities could be identified. Mammograms demonstrated no architectural distortions or microcalcifications. BI-RADS right 1/left 1. PGMI: CC view P; MLO view M (inframammary fold not correctly depicted, pectoralis muscle does not reach nipple line).

### MR Mammography

All presented subtraction images showed pathological multiple enhancement in the outer quadrants of the left breast. The morphology of the enhancing areas was highly pathological and their T2 signal was also suspect (intermediate signal, not shown). Signal–time curves also indicated malignancy (strong initial signal increase, washout; not shown).

**MRI Artifact Category:** 1
**MRI Density Type:** 2

| MRM score | Finding | Points |
|---|---|---|
| **Shape** | irregular | 1 |
| **Border** | ill-defined | 1 |
| **CM Distribution** | rim sign | 2 |
| **Initial Signal Intensity Increase** | strong | 2 |
| **Post-initial Signal Intensity Character** | wash-out | 2 |
| **MRI score (points)** | | **8** |
| **MRI BI-RADS** | | **5** |

### → Preliminary Diagnosis

Extended invasive carcinoma. No differential diagnosis.

| BI-RADS Categorization | | |
|---|---|---|
| Clinical Findings | right 2 | left 2 |
| Ultrasound | right 3 | left 2 |
| Mammography | right 1 | left 1 |
| MR Mammography | right 1 | left 5 |
| **BI-RADS Total** | **right 1** | **left 5** |

### Procedure

Histopathological evaluation of the extensive enhancing areas in the lateral parts of the left breast with MR-guided core biopsy, because ultrasound did not provide clearly corresponding data. MR-guided vacuum biopsy in the upper outer quadrant of the left breast (11 gauge, 12 specimens). Additionally, MR-guided core biopsy in the lower outer quadrant of the left breast (16G, 8 specimens spaced 1 cm apart) to verify multicentricity.

### Histopathology (all specimens)

Tubular breast cancer grade 1–2.

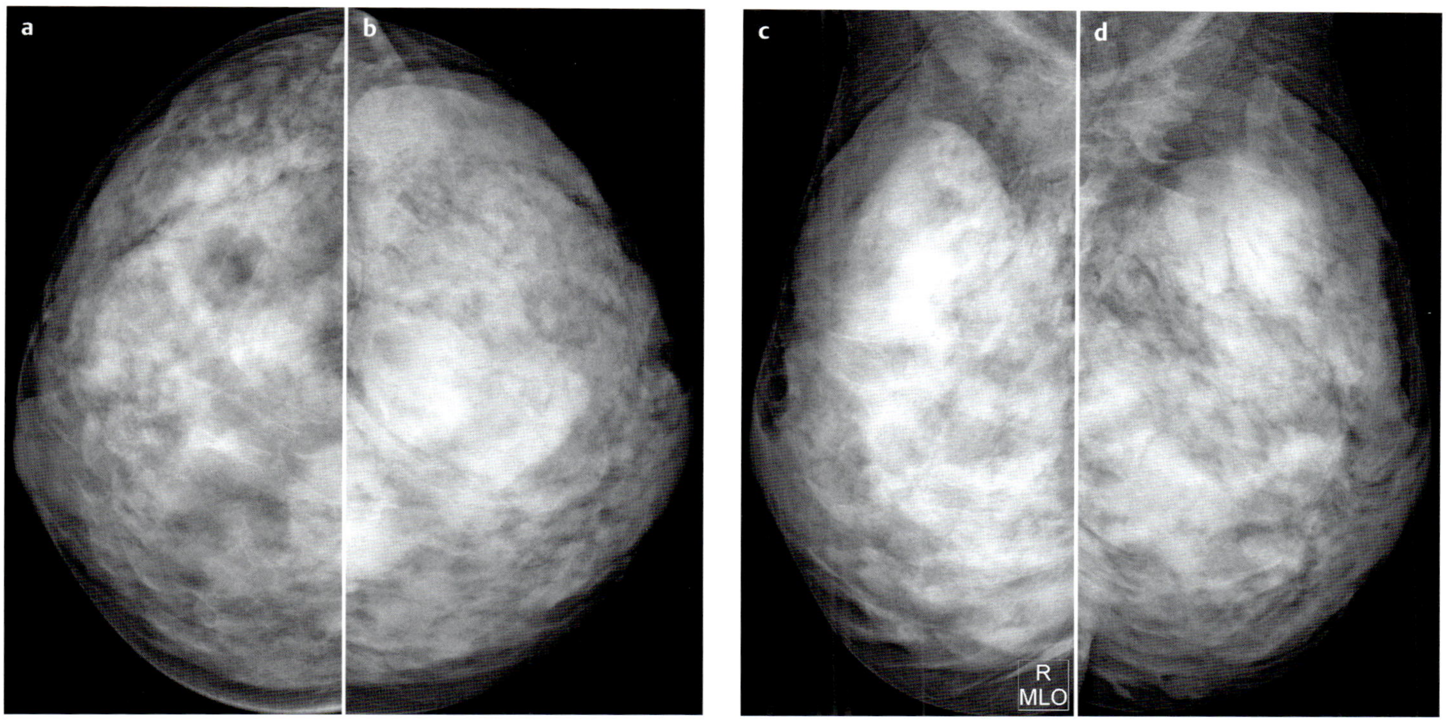


Fig. 23.**6 a – d** Digital mammography in 2 views from screening examination a year earlier, with identical findings.

### Histology

8 cm tubular cancer of the left breast.

TC pT3 pN0, G2.

### Treatment

Mastectomy of the left breast.

This case demonstrates an extensive breast carcinoma that was clinically, mammographically, and sonographically occult and was identified only by the presence of pathological vascularization. Moreover, direct comparison with the mammograms performed one year previously did not help diagnosis, because there were no morphological changes detectable within the dense parenchyma.

**Indication:** Resistance and tenderness in the right breast.
**History:** Unremarkable.
**Risk profile:** No increased risk.
**Age:** 47 years.

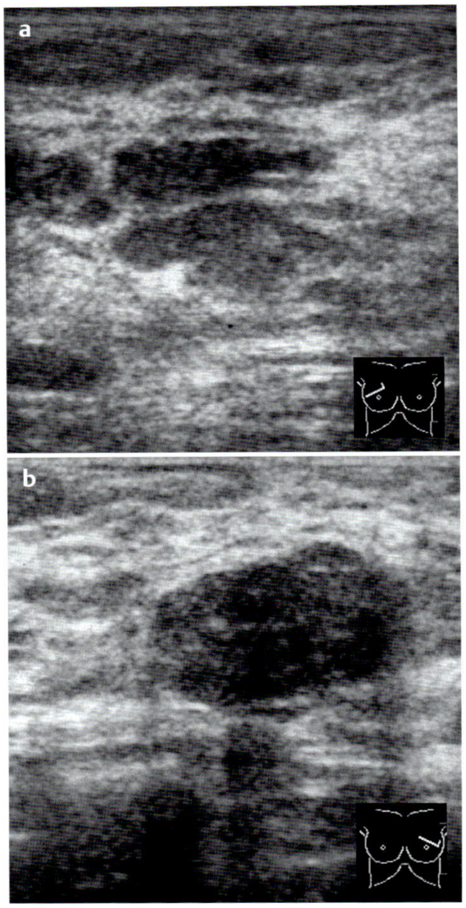


Fig. 24.**1 a, b** Sonography.

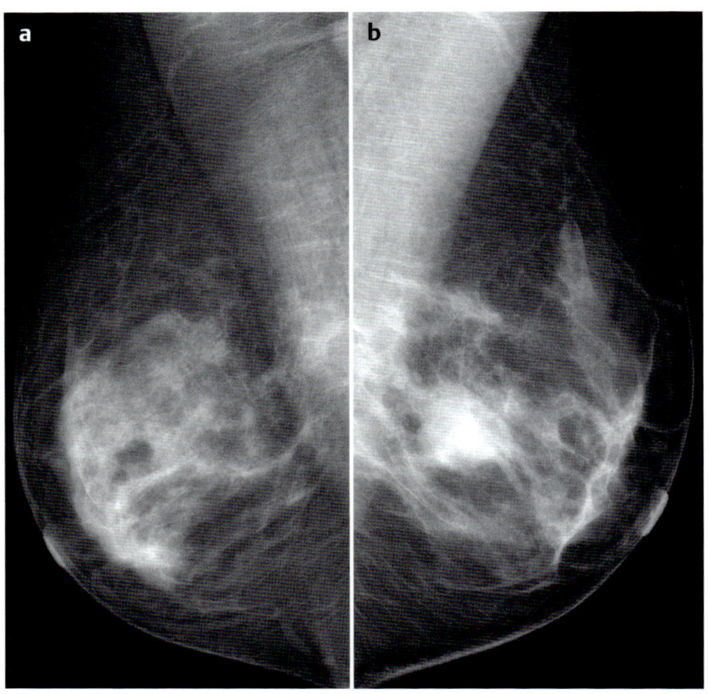


Fig. 24.**2 a, b** Digital mammography, MLO view.

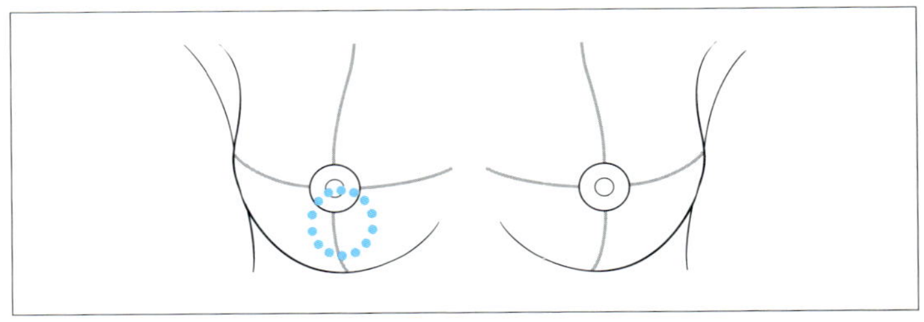

## Clinical Findings

Nodular parenchymal texture with circumscribed resistance of 3 cm between lower quadrants of the right breast.

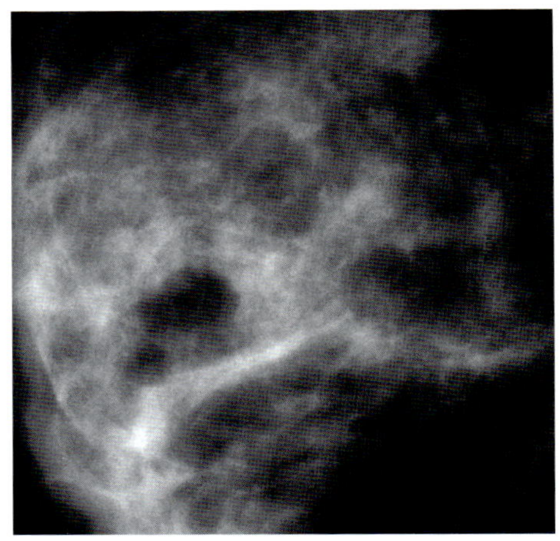

Fig. 24.**3** Magnification view, right breast.

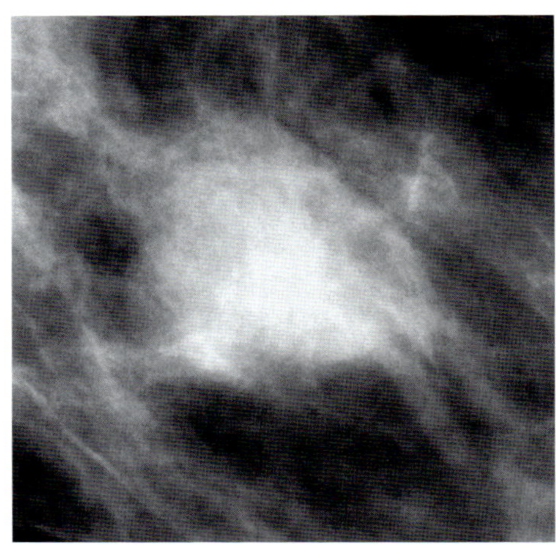

Fig. 24.**4** Magnification view, left breast.

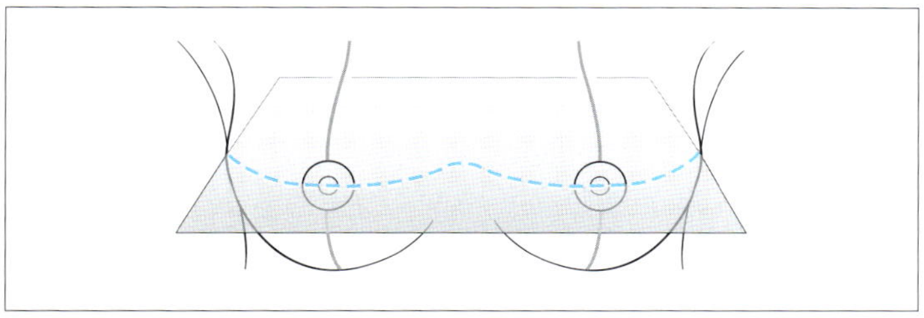

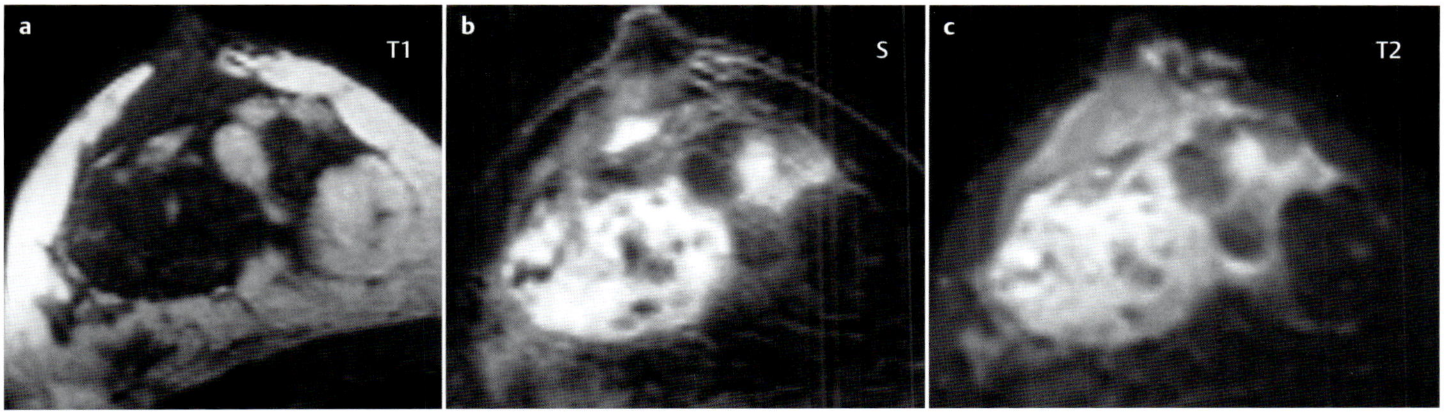


Fig. 24.5 **a – c** Contrast-enhanced MR mammography of the right breast at the level of the nipple.

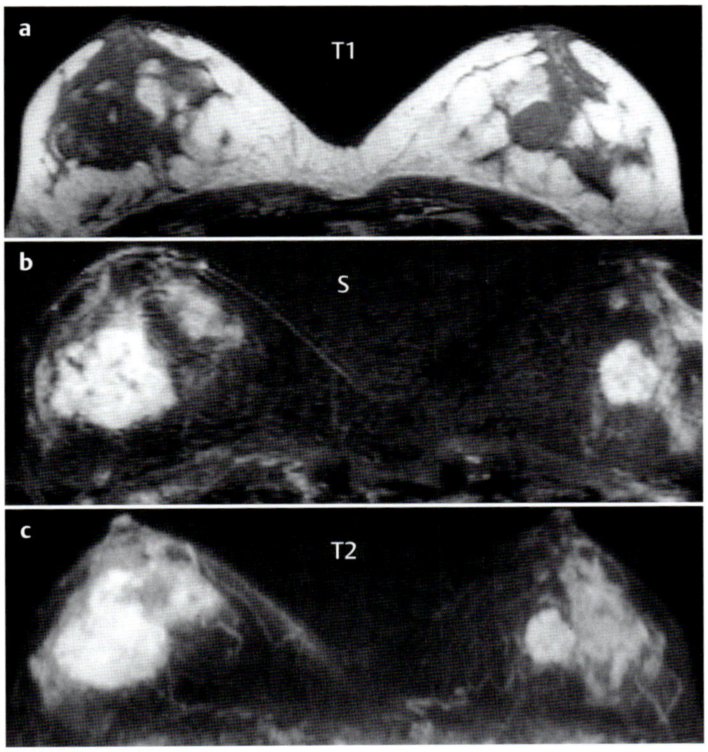


Fig. 24.6 **a – c** Contrast-enhanced MR mammography, just above the level of the nipple.

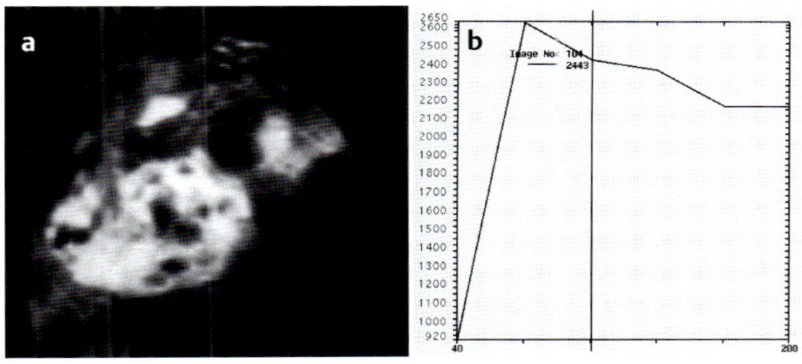


Fig. 24.7 **a, b** Signal-to-time curve, right breast.

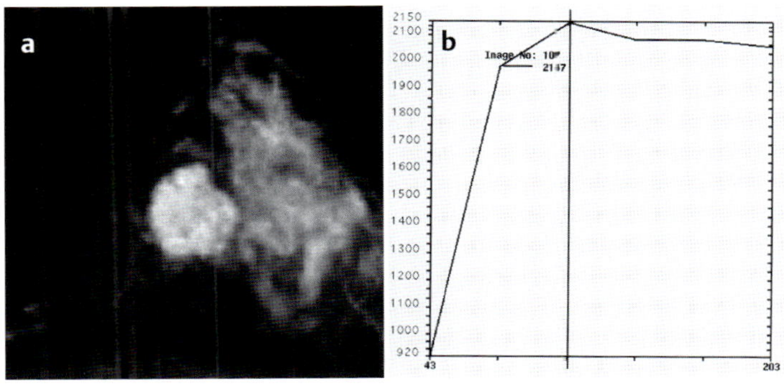


Fig. 24.8 **a, b** Signal-to-time curve; left breast. Signal values in absolute numbers.

Please characterize ultrasound, mammography, and MRI findings.
What is your preliminary diagnosis?
What are your next steps?

These are the imaging studies of a patient with an indistinct palpable mass in the right breast. The left breast did not show any clinical abnormalities.

### Ultrasound

In the area of the clinically observed resistance in the right breast, the echo texture was glandular with lipomatous areas within the parenchyma. No indications of malignancy. The US of the left breast demonstrated a lobulated, well-defined lesion with inhomogeneous acoustic signal and distal shadowing. US BI-RADS right 2/left 3.

### Mammography

Mammograms showed asymmetric, partially extremely dense glandular tissue, ACR type 4. The right breast demonstrated no abnormalities. In the central part of the left breast, mammography showed a lobulated lesion that was partially superimposed but otherwise well defined. There was no architectural distortion; no calcifications. BI-RADS right 1/left 3. PGMI: MLO view G (poor positioning of the nipple on both sides).

### MR Mammography

Corresponding to the palpable mass, MRI demonstrated a large region with hypointense signal and moderate displacement of the surrounding lipomatous tissue. There were some hyperintense focal spots within this hypointense area. These spots did not enhance in postcontrast imaging. Signal-time curves were characterized by strong initial increase and early washout. In the central area of the left breast there was a lobulated, well-defined, hypervascularized lesion with endotumoral septation and nonspecific signal curve.

**MRI Artifact Category:** 2

**MRI Density Type:** 3

| MRM score | Finding right | Points | Finding left | Points |
|---|---|---|---|---|
| **Shape** | oval | 0 | lobulated | 0 |
| **Border** | well-defined | 0 | well-defined | 0 |
| **CM Distribution** | inhomogenous | 1 | inhomogeneous | 1 |
| **Initial Signal Intensity Increase** | strong | 2 | strong | 2 |
| **Post-initial Signal Intensity Character** | wash-out | 2 | plateau | 1 |
| **MRI score (points)** | | **5** | | **4** |
| **MRI BI-RADS** | | **4** | | **4** |

### → Differential Diagnosis

Right breast: Phyllodes tumor, carcinoma (with central necrosis), angiomatous lesion.

Left breast: Fibroadenoma, carcinoma (medullary? mucinous?).

| BI-RADS Categorization | | |
|---|---|---|
| Clinical Findings | right 3 | left 1 |
| Ultrasound | right 2 | left 3 |
| Mammography | right 1 | left 3 |
| MR Mammography | right 4 | left 4 |
| **BI-RADS Total** | **right 4** | **left 4** |

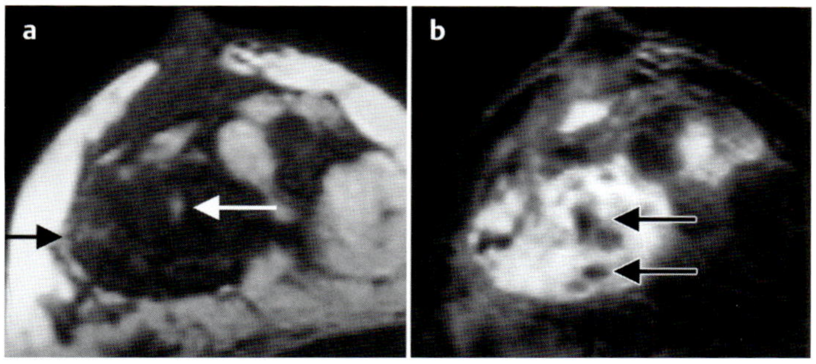


Fig. 24.**9 a, b** Hyperintense spots (white arrows) within the otherwise hypointense lesion in precontrast T1-weighted image (**a**). No enhancement of these spots in subtraction image (black arrows) (**b**).

### Procedure

Histological analysis of the lesion in the right breast. In this case, open biopsy was performed without primary percutaneous core biopsy. The lesion in the left breast was removed simultaneously after US-guided localization.

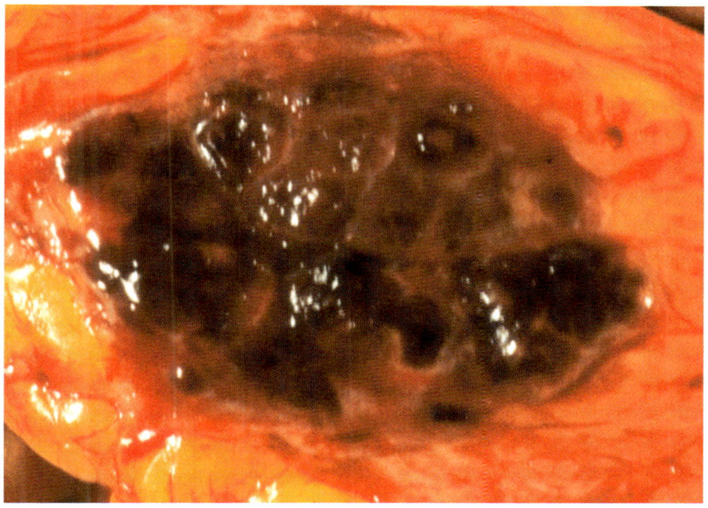

Fig. 24.**10** Histological specimen showing the partially thrombosed vessels of this angiosarcoma (right breast).

### Histology

Right breast: Angiosarcoma
Left breast: Fibroadenoma

### Treatment

BCT of the right breast. Open biopsy of the left breast.

Focal thromboses within angiosarcomas are clearly detectable in MRI. They are characterized by endotumoral spots that are hyperintense in precontrast T1-weighted images and hypointense in T2-weighted imaging., These spots do not enhance after administration of contrast medium.

**Indication:** Resistance between the right upper quadrants.
**History:** Unremarkable.
**Risk profile:** No increased risk.
**Age:** 53 years.

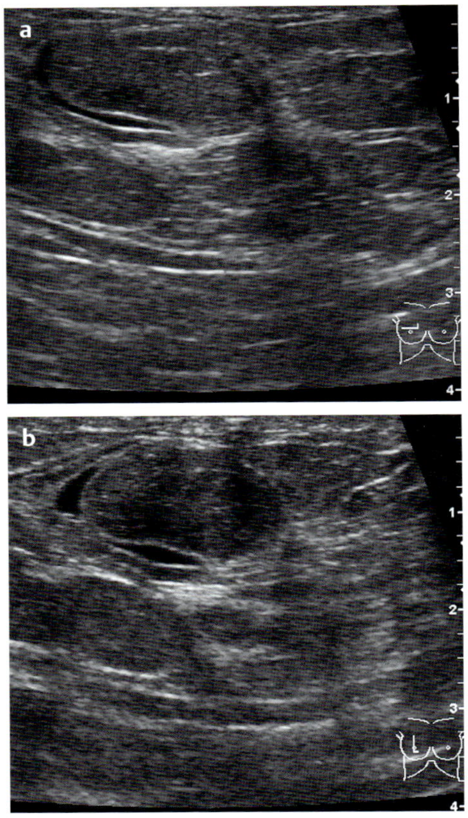


Fig. 25.**1 a, b** Ultrasound.

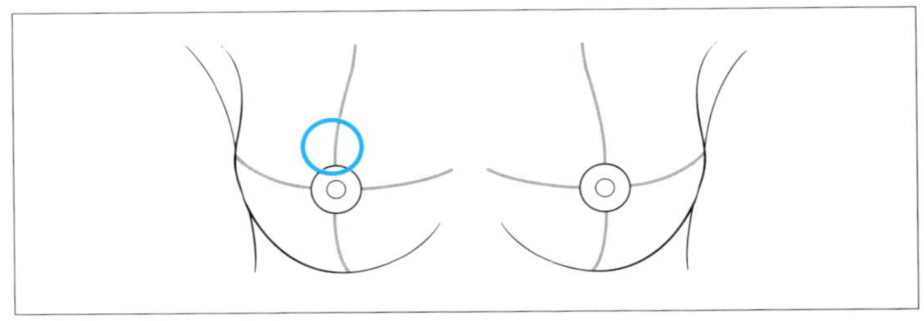

## Clinical Findings

Resistance between the upper quadrants of the right breast, near the areola (diameter 2.5 cm).

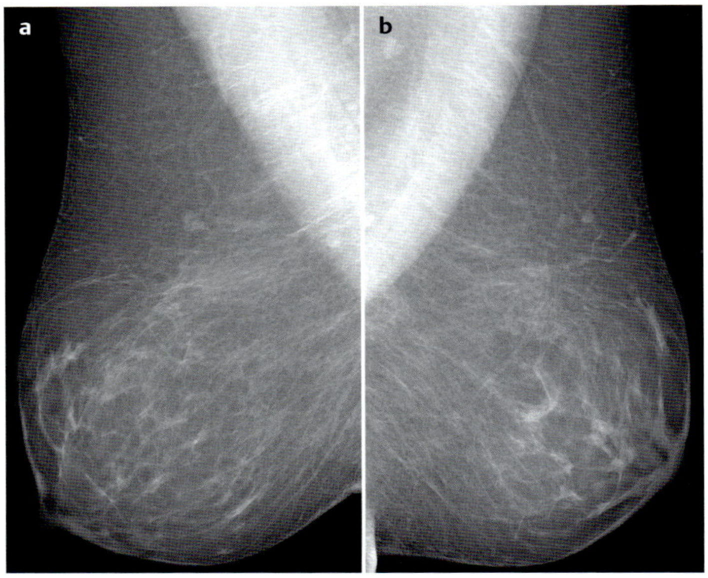


Fig. 25.**2 a, b** Digital mammography, MLO view.

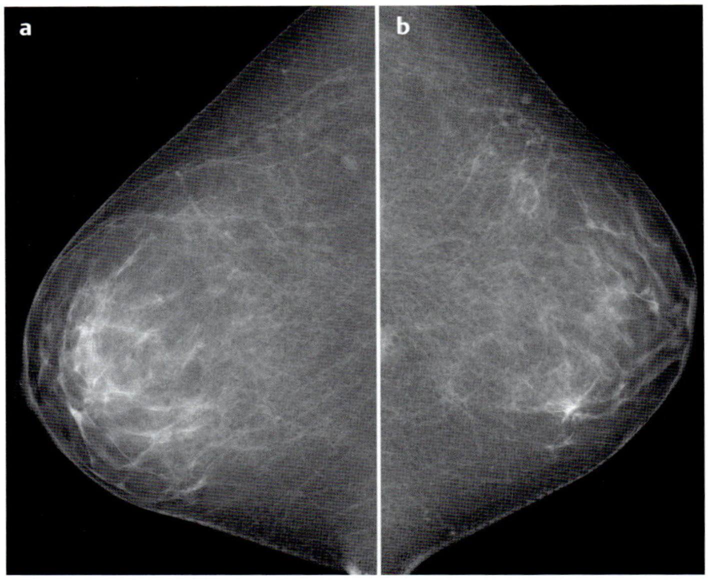


Fig. 25.**3 a, b** Digital mammography, CC view.

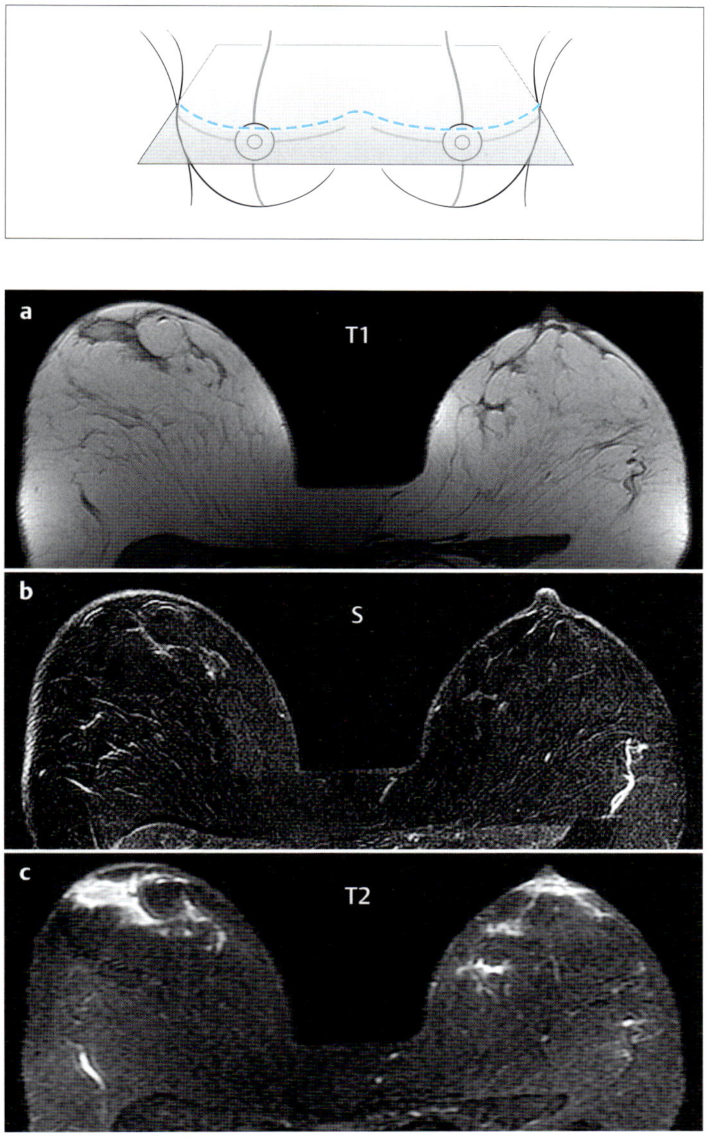


Fig. 25.**4 a–c** Contrast-enhanced MRI of the breasts.

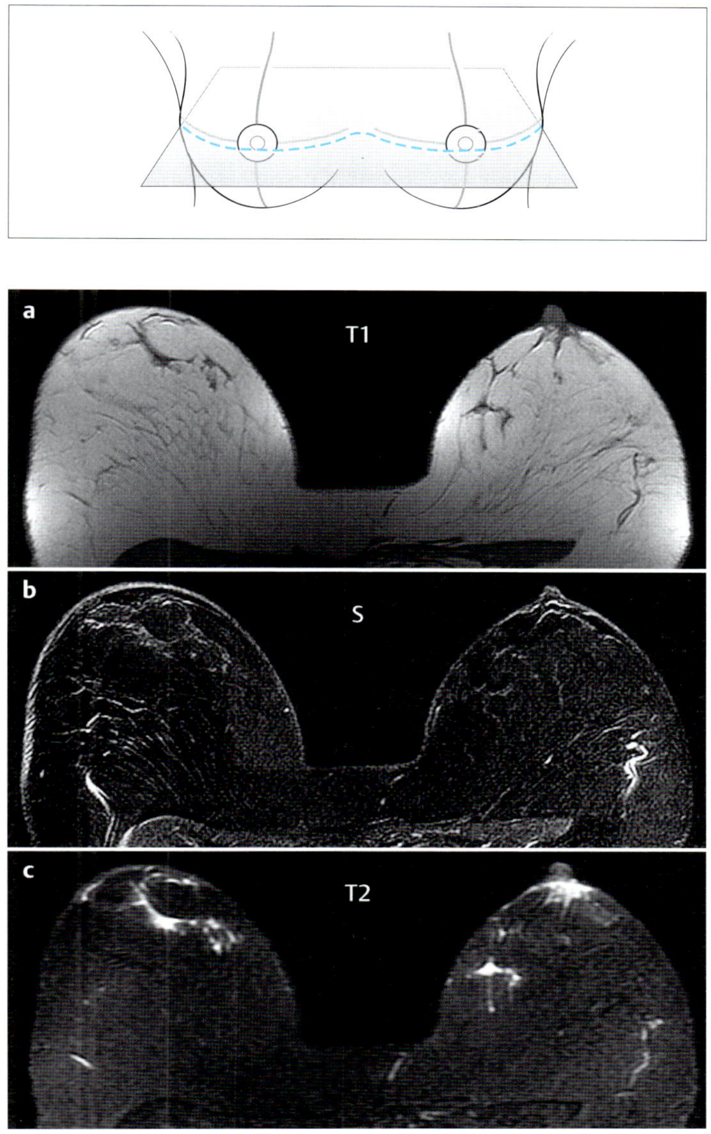


Fig. 25.**5 a–c** Contrast-enhanced MRI of the breasts.

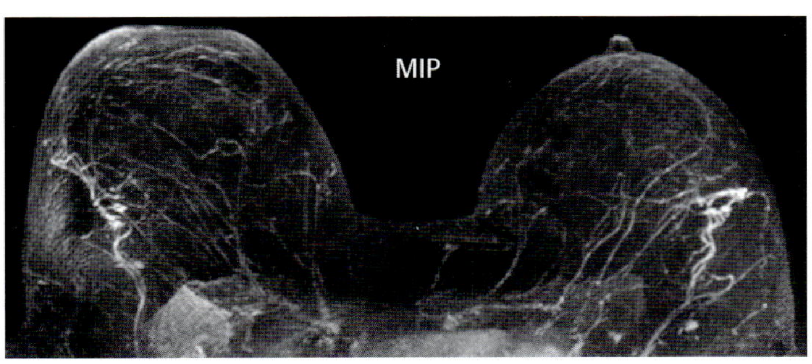


Fig. 25.**6** Contrast-enhanced MR mammography. Maximum intensity projection.

?

Please characterize ultrasound, mammography, and MRI findings.
What is your preliminary diagnosis?
What are your next steps?

These imaging studies were performed to investigate a palpable mass in the patient's right breast.

### Ultrasound

Between the upper quadrants of the right breast near the nipple, sonography demonstrated a well-defined, partially isoechoic, partially hyperechoic lesion of 2.5 cm diameter with indeterminate distal echo behavior. In close proximity to this lesion, lacunar hypoechoic structures with distal signal increase were depicted. US BI-RADS right 2.

### Mammography

Imaging showed predominantly lipomatous parenchyma, ACR type 1. There were no suspicious findings either in the area corresponding to the resistance in the upper part of the right breast or anywhere else. No suspicious densities. Mammograms demonstrated no architectural distortions or microcalcifications. BI-RADS right 1/left 1. PGMI: CC view P; MLO view G (inframammary fold).

### MR Mammography

MRI detected a well-defined lipomatous lesion of 2.5 cm diameter between the upper quadrants of the right breast, with a fat-equivalent signal in T1-weighted and reduced signal in T2-weighted imaging. There was no corresponding enhancement in this region after administration of contrast medium. In addition, MRI showed ectatic milk ducts in the area of the lesion (see T2 images).

**MRI Artifact Category:** 2
**MRI Density Type:** 1

| | |
|---|---|
| No morphological or kinetic analysis due to absence of enhancing lesions in MR imaging. | |
| **MRI score (points)** | **0** |
| **MRI BI-RADS** | **1** |

### → Preliminary Diagnosis

The fat-equivalent behavior of the palpable lesion in all imaging modalities indicates a lipoma.

| BI-RADS Categorization | | |
|---|---|---|
| Clinical Findings | right 3 | left 1 |
| Ultrasound | right 2 | left 1 |
| Mammography | right 1 | left 1 |
| MR Mammography | right 1 | left 1 |
| **BI-RADS Total** | **right 2** | **left 1** |

**Procedure**

No further measures necessary.

## Diagnosis (without histopathological verification)

Lipoma

## Treatment

None.

In breast imaging, evidence of fatty tissue usually indicates a benign lesion.

**Indication:** Screening mammography.
**History:** Unremarkable.
**Risk profile:** No increased risk.
**Age:** 49 years.

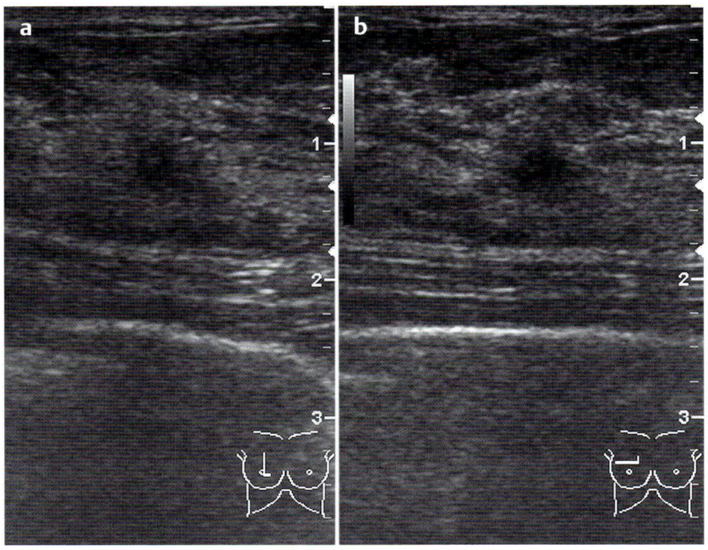


Fig. 26.**1 a, b** Ultrasound.

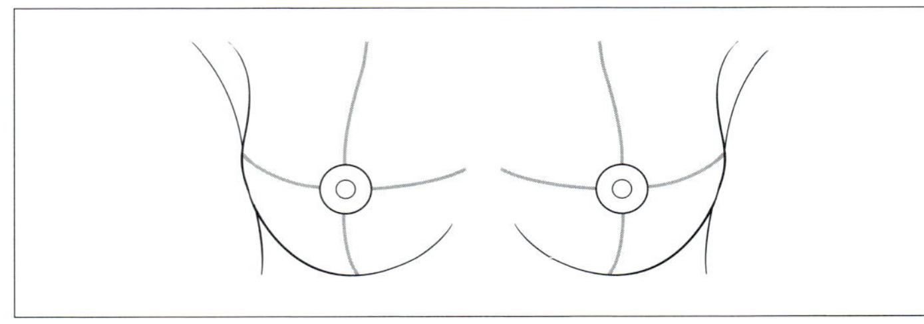

## Clinical Findings

No abnormalities.

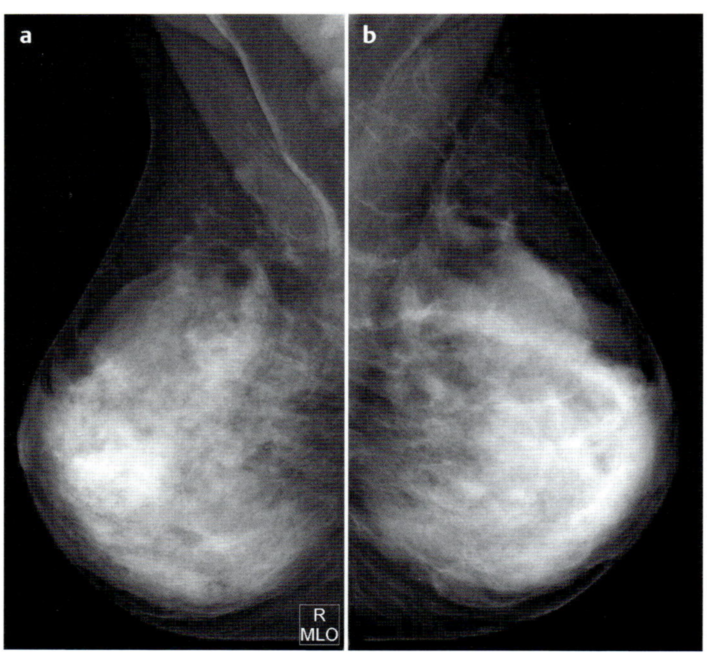


Fig. 26.**2 a, b** Digital mammography, MLO view.

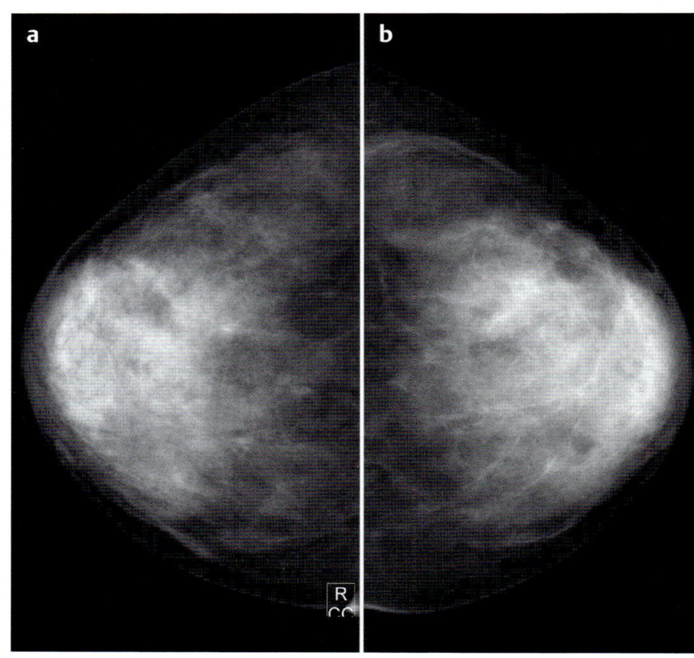


Fig. 26.**3 a, b** Digital mammography, CC view.

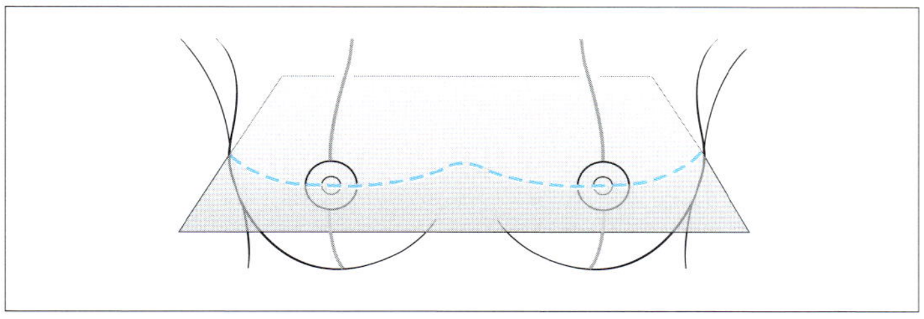

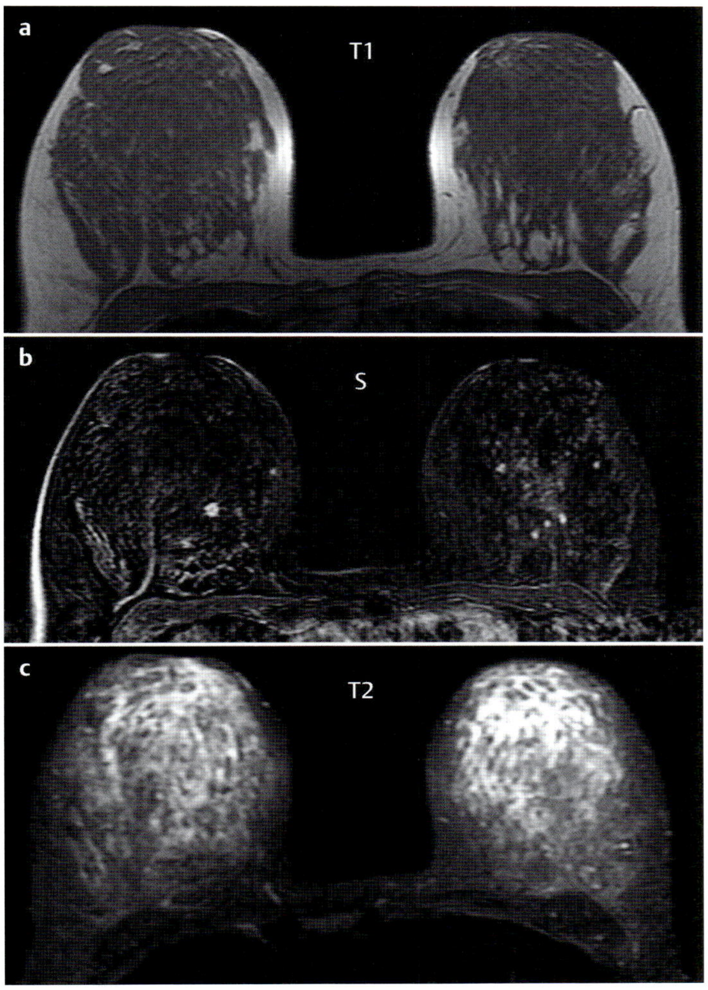


Fig. 26.4 **a–c** Contrast-enhanced MRI of the breasts.

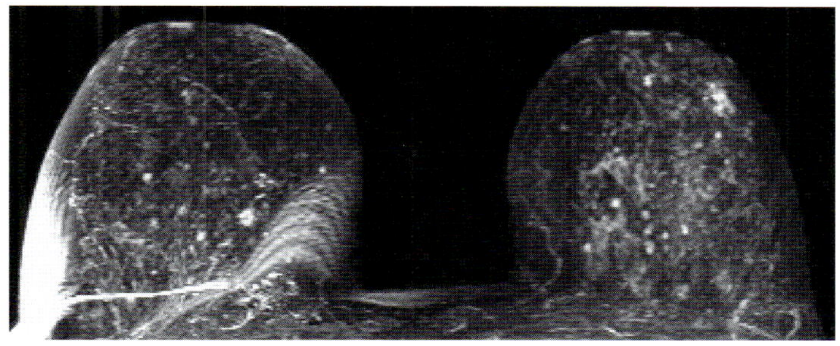

Fig. 26.**5** Contrast-enhanced MR mammography. Maximum intensity projection.

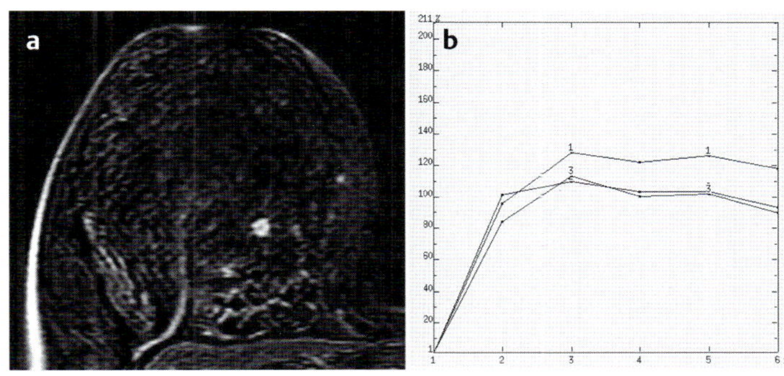


Fig. 26.**6 a, b** Signal-to-time curves.

Please characterize ultrasound, mammography, and MRI findings.
What is your preliminary diagnosis?
What are your next steps?

This case presents the imaging studies of an asymptomatic woman in a screening situation.

### Ultrasound

Retrospectively, in view of the MRI findings, an ill-defined hypoechoic lesion of 5 mm diameter with irregular borders and indeterminate distal echo behavior was depicted by sonography. There was no architectural distortion. US BI-RADS right 3.

### Mammography

Mammography showed bilaterally symmetric, extremely dense parenchyma, ACR type 4. Particularly in the inner quadrants of the right breast, there were no suspicious densities or lesions and no microcalcifications. No architectural distortion (BI-RADS right 1/left 1). PGMI: CC view P; MLO view G (inframammary fold, axillary skin fold).

### MR Mammography

Between the inner quadrants of the right breast, there was an ill-defined, spiculated lesion of approx. 5 mm diameter. This lesion demonstrated ring enhancement, a strong initial signal increase of 140%, and a postinitial plateau. Signal in T2-weighted imaging was indeterminate. No further suspect lesions.

**MRI Artifact Category:** 2
**MRI Density Type:** 2

| MRM score | Finding | Points |
|---|---|---|
| **Shape** | round | 0 |
| **Border** | spiculated | 1 |
| **CM Distribution** | ring | 2 |
| **Initial Signal Intensity Increase** | strong | 2 |
| **Post-initial Signal Intensity Character** | plateau | 1 |
| **MRI score (points)** | | **6** |
| **MRI BI-RADS** | | **5** |

### → Preliminary Diagnosis

Carcinoma.

### Differential Diagnosis

Focal adenosis.

| BI-RADS Categorization | | |
|---|---|---|
| Clinical Findings | right 1 | left 1 |
| Ultrasound | right 3 | left 1 |
| Mammography | right 1 | left 1 |
| MR Mammography | right 5 | left 1 |
| **BI-RADS Total** | **right 5** | **left 1** |

### Consideration

Does the sonographically depicted lesion correspond exactly with the enhancing area in MR mammography? Since the imaging evidence was not conclusive on this point, MR-guided investigation of the lesion was recommended.

### Procedure

MS-guided vacuum biopsy of the lesion in the center of the right breast.

### Histopathology of the biopsy specimen, right breast

Adenosis.

## Diagnosis

Adenosis.

## Treatment

None.

Adenosis is the most frequent cause of false-positive findings in MR imaging of the breast.

**Indication:** Screening.
**History:** Unremarkable.
**Risk profile:** No increased risk.
**Age:** 53 years.

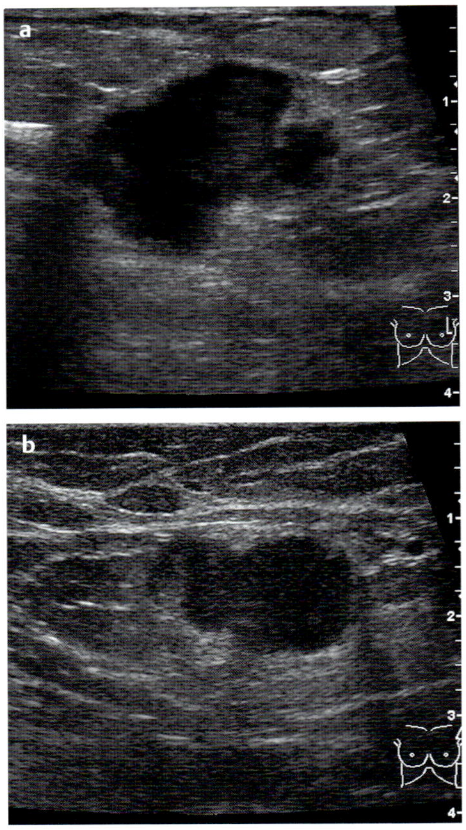


Fig. 27.**1 a, b** Ultrasound.

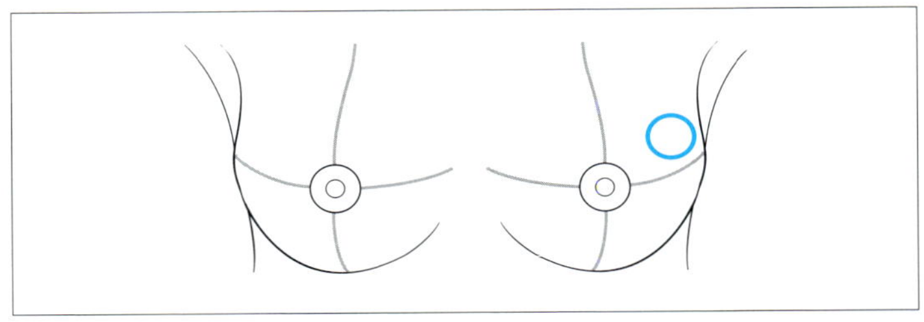

## Clinical Findings

Palpable mass of 2 cm in the upper outer quadrant of the left breast.

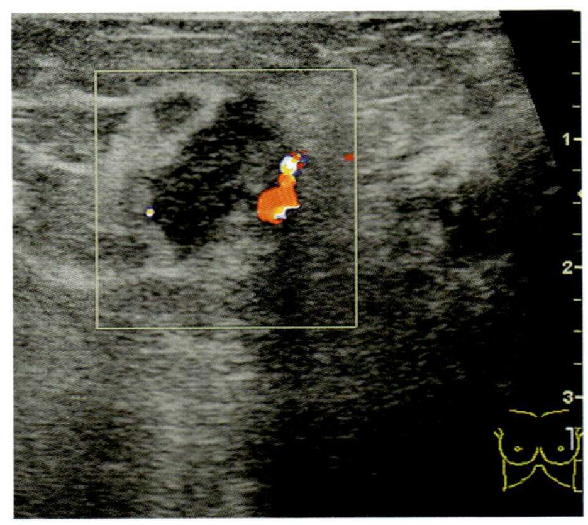

Fig. 27.**2** Color-coded duplex sonography.

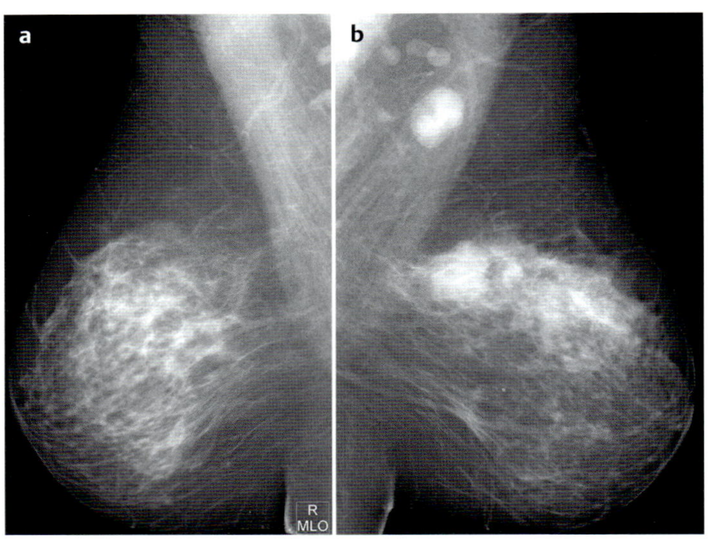


Fig. 27.**3 a, b** Digital mammography, MLO view.

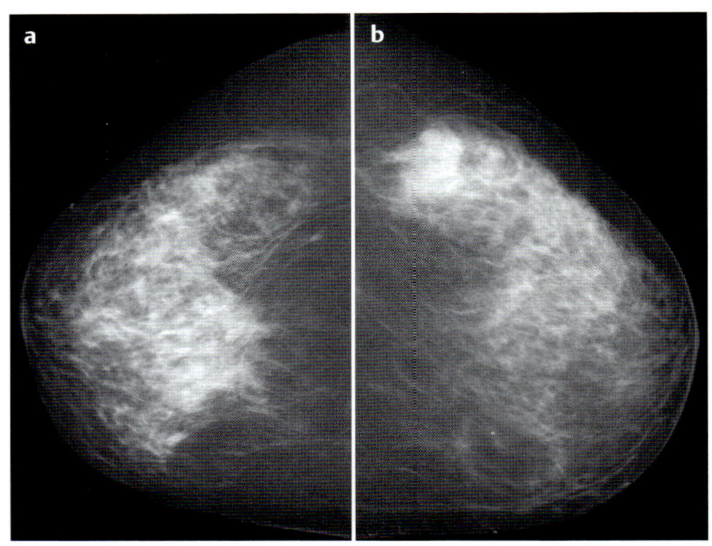


Fig. 27.**4 a, b** Digital mammography, CC view.

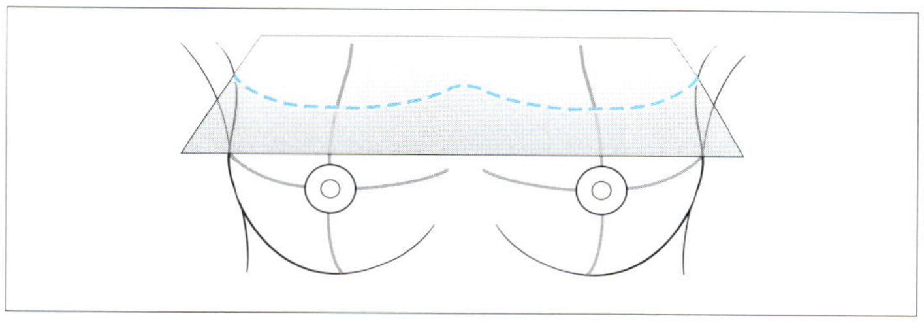

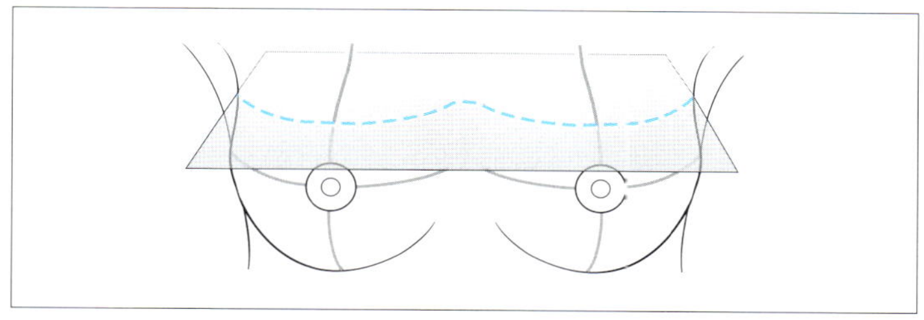

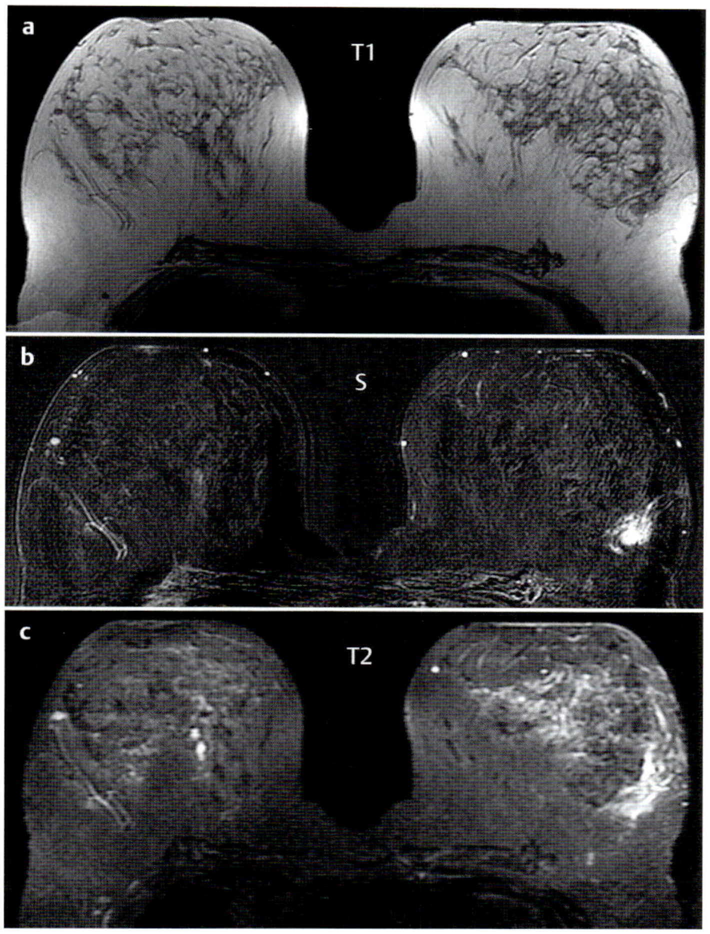


Fig. 27.**5 a – c** Contrast-enhanced MRI of the breasts.

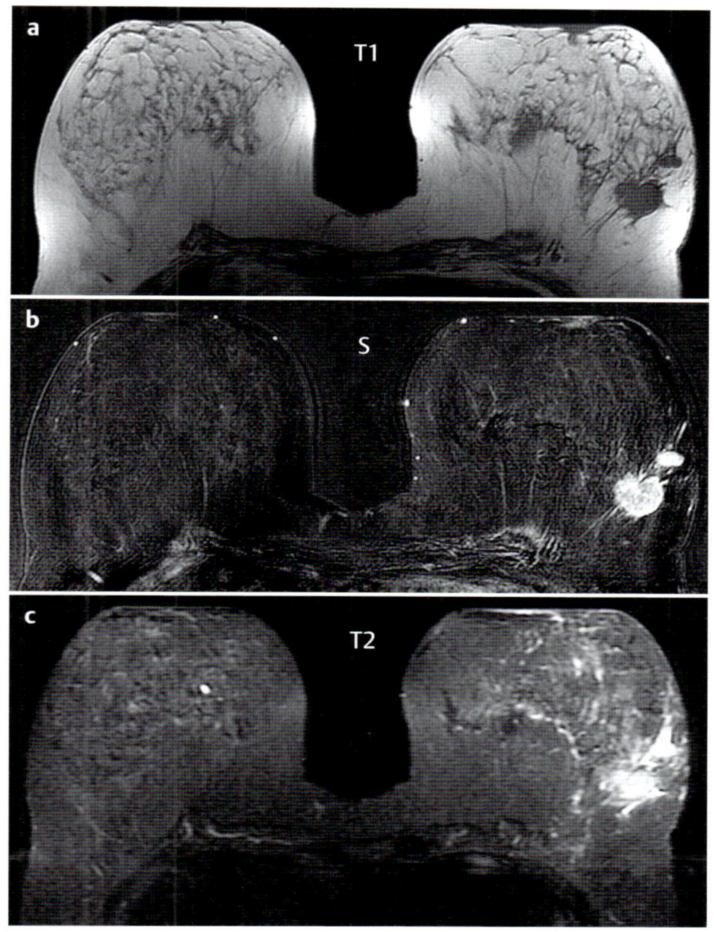


Fig. 27.**6 a – c** Contrast-enhanced MRI of the breasts.

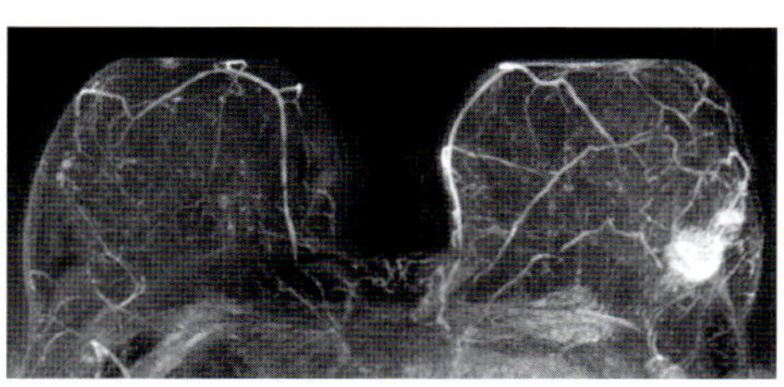

Fig. 27.**7** Contrast-enhanced MR mammography. Maximum intensity projection.

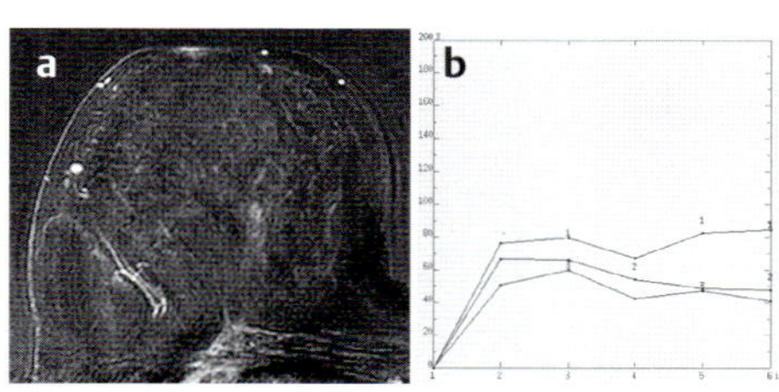


Fig. 27.**8 a, b** Signal-to-time curves, right breast.

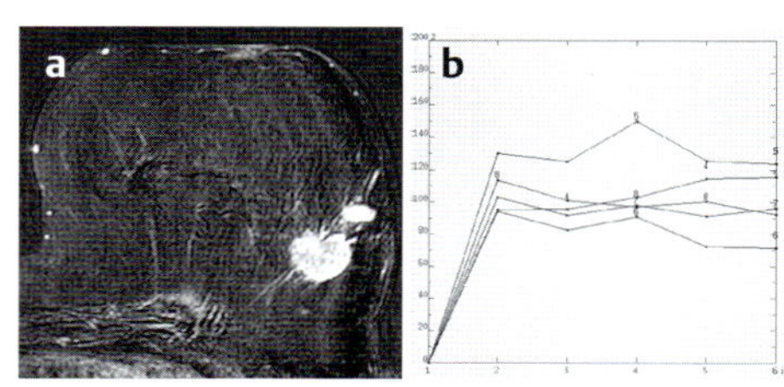


Fig. 27.**9 a, b** Signal-to-time curves, left breast.

?

Please characterize ultrasound, mammography, and MRI findings.
What is your preliminary diagnosis?
What are your next steps?

This case shows the imaging studies of a patient with a palpable mass in the left breast.

## Ultrasound

In the upper outer quadrant of the left breast, sonography detected a hypoechoic, lobulated, partially irregular lesion (diameter 23 mm) with an echoic border. This lesion showed indeterminate distal echo behavior and there was architectural distortion of the surrounding tissue. US BI-RADS left 5. In the right breast there were no suspicious sonographic findings in the upper outer quadrant or elsewhere (not shown).

## Mammography

Imaging demonstrated bilaterally symmetric fibroglandular tissue, ACR type 2. There was a lobulated, isodense, partially ill-defined lesion (diameter 25 mm) in the upper outer quadrant of the left breast. This lesion showed a partial halo sign. Ventral to this lesion, mammograms showed another oval, well-defined, isodense lesion (diameter 10 mm). Pathological enlargement of the axillary lymph nodes. No pathological findings in the right breast. BI-RADS right 1/left 5. PGMI: CC and MLO views P.

## MR Mammography

MRI showed a lobulated, partially ill-defined lesion (diameter 25 mm) in the upper outer quadrant of the left breast. This lesion had pathological contrast enhancement (initial signal increase of 180% and postinitial washout). Imaging depicted further lesions (diameters 10 mm and 5 mm) at distances of 10 mm and 35 mm respectively from the primary lesion. Between the outer quadrants of the right breast there was a round, well-defined lesion (diameter 5 mm) with homogeneous enhancement, initial signal increase of 70%, and postinitial washout as well as increased signal in T2 images.

**MRI Artifact Category:** 1
**MRI Density Type:** 1

| MRM score | Finding right | Points | Finding left | Points |
|---|---|---|---|---|
| **Shape** | round | 0 | lobulated | 1 |
| **Border** | well-defined | 0 | ill-defined | 1 |
| **CM Distribution** | homogeneous | 0 | ring | 2 |
| **Initial Signal Intensity Increase** | moderate | 1 | strong | 2 |
| **Post-initial Signal Intensity Character** | wash-out | 2 | wash-out | 2 |
| **MRI score (points)** | | **3** | | **8** |
| **MRI BI-RADS** | | **3** | | **5** |

## → Differential Diagnosis

Right: Fibroadenoma, papilloma, carcinoma.
Left: Breast cancer with nodal metastases.

| BI-RADS Categorization | | |
|---|---|---|
| Clinical Findings | right 1 | left 5 |
| Ultrasound | right 1 | left 5 |
| Mammography | right 1 | left 5 |
| MR Mammography | right 3 | left 5 |
| **BI-RADS Total** | **right 3** | **left 5** |

**Procedure**

US-guided core biopsy of the mass in the outer part of the left breast.

**Histopathology of the core biopsy specimen**

Medullar carcinoma.

**Further Procedure**

Open biopsy of the lesion in the right breast following preoperative hook-wire localization.

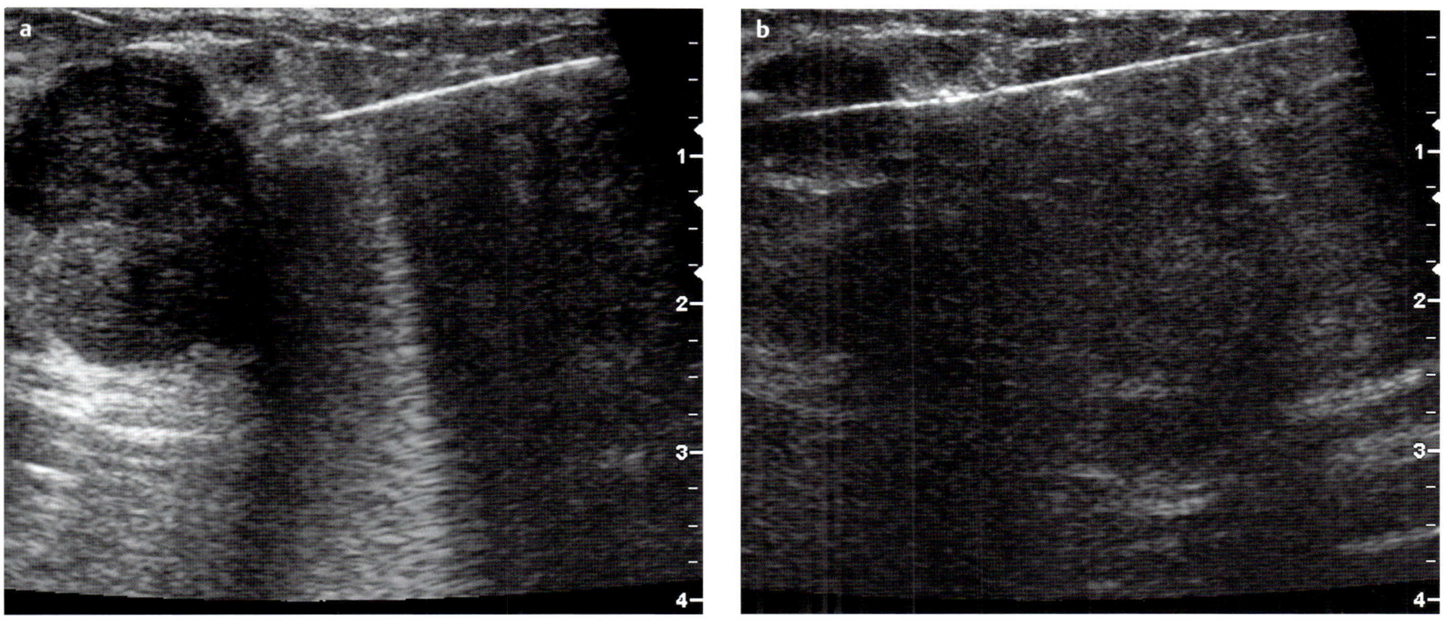

Fig. 27.**10 a, b** US-guided core biopsy (pre-fire (**a**) and post-fire (**b**) imaging).

## Diagnoses

Right breast: Fibroadenoma.

Left breast: Multicentric invasive ductal carcinoma (primary tumor: 27 mm). Contrary to the core biopsy results no medullary carcinoma.

| | |
|---|---|
| Right: | Fibroadenoma. |
| Left: | IDC multicentric pT2, pN1, G2. |

## Treatment

Bilateral mastectomy at patient's request.

The halo sign is *not* a reliable indicator of benign histology.

**Indication:** 2 cm mass between upper quadrants of the left breast.
**History:** Unremarkable.
**Risk profile:** No increased risk.
**Age:** 35 years.

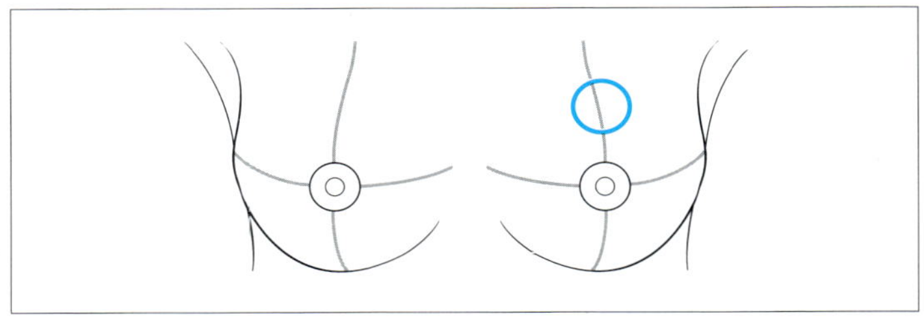

## Clinical Findings

Resistance (diameter 2 cm) between upper quadrants of the left breast.

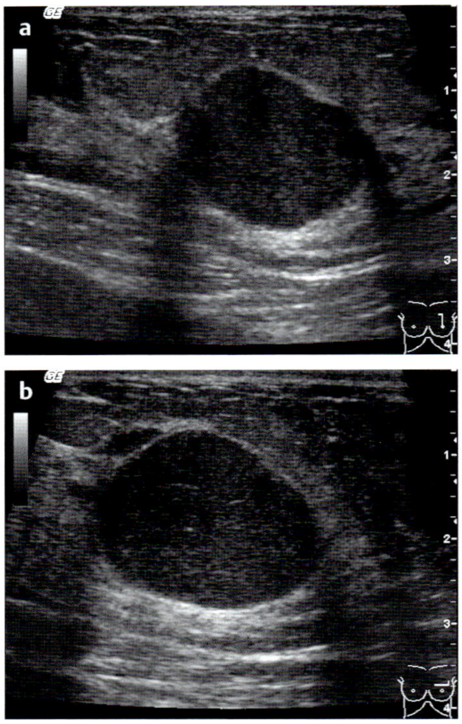


Fig. 28.**1 a, b** Ultrasound.

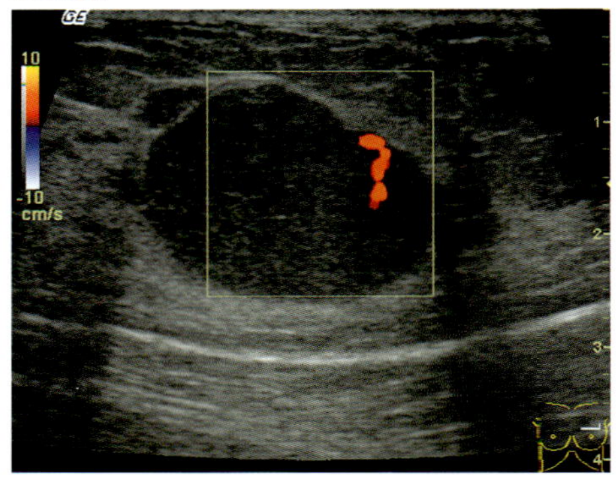


Fig. 28.**2** Color-coded Doppler sonography.

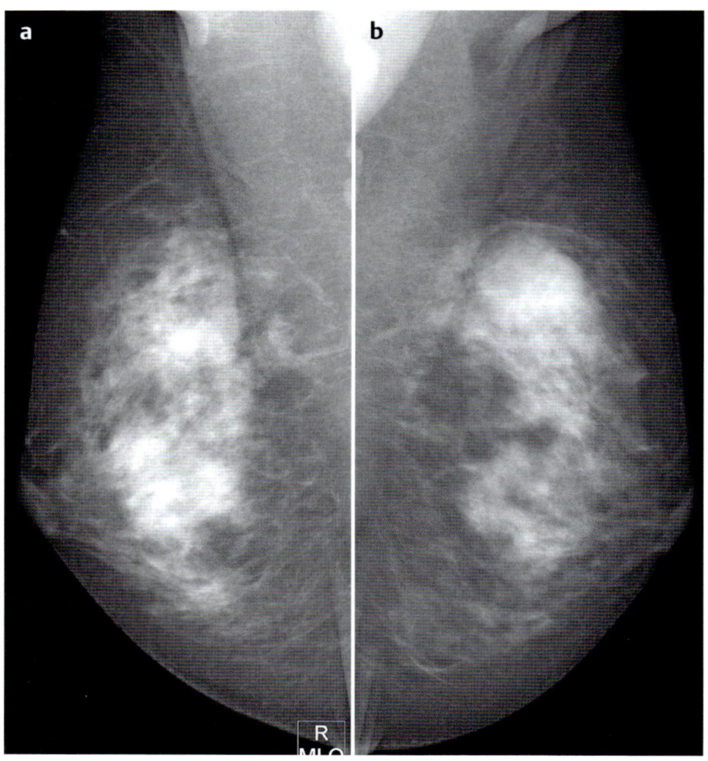


Fig. 28.**3 a, b** Digital mammography, MLO view.

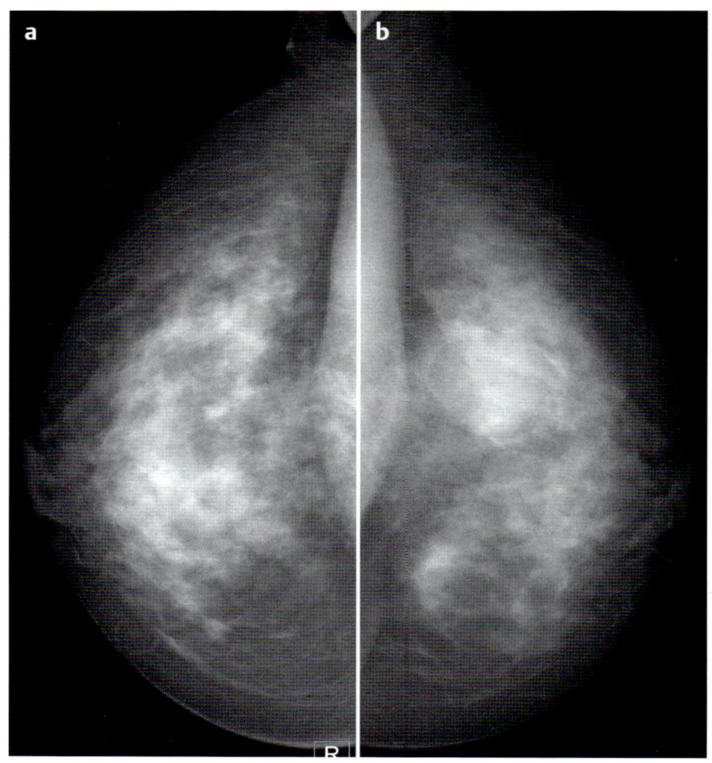


Fig. 28.**4 a, b** Digital mammography, CC view.

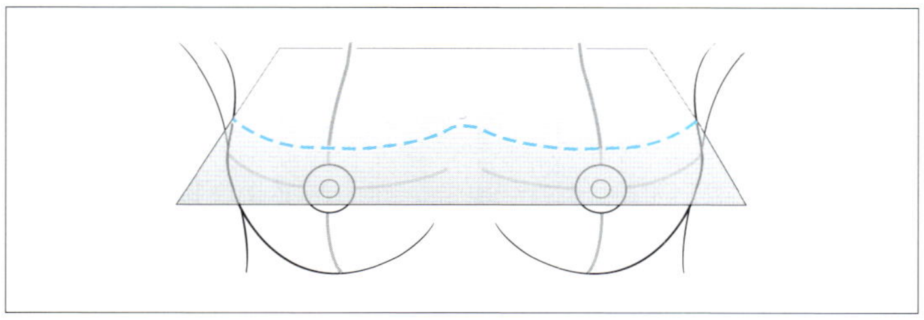

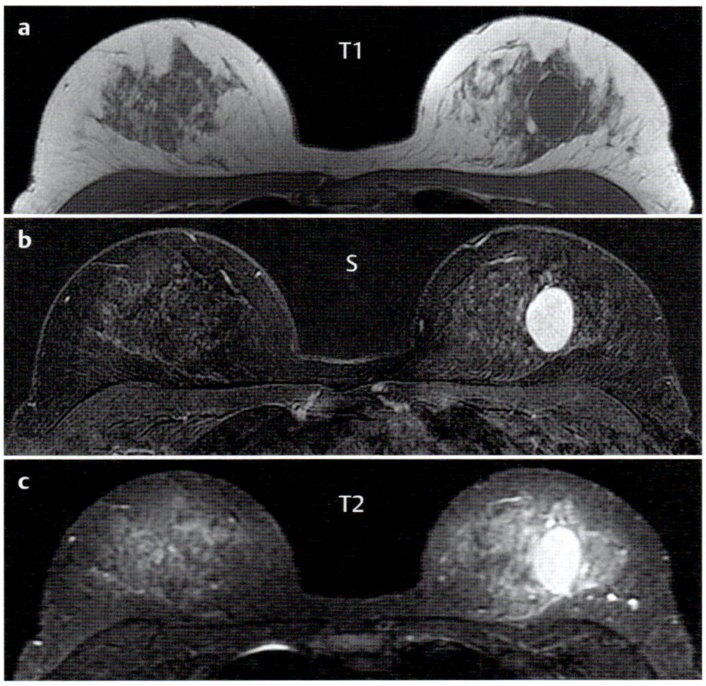


Fig. 28.**5 a – c** Contrast-enhanced MRI of the breasts.

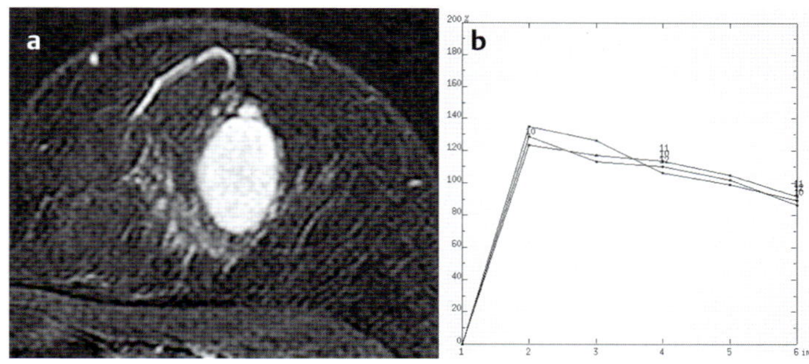


Fig. 28.**7 a, b** Signal-to-time curves.

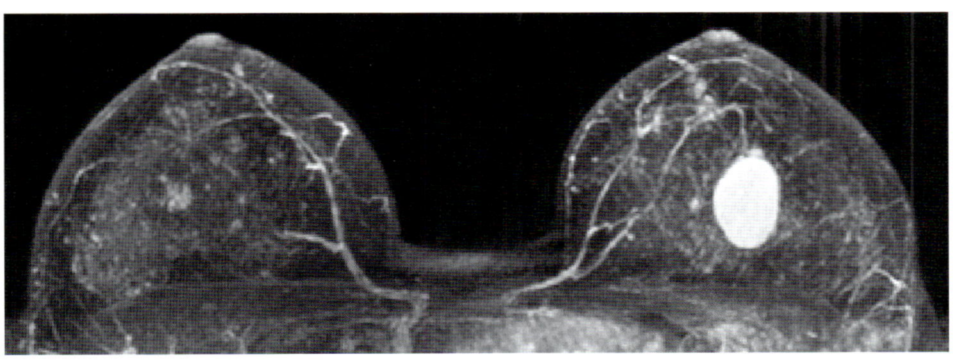

Fig. 28.**6** Contrast-enhanced MR mammography. Maximum intensity projection.

?

Please characterize ultrasound, mammography, and MRI findings.
What is your preliminary diagnosis?
What are your next steps?

This case examines the imaging studies of a young woman with a recently detected resistance between the upper quadrants of the left breast.

### Ultrasound

Corresponding to the resistance between the upper quadrants of the left breast, along a vertical axis from the nipple, the ultrasound depicted an oval hypoechoic lesion (diameter: 2,5 cm) with moderate distal acoustic increase and a lateral echo decrease. US BI-RADS 3.

### Mammography

Mammograms showed inhomogeneous dense parenchyma ACR type 3. Between the upper quadrants of the left breast an isodense, partially ill-defined lesion (diameter 2,5 cm) with a semicircular "Halo sign" was depicted. There were no other suspect densities or architectural distortions and no microcalcifications visible. BI-RADS right 1/left 3. PGMI: P for CC; M for MLO (inframammary fold).

### MR Mammography

In the central region of the left breast MRI demonstrated a well-defined mass (diameter 3 cm) enclosed by a narrow section of lipomatous tissue. After administration of contrast, homogeneous enhancement with strong initial signal increase (120%) followed by washout were visible. Signal in T2-weighted imaging was increased.

**MRI Artifact Category:** 1
**MRI Density Type:** 2

| MRM score | Finding | Points |
|---|---|---|
| **Shape** | oval | 0 |
| **Border** | well-defined | 0 |
| **CM Distribution** | homogeneous | 0 |
| **Initial Signal Intensity Increase** | strong | 2 |
| **Post-initial Signal Intensity Character** | wash-out | 2 |
| **MRI score (points)** | | **4** |
| **MRI BI-RADS** | | **4** |

## → Preliminary Diagnosis

Fibroadenoma.

## Differential Diagnosis

Papilloma, adenoma, phyllodes tumor, medullary carcinoma.

| BI-RADS Categorization | | |
|---|---|---|
| Clinical Findings | right 1 | left 3 |
| Ultrasound | right 1 | left 3 |
| Mammography | right 1 | left 3 |
| MR Mammography | right 1 | left 4 |
| **BI-RADS Total** | **right 1** | **left 4** |

### Procedure

Investigation of the lesion in the left breast by US-guided core biopsy.

### Histology of the specimen

Tubular adenoma.

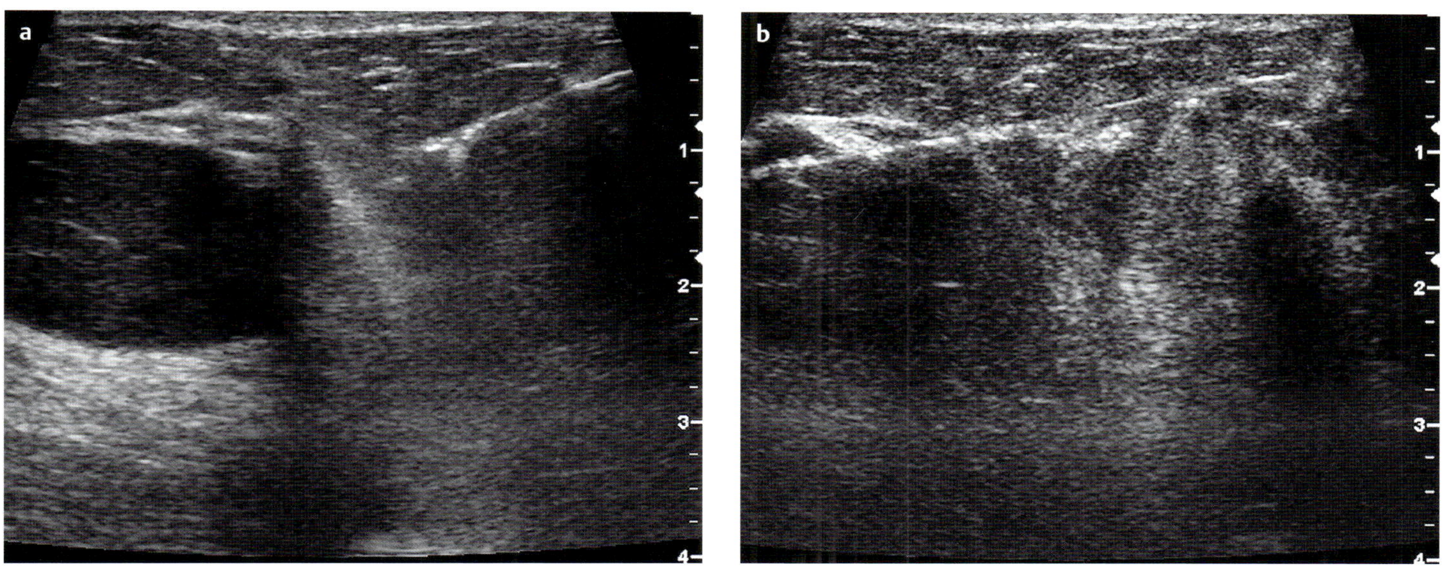


Fig. 28.**8 a, b** US-guided core biopsy. Pre-fire and post-fire documentation.

## Histology

Tubular adenoma.

## Treatment

None.

The question of the role of color-coded duplex sonography in breast diagnostics will probably remain unanswered forever.

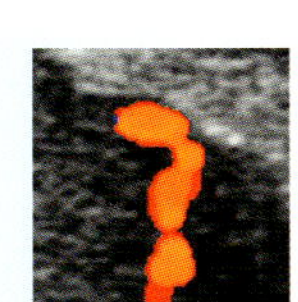

**Indication:** Screening.
**History:** Unremarkable.
**Risk profile:** No increased risk.
**Age:** 54 years.

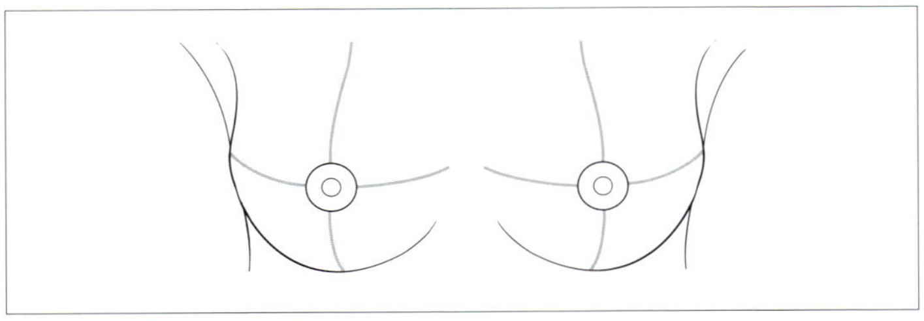

### Clinical Findings

No abnormalities; very firm parenchymal texture in both breasts.

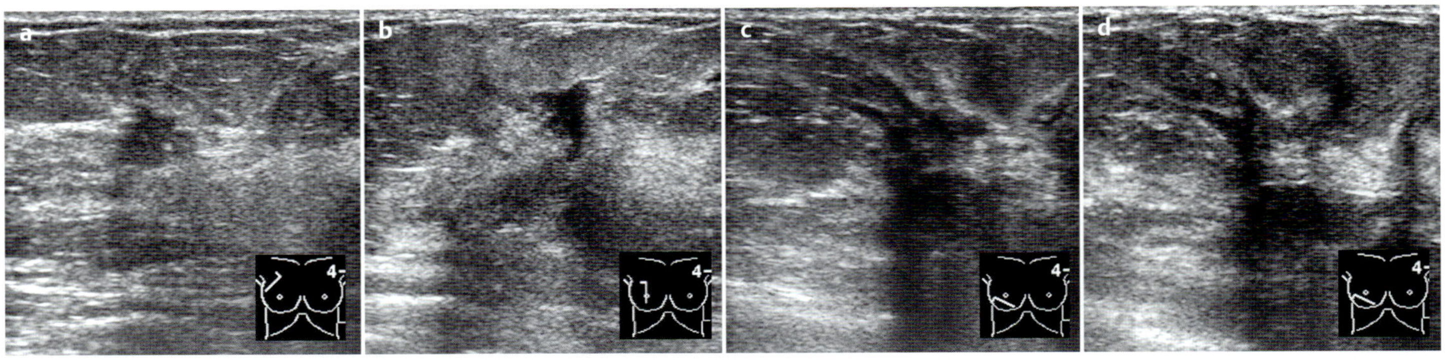


Fig. 29.**1 a–d** Sonography of the right breast.

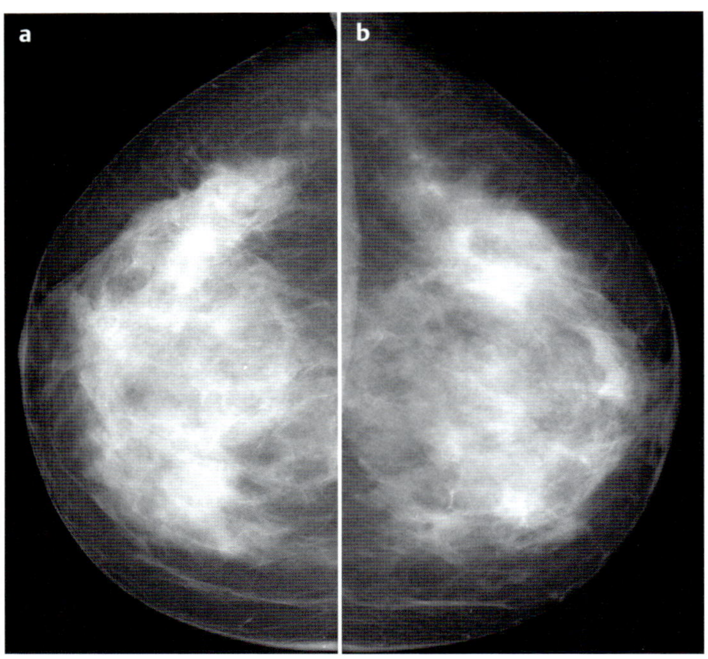


Fig. 29.**2 a, b** Digital mammography, CC view.

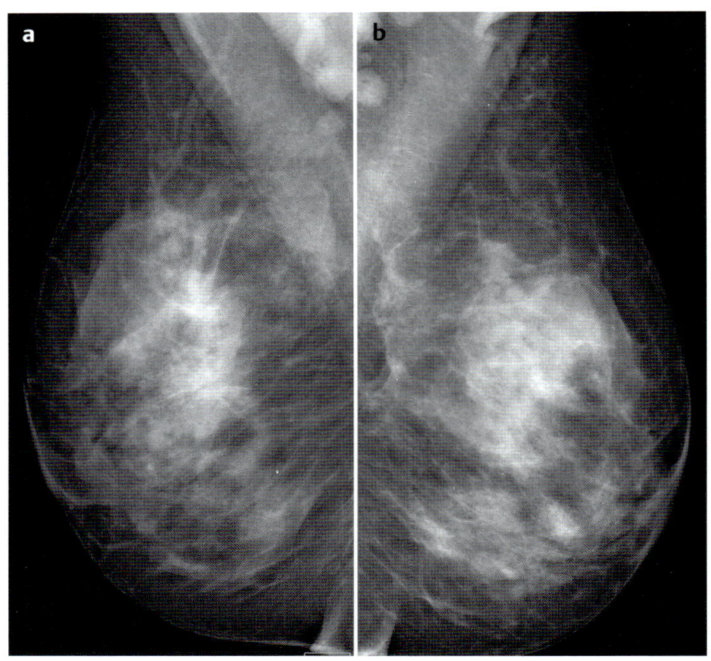


Fig. 29.**3 a, b** Digital mammography, MLO view.

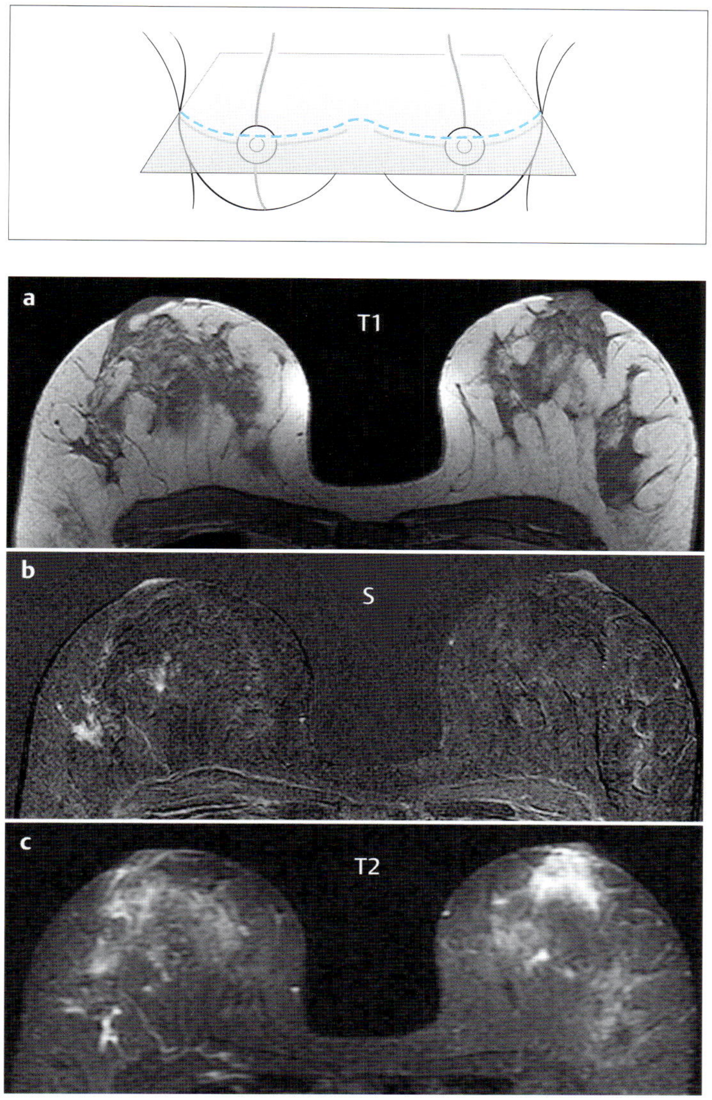


Fig. 29.**4 a – c** Contrast-enhanced MRI of the breasts.

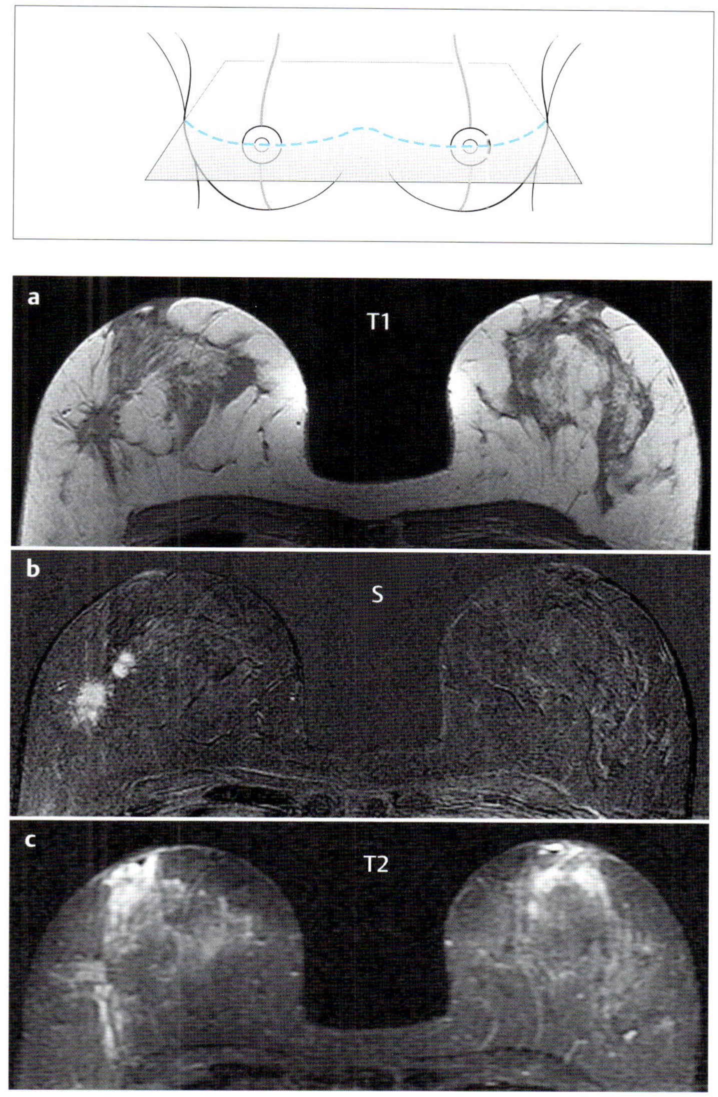


Fig. 29.**5 a – c** Contrast-enhanced MRI of the breasts.

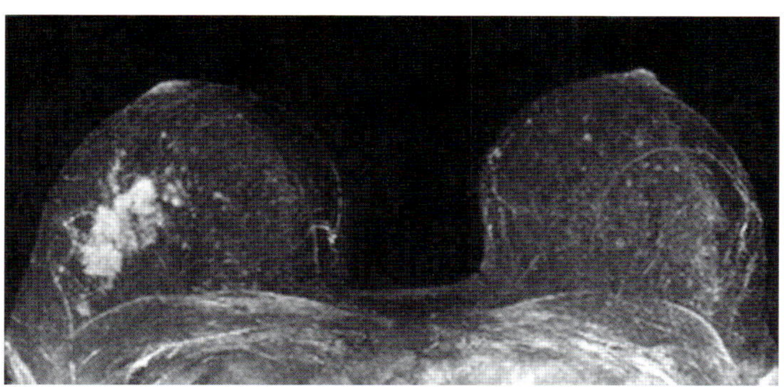

Fig. 29.**6** Contrast-enhanced MR mammography. Maximum intensity projection.

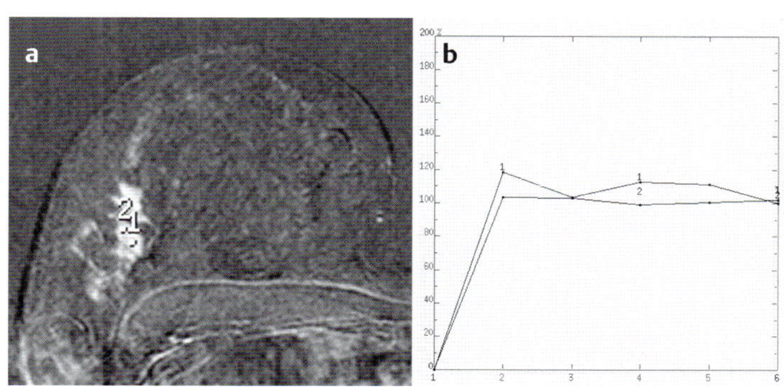


Fig. 29.**7 a, b** Signal-to-time curves.

?

Please characterize ultrasound, mammography, and MRI findings.
What is your preliminary diagnosis?
What are your next steps?

These are the imaging studies of an asymptomatic woman with no increased risk profile.

### Ultrasound

Ultrasound demonstrated suspect irregular lesions with hyperechoic margins in the lateral region of the right breast. These lesions showed individual distal acoustic shadowing and they disrupted adjoining ligamental structures. There was notable architectural distortion in the inferior region of the right breast depicted in ultrasound. US BI-RADS right 5.

### Mammography

Bilaterally extremely dense glandular tissue, ACR type 4. There was an asymmetry of the parenchymal structures with a distortion of the normal architecture and "shrinking sign" in the lateral part of the right breast. Mammography showed no circumscribed mass. No suspicious calcifications. The left breast was normal (BI-RADS right 4/left 1). PGMI: CC view P; MLO view G (inframammary fold incorrectly positioned).

### MR Mammography

In precontrast T1-weighted imaging, MRI reproduced the mammography findings of architectural distortion of the parenchyma and also depicted further nodular formations. Signal in T2-weighted imaging was nonspecific. In the outer quadrants of the right breast, postcontrast imaging depicted partially nodular, partially diffuse multiple enhancing areas with poorly-defined margins and suspect signal behavior.

**MRI Artifact Category:** 2
**MRI Density Type:** 1

| MRM score | Finding | Points |
|---|---|---|
| **Shape** | irregular | 1 |
| **Border** | ill-defined | 1 |
| **CM Distribution** | inhomogenous | 1 |
| **Initial Signal Intensity Increase** | strong | 2 |
| **Post-initial Signal Intensity Character** | plateau | 1 |
| **MRI score (points)** | | **6** |
| **MRI BI-RADS** | | **5** |

### → Preliminary Diagnosis

Extensive carcinoma of the right breast. No differential diagnoses.

| BI-RADS Categorization | | |
|---|---|---|
| Clinical Findings | right 1 | left 1 |
| Ultrasound | right 5 | left 1 |
| Mammography | right 4 | left 1 |
| MR Mammography | right 5 | left 1 |
| **BI-RADS Total** | **right 5** | **left 1** |

**Procedure**

Histological evaluation of the suspect findings in the outer quadrants of the right breast, preferably by US-guided percutaneous core biopsy.

**Histology of the biopsy specimen (right breast)**

Invasive ductal carcinoma.

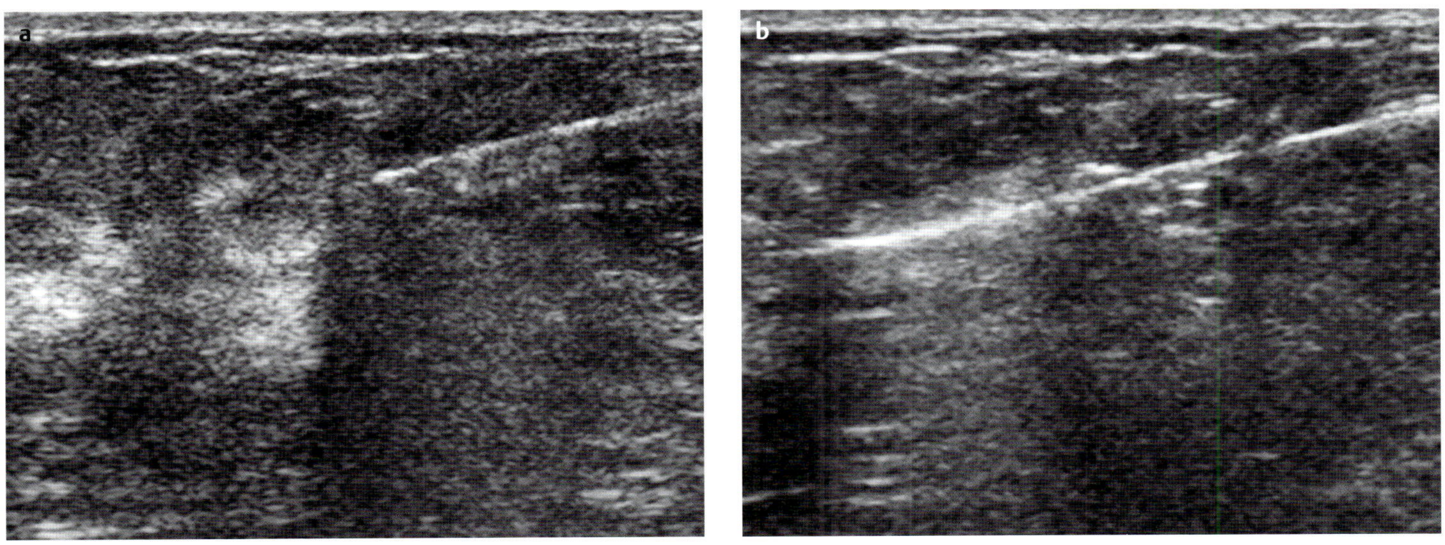


Fig. 29.**8 a, b** US-guided core biopsy. Removal of 5 specimens (14 gauge) using coaxial technique. Pre and post-fire documentation.

## Histology

Invasive ductal carcinoma with extensive intraductal component.

IDC pT2 + EIC, pN0, G2.

## Treatment

Mastectomy of the right breast.

Architectural distortions of the glandular tissue can be seen not only in mammography but also in breast ultrasound and/or MR imaging of the breast (especially in precontrast T1-weighted imaging).

**Indication:** Mastitis in upper outer quadrant of left breast, not responding to antibiotic therapy.
**History:** Open biopsy of abscess after puerperal mastitis and two relapses.
**Risk profile:** No increased risk.
**Age:** 34 years.

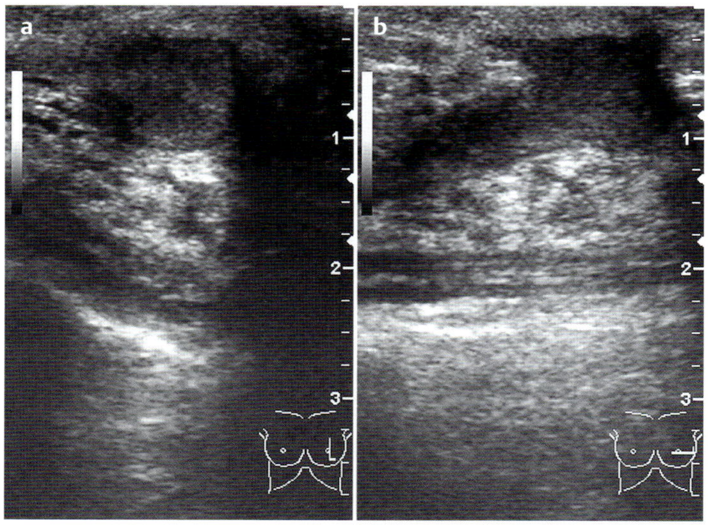


Fig. 30.**1 a, b** Ultrasound.

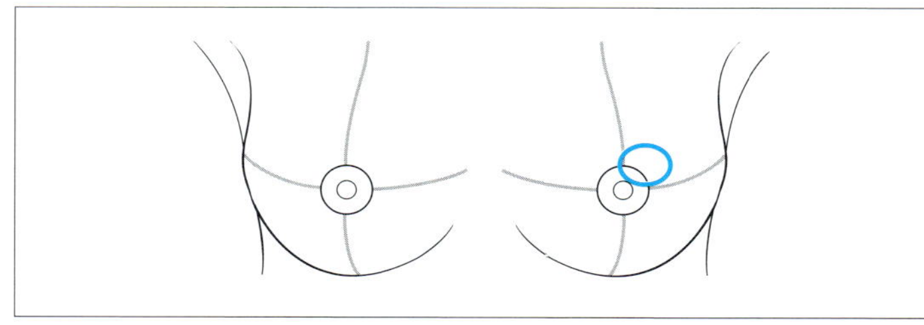

### Clinical Findings

Painful 2 cm resistance in the upper outer quadrant of the left breast, near the nipple. No redness.

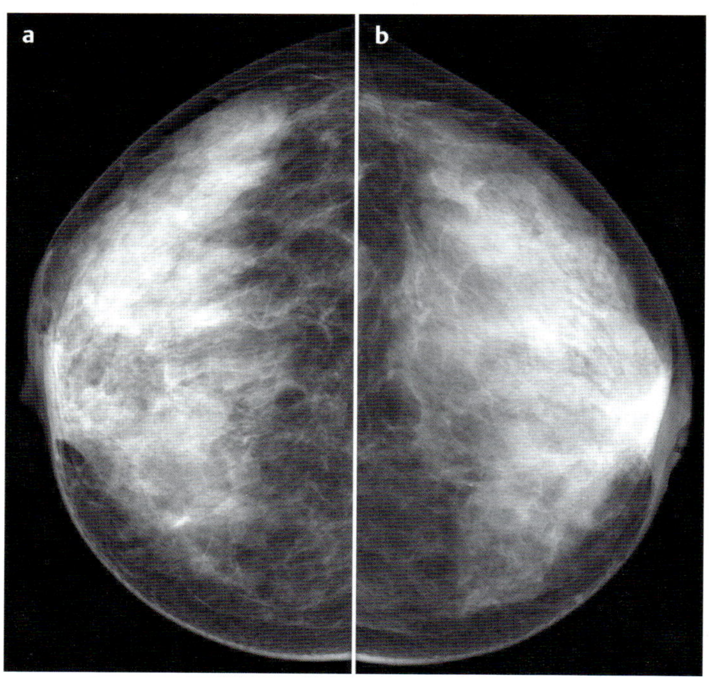


Fig. 30.**2 a, b** Digital mammography, CC view.

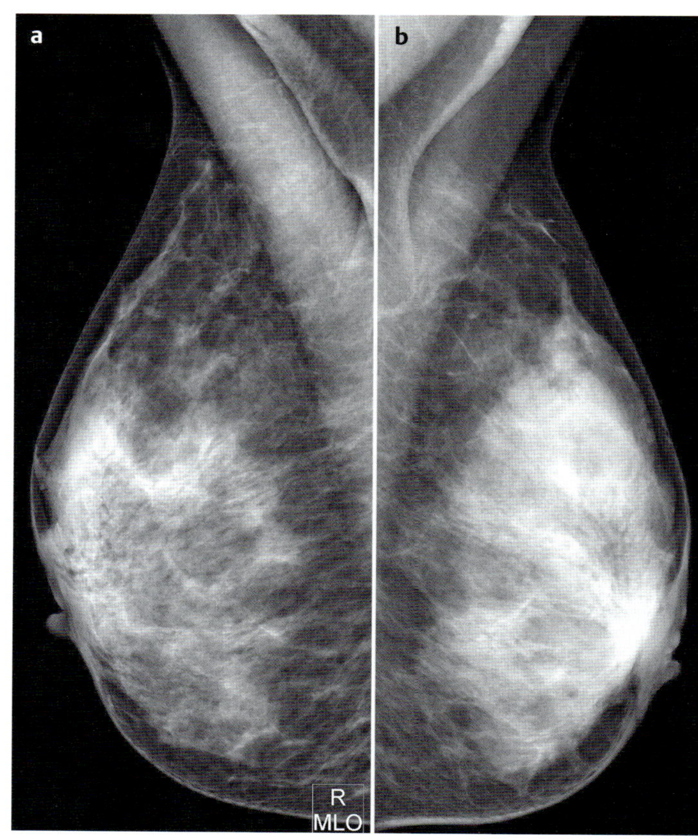


Fig. 30.**3 a, b** Digital mammography, MLO view.

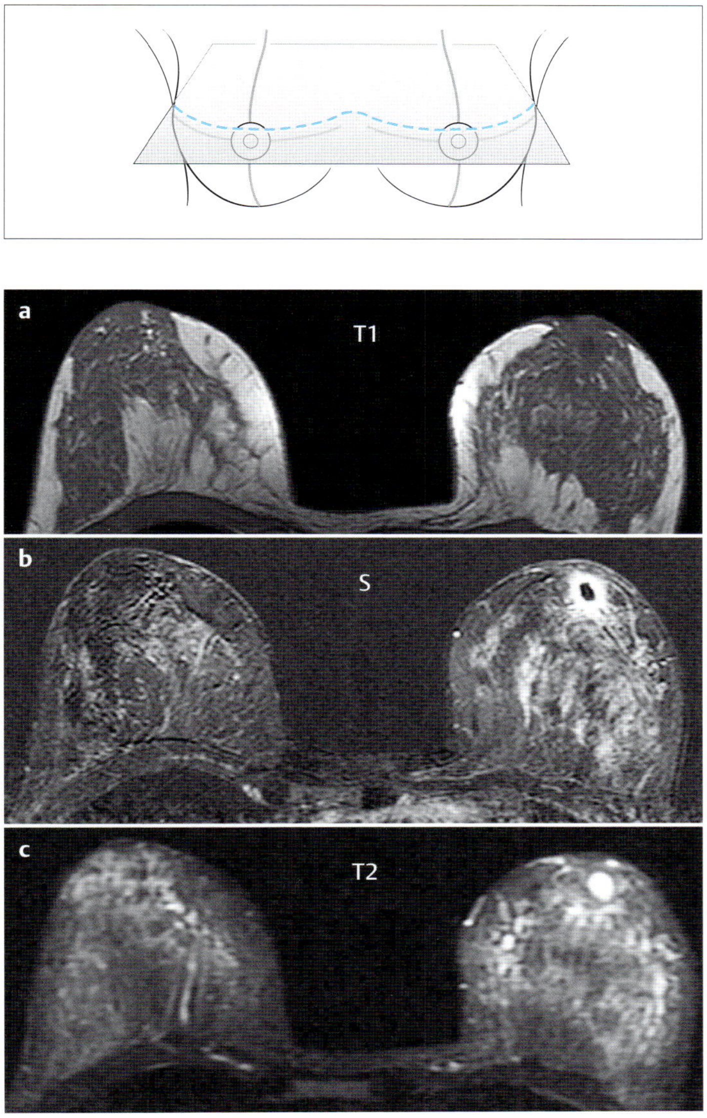


Fig. 30.4 **a – c** Contrast-enhanced MRI of the breasts.

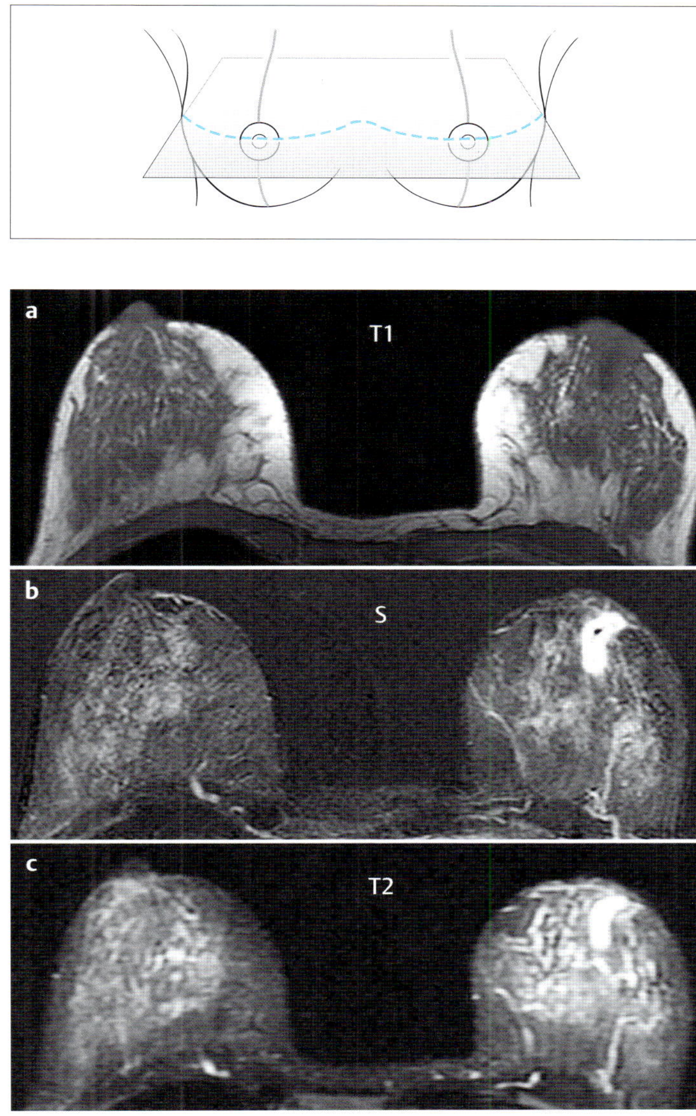


Fig. 30.5 **a – c** Contrast-enhanced MRI of the breasts.

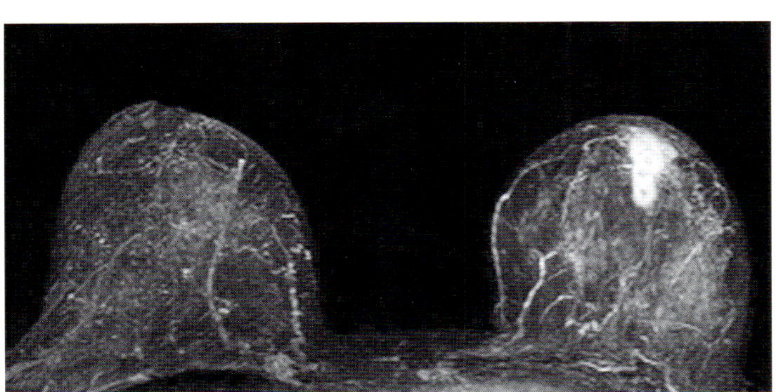

Fig. 30.6 Contrast-enhanced MR mammography. Maximum intensity projection.

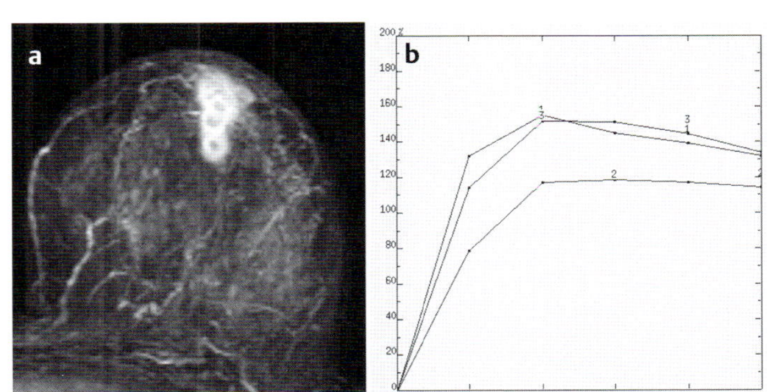


Fig. 30.7 **a, b** Signal-to-time curves.

**?**

Please characterize ultrasound, mammography, and MRI findings.
What is your preliminary diagnosis?
What are your next steps?

These are the imaging studies of a symptomatic woman presenting with a resistance and repeated inflammation of the left breast. Mastitis currently being treated with penicillin.

### Ultrasound

Corresponding to the palpable resistance there was a circumscribed lesion of 1.2 cm diameter with inhomogeneous acoustic signal. This region showed a distal echo increase. US BI-RADS 3.

### Mammography

Mammograms demonstrated a partially extremely dense parenchyma (ACR type 4). There was a slightly increased density of the left breast and a skin thickening of the left areola. Mammography showed no circumscribed densities or masses and no architectural distortion (BI-RADS right 1/left 3). PGMI: MLO view G (incomplete depiction of the inframammary fold); CC view P.

### MR Mammography

In the upper outer quadrant of the left breast–corresponding to the changes found at clinical, mammographic and ultrasound examination–MRI depicted a 3 cm × 1.2 cm tubular lesion with hypervascularization of the wall. The central components of this lesion showed high signal in T2-weighted imaging and did not enhance. No findings of note in the right breast.

**MRI Artifact Category:** 2
**MRI Density Type:** 2

| MRM score | Finding | Points |
|---|---|---|
| **Shape** | round/oval | 0 |
| **Border** | ill-defined | 1 |
| **CM Distribution** | rim sign | 2 |
| **Initial Signal Intensity Increase** | strong | 2 |
| **Post-initial Signal Intensity Character** | plateau | 1 |
| **MRI score (points)** | | **6** |
| **MRI BI-RADS** | | **5** |

## → Preliminary Diagnosis

Chronic mastitis with abscesses and blocked milk ducts, duct ectasia.

## Differential Diagnosis

Inflammatory carcinoma, Paget disease.

| BI-RADS Categorization | | |
|---|---|---|
| Clinical Findings | right 1 | left 3 |
| Ultrasound | right 1 | left 3 |
| Mammography | right 1 | left 3 |
| MR Mammography | right 1 | left 5 |
| **BI-RADS Total** | **right 1** | **left 3** |

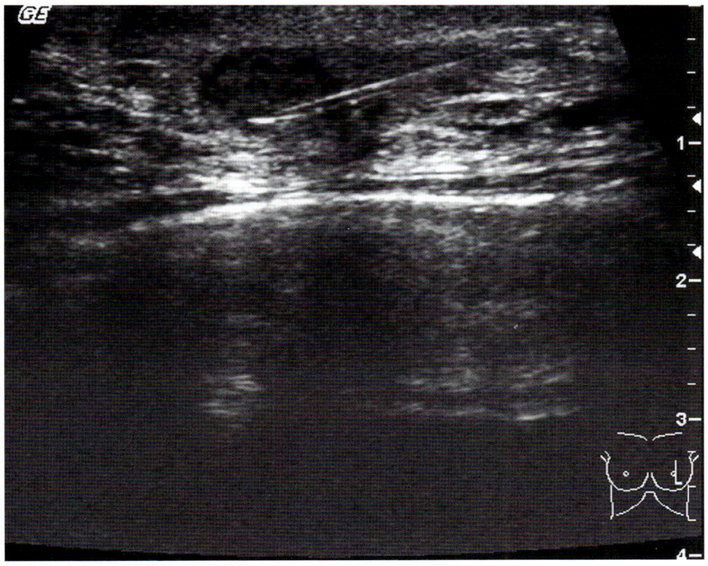


Fig. 30.**8** US-guided FNAP of the abscess.

### Procedure

Fine-needle aspiration of the fluid in the region behind the left areola to verify preliminary diagnosis. Bacteriological analysis of the specimen to identify the pathogen and determine possible resistance to antibiotic therapy.

### Cytology

Infected inspissated cyst.

## Diagnosis

Empyemic abscess in milk duct.

## Treatment

Change of antibiotic therapy to erythromycin due to a resistance to penicillin. Short-term clinical and sonographic follow-up examination after 14 days. Subsequent lumpectomy.

In patients with nonpuerperal mastitis, clinical symptoms should respond to antibiotic therapy within 10–14 days. If there is no response to therapy within this interval, histopathological examination is required.

**Indication:** Palpable mass in the right breast, discovered 2 months previously.
**History:** Unremarkable.
**Risk profile:** No increased risk.
**Age:** 42 years.

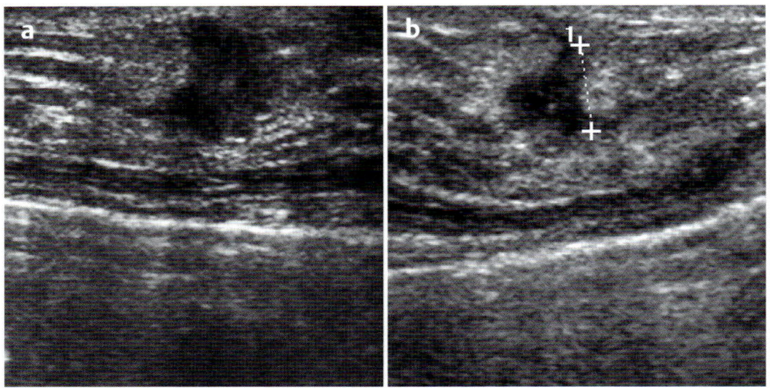


Fig. 31.**1 a, b** Ultrasound image of the region of the resistance.

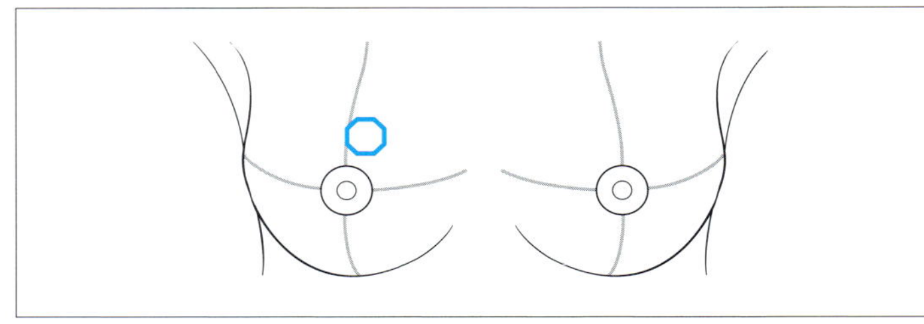

### Clinical Findings

Dense lump 2 cm diameter in the right breast above the nipple.

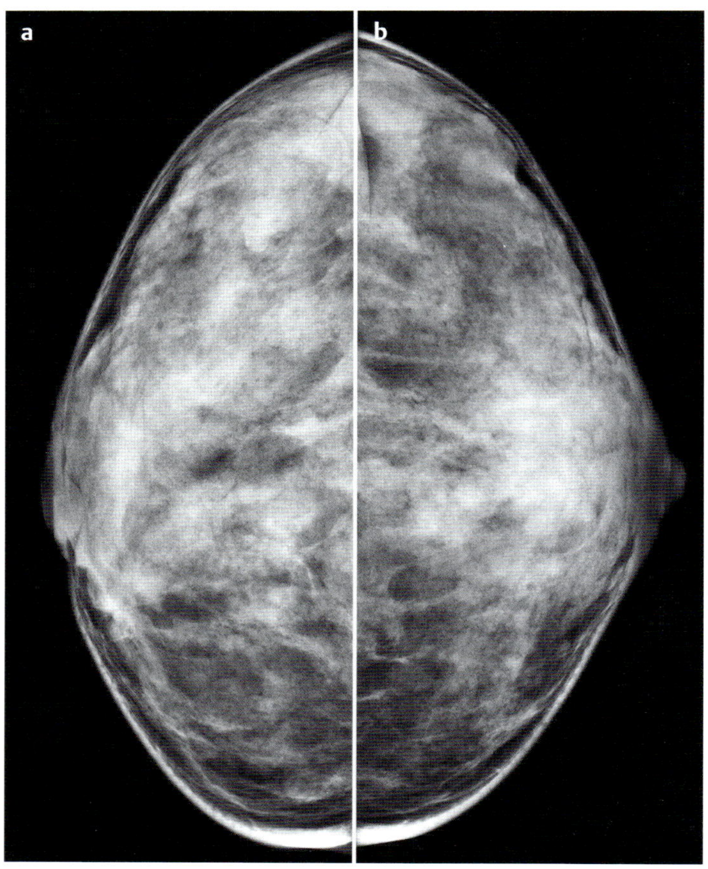


Fig. 31.**2 a, b** Digital mammography, CC view.

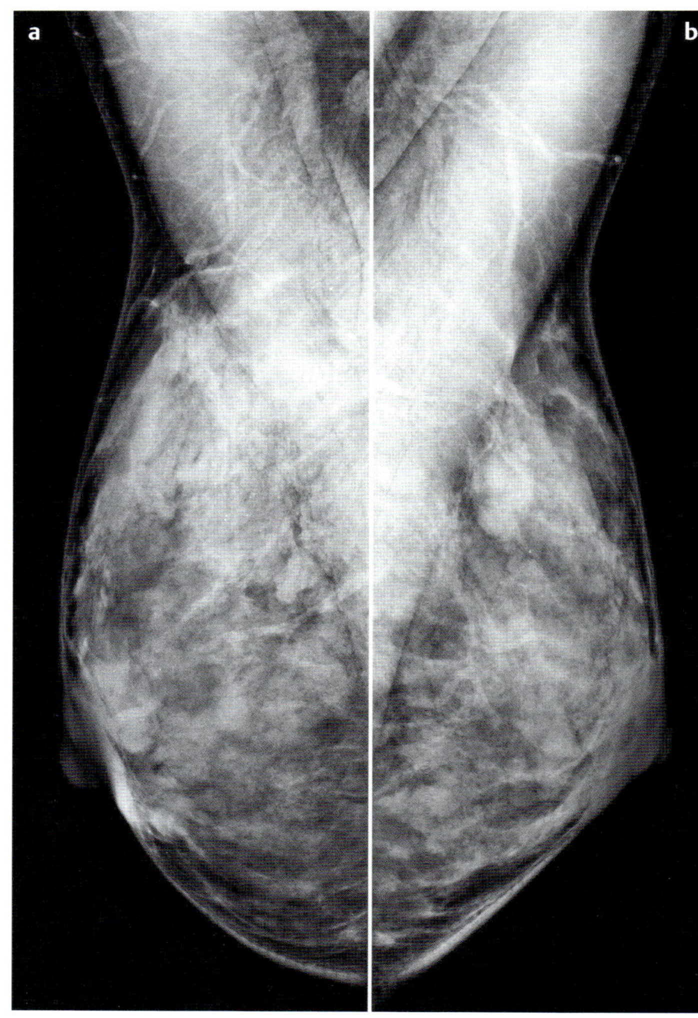


Fig. 31.**3 a, b** Digital mammography, MLO view.

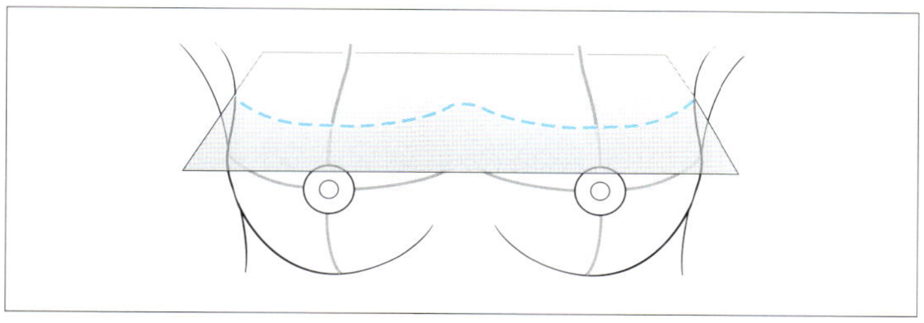

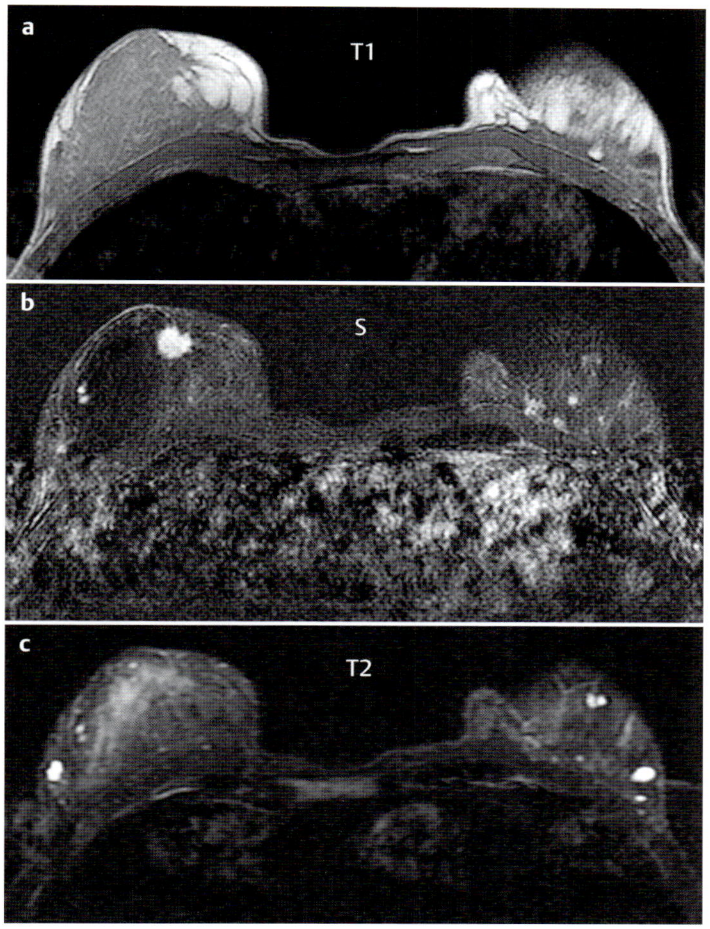


Fig. 31.**4 a – c** Contrast-enhanced MRI of the breasts.

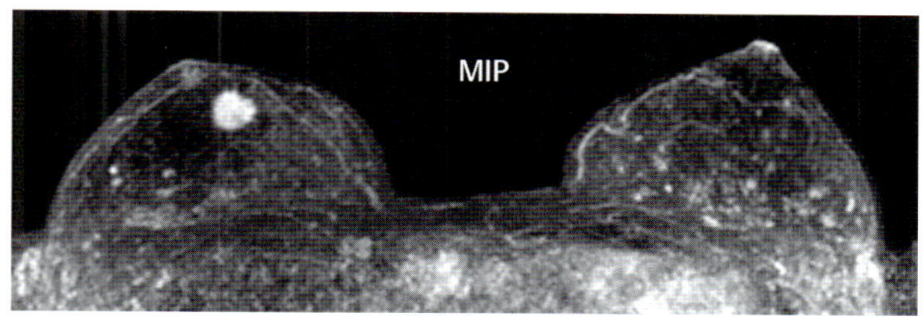


Fig. 31.**5** Contrast-enhanced MR mammography. Maximum intensity projection.

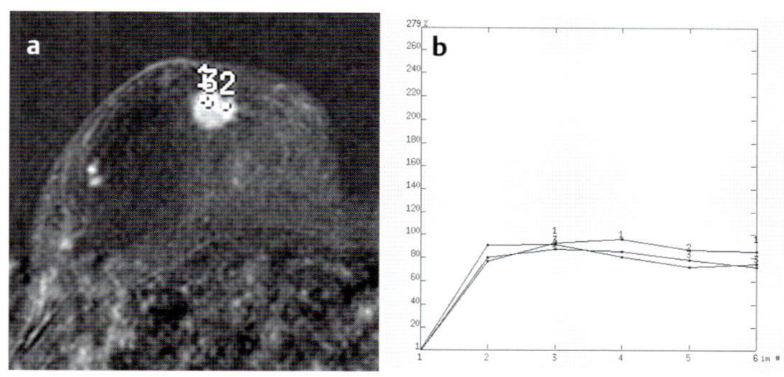


Fig. 31.**6 a, b** Signal-to-time curves.

?

Please characterize ultrasound, mammography, and MRI findings.
What is your preliminary diagnosis?
What are your next steps?

This case shows the imaging studies of a woman presenting with a mass she palpated 2 months previously. The lump has characteristics of a benign glandular sclerosis, but nonetheless was the reason for further investigation.

### Ultrasound

Corresponding to the known lump, ultrasound showed a lobulated and well-defined lesion with a markedly hyperechoic margin and accompanying distortion of the surrounding tissue. US BI-RADS 5 right.

### Mammography

Mammograms showed bilaterally symmetric, extremely dense parenchyma, ACR type 4. Due to the limitations of these conditions, no abnormalities were visible in the area of the palpable mass or elsewhere. There were no architectural distortions or calcifications (BI-RADS right 1/left 1). PGMI: CC view P; MLO view G (inframammary fold).

### MR Mammography

MRI demonstrated a round, hypervascularized lesion about 1 cm in diameter and with partially ill-defined borders in the right breast, cranial to the nipple. This lesion corresponds to the clinical and sonographic findings in the same location and had an intermediate signal in T2 imaging. The nonspecific signal–time curves showed an initial increase of about 70% followed by a plateau. There was also a cyst in the left breast and further spotty enhancing foci in both breasts (see maximum intensity projection, Fig. 31.**5**).

**MRI Artifact Category:** 1
**MRI Density Type:** 2

| MRM score | Finding | Points |
|---|---|---|
| **Shape** | round | 0 |
| **Border** | ill-defined | 1 |
| **CM Distribution** | inhomogenous | 1 |
| **Initial Signal Intensity Increase** | moderate | 1 |
| **Post-initial Signal Intensity Character** | plateau | 1 |
| **MRI score (points)** | | **4** |
| **MRI BI-RADS** | | **4** |

### → Preliminary Diagnosis

Breast cancer.

| BI-RADS Categorization | | |
|---|---|---|
| Clinical Findings | right 3 | left 1 |
| Ultrasound | right 5 | left 1 |
| Mammography | right 1 | left 1 |
| MR Mammography | right 4 | left 2 |
| **BI-RADS Total** | **right 5** | **left 2** |

**Procedure**

Histopathological analysis of the lump, preferably by US-guided percutaneous core biopsy.

**Performed step (departing from guidelines)**

At the patient's request, open biopsy was performed to remove the mass without primary core biopsy analysis.

## Histology

Invasive lobular carcinoma, 12 mm.

ILC pT1c, pN0, G2.

## Treatment

Mastectomy (at patient's request).

This case demonstrates impressively the limitation of conventional mammography in diagnosing noncalcifying carcinomas in patients with extremely dense glandular tissue (ACR type 4). Recent studies indicate that the proportion of carcinomas not detectable in extremely dense breast tissue is 50%.

**Indication:** Screening.
**History:** Bilateral implants 13 years previously.
**Risk profile:** No increased risk.
**Age:** 53 years.

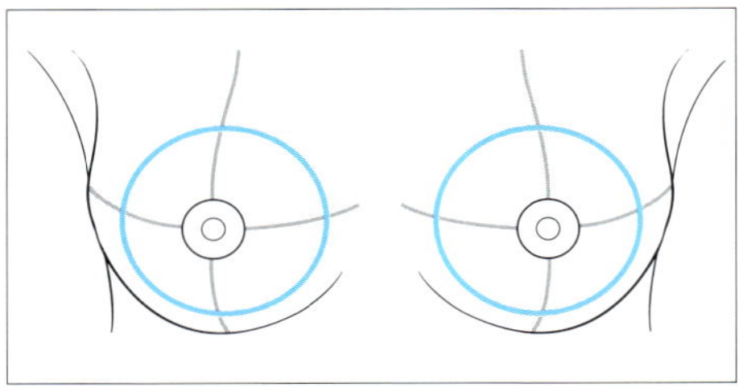

### Clinical Findings

Clinical inspection unremarkable. Implants appear "close-fitting" within the tissue bilaterally. No pathological findings on palpation.

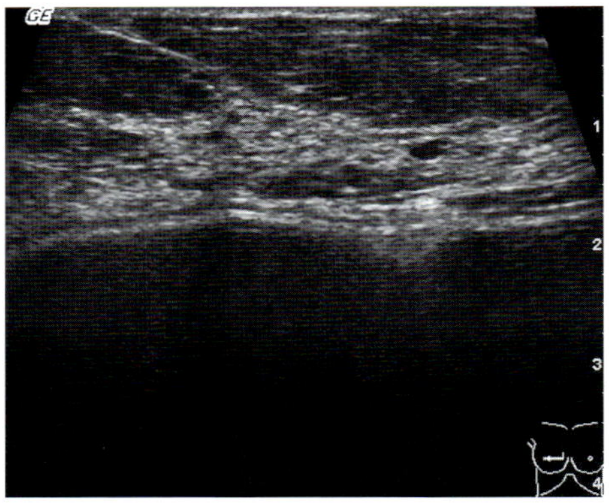

Fig. 32.**1** Sonography, right breast.

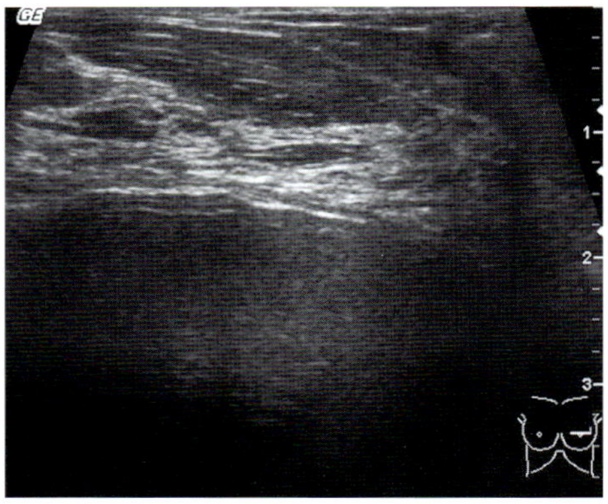

Fig. 32.**2** Sonography, left breast.

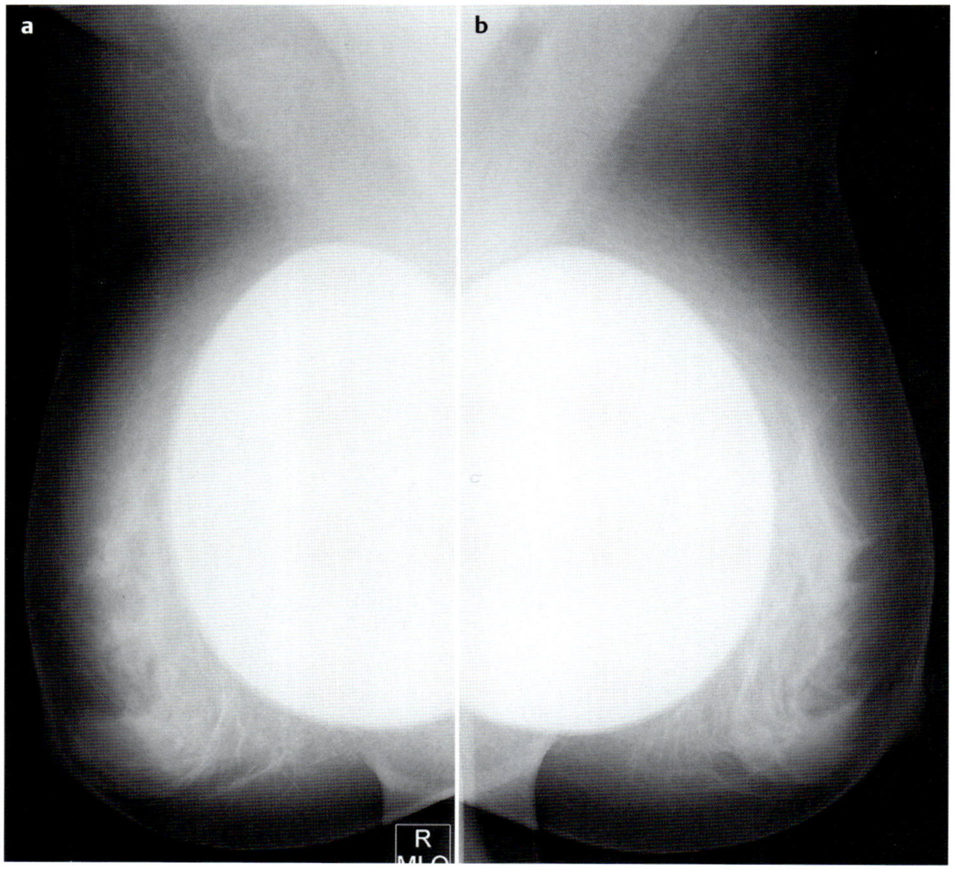


Fig. 32.**3 a, b** Digital mammography, MLO view.

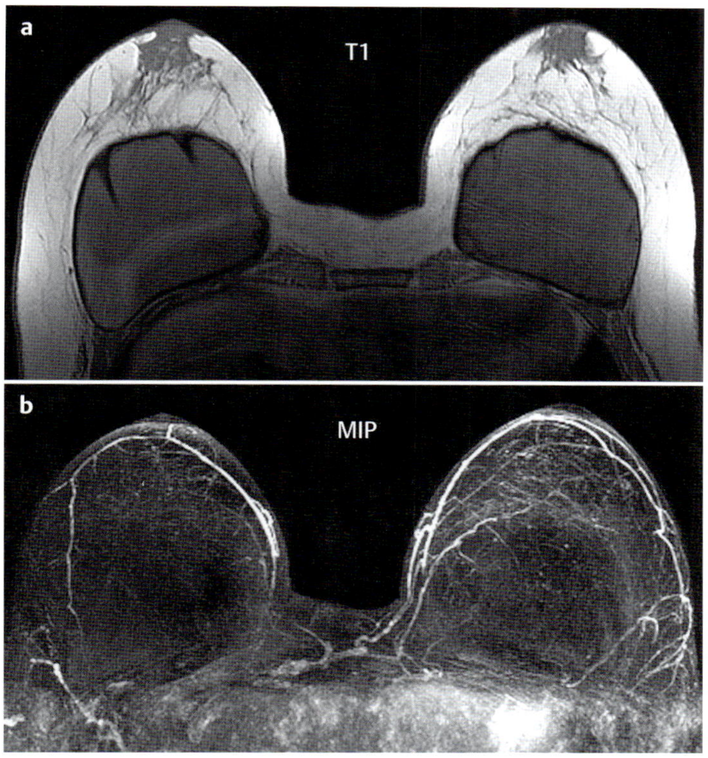


Fig. 32.**4 a, b** Contrast-enhanced MR mammography.

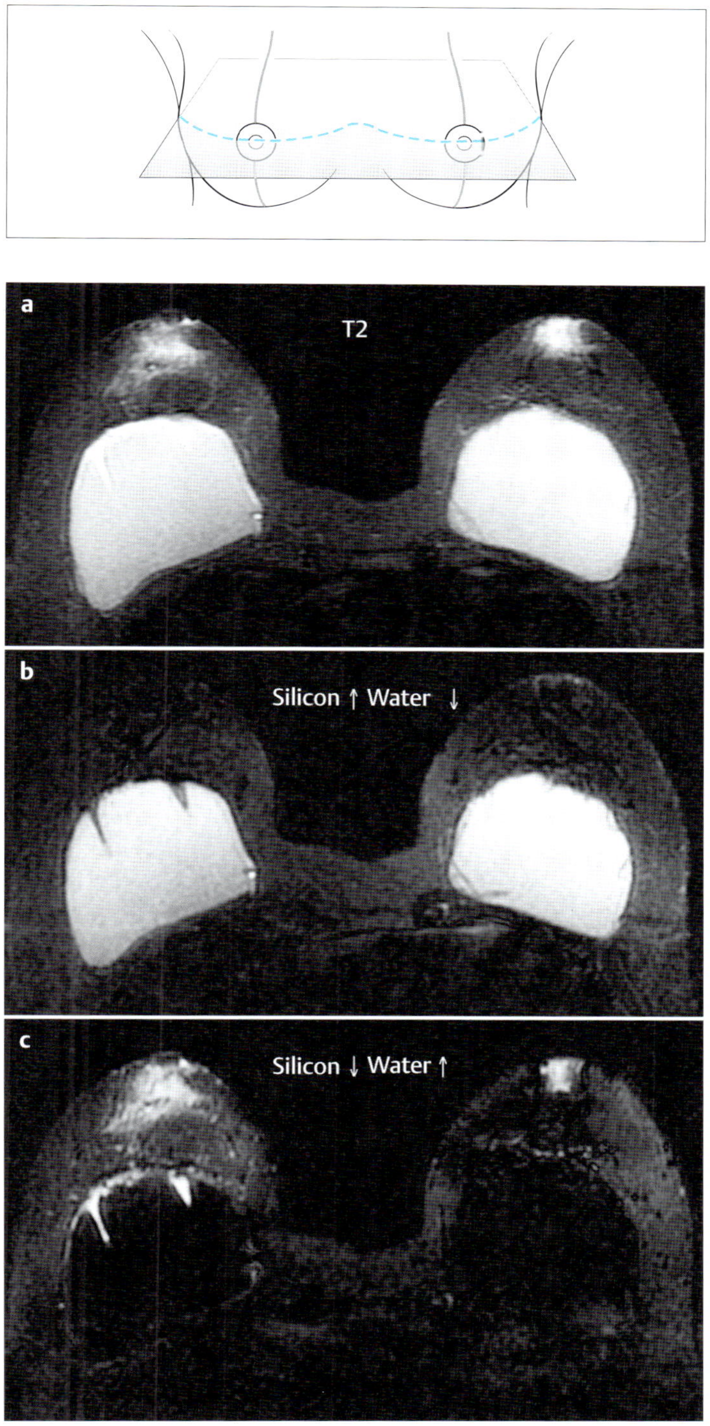


Fig. 32.**5 a – c** MR mammography–prosthesis protocol.

?

Please characterize ultrasound, mammography, and MRI findings.
What is your preliminary diagnosis?
What are your next steps?

This case consists of the imaging studies of an asymptomatic woman with bilateral implants.

### Ultrasound

On the basis of the representative sonograms, no pathological findings. Ultrasound depicted the prepectorally positioned implants with no abnormalities. US BI-RADS right 1/left 1.

### Mammography

Mammography showed the subparenchymal positioning of the implants in both breasts. The surrounding parenchyma could not be adequately assessed. There were, however, no suspicious lesions and no microcalcifications visible (BI-RADS right 1/left 1).

### MR Mammography (contrast-enhanced protocol)

Presentation of both breasts and both prostheses was normal in contrast-enhanced MRI. No pathological enhancement in MIP view after contrast administration.

### MR Mammography (dedicated prosthesis protocol)

MRI showed a single-lumen prosthesis on each side.

**Right breast:** Imaging of implant and the fluid-filled radial folds (no silicone) was normal (Fig. 32.**6 a**).

**Left breast:** Silicone was detected within the radial folds of the implant in all sequences (Fig. 32.**6 b**). This indicates gel bleeding from the prosthesis.

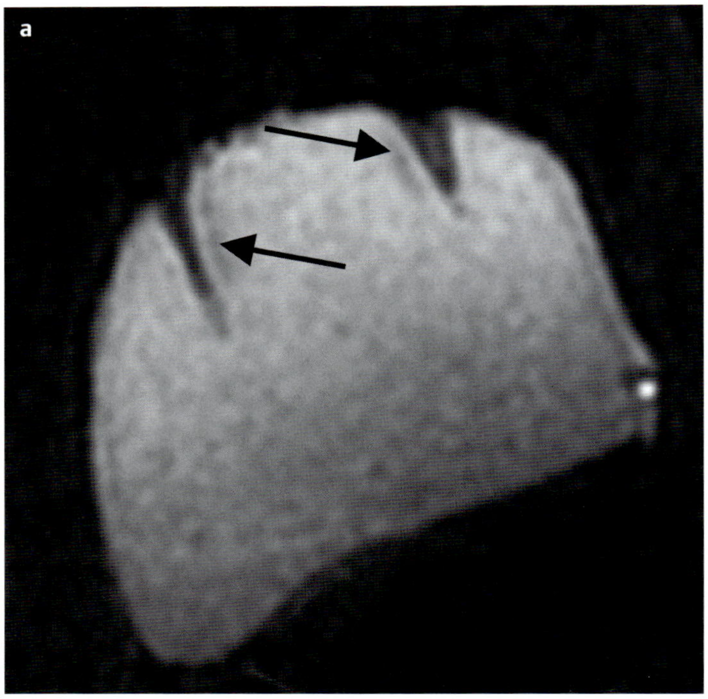


Fig. 32.**6 a** Intact prosthesis with fluid-filled folds (arrows).

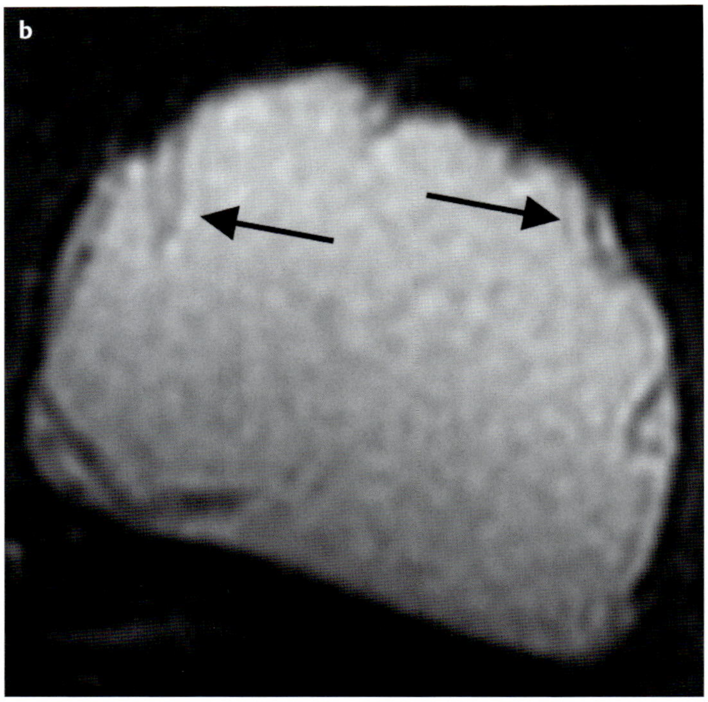


Fig. 32.**6 b** Gel bleeding with signs of silicone within the folds (arrows).

| BI-RADS Categorization | | |
|---|---|---|
| Clinical Findings | right 1 | left 1 |
| Ultrasound | right 1 | left 1 |
| Mammography | right 1 | left 1 |
| MR Mammography | right 1 | left 1 |
| **BI-RADS Total** | **right 1** | **left 1** |

**Assessment**

There is no indication of malignancy in either breast.

## Diagnosis

Gel bleeding of the implant in the left breast.

## Treatment

None.

Gel bleeding can precede intracapsular rupture of prostheses. It can be followed by detachment and rupture of the outer implant envelope.

**Indication:** Resistance in the left upper outer quadrant.
**History:** Unremarkable.
**Risk profile:** Breast cancer in mother at the age of 42 years.
**Age:** 37 years.

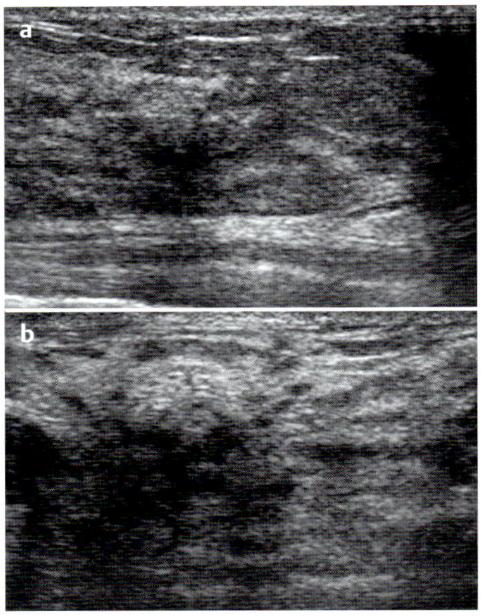

Fig. 33.1 a, b Ultrasound images of the upper outer quadrants of the right (a) and left (b) breasts.

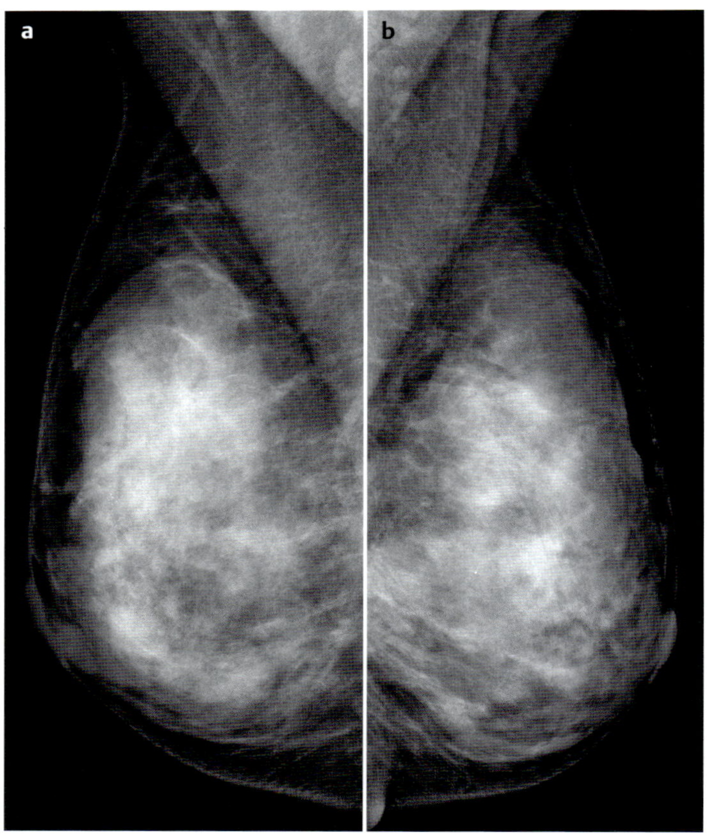

Fig. 33.2 a, b Digital mammography, MLO view.

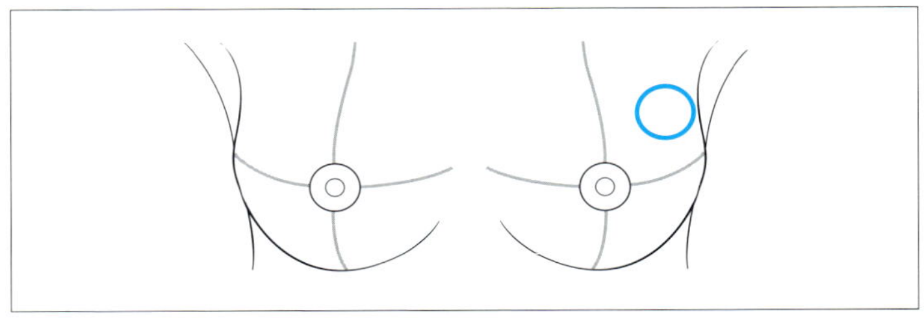

## Clinical Findings

Resistance in the left upper outer quadrant.

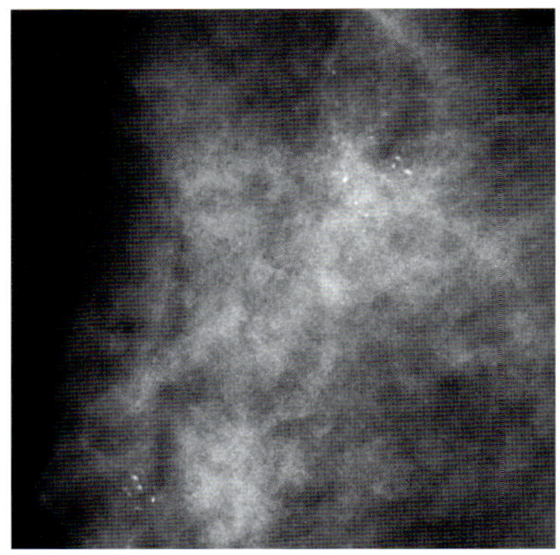

Fig. 33.3 Magnification view of the upper quadrants, right breast.

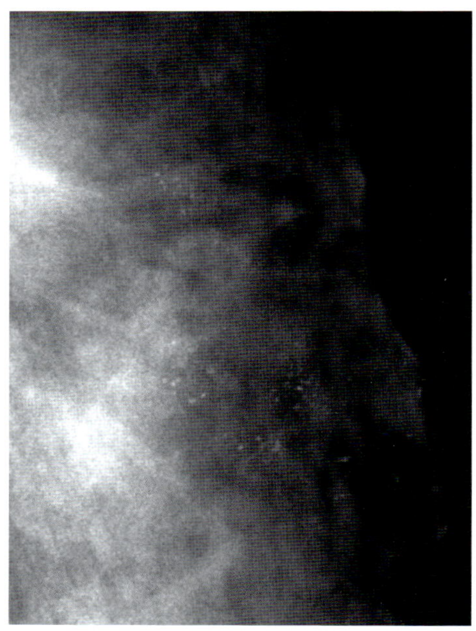

Fig. 33.4 Magnification view of the upper quadrants, left breast.

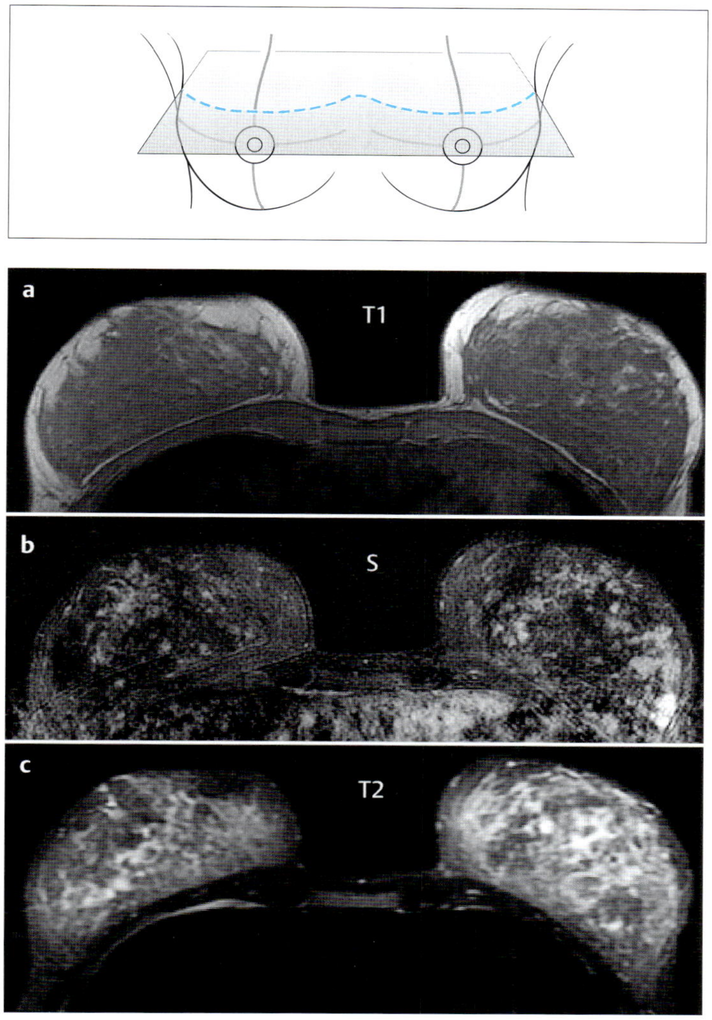


Fig. 33.**5 a – c** Contrast-enhanced MR mammography.

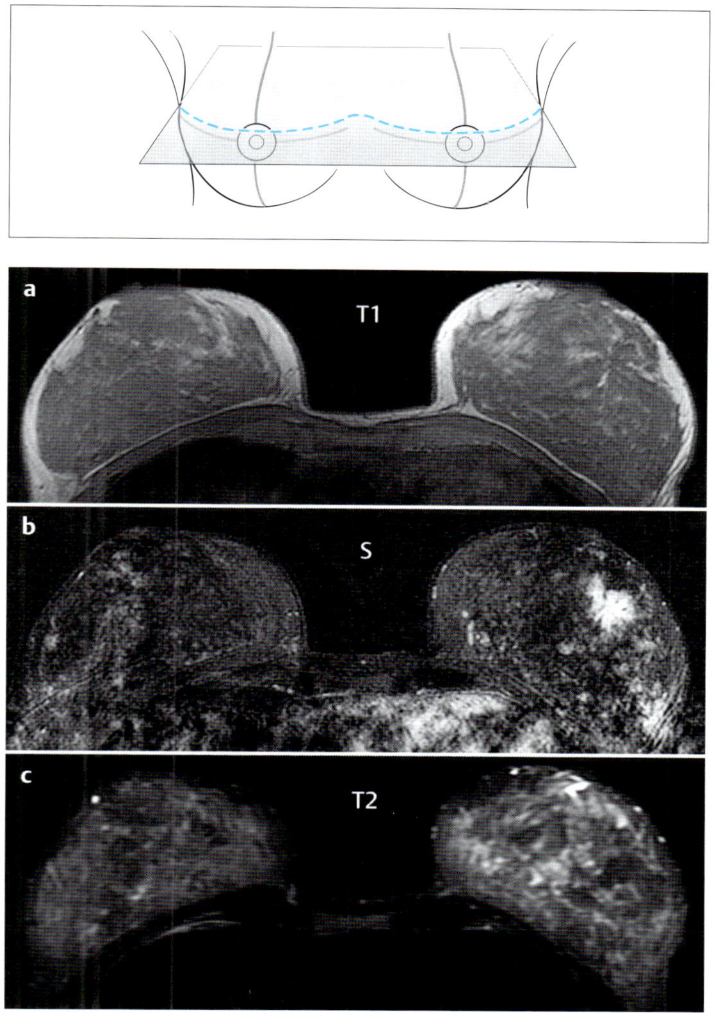


Fig. 33.**6 a – c** Contrast-enhanced MR mammography.

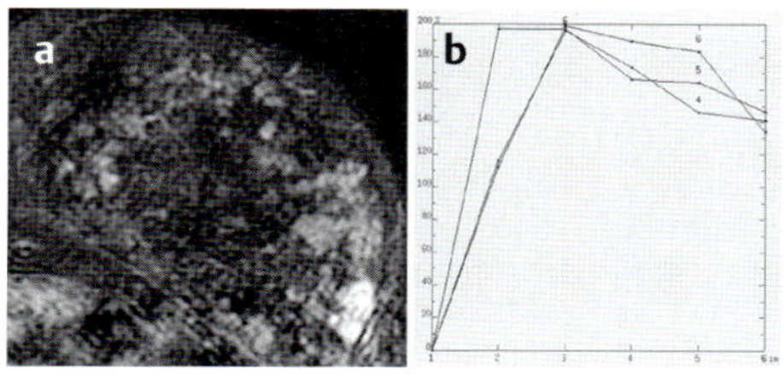


Fig. 33.**7 a, b** Signal-to-time curves.

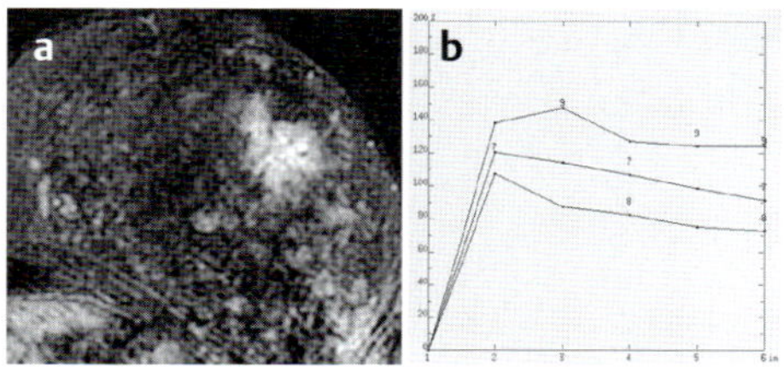


Fig. 33.**8 a, b** Signal-to-time curves.

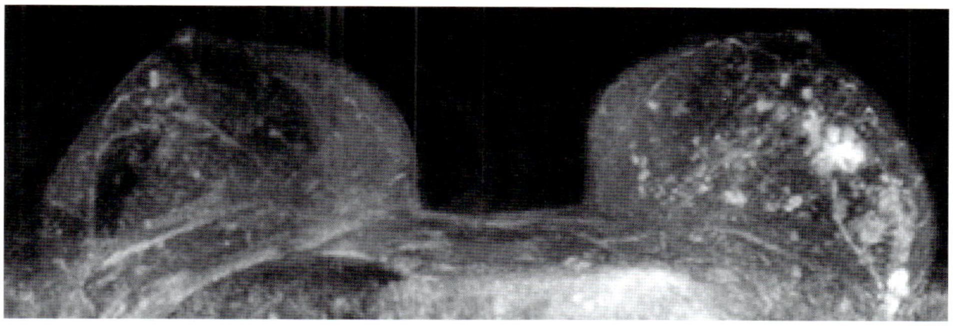

Fig. 33.**9** Contrast-enhanced MR mammography. Maximum intensity projection.

?

Please characterize ultrasound, mammography, and MRI findings.
What is your preliminary diagnosis?
What are your next steps?

This case presents the imaging studies of a symptomatic woman with a resistance in the left breast. The positive family history of breast cancer in the mother at the age of 42 years makes a high familial risk very probable.

### Ultrasound

Corresponding to the palpable resistance, there was an irregular, hypoechoic lesion (diameter 2 cm) with echogenic borders and accompanying architectural distortion of the left breast. The right breast showed very inhomogeneous echogenicity but no firm evidence of suspicious lesions. US BI-RADS right 2/left 4.

### Mammography

Mammograms showed bilaterally symmetric, inhomogeneous dense paremchyma, ACR type 3. In the upper outer quadrant of the left breast–over an area 4.4 cm in length–there were segmentally distributed polymorphous microcalcifications. No accompanying densities were detectable. In the right breast, mammography depicted regionally distributed polymorphous microcalcifications in a central location behind the nipple as well as in the upper outer quadrant. No circumscribed densities (BI-RADS right 4/left 5). PGMI: MLO view G (inframammary fold incorrectly positioned).

### MR Mammography

Corresponding to the sonographic findings, MRI depicted an irregular, inhomogeneously vascularized, spiculated mass between the outer quadrants of the left breast. Signal behavior of this mass was indicative of malignancy. MRI also showed another lesion in the upper outer quadrant of the left breast with clear criteria of malignancy. Both lesions had reduced signal in T2-weighted imaging. There was no suspicious enhancement in the right breast. MRI BI-RADS right 1/left 5 (multicentricity).

**MRI Artifact Category:** 2
**MRI Density Type:** 2

| MRM score | Left breast, upper outer quadrant | Points | Left breast, outer quadrants near nipple | Points |
|---|---|---|---|---|
| **Shape** | irregular | 1 | lobulated | 0 |
| **Border** | spiculated | 1 | ill-defined | 1 |
| **CM Distribution** | inhomogenous | 1 | inhomogeneous | 1 |
| **Initial Signal Intensity Increase** | strong | 2 | strong | 2 |
| **Post-initial Signal Intensity Character** | wash-out | 2 | wash-out | 2 |
| **MRI score (points)** | | **7** | | **7** |
| **MRI BI-RADS** | | **5** | | **5** |

### → Differential Diagnosis

Left: Invasive carcinoma, DCIS.
Right: DCIS, adenosis.

| BI-RADS Categorization | | |
|---|---|---|
| Clinical Findings | right 1 | left 5 |
| Ultrasound | right 2 | left 4 |
| Mammography | right 4 | left 5 |
| MR Mammography | right 1 | left 5 |
| **BI-RADS Total** | **right 4** | **left 5** |

### Procedure

**Left breast:** US-guided core biopsy of ultrasound finding for histological analysis.

**Right breast:** Stereotactic vacuum core biopsy of the microcalcifications for histological analysis. (Figs. 33.**10** and 33.**11**)

### Histology of the specimens

**Left breast:** Invasive ductal carcinoma.

**Right breast:** Ductal carcinoma in situ (Fig. 33.**11**).

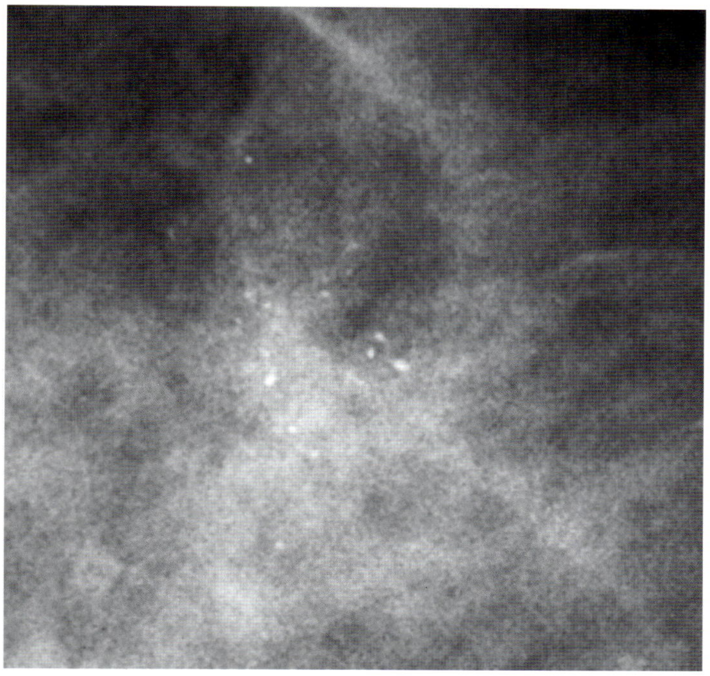

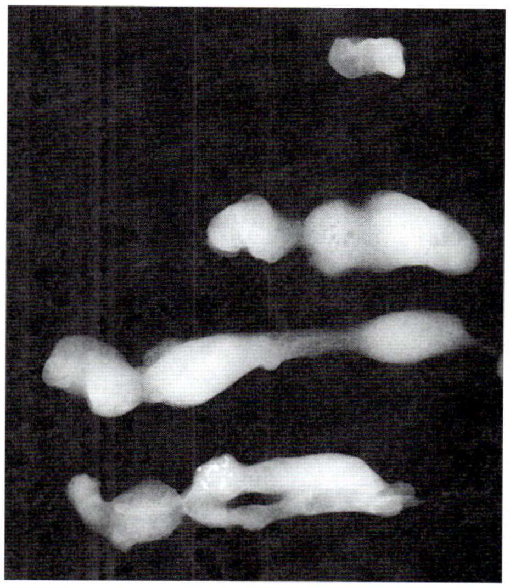

Fig. 33.**11** Specimen radiography with positive findings of microcalcifications.

## Histology

Left breast: Multicentric, invasive ductal carcinoma, axillary lymph node status normal.
Right breast: Ductal carcinoma in situ (van Nuys score 2).

Left: IDC pT1b (multicentric), pN0, G2.
Right: DC pTis, pN0, G2.

## Treatment

Bilateral mastectomy was indicated because of the high risk associated with bilateral carcinoma and positive family history.

Approximately 5 % of women with breast cancer also have contralateral carcinomas.

**Indication:** Screening.
**History:** Bilateral implants 30 years previously to correct anisomastia.
**Risk profile:** Not increased.
**Age:** 53 years.

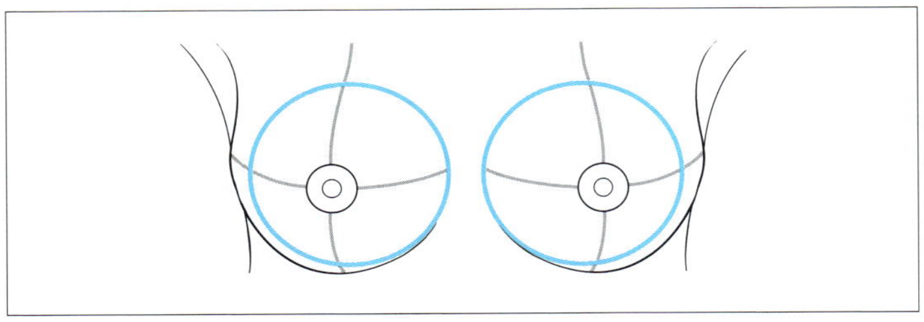

### Clinical Findings

Regular asymptomatic scars bilaterally.

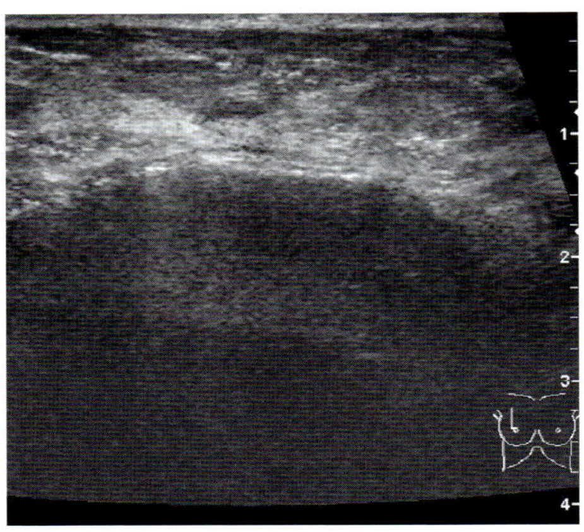


Fig. 34.**1** Ultrasound image, right breast.

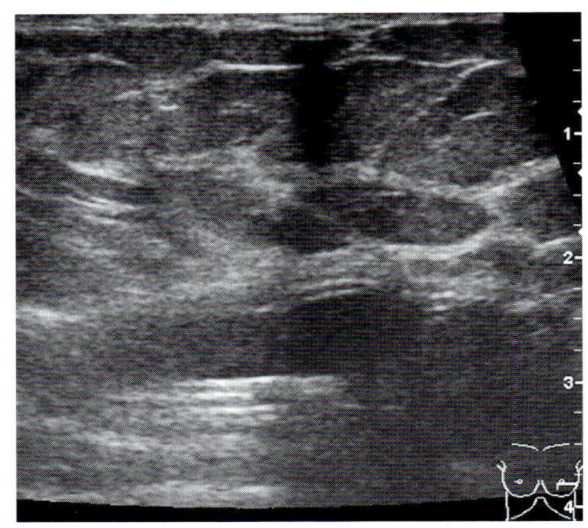


Fig. 34.**2** Ultrasound image, left breast.

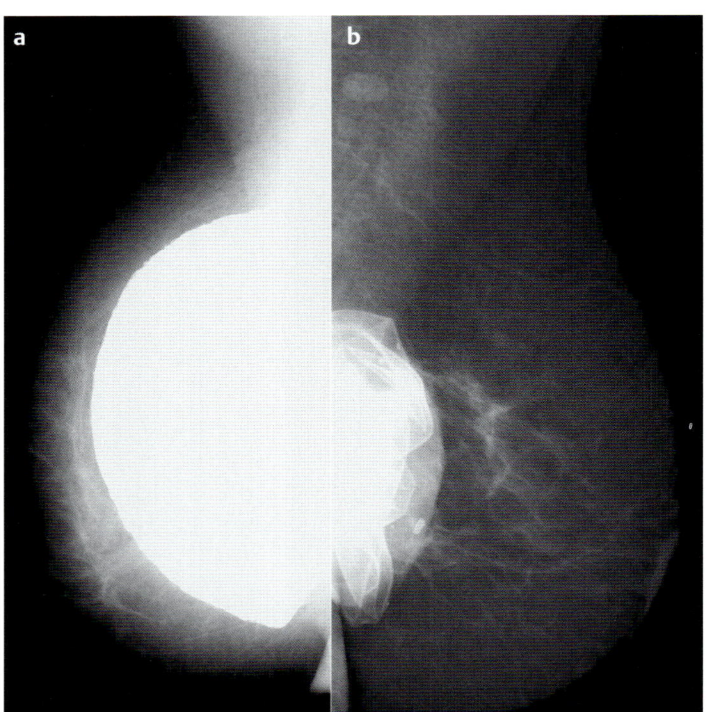


Fig. 34.**3 a, b** Digital mammograpy, MLO view.

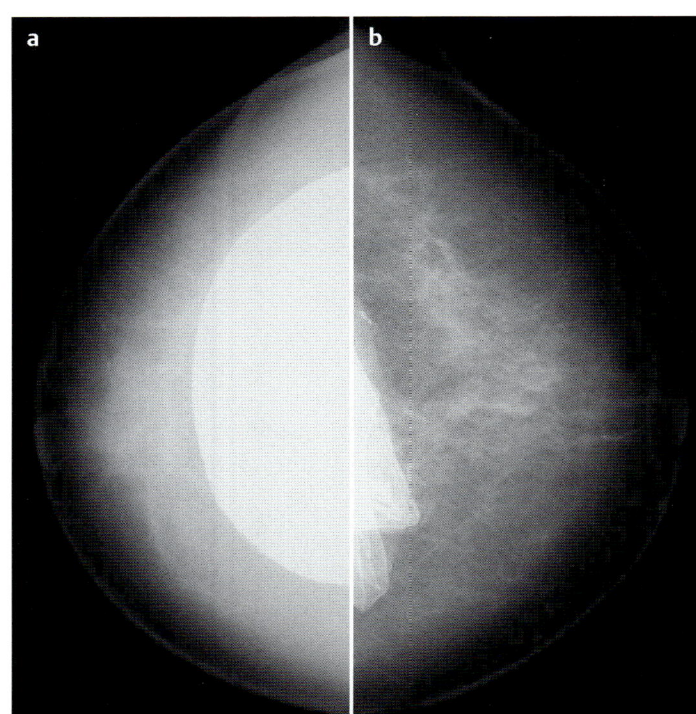


Fig. 34.**4 a, b** Digital mammography, CC view.

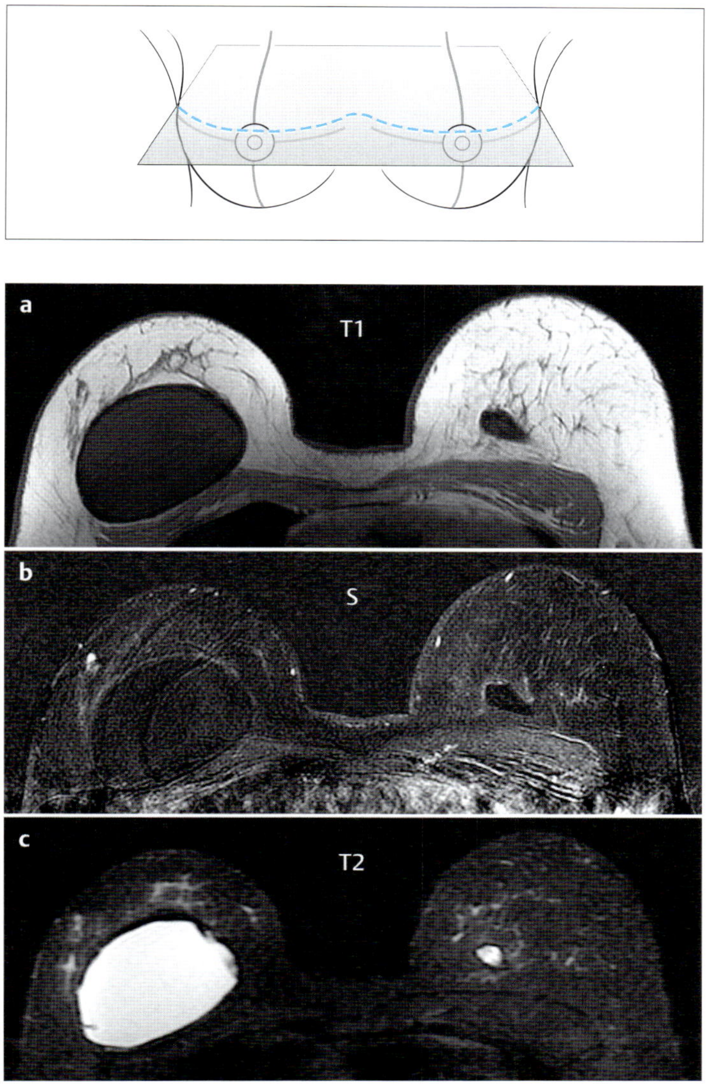


Fig. 34.5 **a – c** Contrast-enhanced MRI of the breasts.

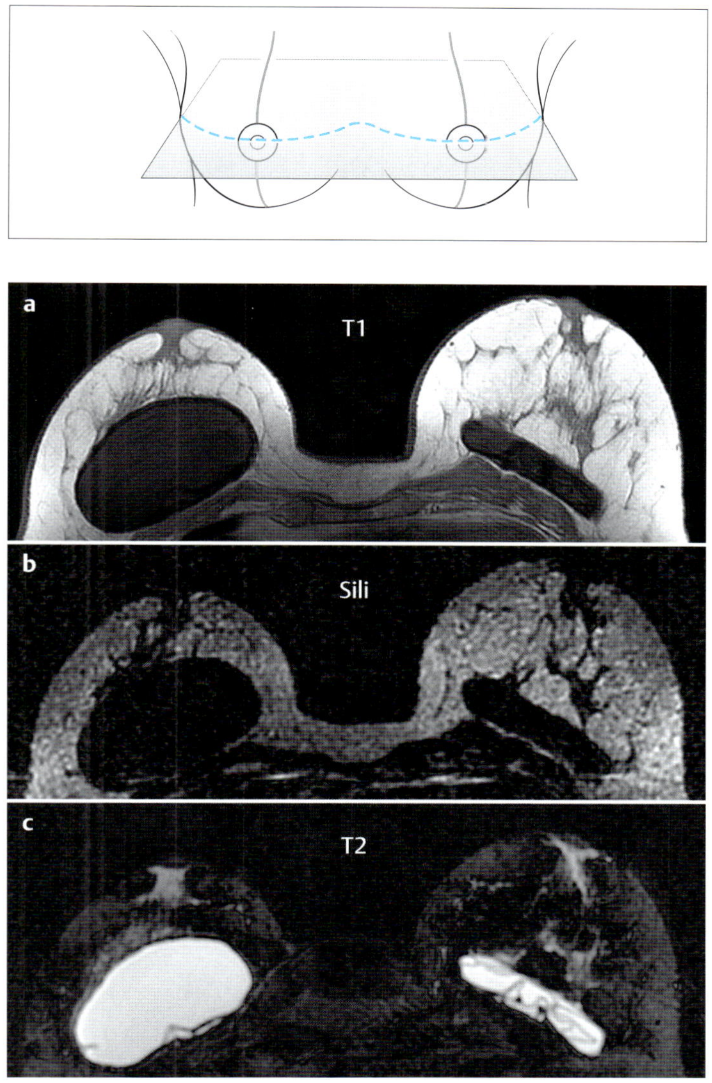


Fig. 34.6 **a – c** Contrast-enhanced MRI of the breasts.

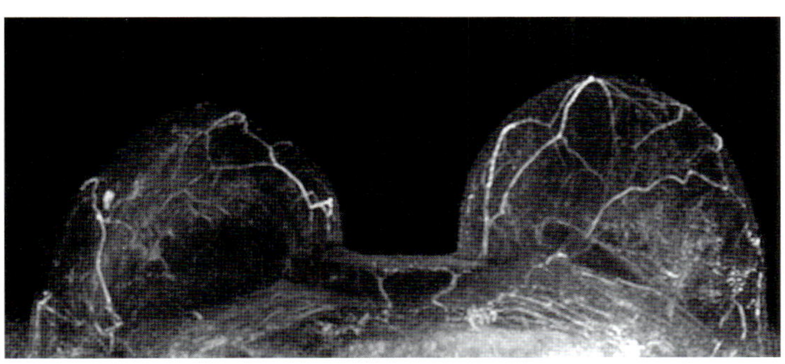

Fig. 34.**7** Contrast-enhanced MR mammography. Maximum intensity projection.

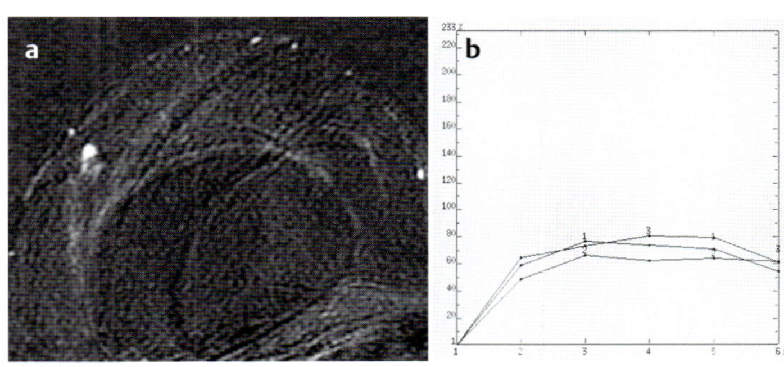


Fig. 34.**8 a, b** Signal-to-time curves.

?

Please characterize ultrasound, mammography, and MRI findings.
What kind of implants do you see?
What is your preliminary diagnosis?
What are your next steps?

Imaging of an asymptomatic woman with bilateral prostheses inserted 30 years previously to correct anisomastia.

### Ultrasound

Ultrasound showed that the left prosthesis had a markedly smaller volume than the right. There were no other unusual findings. US BI-RADS right 1/left 1.

### Mammography

Images showed a fibroglandular parenchyma, ACR type 2. There were no suspicious lesions and no architectural distortions. Mammography demonstrated no suspicious microcalcifications. Left mammography showed a collapsed prosthesis with clumped calcifications. BI-RADS right 1/left 1. PGMI is not defined for implant images.

### MR Mammography

MRI documented the collapsed left implant. It depicted a single-lumen saline-filled implant (no adequate signal in silicon sequences, Fig. 34.**6 b**). MRI also depicted a well-defined, hypervascularized focus of 1 cm diameter in the upper outer quadrant of the right breast, which showed nonspecific signal behavior after contrast administration. T2 signal in the focal area was increased. This focus had a lipomatous central area in precontrast T1-weighted imaging.

Have you been able to determine the type of prosthesis involved here?

**MRI Artifact Category:** 2
**MRI Density Type:** 1

| MRM score | Finding right | Points |
|---|---|---|
| **Shape** | round | 0 |
| **Border** | well-defined | 0 |
| **CM Distribution** | homogenous | 0 |
| **Initial Signal Intensity Increase** | moderate | 1 |
| **Post-initial Signal Intensity Character** | plateau | 1 |
| **MRI score (points)** | | **2** |
| **MRI BI-RADS** | | **2** |

### → Diagnosis

Left breast: Complete rupture of the implant (envelope and capsule). No differential diagnosis.

Right breast: Nonspecific lymphadenitis. No differential diagnosis.

| BI-RADS Categorization | | |
|---|---|---|
| Clinical Findings | right 1 | left 1 |
| Ultrasound | right 1 | left 1 |
| Mammography | right 1 | left 1 |
| MR Mammography | right 2 | left 1 |
| **BI-RADS Total** | **right 2** | **left 1** |

### Procedure

None. This woman had saline-only prostheses in both breasts. No intervention was necessary following the complete rupture of the left implant, since the saline content was completely resorbed. The hypervascularized focus in the right breast could be clearly identified as a lymph node due to the fatty hilum visible at its center in MRI. This is therefore categorized as a harmless ancillary finding.

### Remark

Luckily the rupture occurred in the larger breast. Aesthetically, no intervention was required. The uneven calcifications within the capsule did not show criteria of malignancy.

### Diagnosis (without operative or histopathological verification)

Left: Complete rupture of saline implant.
Right: Lymphadenitis.

### Consequences

None.

MR Mammography allows accurate differentiation of the components of breast implants (particularly saline and silicone) by means of specific prosthesis protocols.

**Indication:** Screening.
**History:** Unremarkable; currently undergoing hormone replacement therapy.
**Risk profile:** Breast cancer in an aunt and two cousins.
**Age:** 53 years.

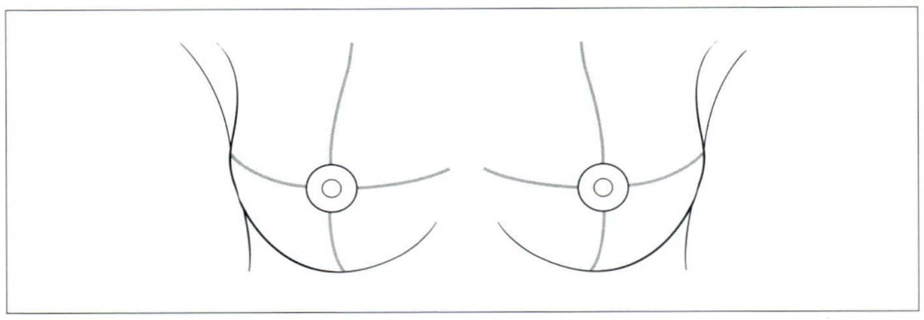

## Clinical Findings

Normal.

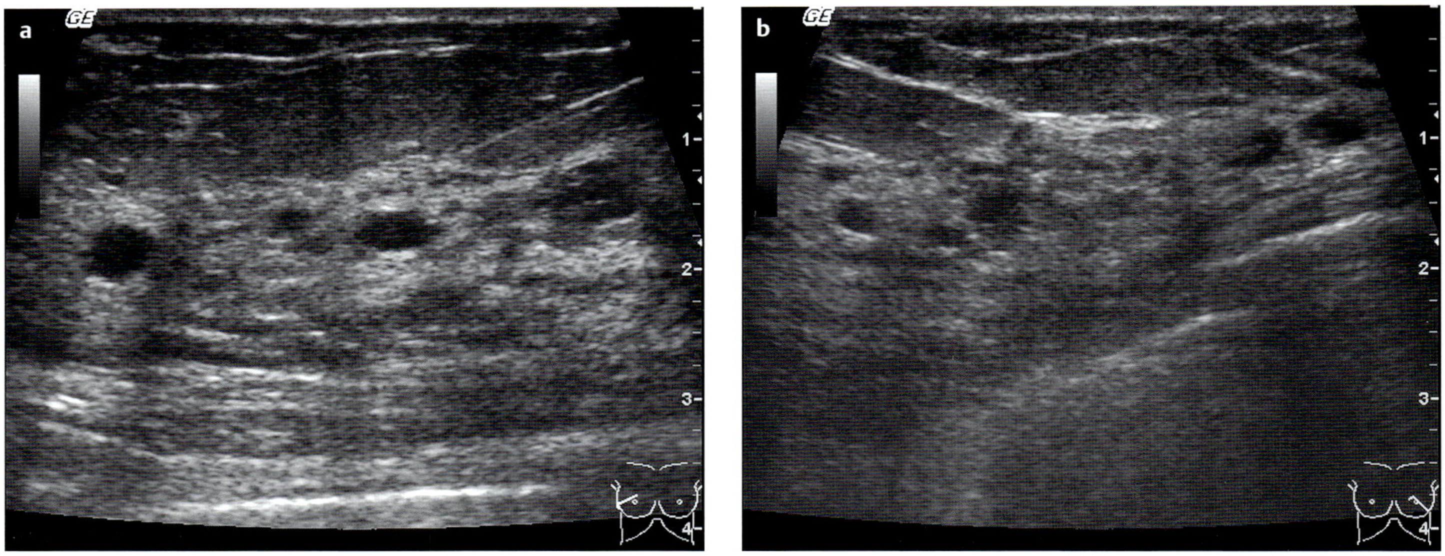

Fig. 35.**1 a, b** Sonography.

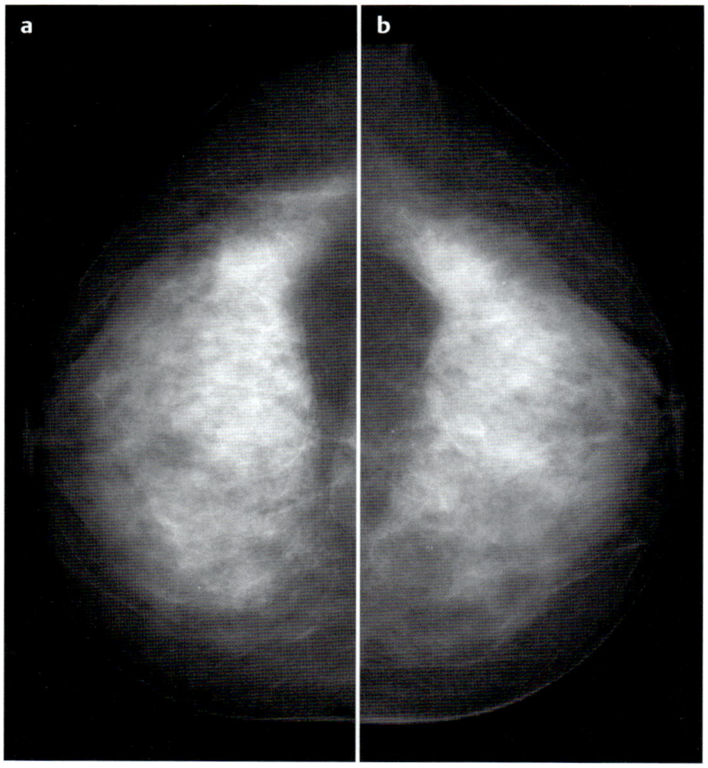

Fig. 35.**2** Digital mammography, CC view.

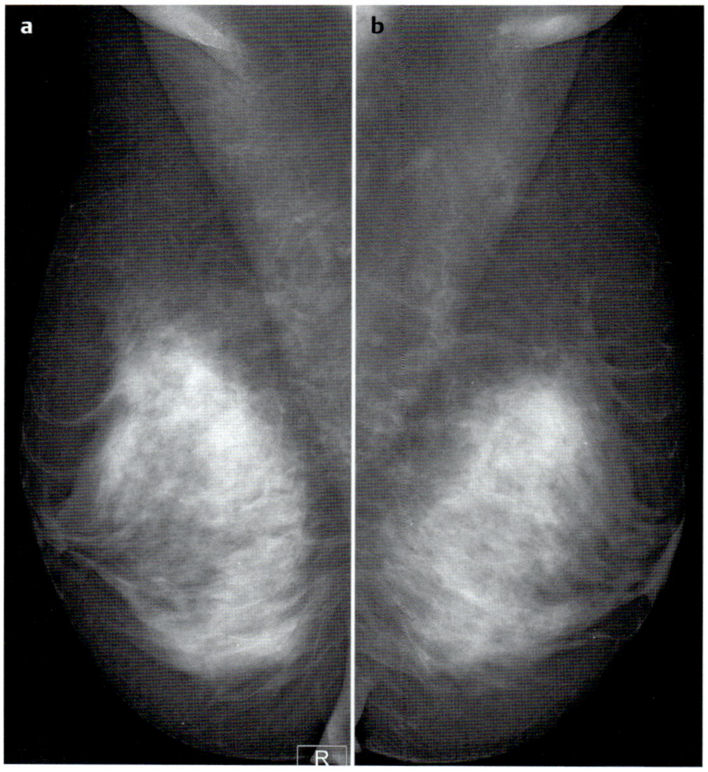

Fig. 35.**3** Digital mammography, MLO view.

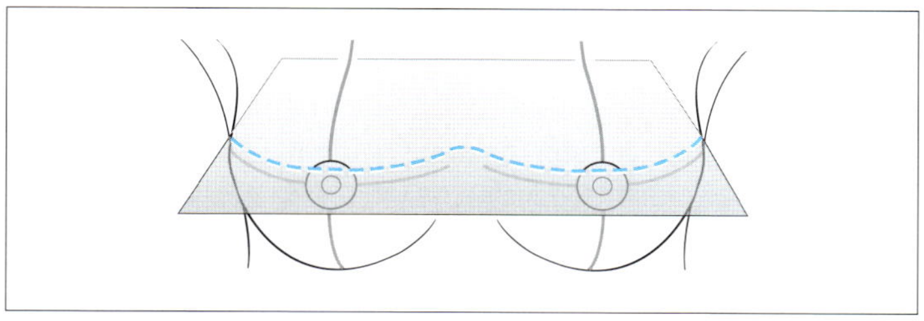

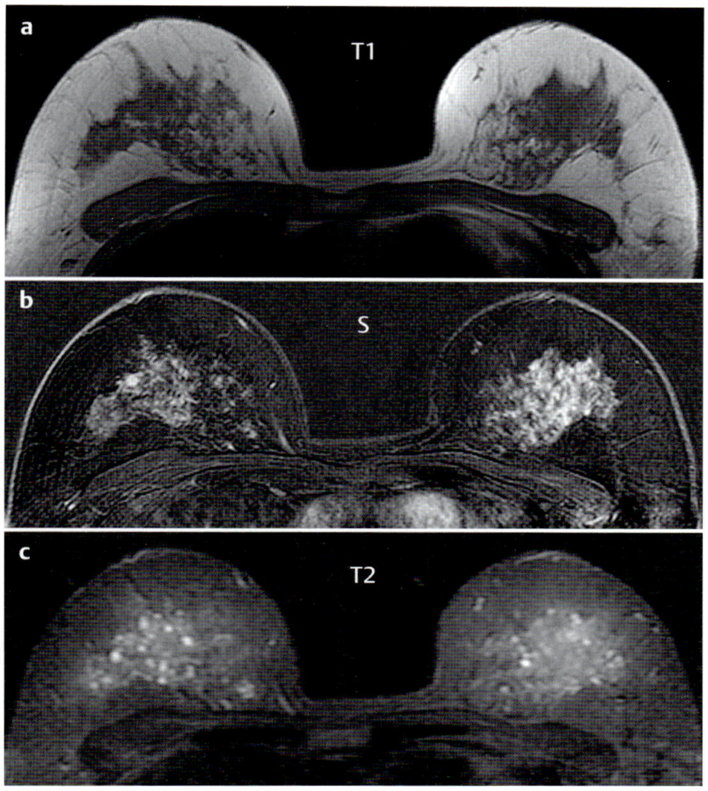


Fig. 35.**4 a – c** Contrast-enhanced MRI of the breasts.

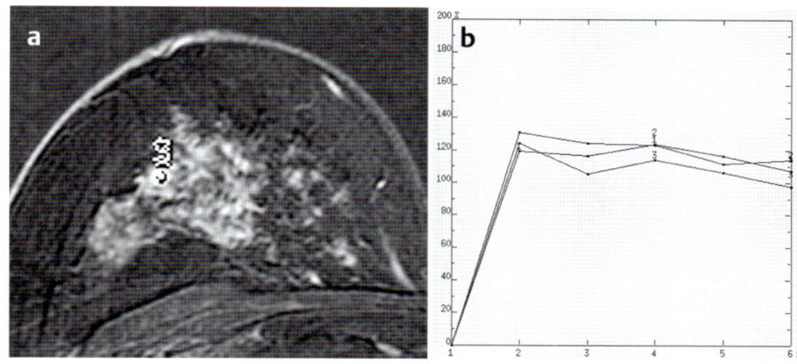


Fig. 35.**6 a, b** Signal-to-time curves.

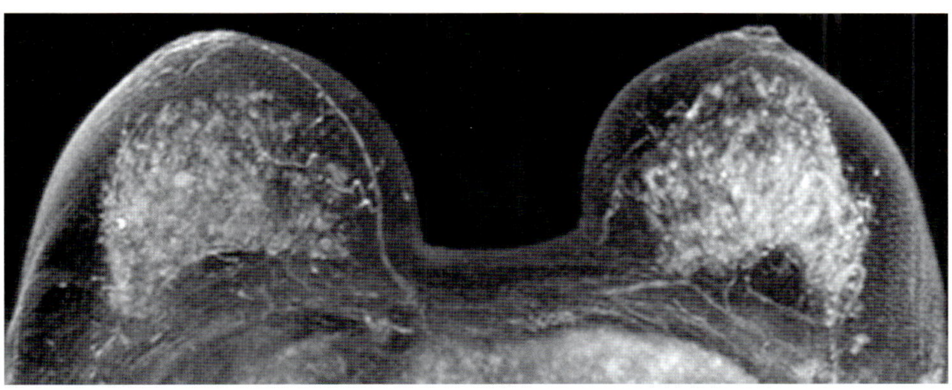

Fig. 35.**5** Contrast-enhanced MR mammography. Maximum intensity projection.

?

Please characterize ultrasound, mammography, and MRI findings.
What is your preliminary diagnosis?
What are your next steps?

Imaging in a screening situation is represented. MRI was performed because the very dense tissue meant that mammograms were inconclusive, and because of the slight familial risk.

### Ultrasound

Ultrasound showed several cysts in the upper outer quadrants of both breasts. There were no suspicious findings. US BI-RADS right 2/left 2.

### Mammography

Mammograms showed bilaterally symmetric, extremely dense tissue, ACR type 4. Under the limitations imposed by these conditions, no abnormalities were visible (no density, no mass, no microcalcifications, no architectural distortion). BI-RADS right 1/left 1. PGMI: CC view I (incomplete presentation of the left inner quadrant); MLO view G (inframammary fold and left nipple incorrectly positioned).

### MR Mammography

Both breasts showed generally strong enhancement of the glandular tissue. In the upper outer quadrant of the right breast there was a circumscribed enhancing lesion of 5 mm diameter with multiple criteria of malignancy (Fig. 35.**7**).

**MRI Artifact Category:** 2
**MRI Density Type:** 4

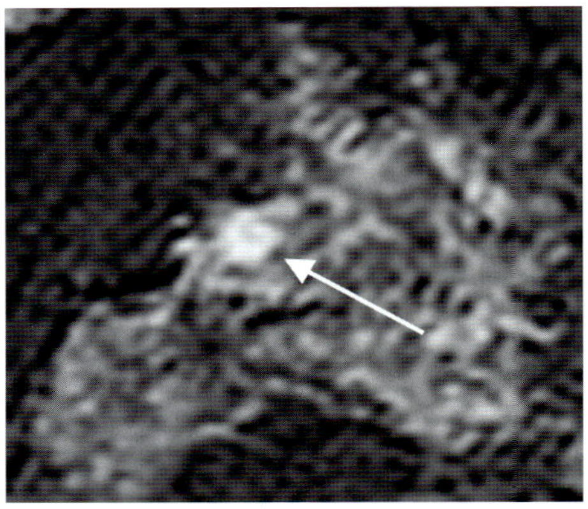

Fig. 35.**7** Lesion in the upper outer quadrant of the right breast.

| MRM score | Finding | Points |
|---|---|---|
| **Shape** | round | 0 |
| **Border** | well-defined | 1 |
| **CM Distribution** | rimsign | 2 |
| **Initial Signal Intensity Increase** | strong | 2 |
| **Post-initial Signal Intensity Character** | wash-out | 2 |
| **MRI score (points)** | | **7** |
| **MRI BI-RADS** | | **5** |

### → Differential Diagnosis

Adenosis (hormonally induced?), carcinoma.

| BI-RADS Categorization | | |
|---|---|---|
| Clinical Findings | right 1 | left 1 |
| Ultrasound | right 2 | left 2 |
| Mammography | right 1 | left 1 |
| MR Mammography | right 5 | left 1 |
| **BI-RADS Total** | **right 5** | **left 1** |

**Procedure (Option 1)**

MR-guided percutaneous vacuum biopsy of the focal enhancing lesion in the upper outer quadrant of the right breast.

**Alternative (Option 2)**

Repeat imaging studies 4 – 6 weeks after stopping the hormone replacement therapy (Figs. 35.**8**–35.**10**).

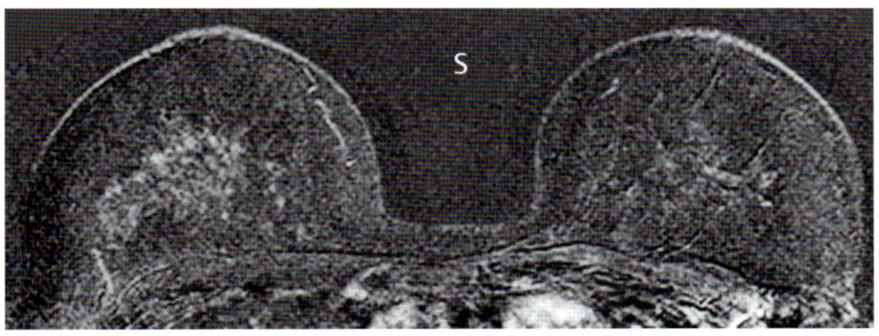


Fig. 35.**8** MR imaging six weeks after cease of hormone replacement therapy.

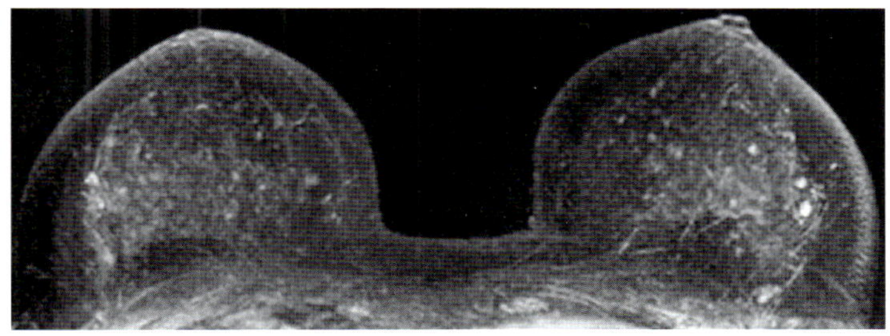

Fig. 35.**9** Maximum intensity projection after cease of hormone replacement therapy.

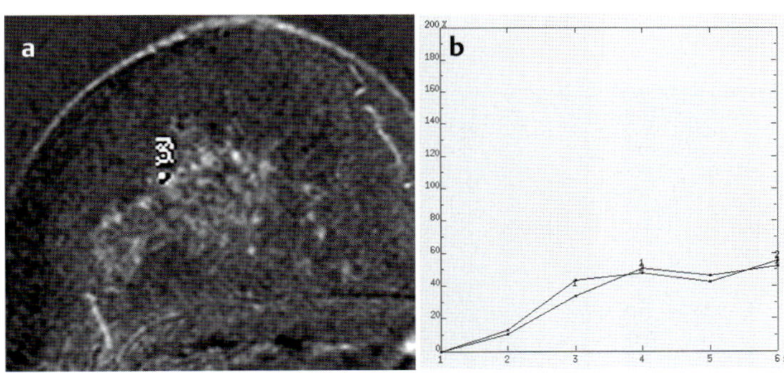


Fig. 35.**10 a, b** Signal-to-time curves after cease of hormone replacement therapy.

## Diagnosis (without histopathological verification)

Hormonally-induced focal enhancement in the right breast. Normalization after stopping hormone replacement therapy.

## Treatment

None.

Hormonally-induced spotty enhancement in MRI can mimic malignant tumors.

**Indication:** Resistance in the right breast.
**History:** Unremarkable.
**Risk profile:** No increased risk.
**Age:** 39 years.

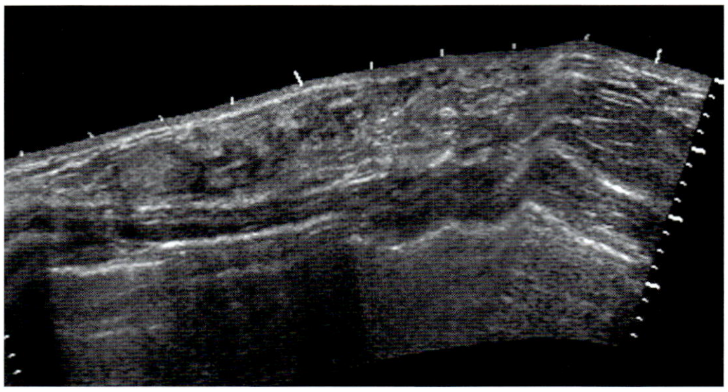

Fig. 36.1 Sonography of the right breast. Panoramic view.

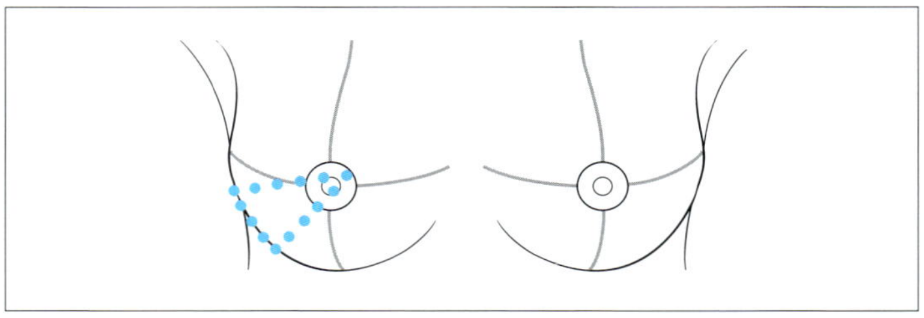

## Clinical Findings

Segmental resistance in the lower outer quadrant of the right breast.

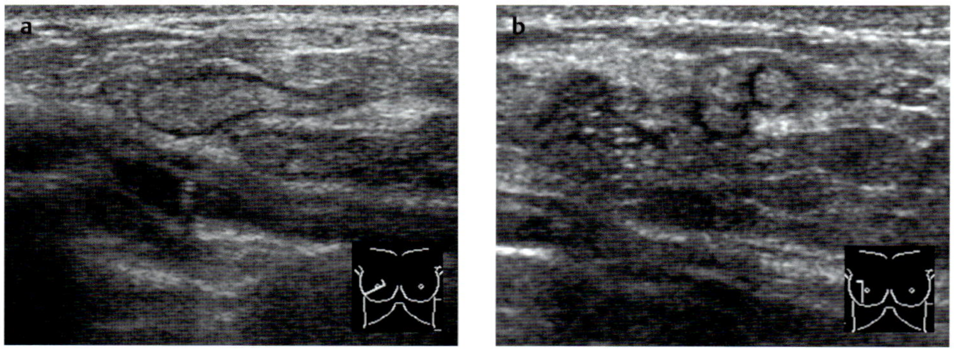

Fig. 36.2 a, b Sonography.

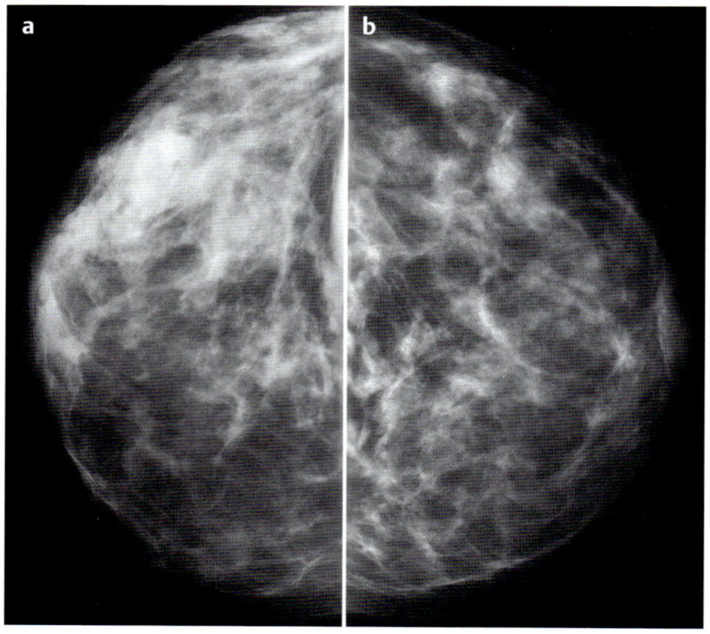

Fig. 36.3 a, b Conventional mammography, CC view [imaging not performed by authors].

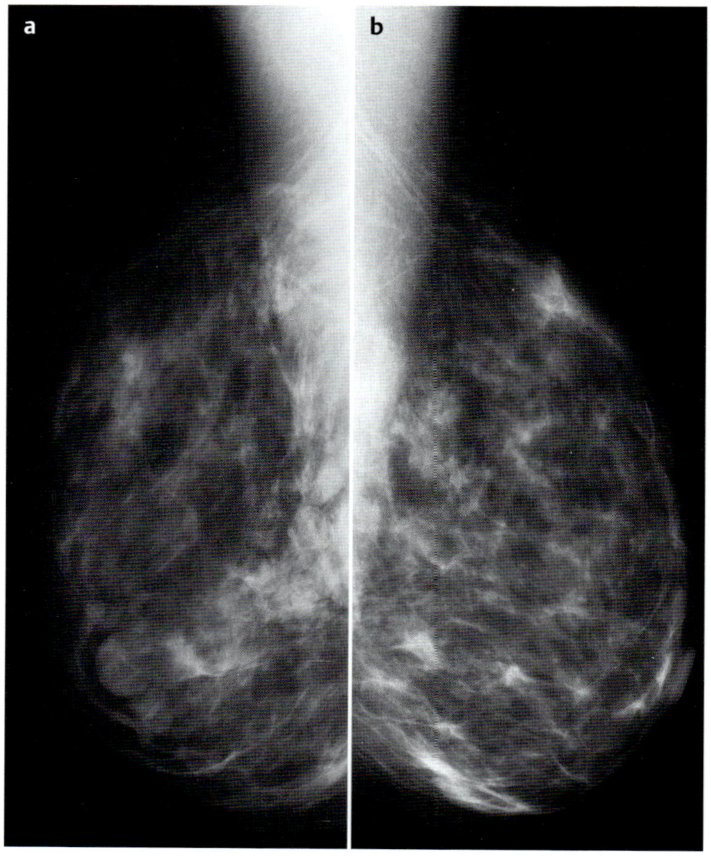

Fig. 36.4 a, b Conventional mammography, MLO view [imaging not performed by authors].

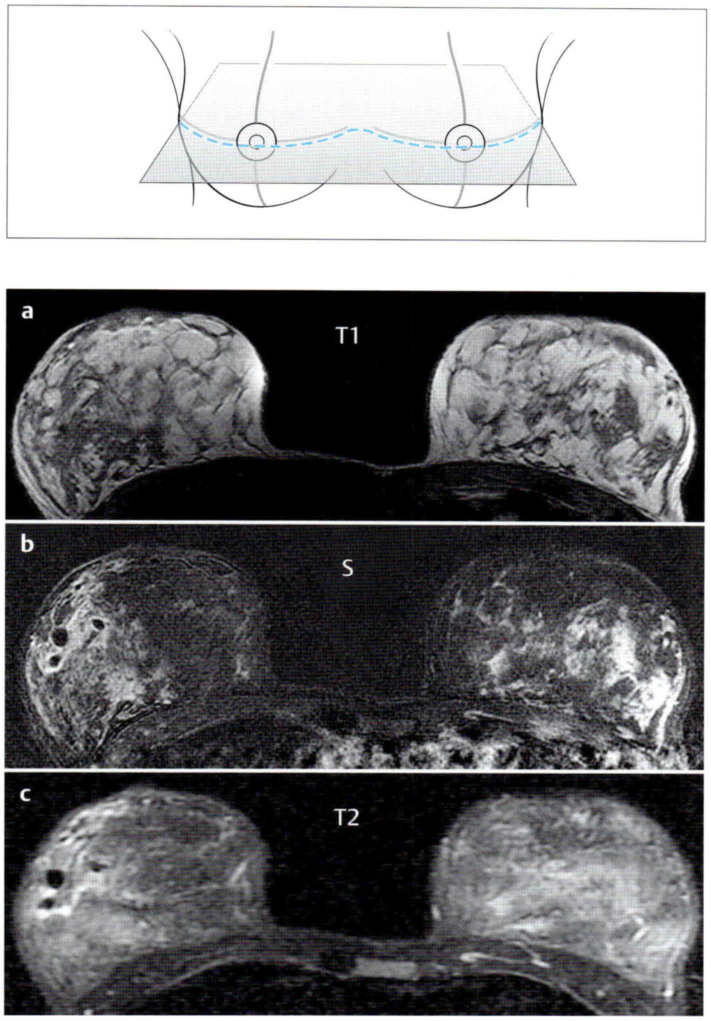


Fig. 36.**5 a – c** Contrast-enhanced MRI of the breasts.

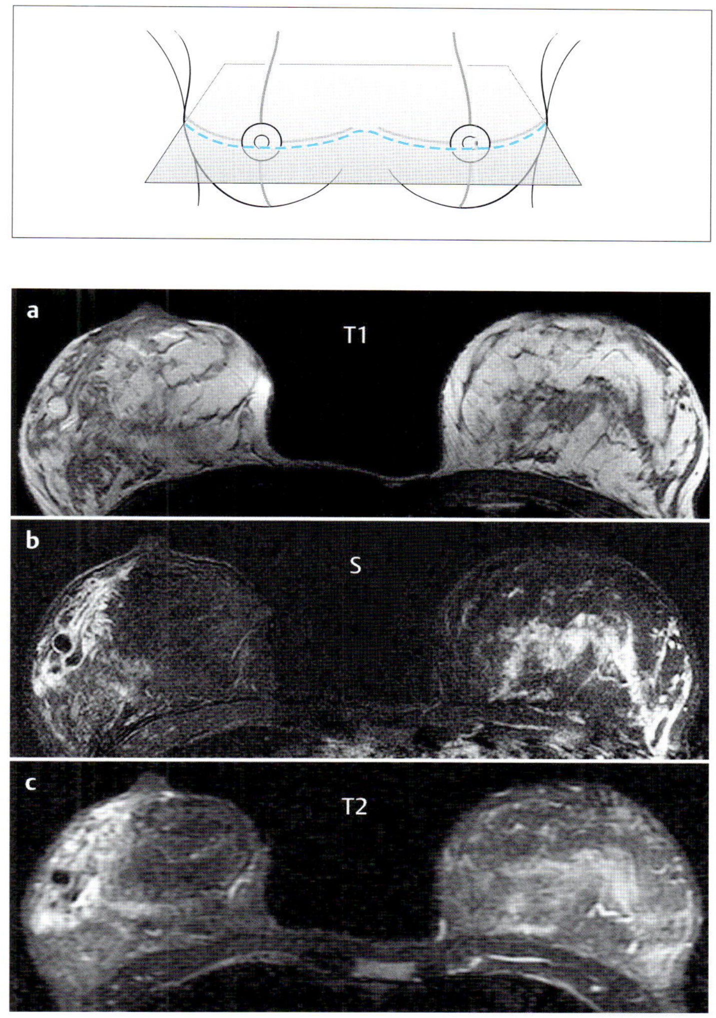


Fig. 36.**6 a – c** Contrast-enhanced MRI of the breasts.

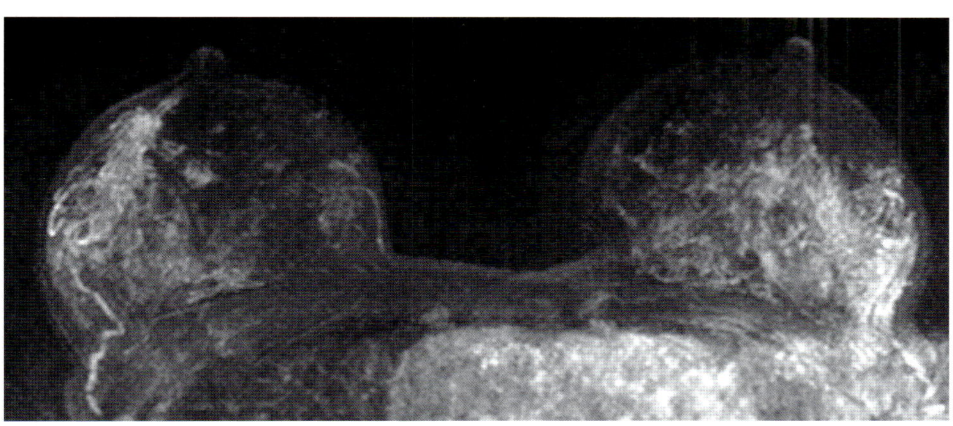

Fig. 36.**7** Contrast-enhanced MR mammography. Maximum intensity projection.

?

Please characterize ultrasound, mammography, and MRI findings.
What is your preliminary diagnosis?
What are your next steps?

This case illustrates the imaging of a symptomatic woman with a palpable segmental resistance of the right breast.

## Ultrasound

In the same area as the palpable segmental mass, US demonstrated multiple round lesions of varying sizes, all with homogeneous internal echo pattern and well-defined margins. There were linear hypoechoic structures surrounding each lesion, denoting their intraductal position. US BI-RADS right 3.

## Mammography

Mammograms demonstrated bilaterally, mainly symmetric, inhomogeneous dense tissue, ACR type 3. Positioning of the right breast was inadequate, but round lesions were visible in the lower outer quadrant. There were no densities or architectural distortions. There were no calcifications. BI-RADS right 3/left 1. PGMI: CC view G (nipple not in profile); MLO view I (inadequate positioning of the entire right breast; parenchyma superimposed over the nipple).

## MR Mammography

MRI showed multiple hyperintense round lesions in a segmental orientation in the right breast, consistent with ultrasound and clinical findings. Postcontrast images verified a marked enhancement of the milk duct walls in this area, while the intraductal lesions showed no contrast uptake. These lesions were hypointense in T2-weighted images.

In this case a signal–time curve analysis was not performed, because the intraductal lesions showed no enhancement. It seemed more relevant to perform an accurate analysis of the structures' signal across the different sequences.

| | Signal of the intraductal "lesions" |
|---|---|
| **T1-weighted imaging** | hyperintense |
| **T2-weighted imaging** | hypointense |
| **Enhancement (intraductal)** | none |
| **Enhancement (duct wall)** | strong |

## → Differential Diagnostic Considerations

Intraductal blood pooling (T1 signal ↑, T2 signal ↓)? Intraductal milk retention?

Stenosing milk duct near the nipple? Focal inflammation?

A malignant tumor can be excluded (no enhancement of the intraductal structures, T2 signal ↓).

| BI-RADS Categorization | | |
|---|---|---|
| Clinical Findings | right 4 | left 1 |
| Ultrasound | right 3 | left 1 |
| Mammography | right 3 | left 1 |
| MR Mammography | right 3 | left 1 |
| **BI-RADS Total** | **right 3** | **left 1** |

### Procedure

US-guided fine-needle aspiration cytology to identify the intraductal process in the lower outer quadrant of the right breast.

### Cytology of the right breast

Eosinophilic protein-rich precipitate incorporating copious fat. Also, signs of a focal granulomatous inflammation.

### Further procedure

At the express wish of the young patient, a wait-and-see approach was followed and follow-up sonography was performed at intervals of 2, 6, and 12 weeks. The patient declined repeat mammography to obtain better-quality images of the right breast.
Finding after 20 weeks: Complete resorption of the intraductal fluid.

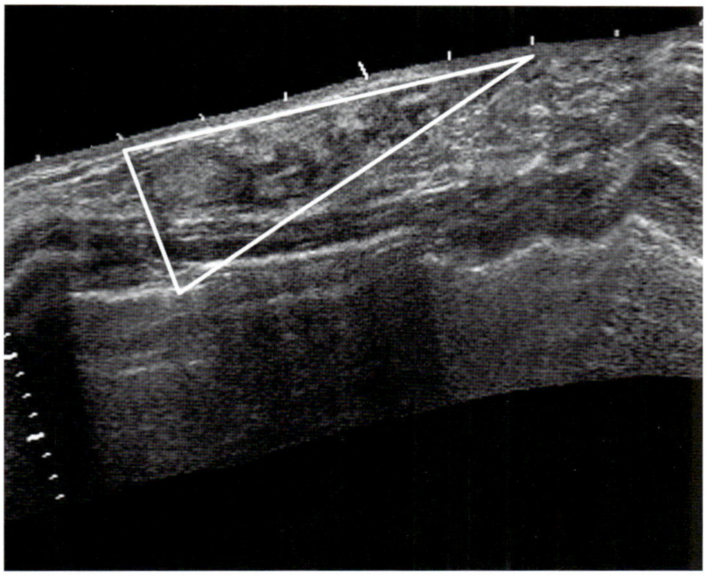

Fig. 36.**8** Segmental distribution of the changes in panoramic view.

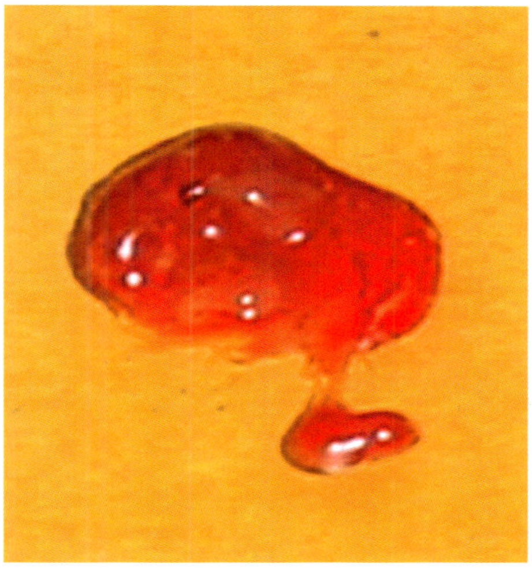

Fig. 36.**9** Viscous fluid in aspirated specimen from the right breast.

## Diagnosis (without histopathological verification)

Segmental inflammation of a milk duct with intraductal fluid retention.

## Treatment

None.

Mammographic images of PGMI category I (inadequate) can result in a few cases. In this event, mammography should always be repeated to obtain better-quality images.

**Indication:** Follow-up after mastectomy.
**History:** Mastectomy of the right breast 4 years previously. Reconstructive surgery.
**Risk profile:** Increased due to earlier breast cancer.
**Age:** 49 years.

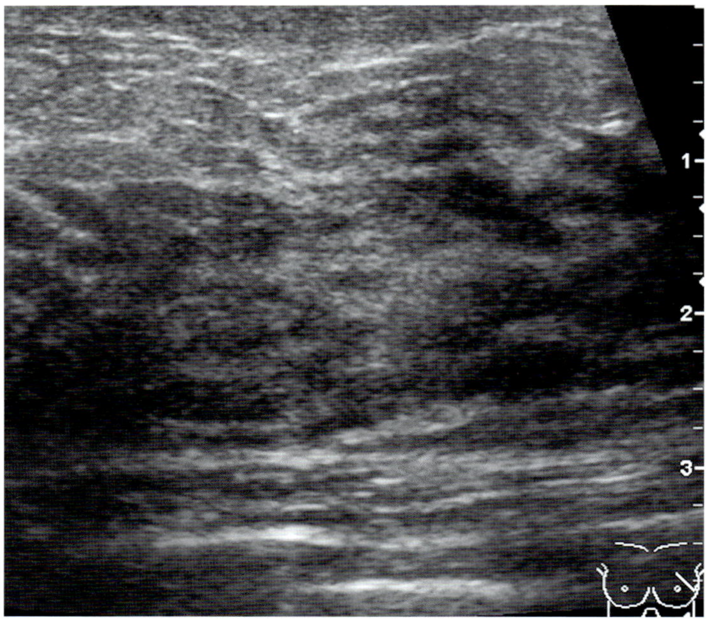


Fig. 37.1 Sonography.

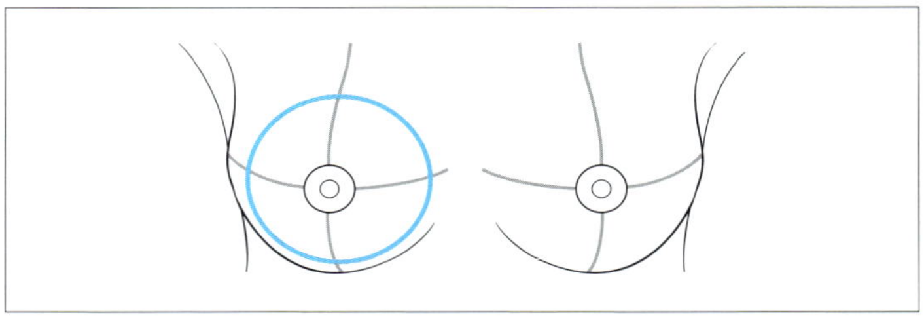

## Clinical Findings

Implant in right breast. No palpable findings in left breast.

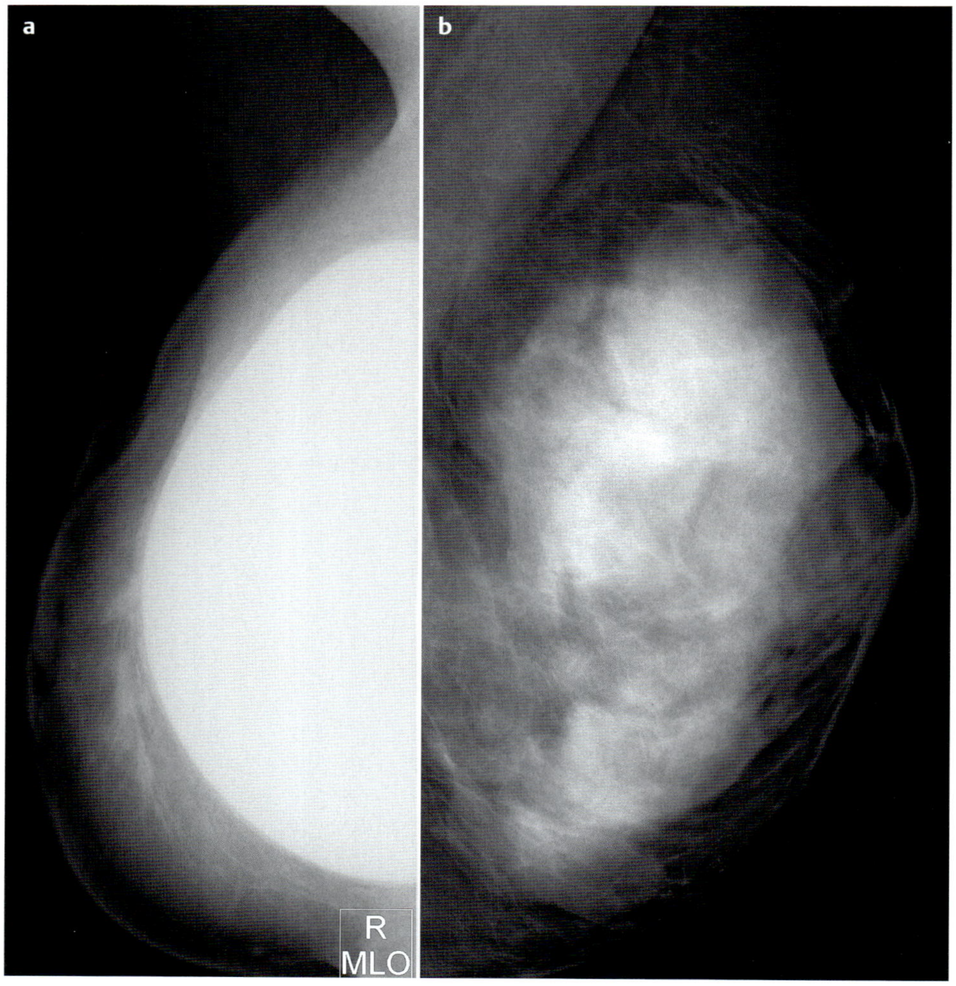


Fig. 37.2 a, b Digital mammography, MLO view.

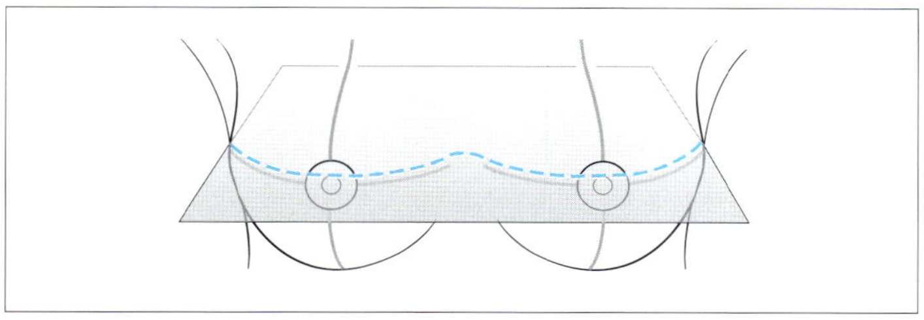

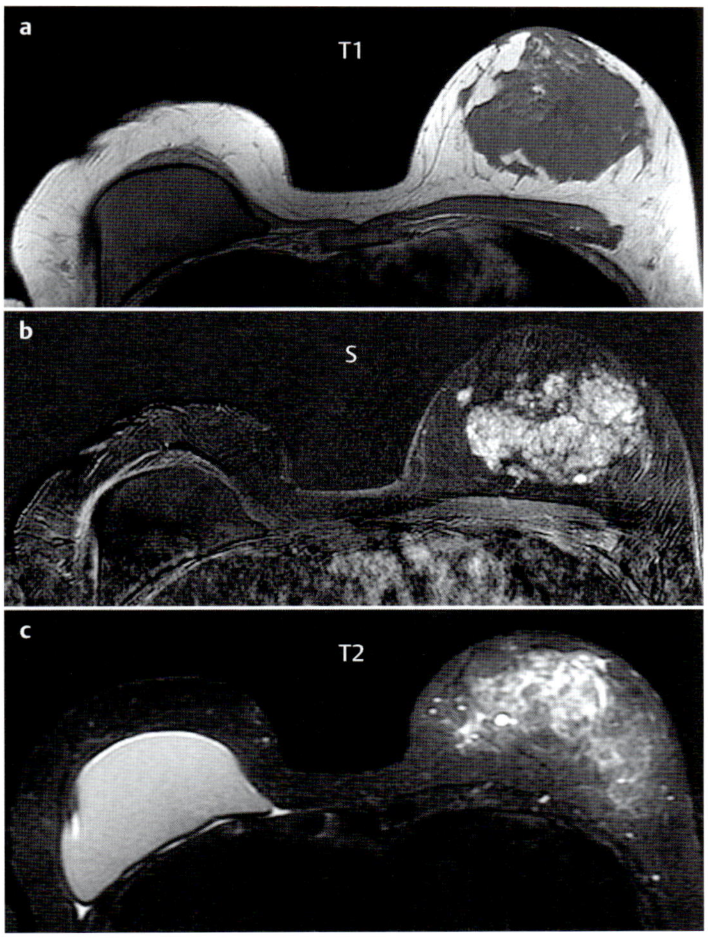


Fig. 37.3 **a–c** Contrast-enhanced MRI of the breasts.

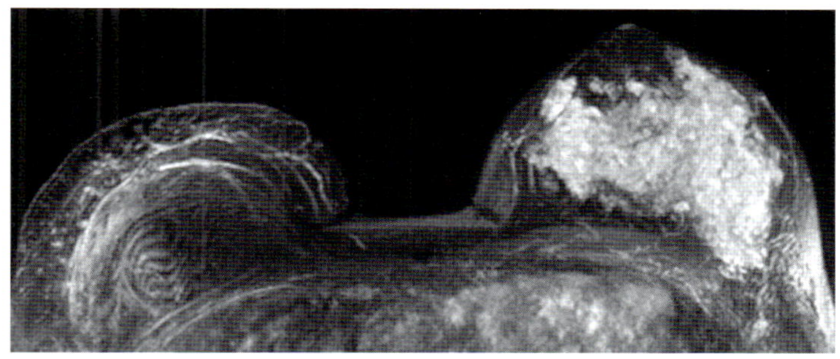

Fig. 37.4 **a–c** Contrast-enhanced MR mammography. Maximum intensity projection.

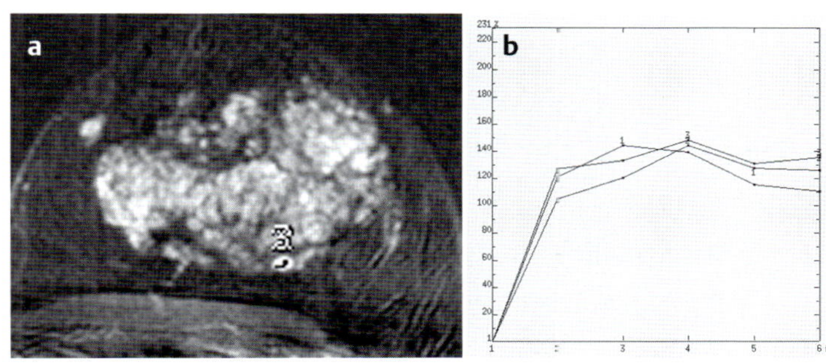


Fig. 37.5 **a, b** Signal-to-time curves.

Please characterize ultrasound, mammography, and MRI findings.
What is your preliminary diagnosis?
What are your next steps?

This case shows the follow-up imaging of an asymptomatic woman who underwent mastectomy and reconstructive surgery of the right breast, and therefore has an increased risk profile.

### Ultrasound

Sonography showed normal glandular tissue in the upper outer quadrant of the left breast, with no unusual findings. US BI-RADS left 1.

### Mammography

The implant in the right breast limited evaluation. No densities or calcifications were visible. The tissue of the left breast was extremely dense, ACR type 4. Under these limiting conditions, no circumscribed densities and no architectural distortion were detected. No calcifications. BI-RADS right 1/left 1. PGMI is not defined for mammograms including implants.

### MR Mammography

Normal MRI of the subpectorally located implant in the right breast.
The parenchyma of the left breast showed diffuse, fine-textured, lobulated enhancement post contrast. Limited by this high vascularization, no circumscribed hypervascularized lesions were visible. Representative signal–time curves in some nodular spotty areas showed a strong initial signal increase followed by a mild washout.

**MRI Artifact Category:** 2
**MRI Density Type:** 4

| MRM score | Finding | Points |
|---|---|---|
| **Shape** | round | 0 |
| **Border** | well-defined | 0 |
| **CM Distribution** | inhomogenous | 1 |
| **Initial Signal Intensity Increase** | strong | 2 |
| **Post-initial Signal Intensity Character** | wash-out | 2 |
| **MRI score (points)** | | **5** |
| **MRI BI-RADS** | | **4** |

## → Preliminary Diagnosis

Extensive adenosis of the left breast.

## Differential Diagnosis

Diffuse breast cancer.

| BI-RADS Categorization | | |
|---|---|---|
| Clinical Findings | right – | left 1 |
| Ultrasound | right – | left 1 |
| Mammography | right – | left 1 |
| MR Mammography | right – | left 4 |
| **BI-RADS Total** | **right –** | **left 4** |

### Procedure

Follow-up MRI in a more suitable week of the menstrual cycle.

### Next Step

US-guided blind biopsy (14 gauge) of the left breast at 1-o'clock, 3-o'clock and 5-o'clock positions.

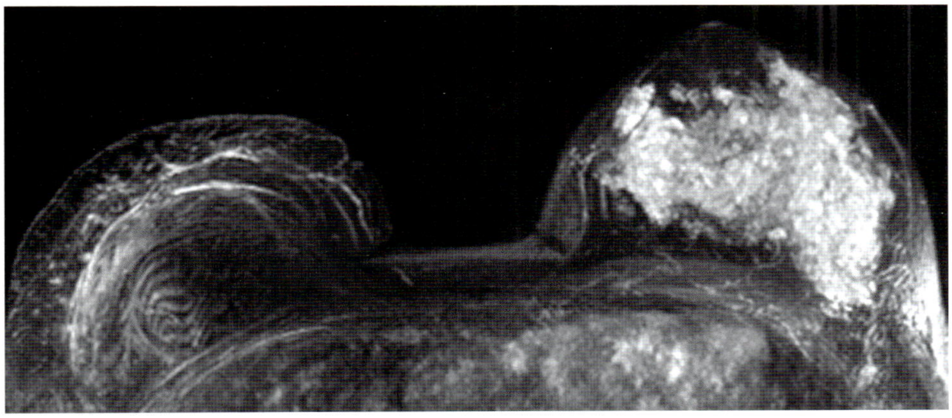

Fig. 37.**6** Original MR mammography. Menstrual cycle week 4.

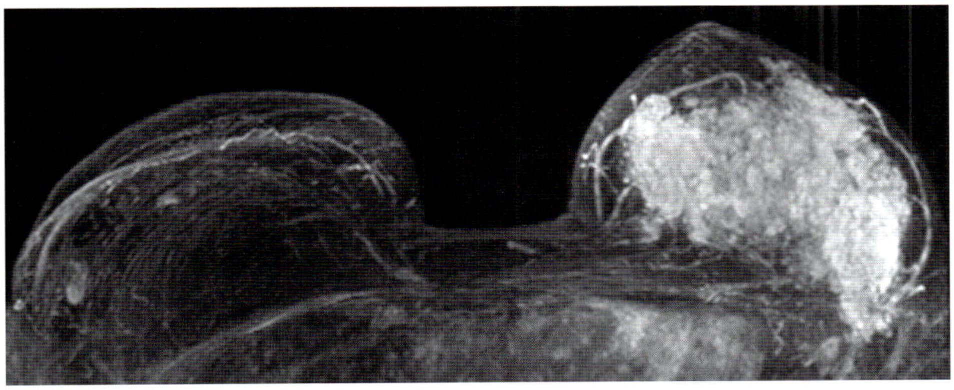

Fig. 37.**7** Follow-up MR mammography. Menstrual cycle week 2. Enhancement pattern identical to primary MRI.

### Histology of the left breast (3 biopsy specimens)

Adenosis.

### Treatment

None. Continued aftercare monitoring for original cancer.

In some rare cases MR imaging shows early, diffuse, strong contrast uptake, which inhibits accurate detection and characterization of suspicious lesions. This situation (MRI density type 4) is comparable to the problems with mammograms of extremely dense tissue (ACR type 4).

**Indication:** Screening.
**History:** Unremarkable.
**Risk profile:** No increased risk.
**Age:** 57 years.

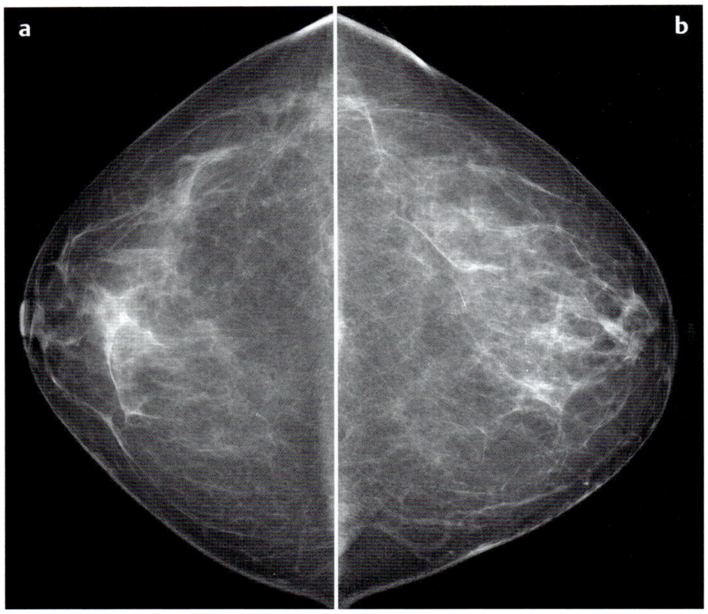

Fig. 38.**1 a, b** Digital mammography, CC view.

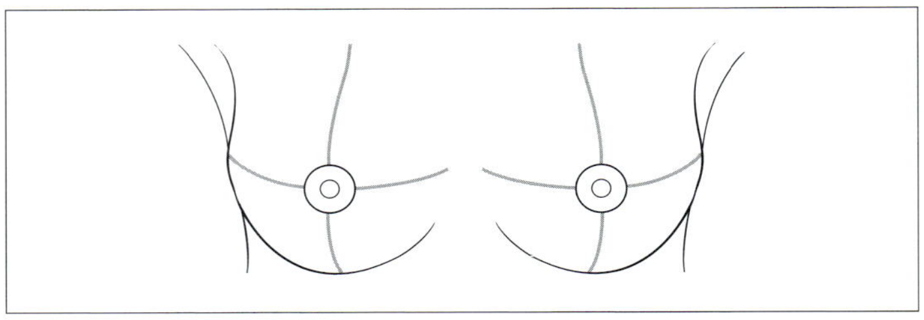

### Clinical Findings

No findings.

### Ultrasound

Unremarkable (not shown).

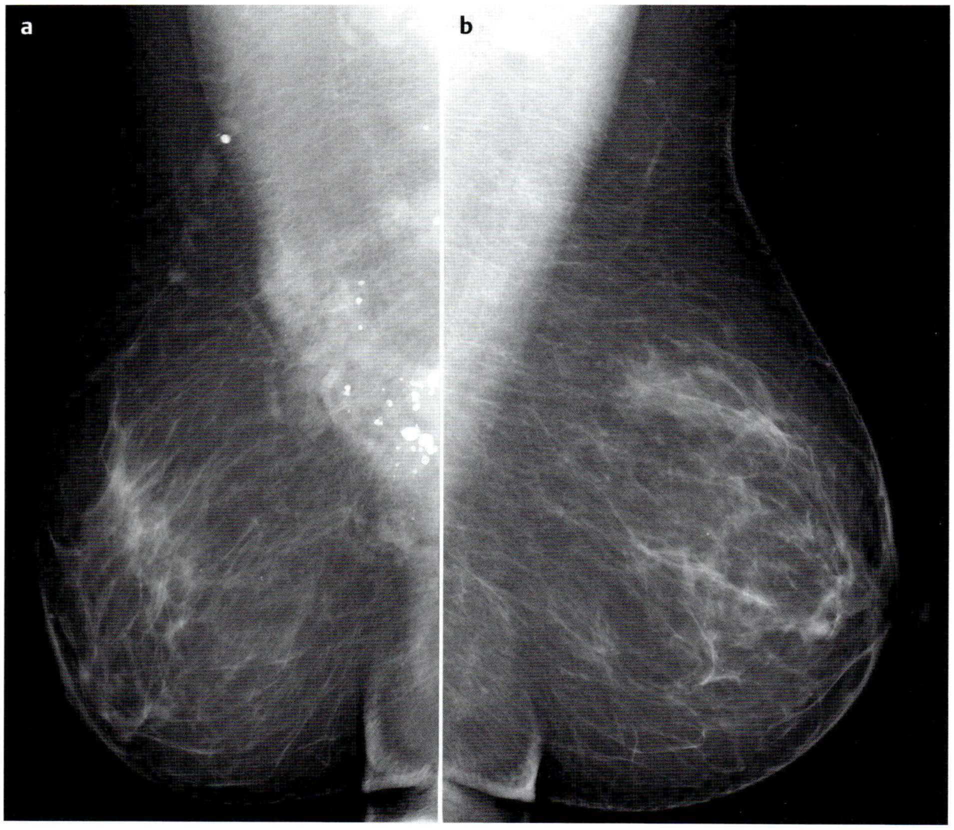

Fig. 38.**2 a, b** Digital mammography, MLO view.

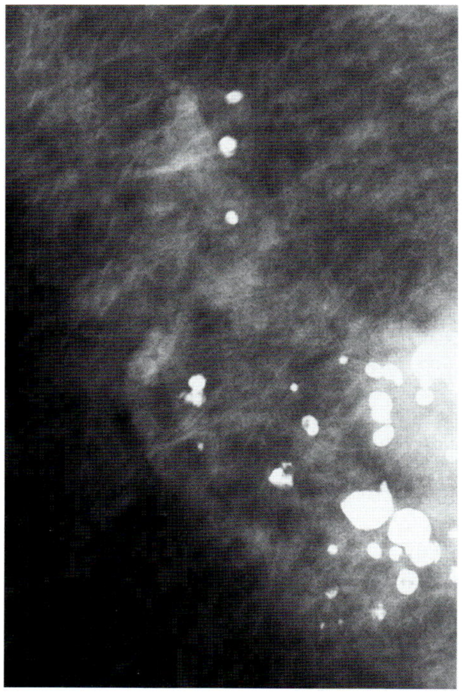

Fig. 38.**3** Magnification view of the right breast.

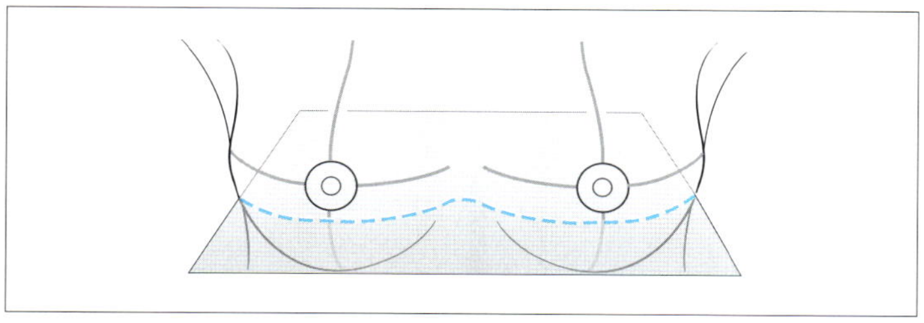

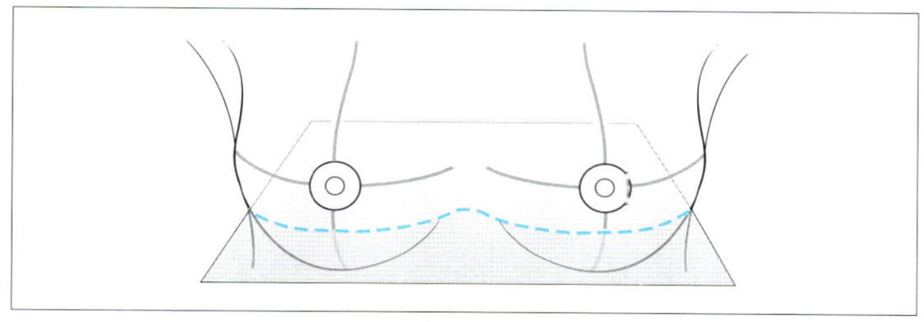

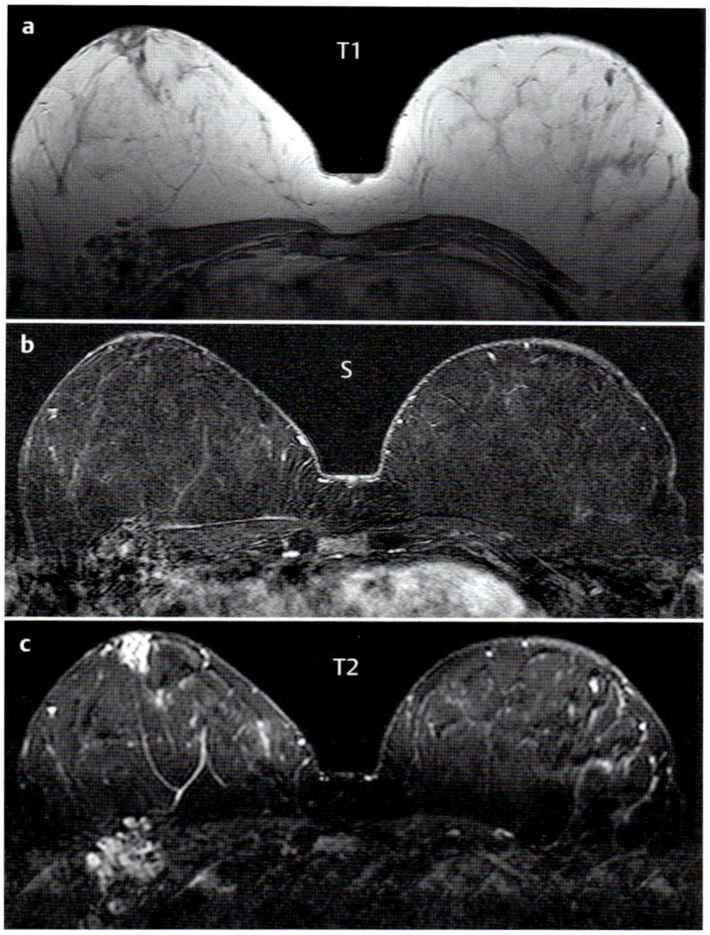


Fig. 38.**4 a – c** Contrast-enhanced MR mammography.

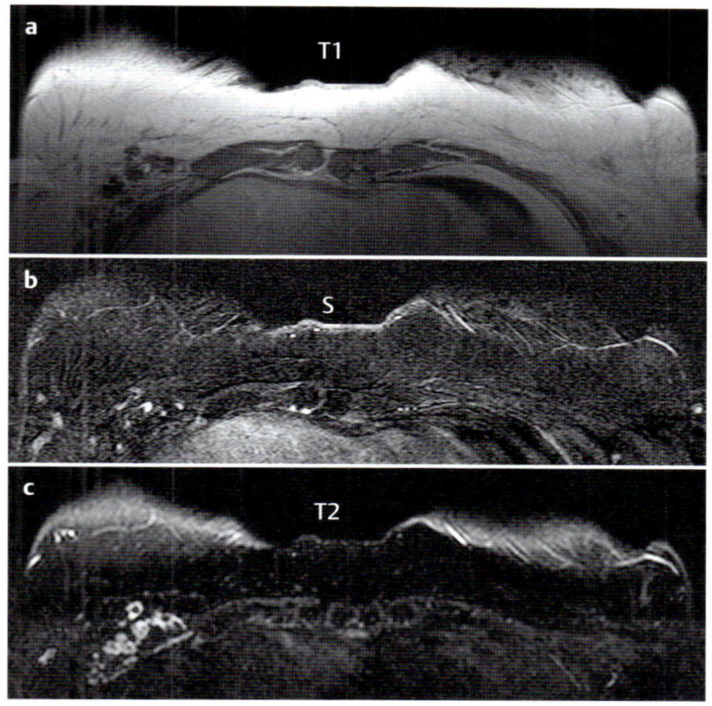


Fig. 38.**5 a – c** Contrast-enhanced MR mammography.

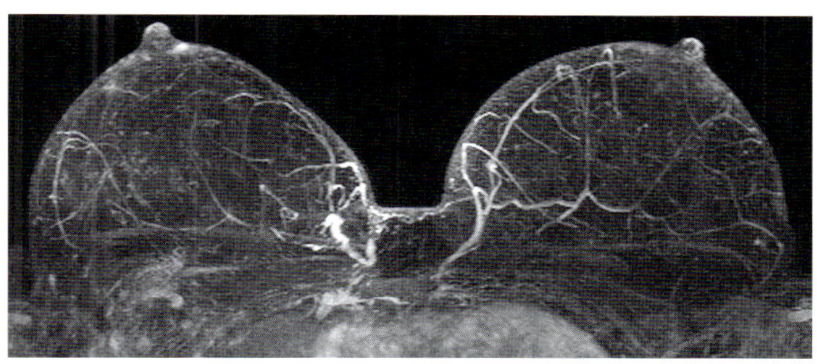

Fig. 38.**6** Contrast-enhanced MR mammography. Maximum intensity projection.

?

Please characterize mammography and MRI findings.
What is your preliminary diagnosis?
What are your next steps?

This case illustrates the imaging studies of an asymptomatic woman presenting for stereotactic vacuum core biopsy of "suspicious macro- and microcalcifications" in the lower outer quadrant of the right breast.

### Ultrasound

Particularly in the lower outer quadrant of the right breast, there were no findings consistent with the macro- and microcalcifications. US BI-RADS 1.

### Mammography

Mammography showed bilaterally symmetric fibroglandular parenchyma, ACR type 2. Multiple monomorphous macrocalcifications were visible in regional distribution in the lower outer quadrant, close to the chest wall. There were no microcalcifications. Mammograms showed no mass or density and no architectural distortion. BI-RADS right 3/left 1. PGMI: CC view G (nipple not in profile); MLO view G (inframammary fold not correctly positioned; superimposition of abdominal wall on parenchyma).

### MR Mammography

In precontrast T1-weighted imaging, MRI documented an area near the chest wall of approx. 3 cm × 3 cm containing multiple foci up to 5 mm in diameter with hypointense signal. After administration of contrast there were individual enhancing spots within this area. Signal in T2-weighted imaging was increased. No other unusual findings.

**MRI Artifact Category:** 1
**MRI Density Type:** 1

| No evaluable enhancement | |
|---|---|
| **MRI score (points)** | **0** |
| **MRI BI-RADS** | **1** |

## → Preliminary Diagnosis

Hematoma with calcifications.

## Differential Diagnosis

Hamartoma, fat necrosis (previous trauma?), hemangioma, angiosarcoma.

| BI-RADS Categorization | | |
|---|---|---|
| Clinical Findings | right 1 | left 1 |
| Ultrasound | right 1 | left 1 |
| Mammography | right 3 | left 1 |
| MR Mammography | right 1 | left 1 |
| **BI-RADS Total** | **right 3** | **left 1** |

### Limit of the Requested Stereotactic Vacuum Core Biopsy

In this specific case the stereotactic table (manufacturer: Fischer Imaging) required the use of a diagonal needle angle, in the direction of the chest wall, to access findings close to the chest wall. Therefore, the requested stereotactic biopsy was not performed because of the risk of thoracic injury. At the patient's request, and despite the BI-RADS 3 categorization of the mammography findings (because of the rare differential diagnosis of angiosarcoma), an open biopsy of this lesion was performed after hook-wire localization.

### Macroscopic Findings

Circumscribed vascular tumor with focal ectasia and partial thrombosis as well as bulletlike calcifications. (Fig. 38.**7**).

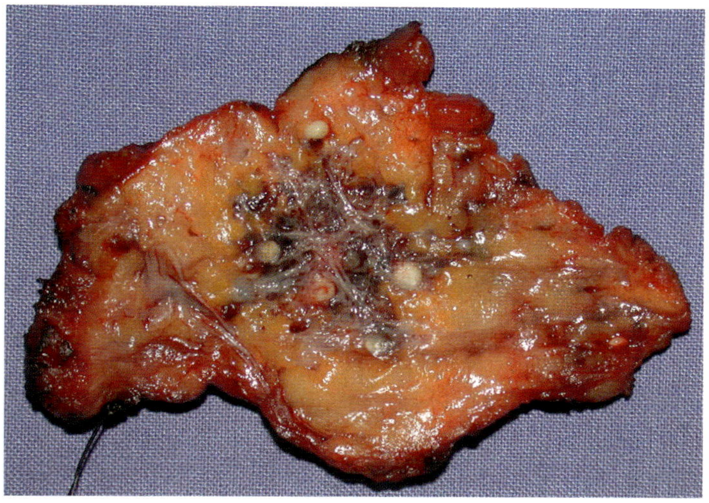

Fig. 38.**7** Excised specimen.

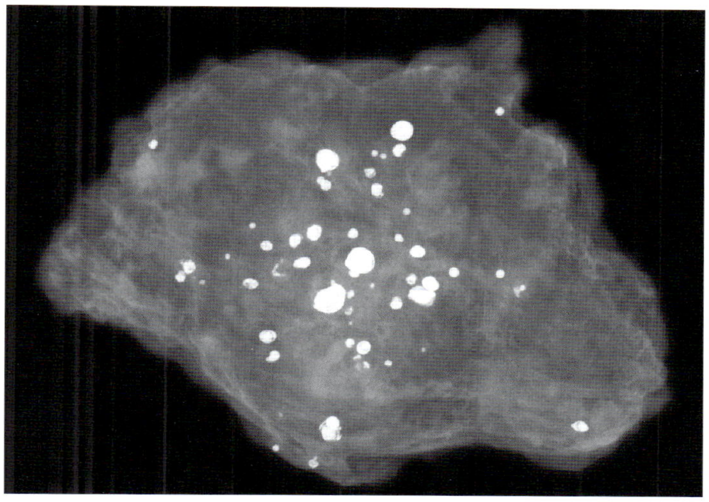

Fig. 38.**8** Specimen radiography.

## Histology

Intramammary hemangioma

## Treatment

Excisional biopsy. No further consequences.

In the absence of accompanying microcalcifications, macrocalcifications almost always represent benign lesions.

**Indication:** Painful resistance in the left breast.
**History:** Unremarkable.
**Risk profile:** No increased risk.
**Age and sex:** 62 years, *male*.

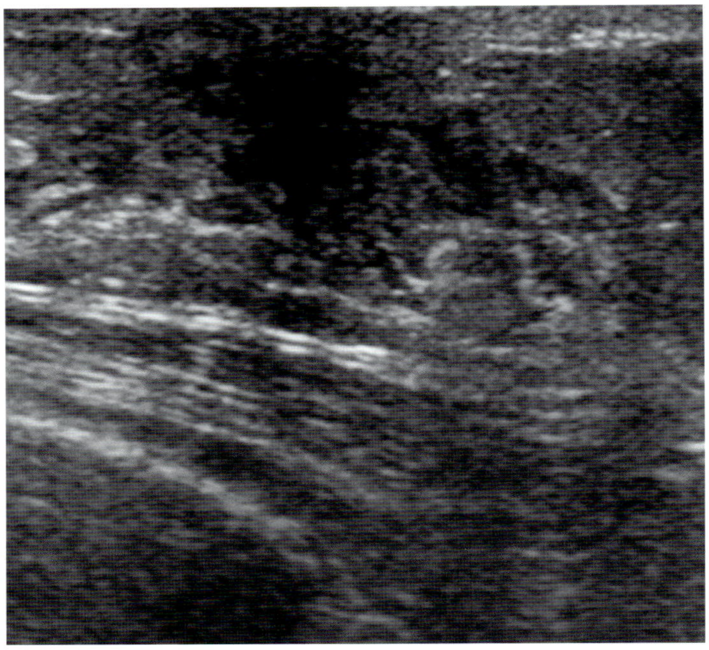

Fig. 39.**1** Ultrasound.

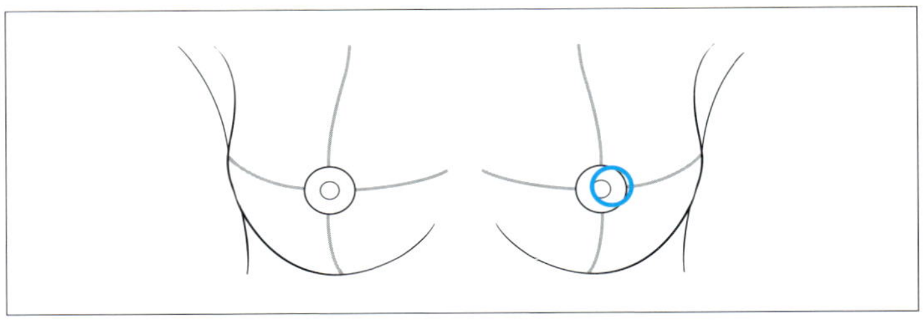

## Clinical Findings

Painful resistance 1 cm in diameter behind the areola of the left breast. Bilateral gynecomastia.

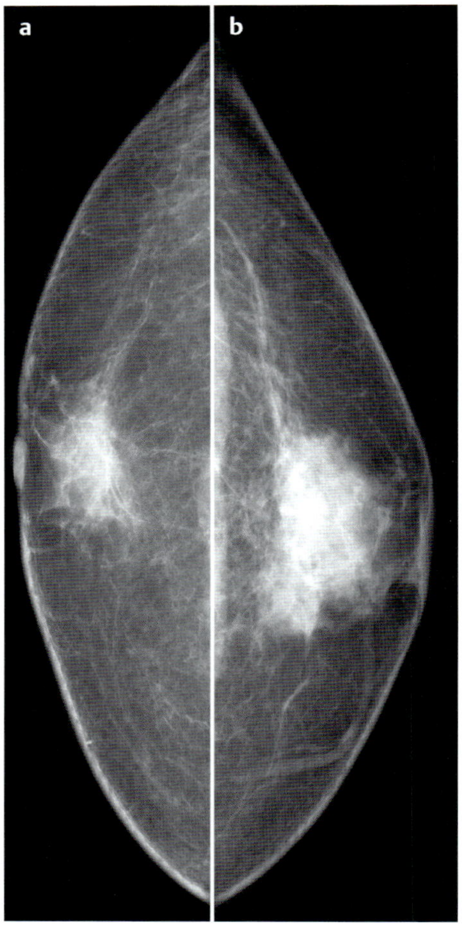

Fig. 39.**2 a, b** Digital mammography, CC view.

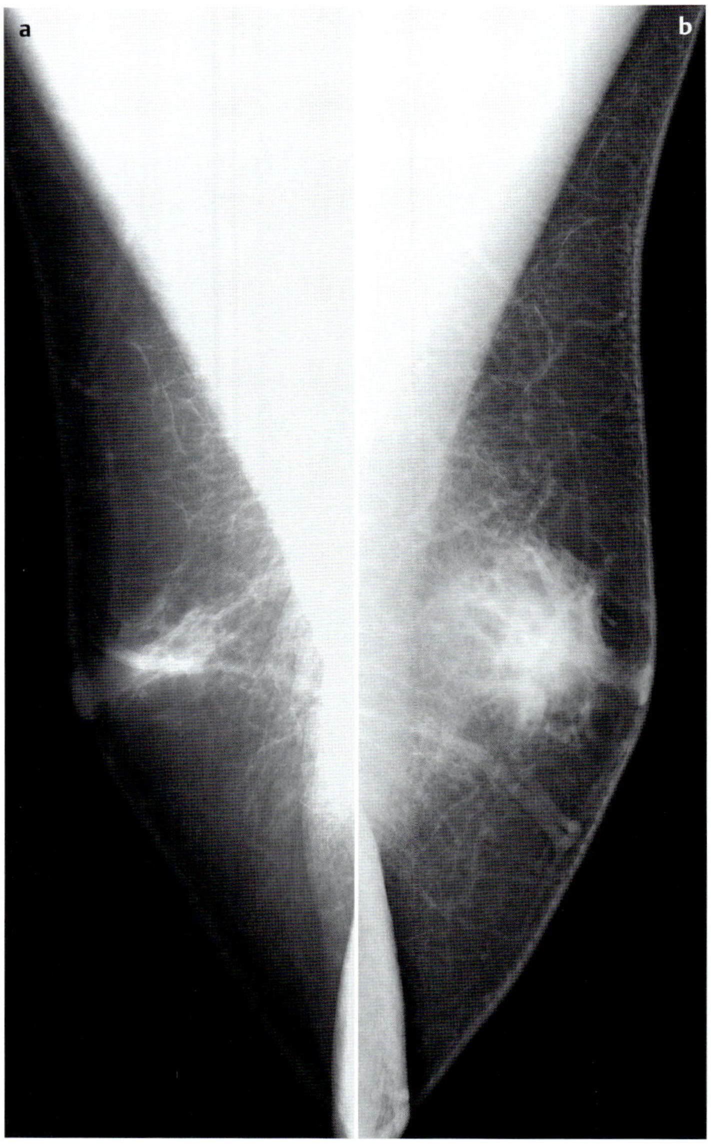

Fig. 39.**3 a, b** Digital mammography, MLO view.

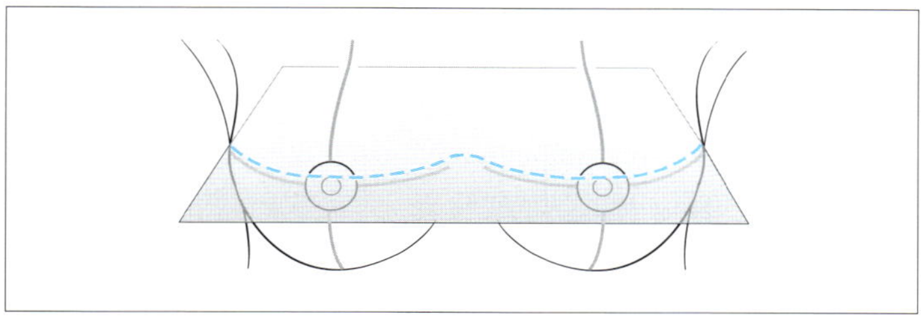

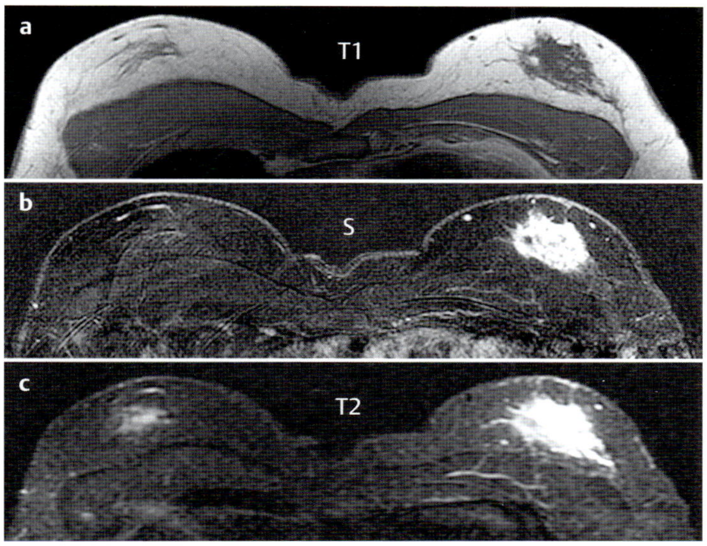


Fig. 39.**4 a – c** Contrast-enhanced MR mammography.

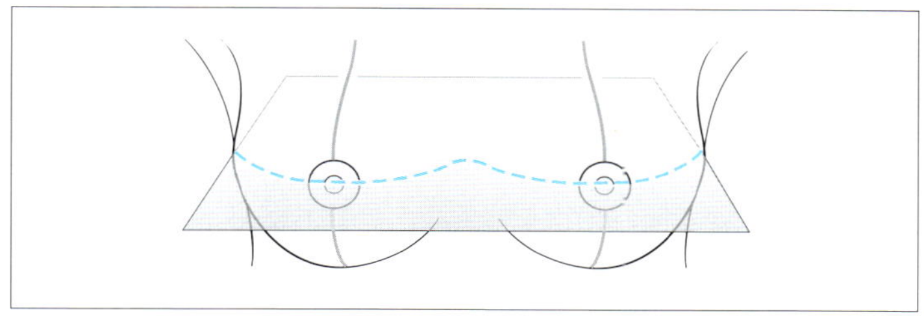

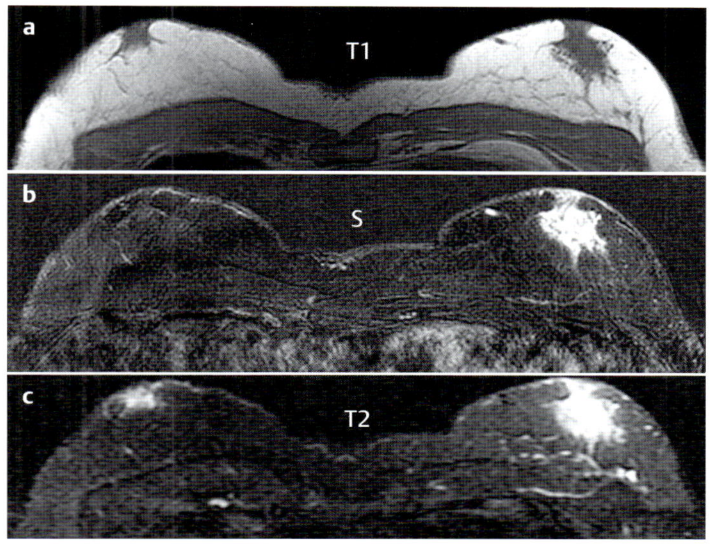


Fig. 39.**5 a – c** Contrast-enhanced MR mammography.

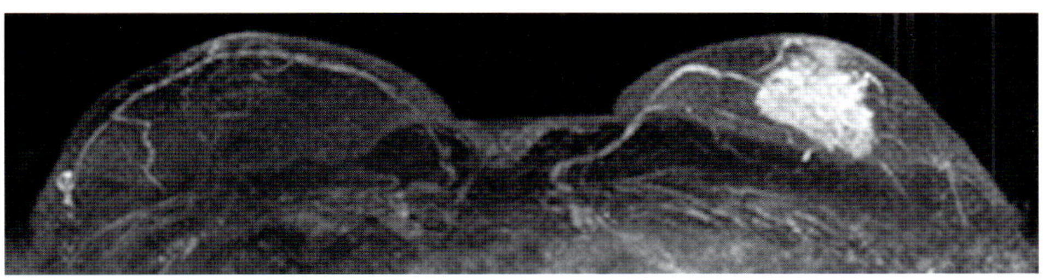

Fig. 39.**6** Contrast-enhanced MR mammography. Maximum intensity projection.

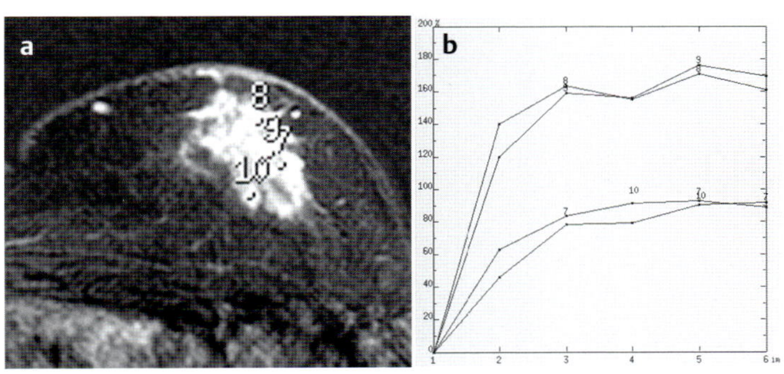


Fig. 39.**7 a, b** Signal-to-time curves.

Please characterize ultrasound, mammography, and MRI findings.
What is your preliminary diagnosis?
What are your next steps?

These are the imaging studies of a symptomatic man.

### Ultrasound

In the area of the resistance in the left breast, ultrasound showed a hypoechoic, lobulated mass (diameter 1 cm) with indeterminate distal echo pattern. US BI-RADS left 4.

### Mammography

Mammograms demonstrated asymmetry of the parenchyma (left > right). There were no densities, architectural distortion, or microcalcifications. No circumscribed lesions. BI-RADS right 2/left 3. PGMI is not defined for imaging of men.

### MR Mammography

MRI showed asymmetric parenchyma with partially ill-defined periphery. There was a notable unilateral enhancement of the left side after contrast administration, with a nonspecific signal curve. There were no unusual findings contralaterally.

**MRI Artifact Category:** 1
**MRI Density Type:** 1

| MRM score | Finding | Points |
|---|---|---|
| **Shape** | irregular | 1 |
| **Border** | ill-defined | 1 |
| **CM Distribution** | inhomogenous | 1 |
| **Initial Signal Intensity Increase** | strong | 2 |
| **Post-initial Signal Intensity Character** | plateau | 1 |
| **MRI score (points)** | | **6** |
| **MRI BI-RADS** | | **5** |

### → Preliminary Diagnosis

Right: Gynecomastia.
Left: Gynecomastia (asymmetrically to the other breast), mastitis, diffuse invasive carcinoma.

| BI-RADS Categorization | | |
|---|---|---|
| Clinical Findings | right 2 | left 3 |
| Ultrasound | right 1 | left 4 |
| Mammography | right 2 | left 3 |
| MR Mammography | right 1 | left 5 |
| **BI-RADS Total** | **right 1** | **left 5** |

### Procedure

US-guided core biopsy.

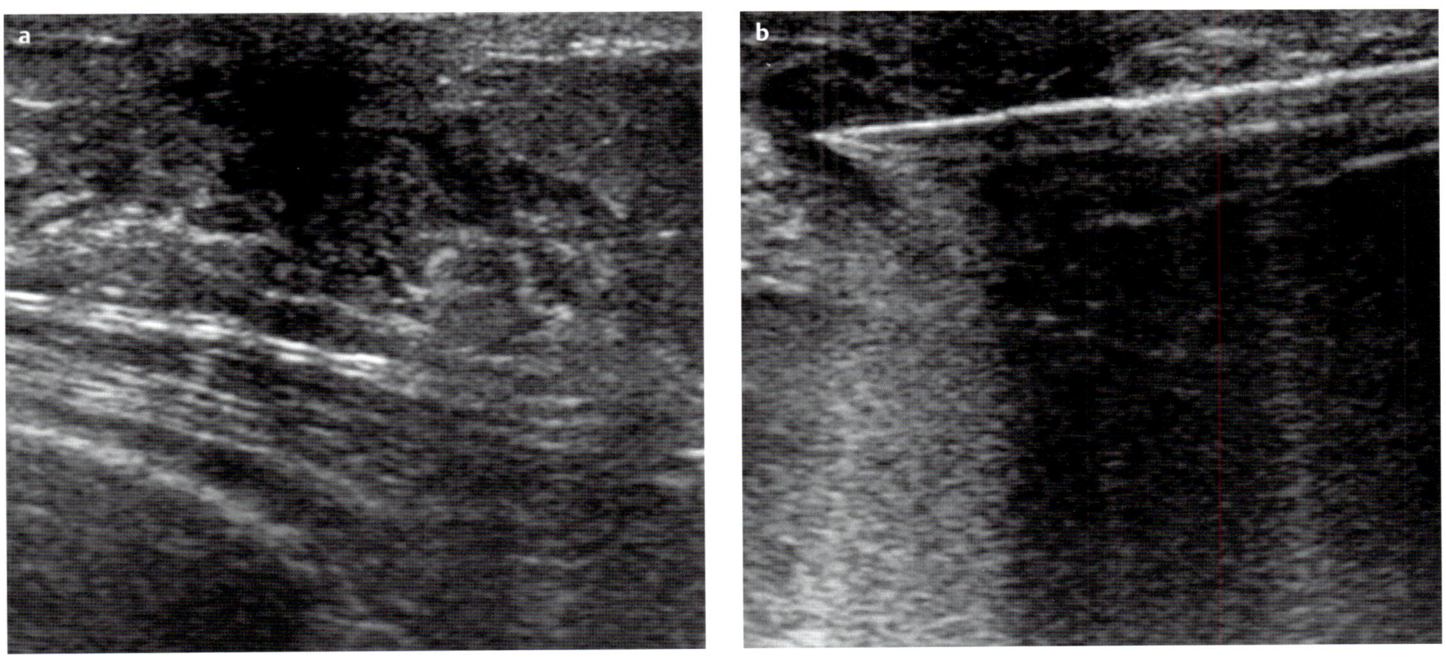

Fig. 39.**8 a, b** Pre-fire and post-fire documentation of US-guided core biopsy.

## Histology

Adenosis.

## Treatment

None.

The most important differential diagnosis of invasive carcinoma in MR mammography is adenosis.
T2 signal usually is high in adenosis and low in breast cancer. There are, however, exceptions in both entities.

**Indication:** Resistance in the left breast.
**History:** Unremarkable.
**Risk profile:** Premenopausal breast cancer in a sister.
**Age:** 47 years.

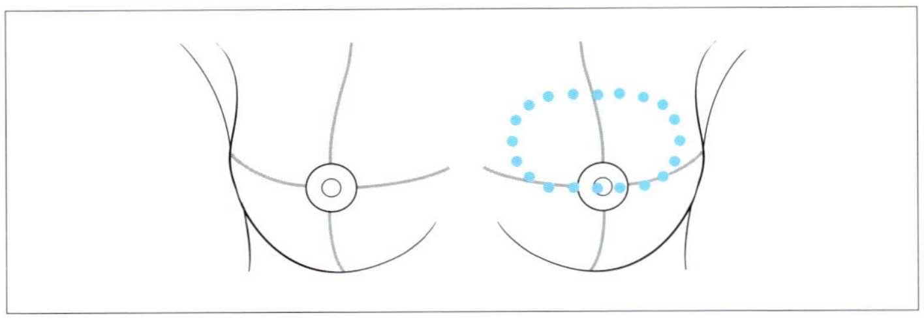

## Clinical Findings

Increased resistance of the upper half of the left breast.

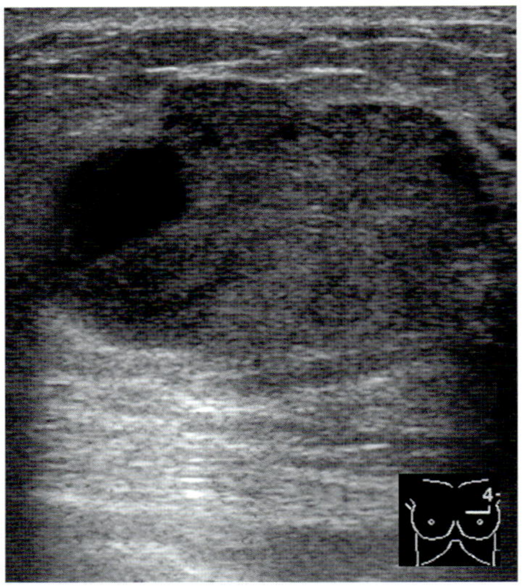

Fig. 40.**1** Sonography.

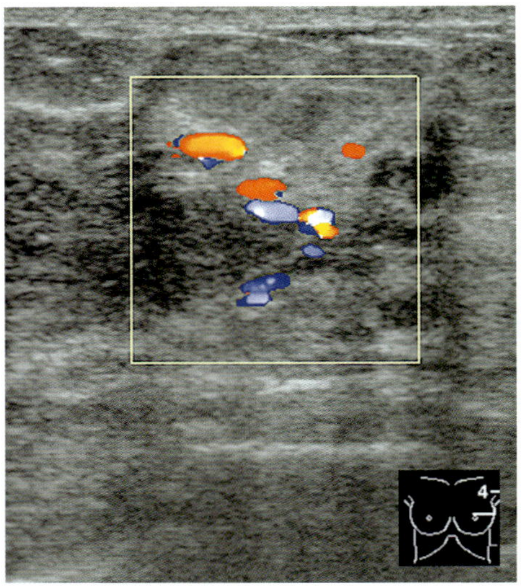

Fig. 40.**2** Color-coded Doppler sonography.

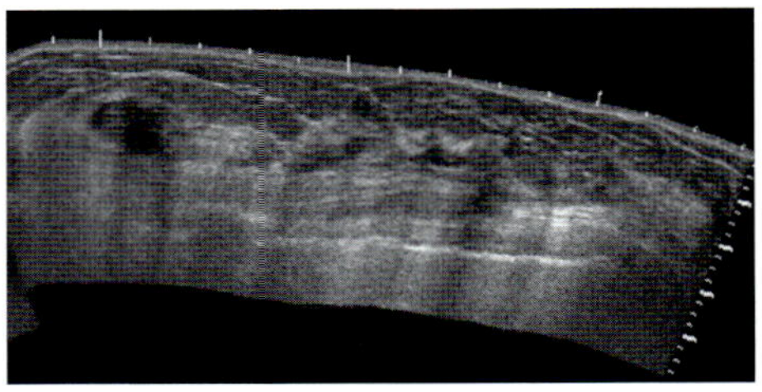

Fig. 40.**3** Sonography. Panoramic view of the left breast.

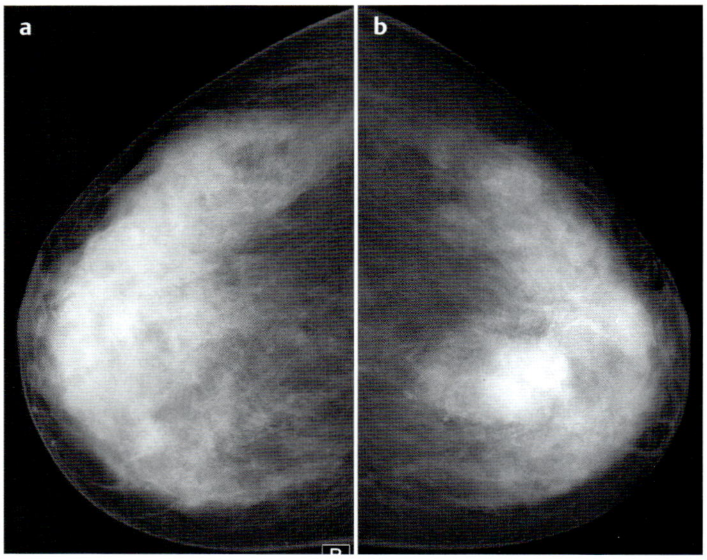

Fig. 40.**4 a, b** Digital mammography, CC view.

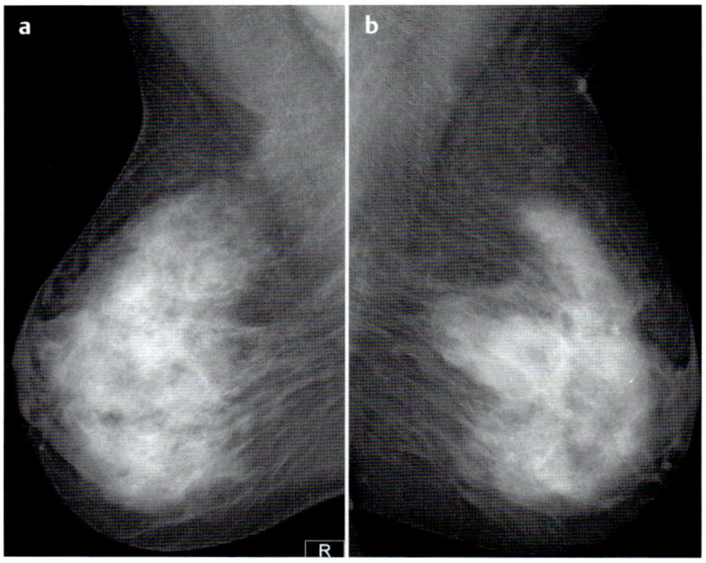

Fig. 40.**5 a, b** Digital mammography, MLO view.

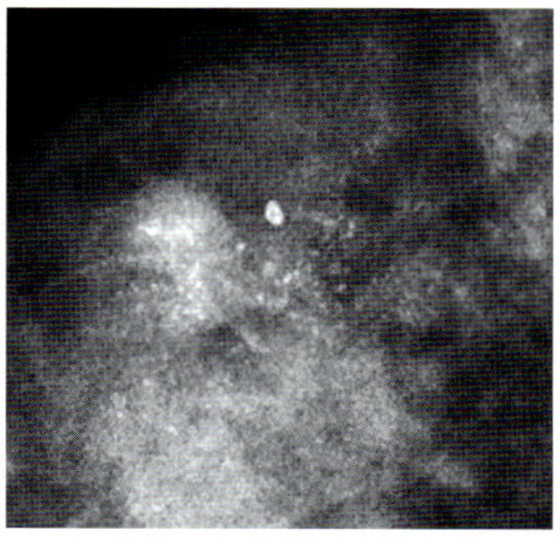

Fig. 40.**6** Magnification view of the central region of the right breast.

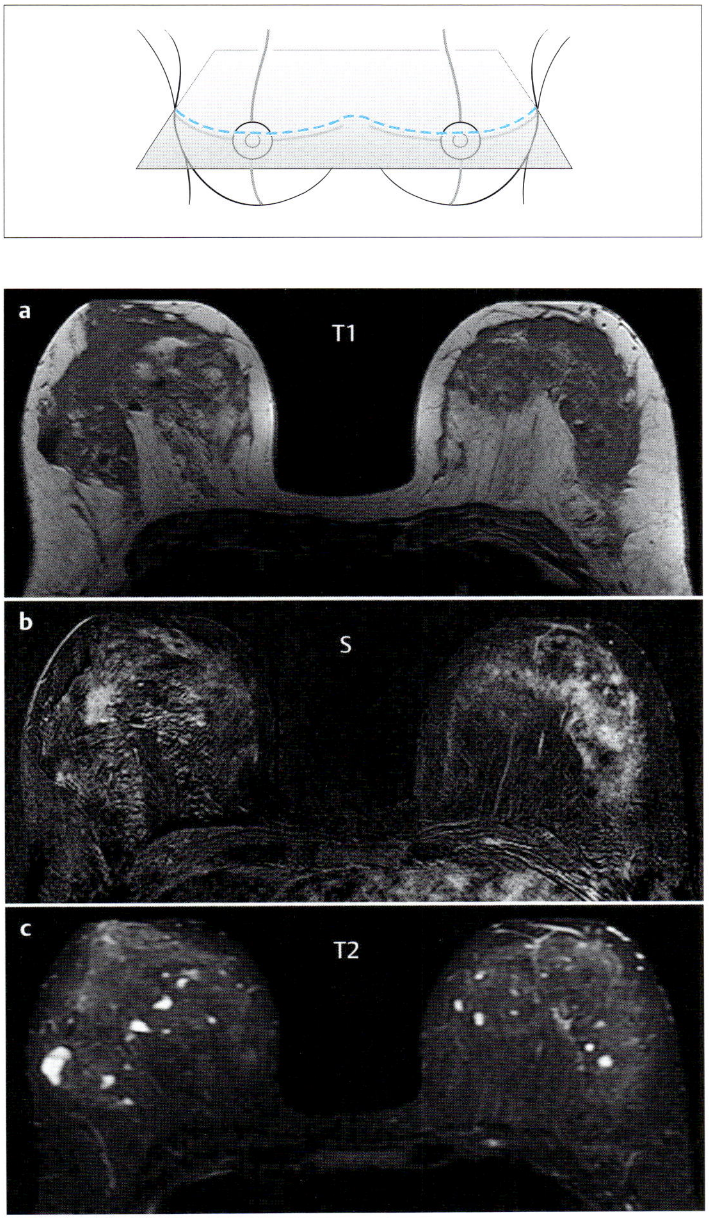


Fig. 40.**7 a–c** Contrast-enhanced MRI of the breasts.

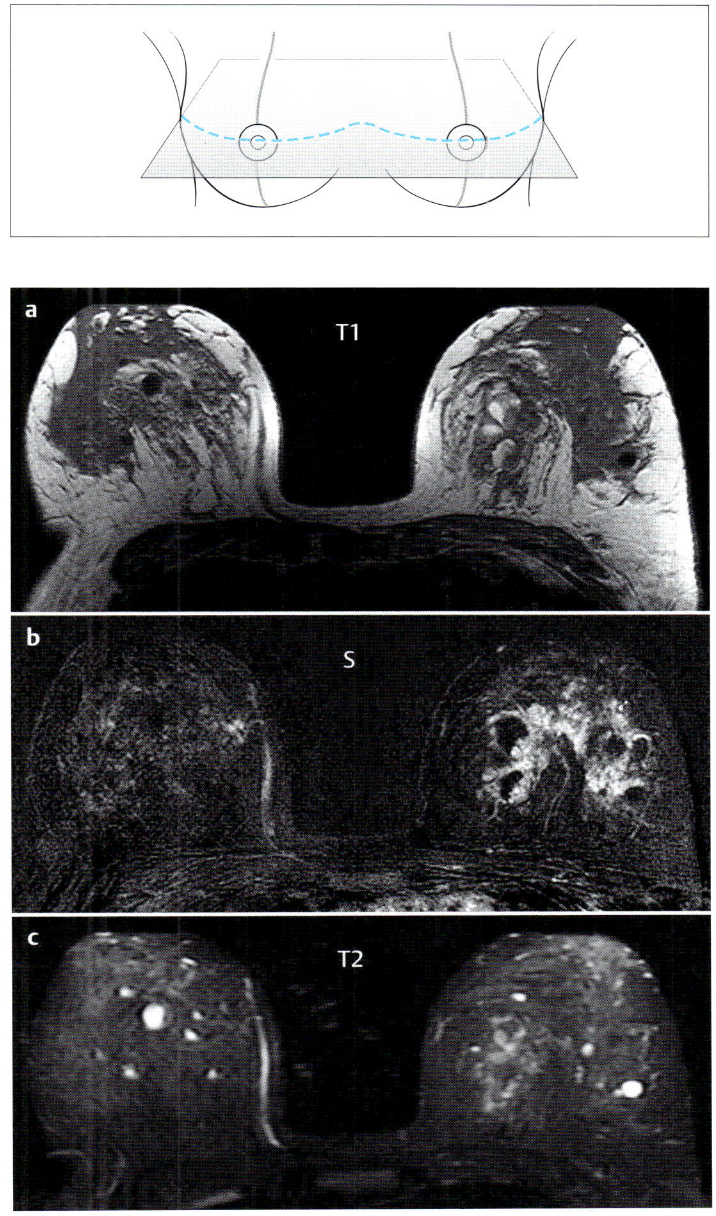


Fig. 40.**8 a–c** Contrast-enhanced MRI of the breasts.

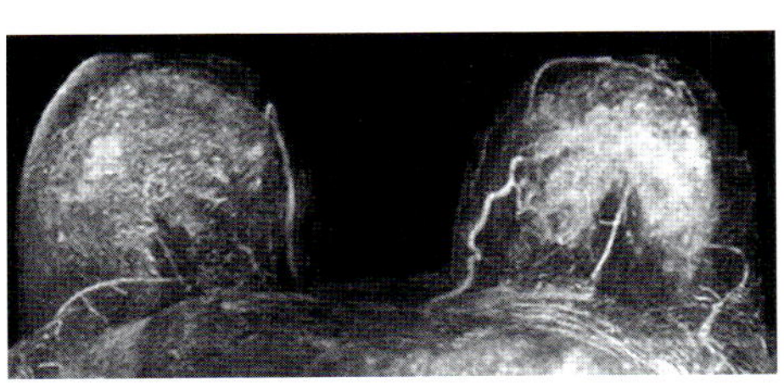

Fig. 40.**9** Contrast-enhanced MR mammography. Maximum intensity projection.

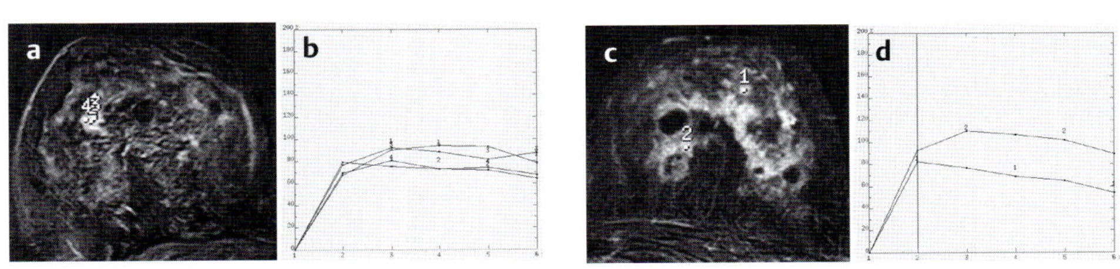


Fig. 40.**10 a–d** Signal-to-time curves of right (**a**) and left (**b**) breasts.

?

Please characterize ultrasound, mammography, and MRI findings.
What is your preliminary diagnosis?
What are your next steps?

This case shows the imaging studies of a symptomatic patient with increased resistance in the upper quadrants of the left breast.

### Ultrasound

The imaging of the right breast was normal. In the upper inner quadrant of the left breast there was a well-defined, homogeneous hypoechoic area, within which cysts were visible. Distal echo increase was slight. In the upper outer quadrant of the left breast, US demonstrated patchy hypoechoic lesions with distal echo shadowing. In this area color-coded Doppler sonography clearly showed increased vascularization. Multiple cysts bilaterally. US BI-RADS right 1, left inner quadrant 3, left outer quadrant 4.

### Mammography

Mammography showed a very dense, asymmetric parenchyma ACR type 4, In the central part of the left breast there was a circumscribed lobulated area with well-defined margins. There were no calcifications in the left breast. In the central part of the right breast, the mammogram showed regionally distributed polymorphous microcalcifications (BI-RADS right 4/left 4).

### MR Mammography

In the upper outer quadrant of the right breast there was a poorly-defined area with increased vascularization in comparison with the surrounding tissue There was also pathologically increased vascularization in the upper quadrants of the left breast. In the upper inner quadrant, there were multiple cysts, partially infiltrated with hypervascularized tissue (Fig. 40.**11**). Multiple cysts bilaterally.

**MRI Artifact Category:** 2
**MRI Density Type:** 3

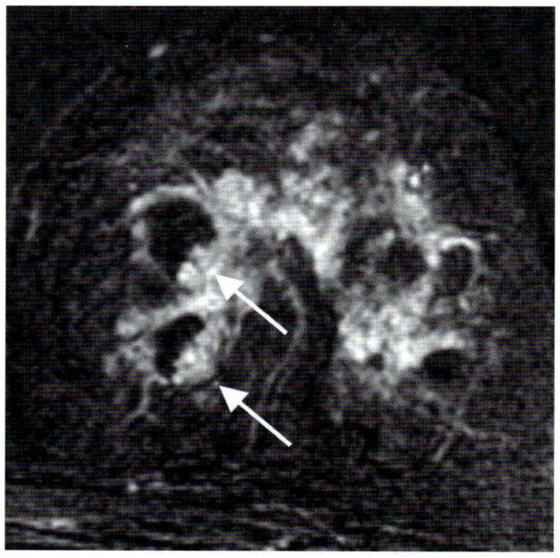

Fig. 40.**11** Intracystic tumor infiltration.

| MRM score | right | Points | left | Points |
|---|---|---|---|---|
| **Shape** | irregular | 1 | irregular | 1 |
| **Border** | ill-defined | 1 | ill-defined | 1 |
| **CM Distribution** | inhomogenous | 1 | inhomogenous | 1 |
| **Initial signal Intensity Increase** | moderate | 1 | strong | 2 |
| **Post-initial Signal Intensity Character** | plateau | 1 | wash-out | 2 |
| **MRI score (points)** | | **5** | | **7** |
| **MRI BI-RADS** | | **4** | | **5** |

### → Differential Diagnosis

Right breast: Focal adenosis, DCIS, invasive carcinoma.
Left breast: Carcinoma (invasive papillary?), DCIS, adenosis.

| BI-RADS Categorization | | |
|---|---|---|
| Clinical Findings | right 1 | left 4 |
| Ultrasound | right 1 | left 4 |
| Mammography | right 4 | left 4 |
| MR Mammography | right 4 | left 5 |
| **BI-RADS Total** | **right 4** | **left 5** |

### Procedure

Histological analysis of the microcalcifications in the right breast after stereotactic vacuum biopsy. Histological evaluation of the cranial quadrants of the left breast–separate specimens from inner and outer quadrants–by US-guided core biopsy.

### Histology of the biopsy specimens

**Right:** Extensive intraductal, minimally invasive carcinoma.
Left upper inner quadrant: Intraductal papilloma.
**Left upper outer quadrant:** Cribriform papillary intraductal carcinoma.

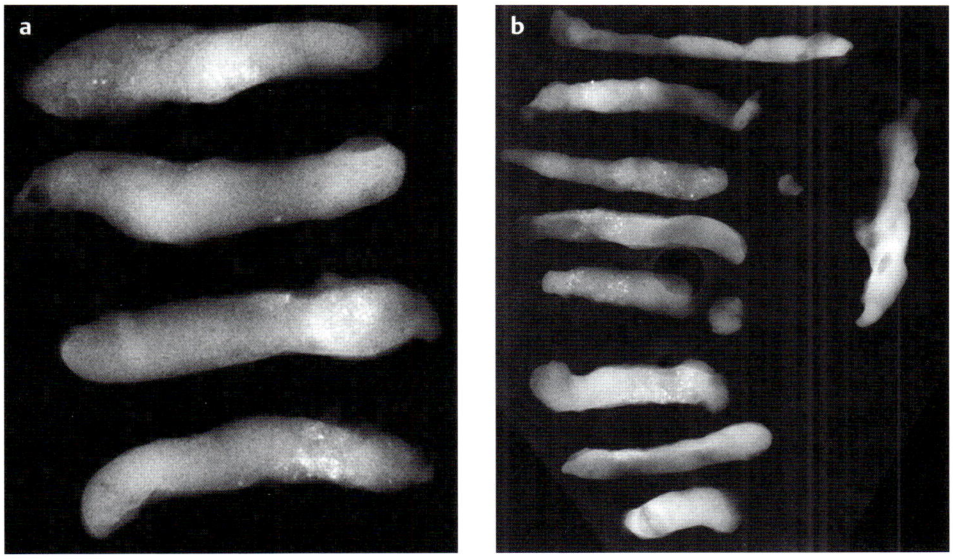

Fig. 40.**12 a, b** Radiography of the specimens from the right breast.

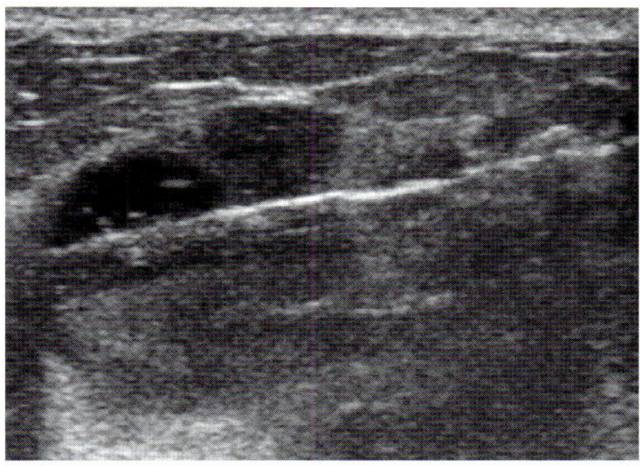

Fig. 40.**13** US-guided core biopsy of the left breast, upper inner quadrant.

## Histology (after open biopsy)

Right: Invasive ductal carcinoma (7 mm) with extensive DCIS (5 cm).
Left: Partially papillary, partially cribriform ductal carcinoma in situ.

Right: IDC pT1b, pN0 (0/2 SN), G1 + DCIS.
Left: DCIS pTis (van Nuys score 8), pN0, G2.

## Treatment

Bilateral mastectomy.

This case shows what is probably the malignant transformation of a papilloma to a papillary breast cancer.

**Indication:** Palpable mass in the left breast.
**History:** Unremarkable.
**Risk profile:** No increased risk.
**Age:** 45 years.

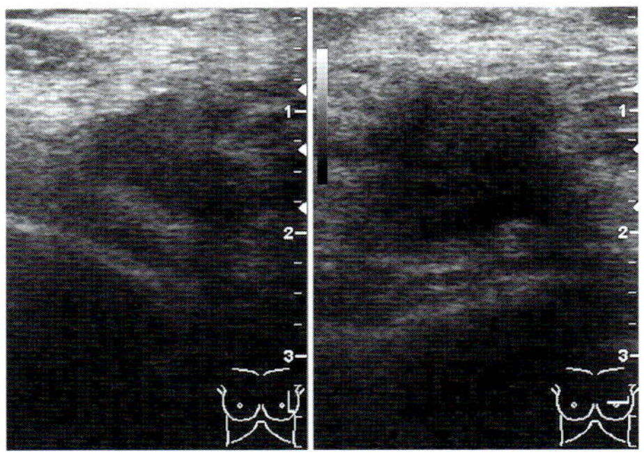

Fig. 41.**1** Ultrasound.

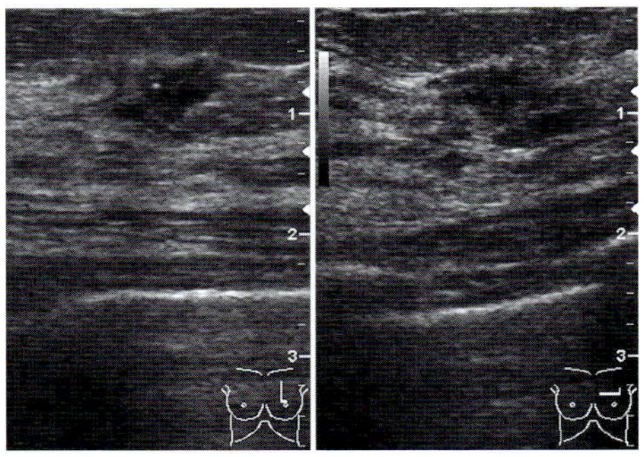

Fig. 41.**2** Ultrasound.

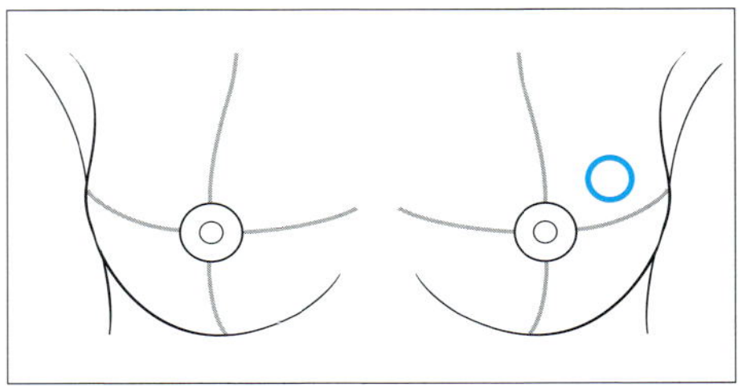

**Clinical Findings**

Resistance in the upper outer quadrant of the left breast.

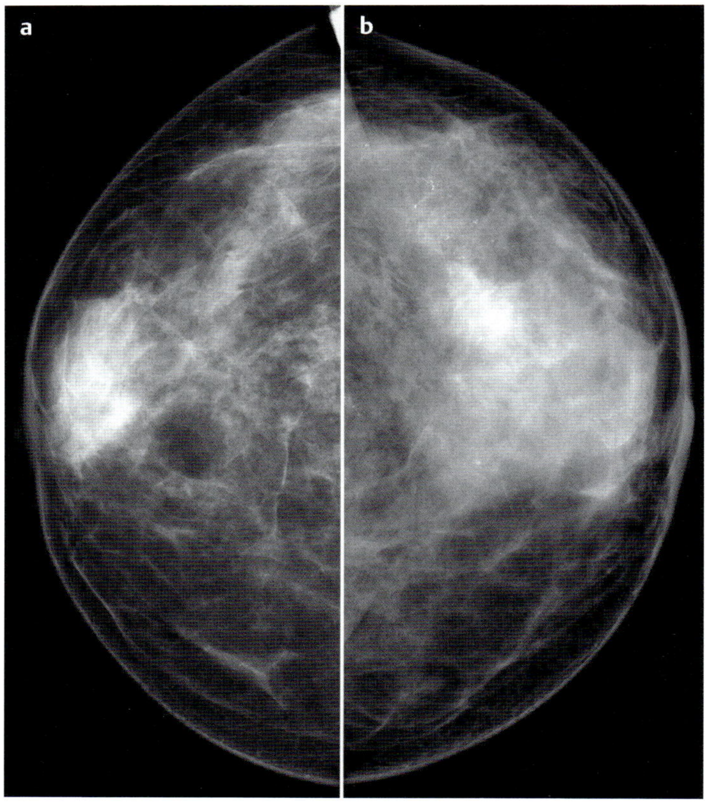


Fig. 41.**3 a, b** Digital mammography, CC view.

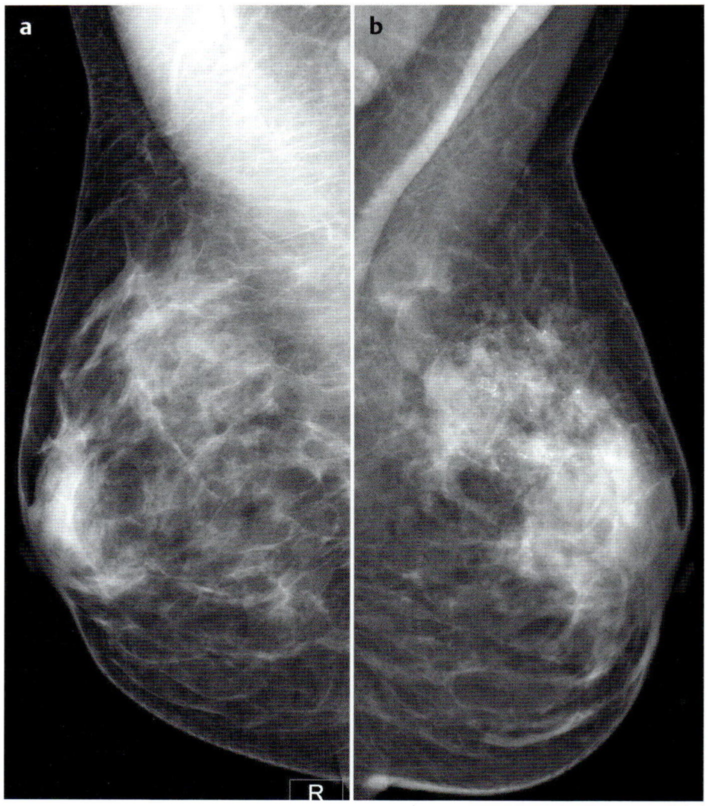


Fig. 41.**4 a, b** Digital mammography, MLO view.

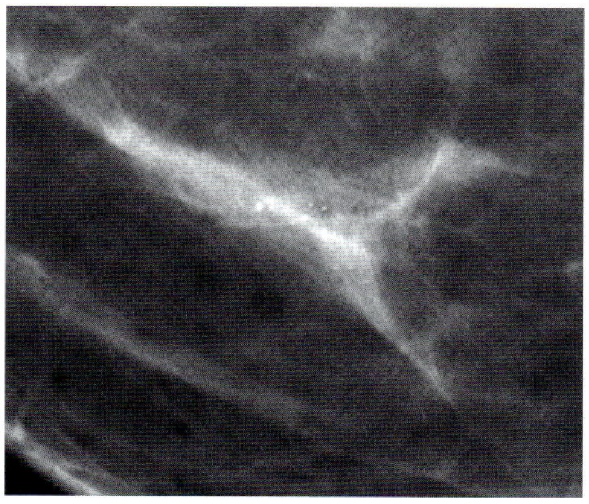

Fig. 41.**5** Magnification view, inner quadrants of right breast.

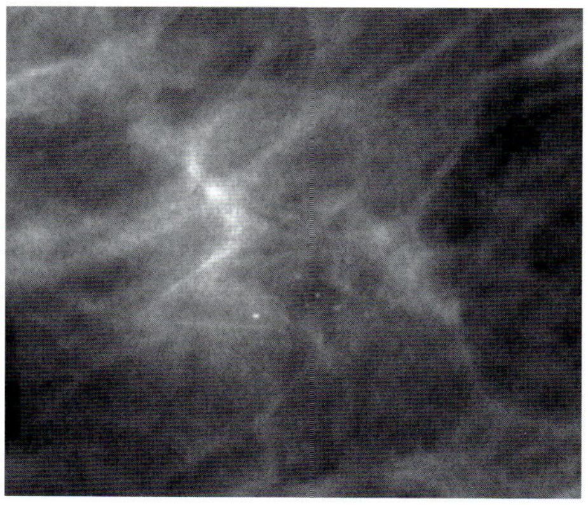

Fig. 41.**6** Magnification view, lower quadrants of right breast.

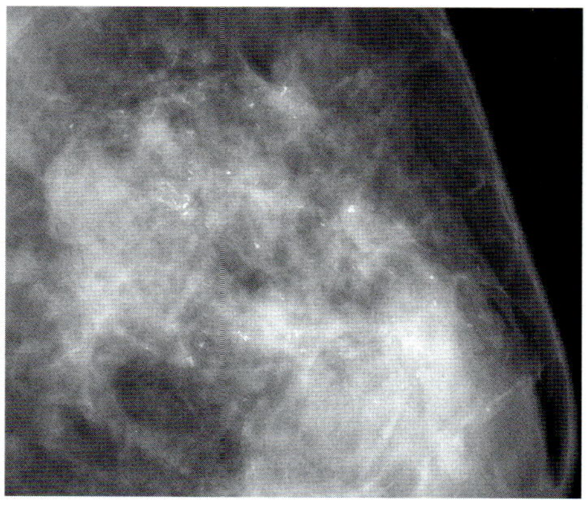

Fig. 41.**7** Magnification view, upper outer quadrants of left breast.

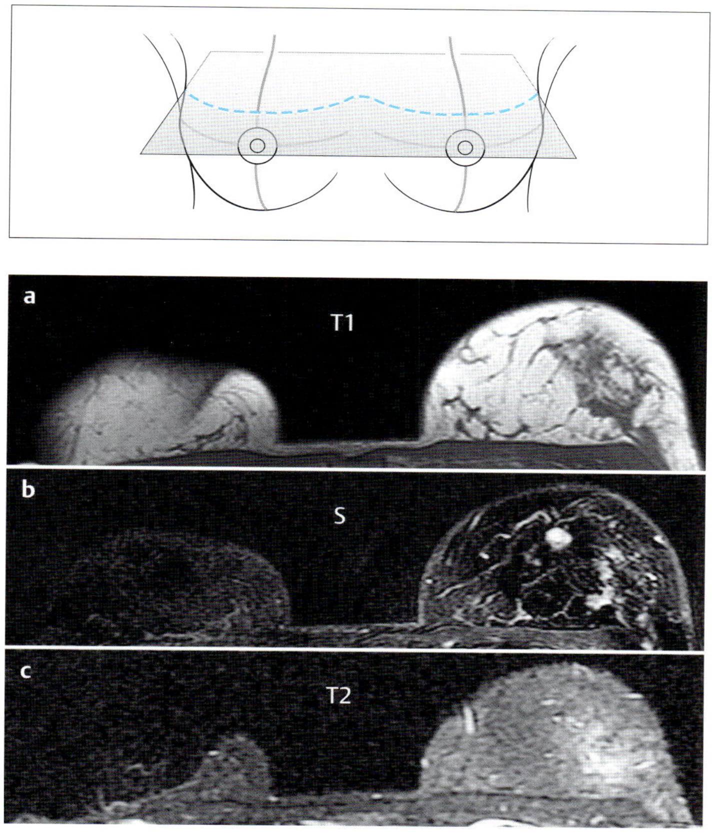


Fig. 41.8 **a–c** Contrast-enhanced MR mammography.

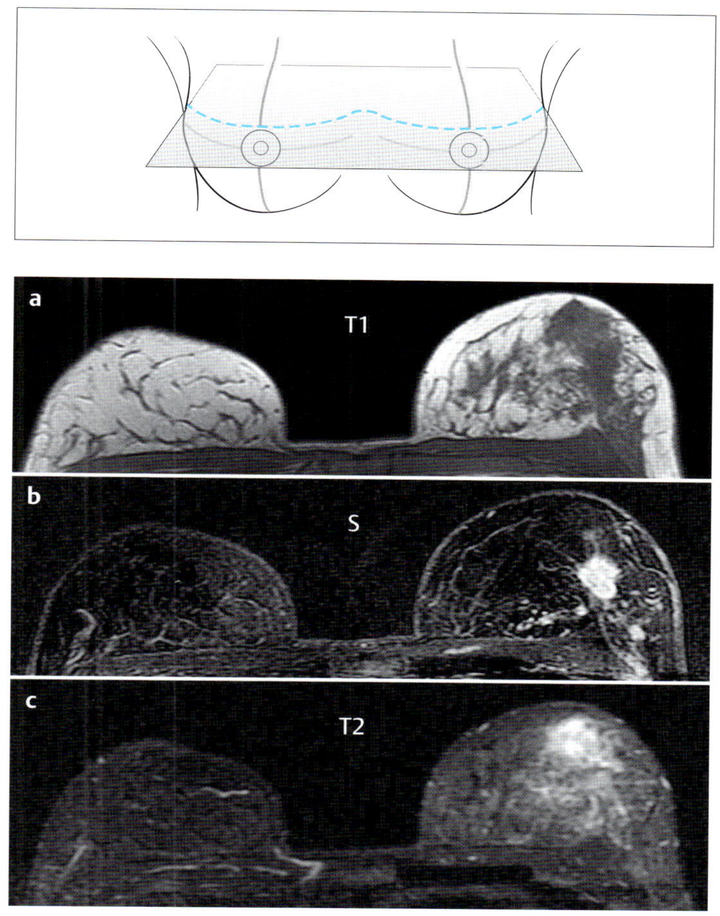


Fig. 41.9 **a–c** Contrast-enhanced MR mammography.

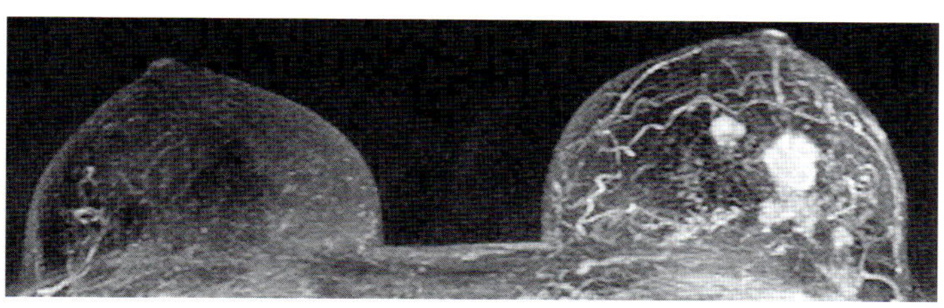

Fig. 41.**10** Contrast-enhanced MR mammography. Maximum intensity projection.

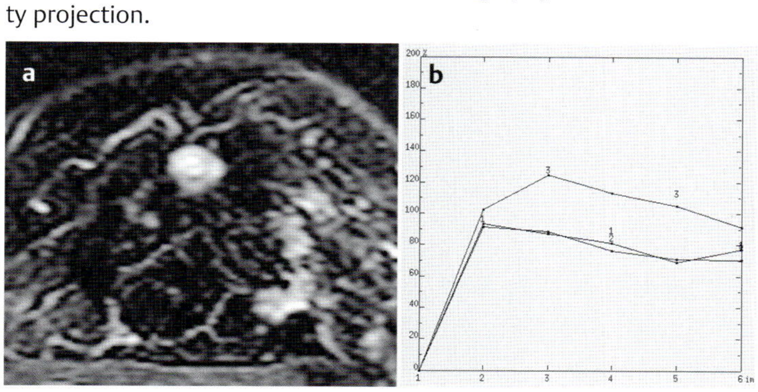


Fig. 41.**11 a, b** Signal-to-time curves.

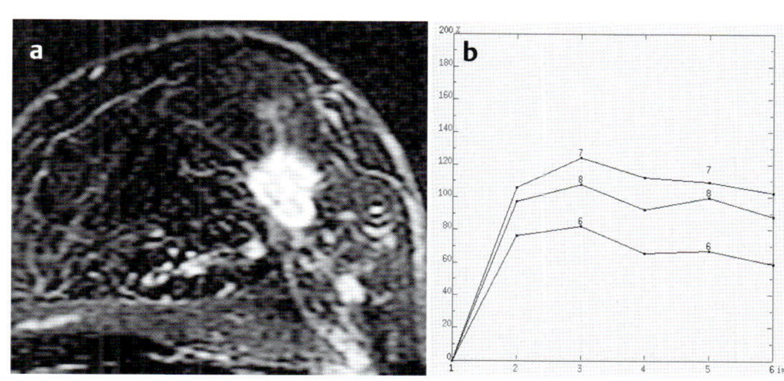


Fig. 41.**12 a, b** Signal-to-time curves.

?

Please characterize ultrasound, mammography, and MRI findings.
What is your preliminary diagnosis?
What are your next steps?

This case demonstrates the imaging studies of a symptomatic woman with a resistance in the left breast. The patient had not previously been screened until the present examination at the age of 45 years.

### Ultrasound

Ultrasound showed a hypoechoic lesion of 1.7 cm diameter with irregular, hyperechoic margins, distal shadowing and accompanying architectural distortion. Another hypoechoic lesion of 8 mm diameter was detected between the upper quadrants of the left breast. This lesion showed indeterminate distal echo behavior and no architectural distortion. US BI-RADS 5 with signs of multicentricity.

### Mammography

Asymmetric, inhomogeneous parenchyma (left > right), ACR type 3. Mammography showed a vague, isodense, ill-defined mass (diameter 1.8 mm) in the upper outer quadrant of the left breast, and polymorphous microcalcifications in a segmental distribution in the same quadrant. There was a cluster of monomorphous microcalcifications in the lower inner quadrant of the right breast (BI-RADS right 3/left 5). PGMI: CC view G (superimposition of the parenchyma of right breast); MLO view G (axillary skin fold, inframammary fold).

### MR Mammography

Lobulated, partially ill-defined mass (diameter 2 cm) in the left upper outer quadrant with clear criteria of malignancy. This lesion had hypointense signal in T2-weighted sequences. Between the upper quadrants of the left breast, there was a lobulated, partially ill-defined mass of 1 cm diameter, also with evident criteria of malignancy and reduced signal in T2-weighted imaging.

**MRI Artifact Category:** 2
**MRI Density Type:** 1

| MRM score | Left breast, upper outer quadrant | Points | Left breast, between upper quadrants | Points |
|---|---|---|---|---|
| **Shape** | lobulated | 0 | round | 0 |
| **Border** | spiculated | 1 | well-defined | 0 |
| **CM Distribution** | ring | 2 | ring | 2 |
| **Initial Signal Intensity Increase** | strong | 2 | strong | 2 |
| **Post-initial Signal Intensity Character** | wash-out | 2 | wash-out | 2 |
| **MRI score (points)** | | **7** | | **6** |
| **MRI BI-RADS** | | **5** | | **5** |

### → Preliminary Diagnosis

Multicentric carcinoma in the left breast.

### Differential Diagnosis

Carcinoma in the outer quadrants; fibroadenoma between the upper quadrants of the left breast.

| BI-RADS Categorization | | |
|---|---|---|
| Clinical Findings | right 1 | left 4 |
| Ultrasound | right 1 | left 5 (MCC) |
| Mammography | right 3 | left 5 |
| MR Mammography | right 1 | left 5 (MCC) |
| **BI-RADS Total** | **right 3** | **left 5 (MCC)** |

### Procedure

US-guided core biopsy of the palpable mass in the upper outer quadrant of the left breast for histopathological analysis. Additional evaluation of the lesion between the upper quadrants to establish multicentricity.

### Histology of the core biopsy–left

**Left upper outer quadrant:** invasive ductal carcinoma.
Between left upper quadrants: invasive ductal carcinoma.

### Further procedure

Stereotactic vacuum core biopsy of the microcalcifications in the lower inner quadrant of the right breast, despite their BI-RADS 3 categorization. Risk of contralateral cancer increased by carcinoma in the left breast.

### Histology of the vacuum core biopsy–right

Right lower inner quadrant: sclerosing adenosis.

### Histology

Multicentric ductal invasive carcinoma (diameter 22 mm and 14 mm). Lymph nodes positive (1/17).

Left: IDC pT2 multicentric pN1, G2.
Right: Sclerosing adenosis.

### Treatment

Mastectomy of the left breast. No further intervention at the right breast.

10–20% of breast cancers are multicentric. In these cases mastectomy is usually recommended.

**Indication:** Screening mammography.
**History:** Unremarkable.
**Risk profile:** Normal.
**Age:** 54 years.

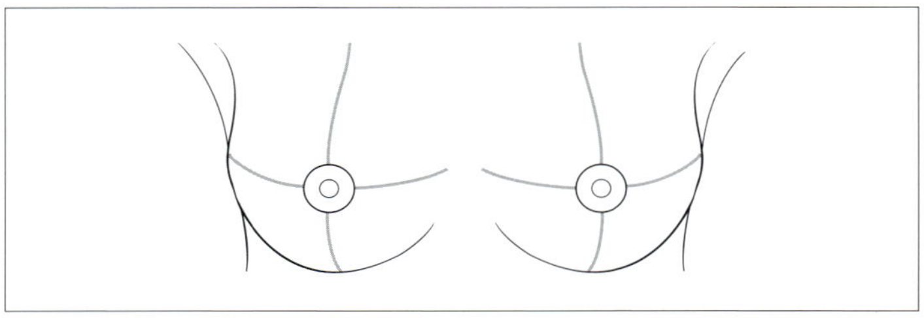

## Clinical Findings

No findings.

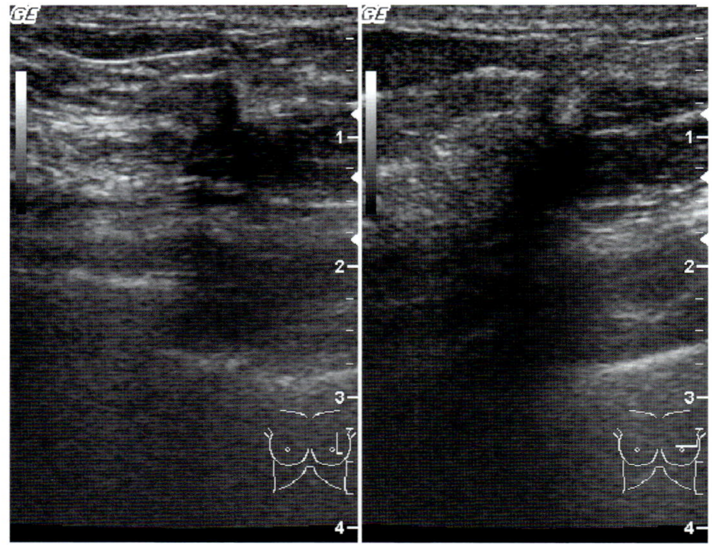

Fig. 42.**1** Ultrasound.

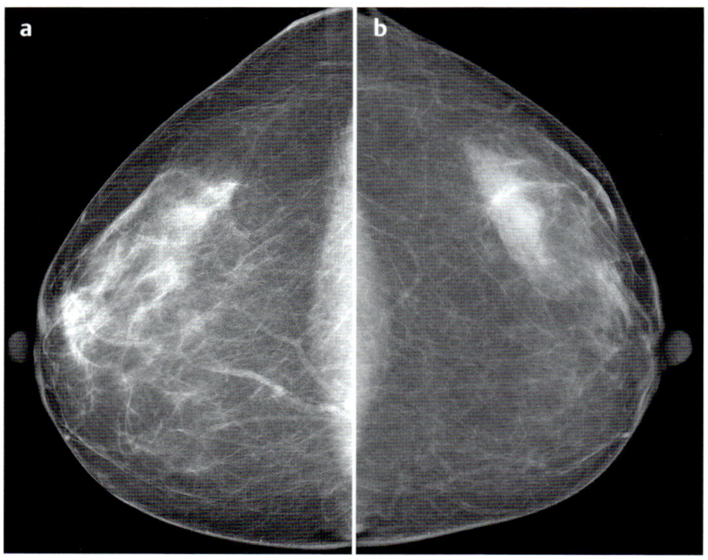

Fig. 42.**2 a, b** Digital mammography, CC view.

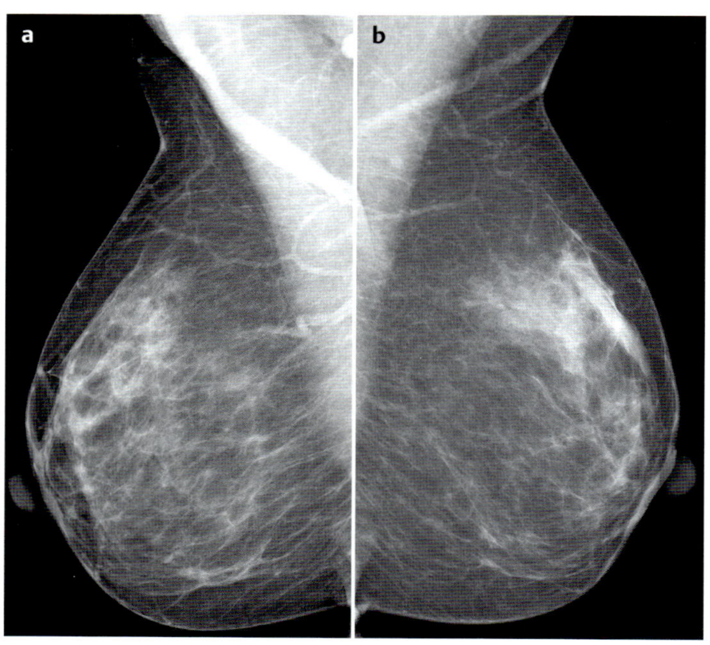

Fig. 42.**3 a, b** Digital mammography, MLO view.

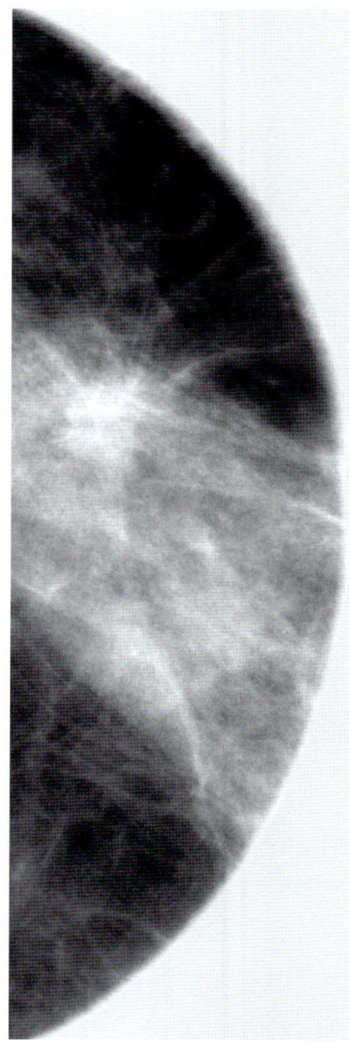

Fig. 42.**4** Spot compression, left breast.

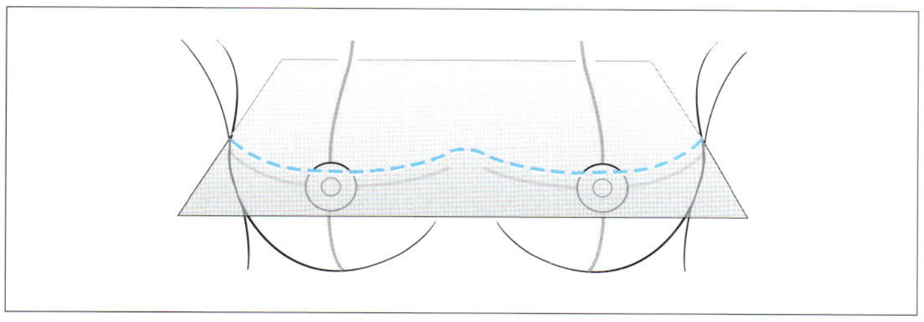

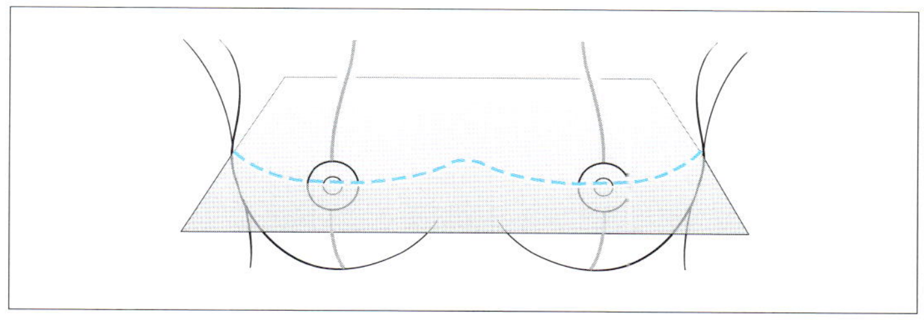

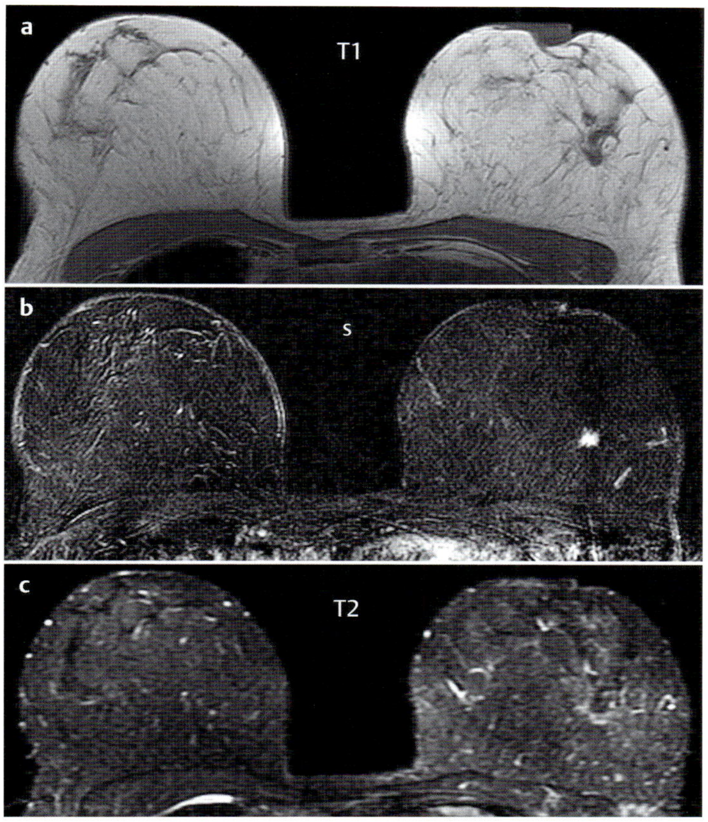


Fig. 42.**5 a – c** Contrast-enhanced MRI of the breasts.

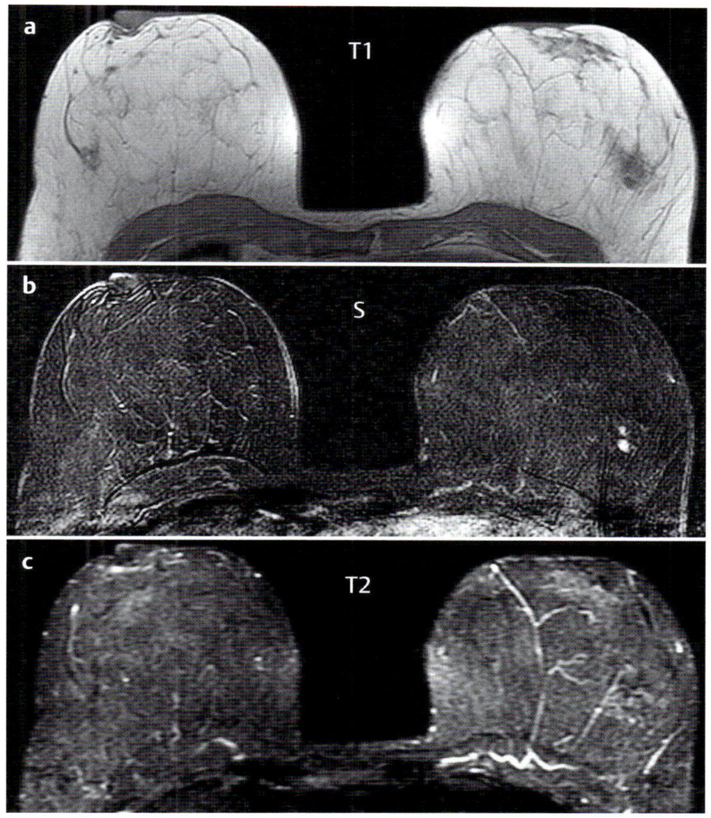


Fig. 42.**6 a – c** Contrast-enhanced MRI of the breasts.

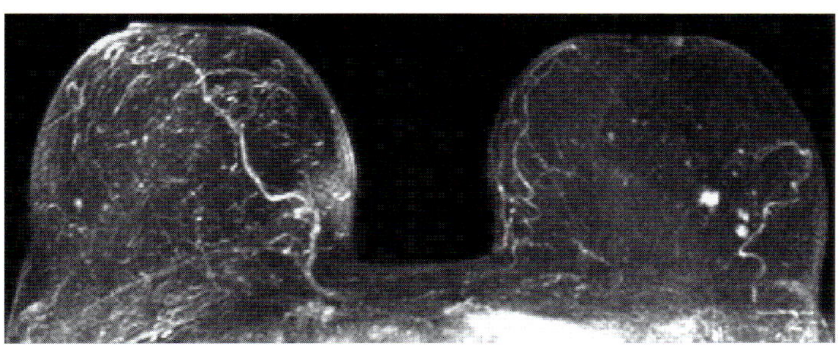

Fig. 42.**7** Contrast-enhanced MR mammography. Maximum intensity projection.

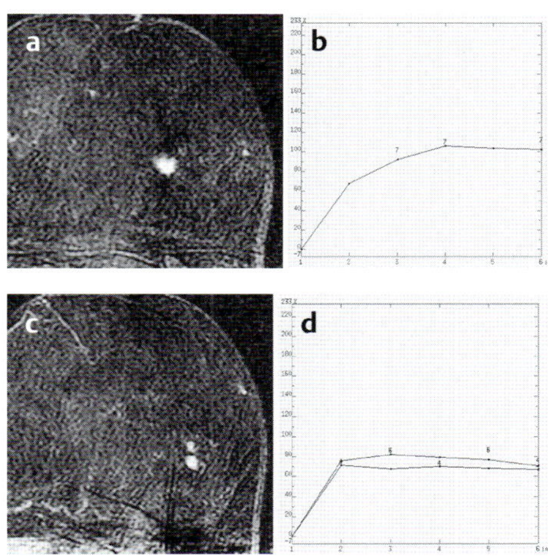


Fig. 42.**8 a – d** Signal-to-time curves.

Please characterize ultrasound, mammography, and MRI findings.
What is your preliminary diagnosis?
What are your next steps?

This case demonstrates the imaging studies of an asymptomatic woman presenting for screening.

### Ultrasound

In the upper outer quadrant of the left breast there was an irregular, hypoechoic lesion with distal acoustic shadowing (diameter 8 mm). US BI-RADS left 4.

### Mammography

Imaging showed an asymmetric (right > left), partially inhomogeneous dense parenchyma, ACR type 3. There was an isodense, slightly spiculated mass (diameter 1 cm) in the upper outer quadrant of the left breast. Spot compression obtained a more precise depiction of the spiculated quality of this lesion. BI-RADS right 1/ left 4. PGMI: CC view P; MLO view G (inframammary fold).

### MR Mammography

MRI demonstrated a spiculated, ill-defined mass (diameter: 1 cm) in the upper outer quadrant with strong initial signal increase and postinitial plateau as well as a reduced signal in T2-weighted imaging. 1.2 cm caudal of this mass there were two homogeneously enhancing lesions, each of 5 mm diameter, with initial signal increase of 80% and postinitial plateau as well as reduced signal in T2-weighted imaging (MRI BI-RADS 3).

### Note

The lesion in the upper outer quadrant of the left breast was visible, at a similar size, in MR images produced 3 years previously in another clinic (Fig. 42.**9**).

**MRI Artifact Category:** 2
**MRI Density Type:** 1

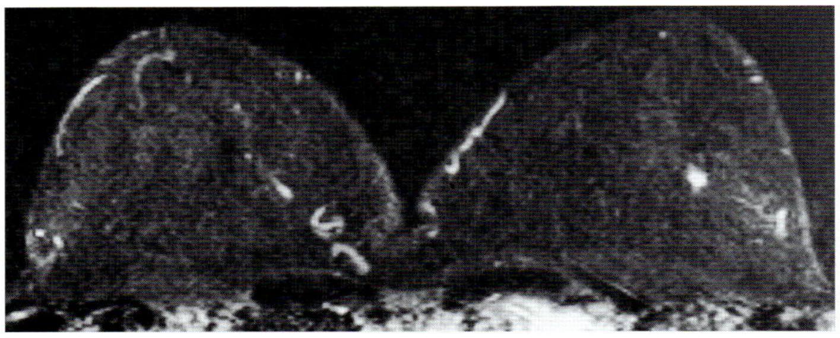

Fig. 42.**9** MR mammography three years earlier demonstrated a hypervascularized lesion in the left breast [imaging not performed by authors]. 256 matrix.

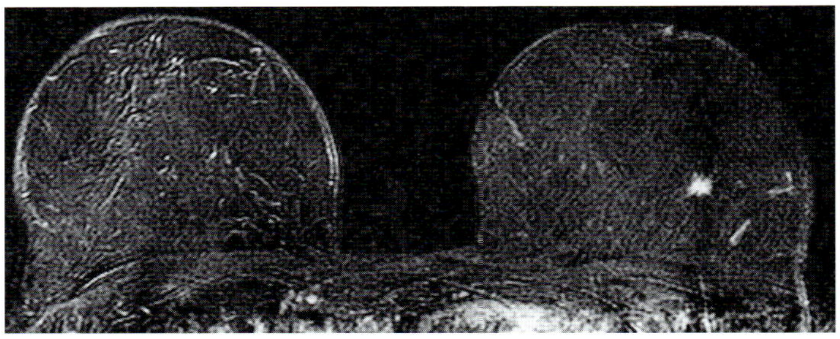

Fig. 42.**10** Current MR mammography for comparison. 512 matrix.

| MRM score | Finding upper outer quadrant, left breast | Points | Finding between outer quadrants, left breast | Points |
|---|---|---|---|---|
| **Shape** | irregular | 1 | round | 0 |
| **Border** | spiculated | 1 | well-defined | 0 |
| **CM Distribution** | homogeneous | 0 | homogeneous | 0 |
| **Initial Signal Intensity Increase** | strong | 2 | moderate | 1 |
| **Post-initial Signal Intensity Character** | plateau | 1 | plateau | 1 |
| **MRI score (points)** | | **5** | | **2** |
| **MRI BI-RADS** | | **4** | | **2** |

### → Preliminary Diagnosis

Left upper outer quadrant: Carcinoma.
Left between outer quadrants: Fibroadenoma.

### → Differential Diagnosis

Adenosis, papilloma.

| BI-RADS Categorization | | |
|---|---|---|
| Clinical Findings | right 1 | left 1 |
| Ultrasound | right 1 | left 4 |
| Mammography | right 1 | left 4 |
| MR Mammography | right 1 | left 4 |
| **BI-RADS Total** | **right 1** | **left 4** |

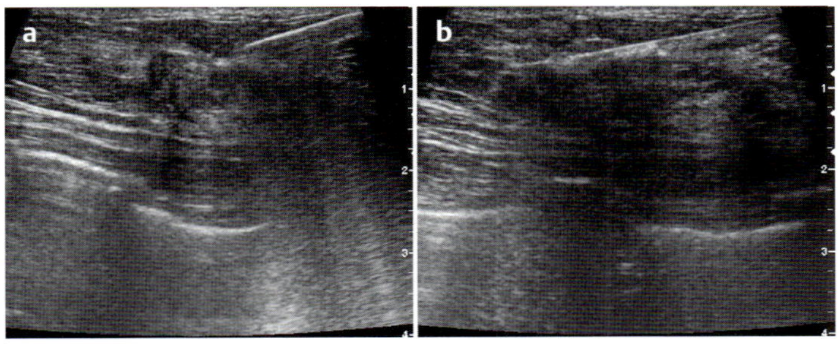

Fig. 42.**11 a, b** US-guided core biopsy of the left breast. Pre-fire and post-fire documentation.

### Procedure

US-guided core biopsy and histopathological evaluation of the lesion in the upper outer quadrant of the left breast (Fig. 42.**11**a,b).

### Histopathology of the core biopsy specimen

Tubular carcinoma.

### Further procedure

Open biopsy of the tubular carcinoma as well as of the secondary lesions in the left breast after MRI-guided hook-wire localization (Fig. 42.**12**).

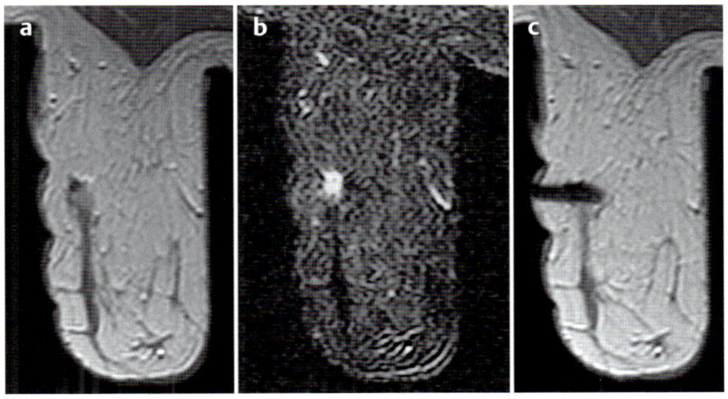

Fig. 43.**12 a – c** MR-guided preoperative hook-wire localization. Precontrast image, subtraction image and documentation of the wire in position.

## Histology

Tubular carcinoma (diameter 12 mm) accompanied by focal adenosis.

TC pT1c, pN1, G1.

## Treatment

Breast conservation therapy.

Tubular carcinomas usually have very slow tumor growth, often barely increasing in size over several years.

**Indication:** Sanguineous secretion from the left nipple.
**History:** Breast conservation therapy of the right breast 7 years previously.
**Risk profile:** Increased by earlier occurrence of breast cancer.
**Age:** 67 years.

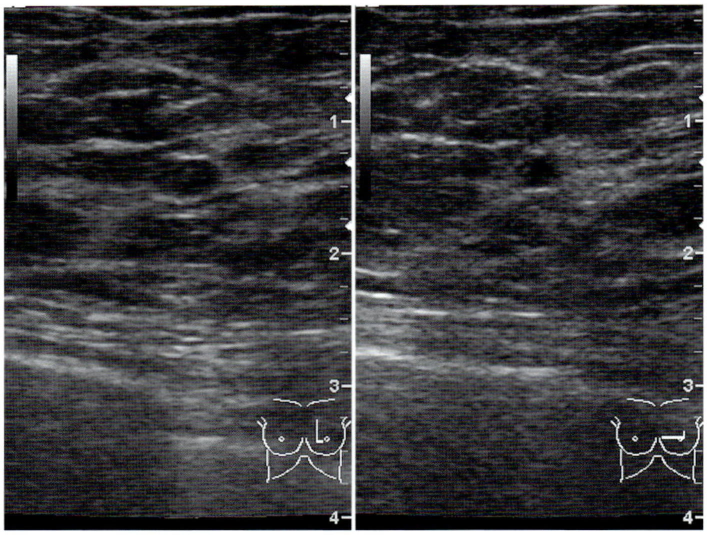

Fig. 43.**1** Sonography.

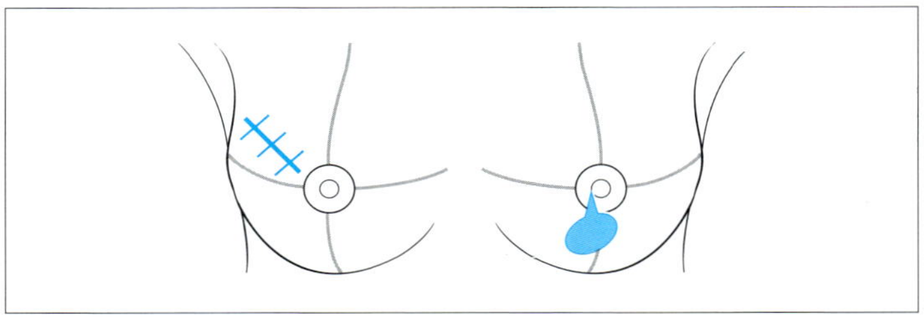

## Clinical Findings

No findings at palpation. Sanguineous secretion from one duct of the left breast.

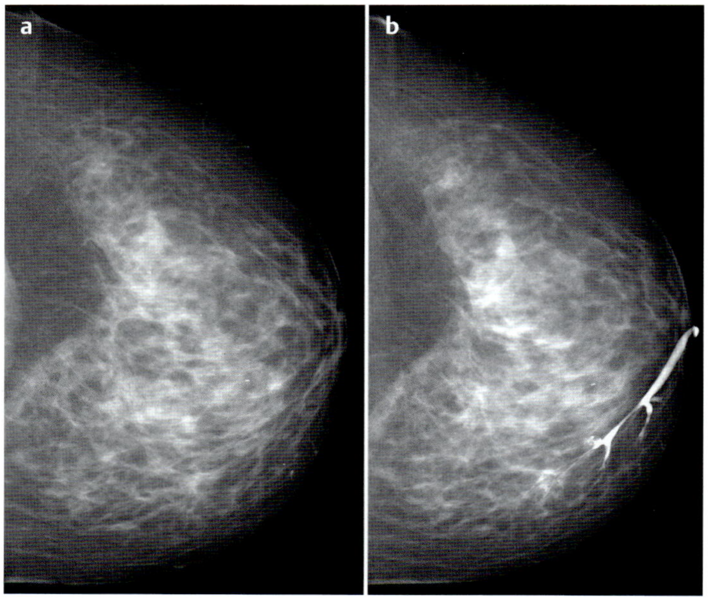


Fig. 43.**2 a, b** Digital mammography and galactography of the left breast, CC view.

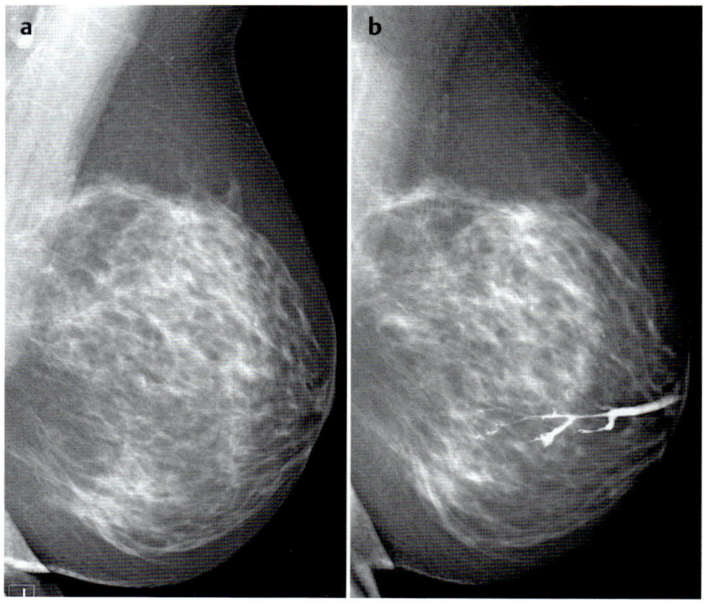


Fig. 43.**3 a, b** Digital mammography and galactography of the left breast, ML view.

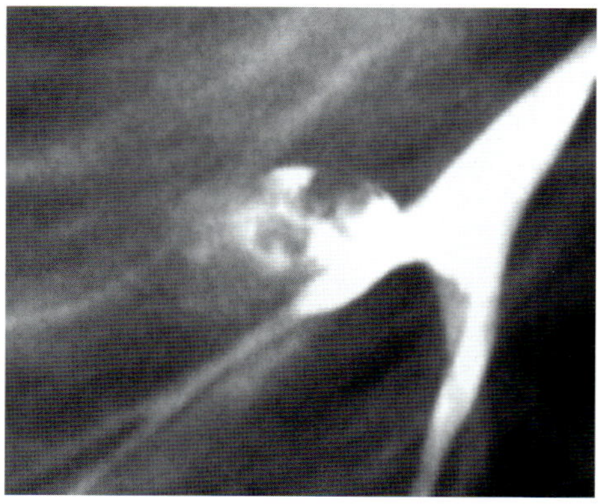

Fig. 43.**4** Magnification view of galactography of the left breast (CC).

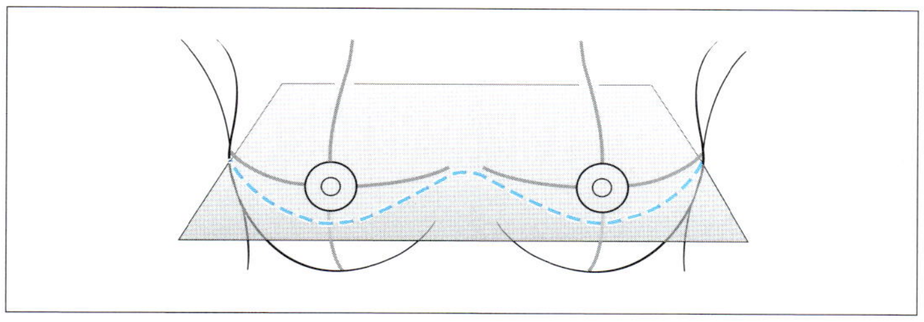

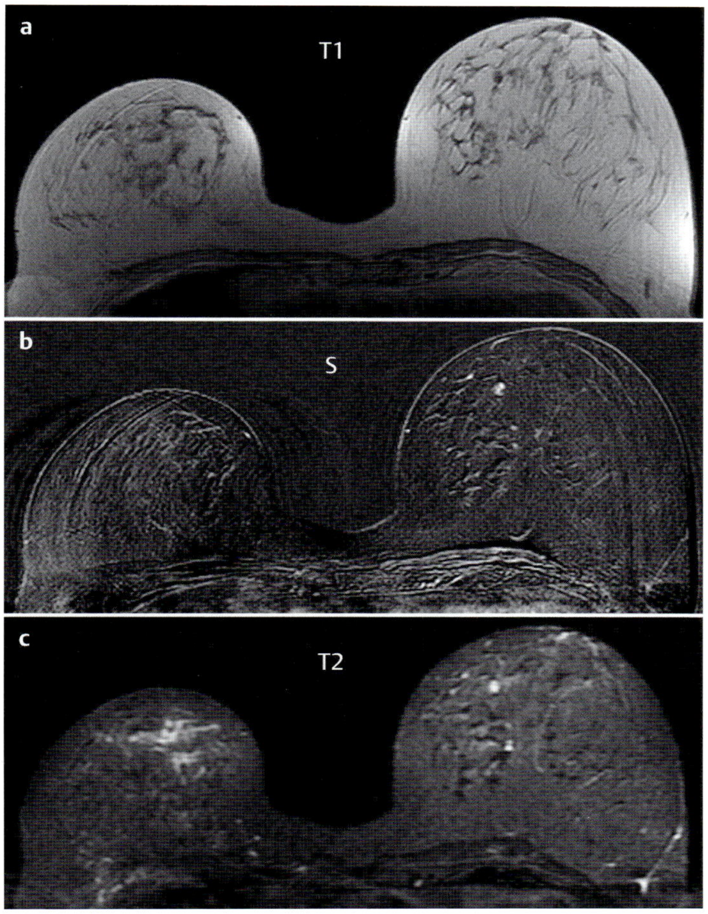


Fig. 43.**5 a–c** Contrast-enhanced MR mammography.

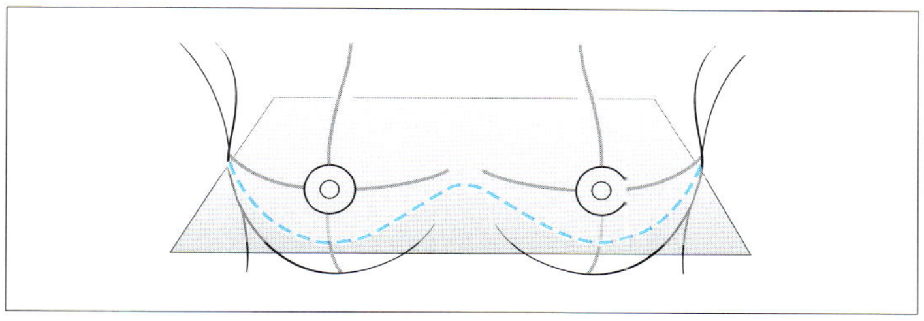

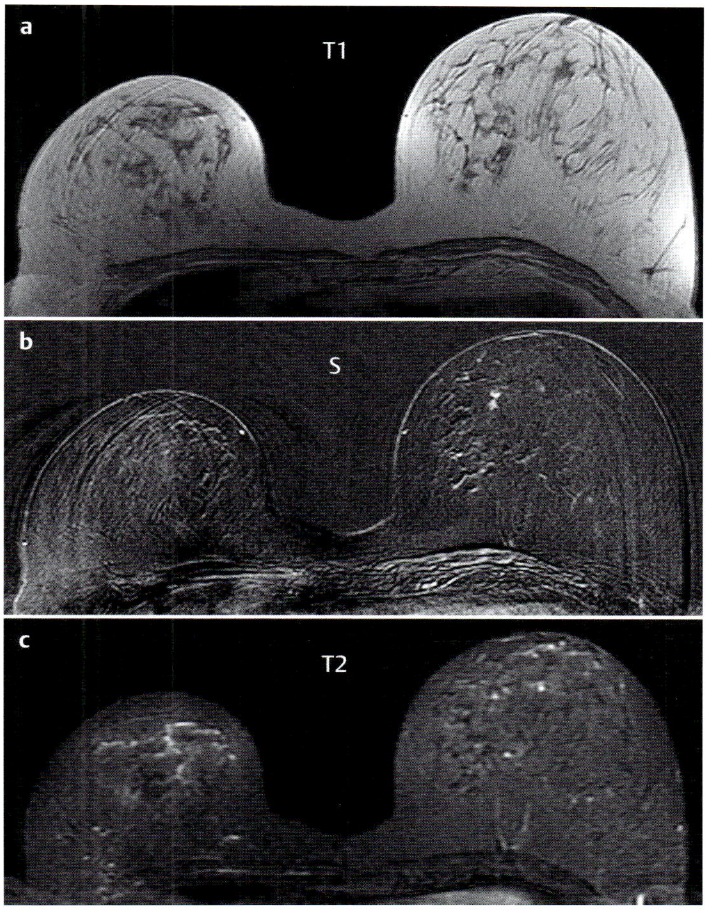


Fig. 43.**6 a–c** Contrast-enhanced MR mammography.

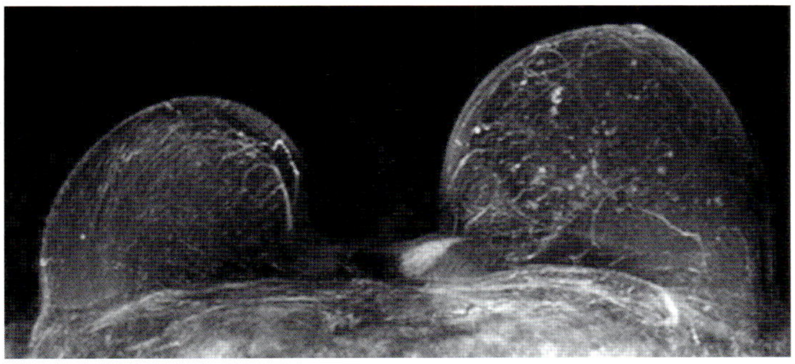

Fig. 43.**7** Contrast-enhanced MR mammography. Maximum intensity projection.

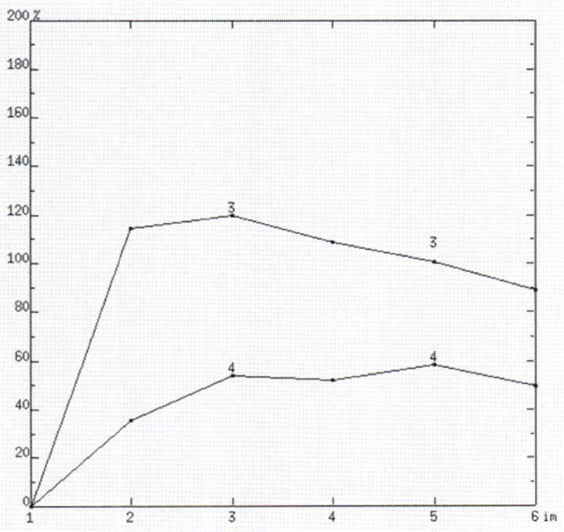


Fig. 43.**8** Signal-to-time curves of the lesion in the left breast.

Please characterize ultrasound, mammography, and MRI findings.
What is your preliminary diagnosis?
What are your next steps?

This is the imaging study of a symptomatic woman with a high risk profile presenting with pathological secretion from the left nipple.

### Ultrasound

Following an ectatic duct in the lower inner quadrant of the left breast, ultrasound showed vague indications of a hypoechoic mass, 3 mm in diameter, with indeterminate distal signal behavior. US BI-RADS 3.

### Mammography

Imaging showed inhomogeneous dense parenchyma, ACR type 3. There were no suspicious masses or densities, particularly in the lower inner quadrant of the left breast, and no microcalcifications. No architectural distortion. Galactography demonstrated a 3 mm contrast-filling defect in the lower inner quadrant of the left breast. BI-RADS right 1/left 3. PGMI is not defined for unilateral imaging.

### MR Mammography

Consistent with the lesion found in galactography, there was a hypervascularized, partially ill-defined lesion of 3 mm diameter in the lower inner quadrant of the left breast, with an increased signal in T2-weighted imaging. The lesion showed initial signal increase of 120% followed by washout.

**MRI Artifact Category:** 2
**MRI Density Type:** 1

| MRM score | Finding | Points |
|---|---|---|
| **Shape** | round | 0 |
| **Border** | ill-defined | 1 |
| **CM Distribution** | homogenous | 0 |
| **Initial Signal Intensity Increase** | strong | 2 |
| **Post-initial Signal Intensity Character** | wash-out | 2 |
| **MRI score (points)** | | **5** |
| **MRI BI-RADS** | | **4** |

### → Differential Diagnosis

Papilloma, adenoma, fibroadenoma, carcinoma.

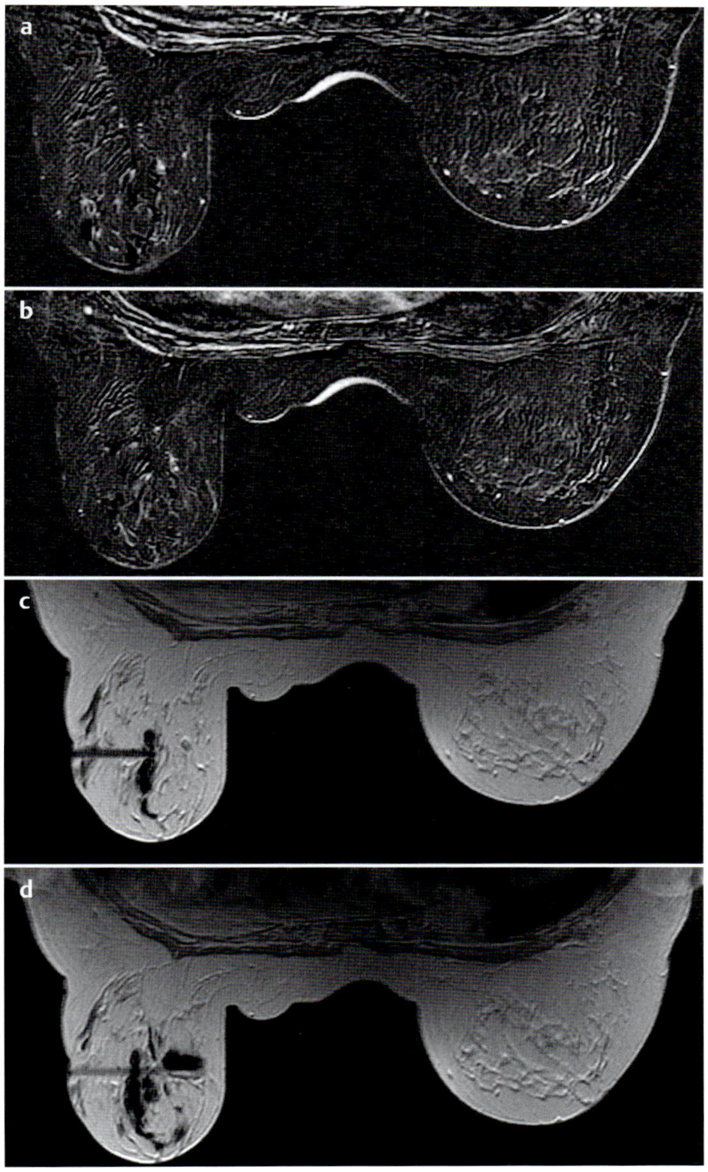


| BI-RADS Categorization | | |
|---|---|---|
| Clinical Findings | right 1 | left 3 |
| Ultrasound | right 1 | left 3 |
| Mammography | right 1 | left 3 |
| MR Mammography | right 1 | left 4 |
| **BI-RADS Total** | **right 1** | **left 4** |

**Procedure**

Histological analysis of the galactography findings in the lower inner quadrant of the left breast. MR-guided percutaneous vacuum biopsy with the objective of complete extraction of the lesion as a diagnostic and therapeutic intervention (Figs. 43.**9** and 43.**10**).

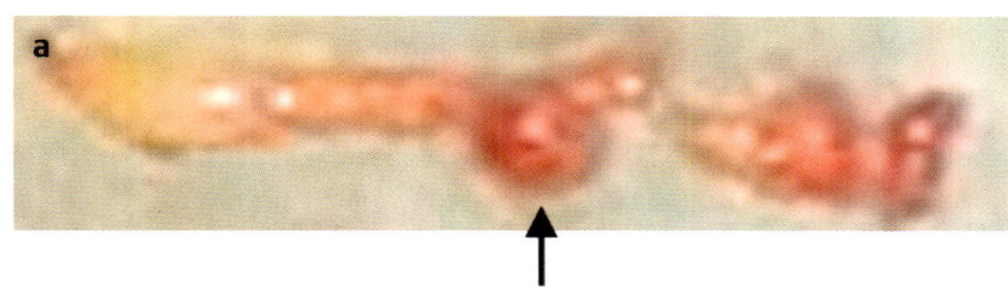


Fig. 43.**10 a** First biopsy specimen containing a round nodular structure (arrow).

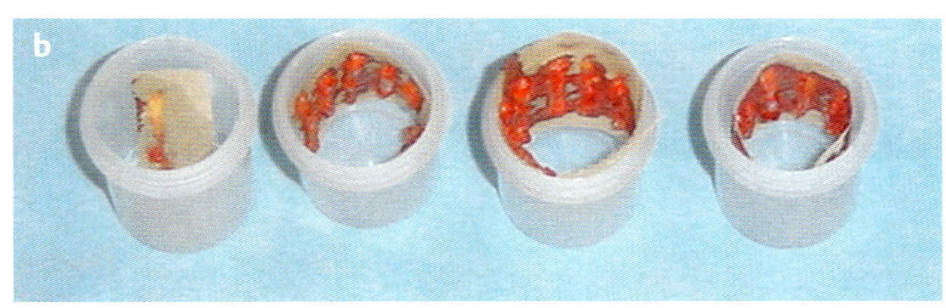


Fig. 43.**10 b** Complete set of 20 biopsy specimens ready for dispatch to histology lab.

## Histology

Completely removed intraductal papilloma (extracted in the very first core specimen (see Fig. 43.**10 a**). No malignancy.

Intraductal papilloma.

## Treatment

No additional therapy required due to the complete resection of the papilloma. Nipple bleeding ceased after core biopsy.

The risk of solitary intraductal papillomas becoming malignant is about 3–7%. In the case of multiple peripheral papillomas the relative risk of breast cancer is 10–33%. For this reason, the resection of papillomas is recommended. This can be achieved by vacuum biopsy in the case of small papillomas.

**Indication:** Palpable mass in the right breast.
**History:** Unremarkable.
**Risk profile:** No increased risk.
**Age:** 28 years.

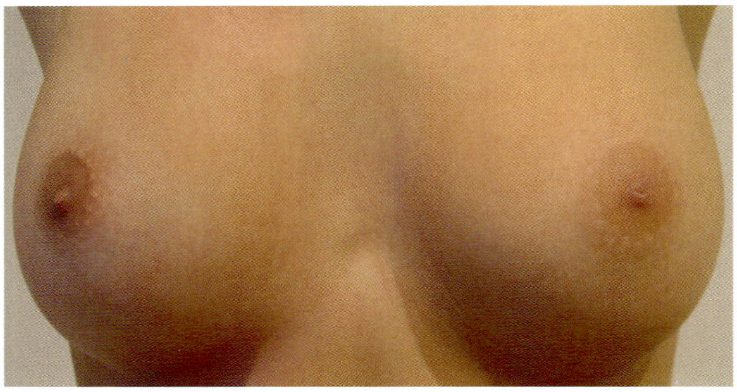

Fig. 44.**1** Clinical examination. Well-defined, mobile lump between the outer quadrants of the right breast.

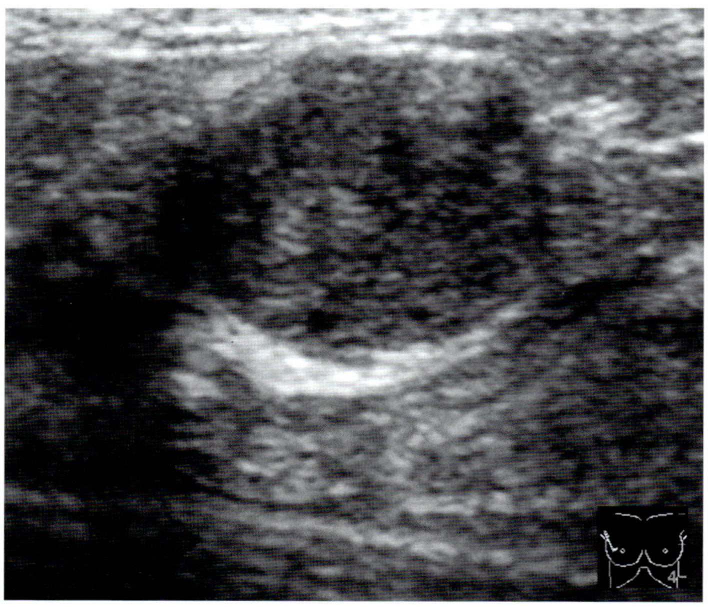

Fig. 44.**2** Sonography.

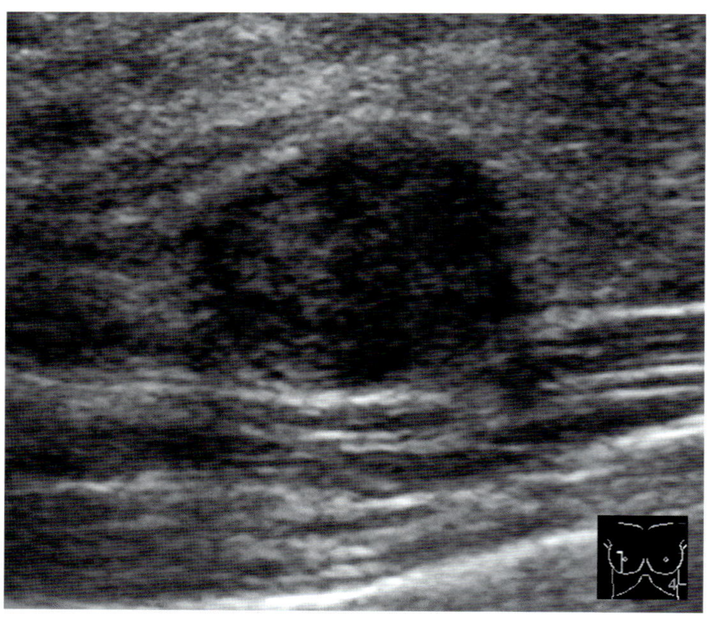

Fig. 44.**3** Sonography.

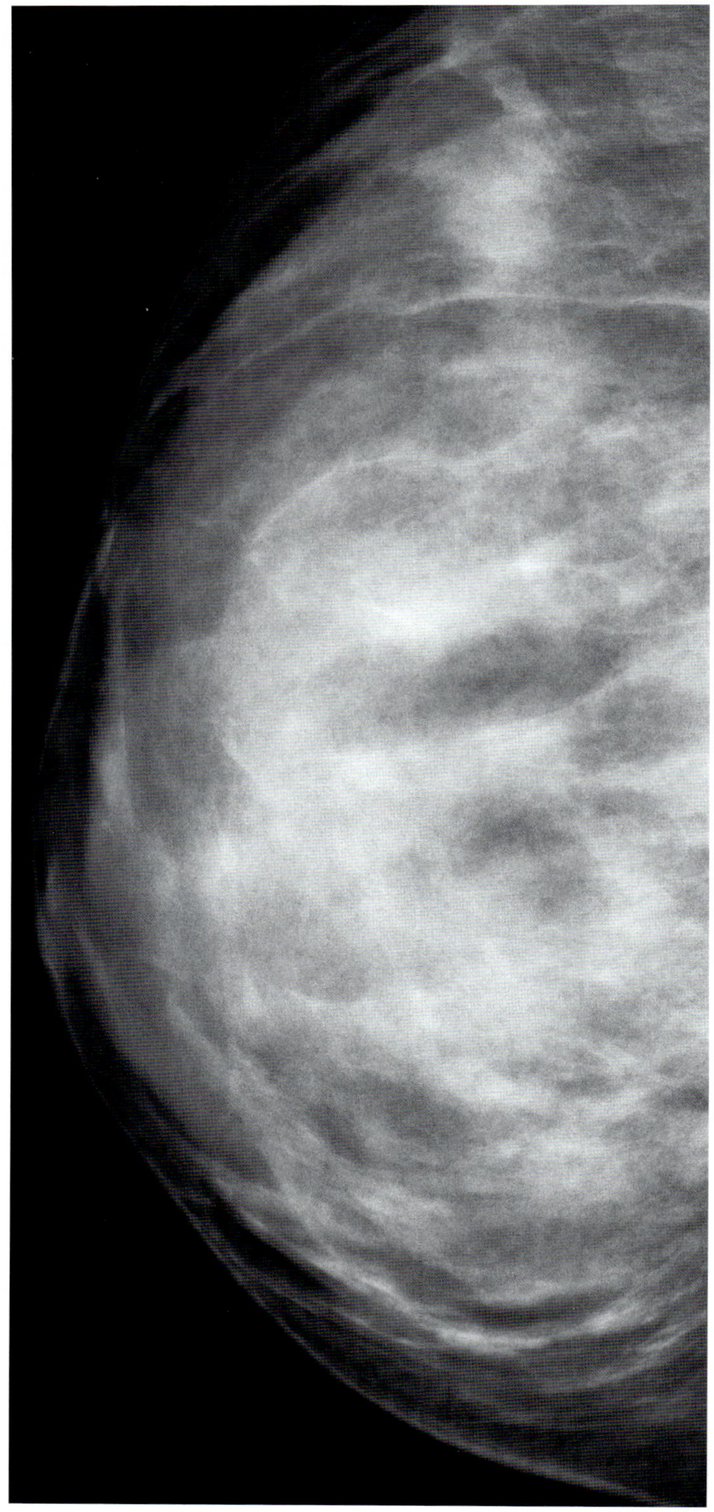

Fig. 44.**4** Digital mammography, CC view.

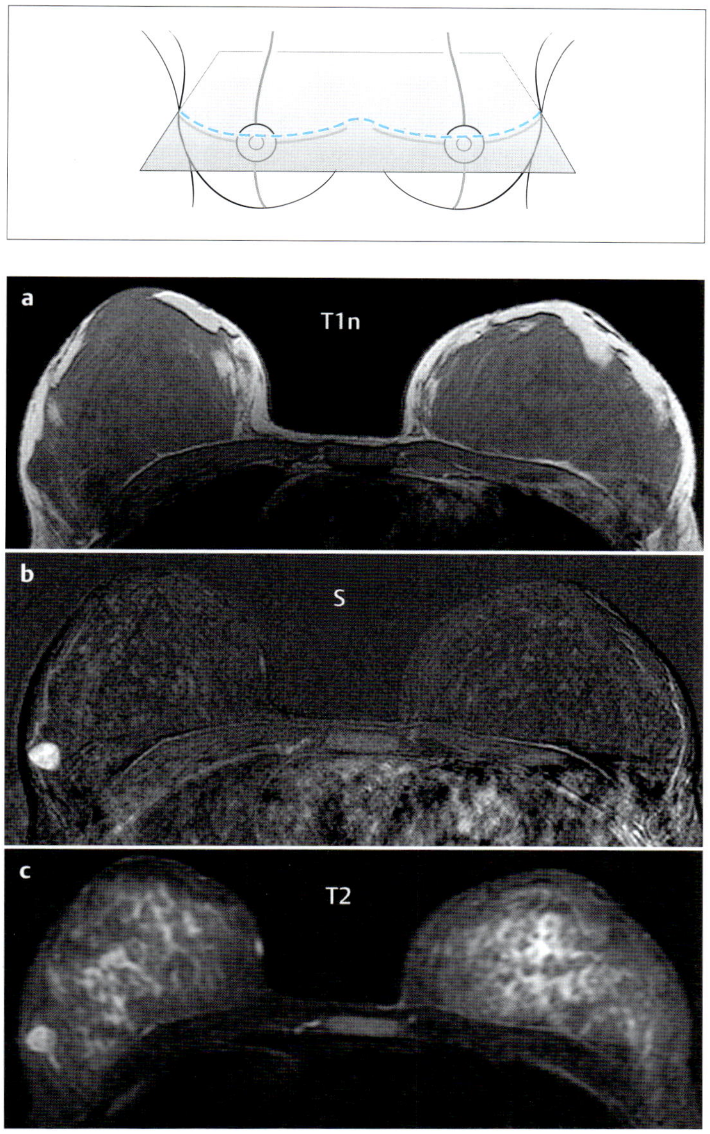


Fig. 44.5 **a – c** Contrast-enhanced MR mammography.

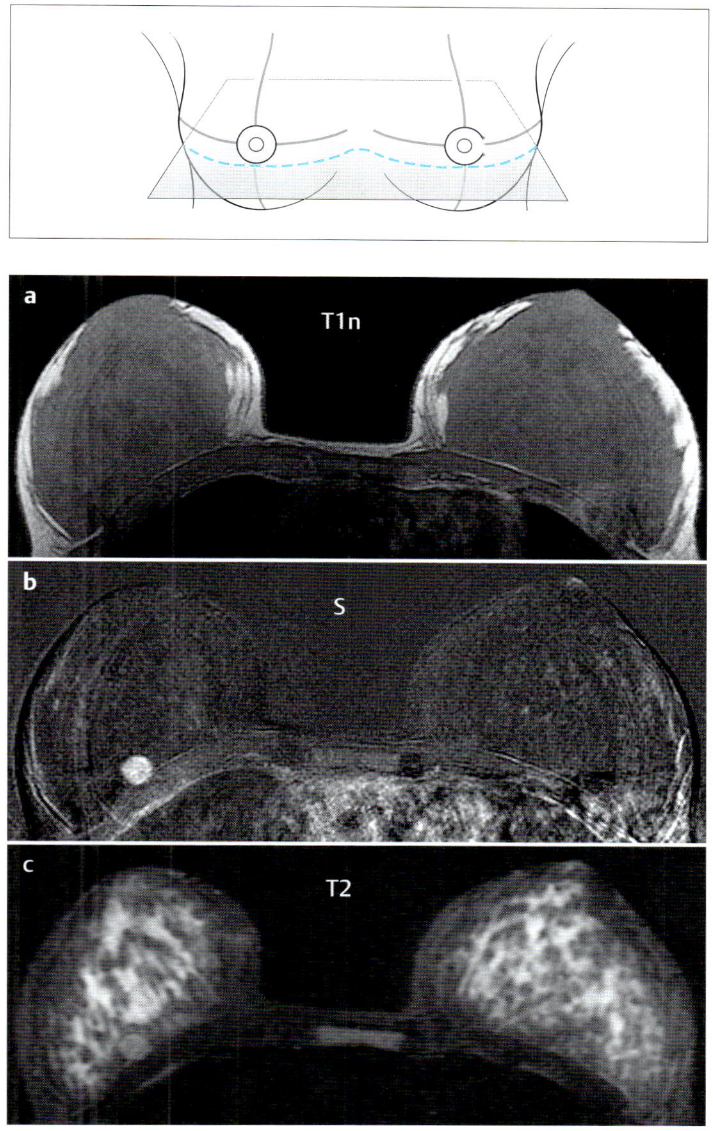


Fig. 44.6 **a – c** Contrast-enhanced MR mammography.

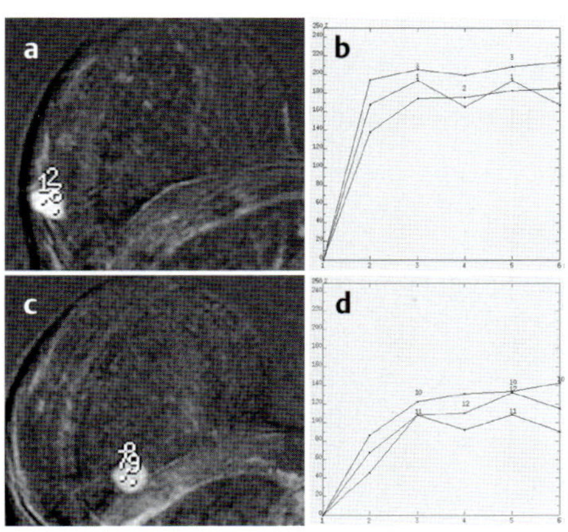


Fig. 44.7 **a – d** Signal-to-time curves.

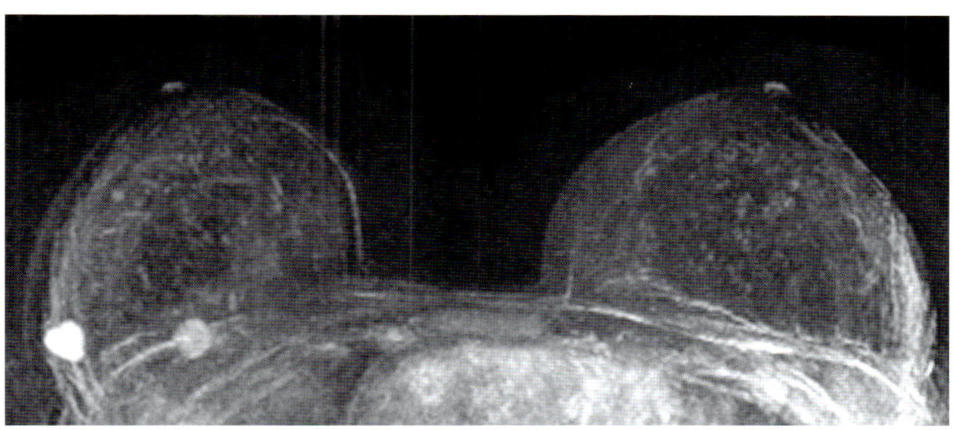

Fig. 44.8 Contrast-enhanced MR mammography. Maximum intensity projection.

?

Please characterize ultrasound, mammography, and MRI findings.
What is your preliminary diagnosis?
What are your next steps?

The imaging was carried out to clarify the situation in a very young patient with a newly discovered palpable mass in her right breast. Because of the symptoms present–the lump in the right breast–dose-reduced digital mammography (one-view) was performed to exclude possible microcalcifications.

### Ultrasound

Consistent with the palpable lump, ultrasound showed a round lesion with well-defined margins and an inhomogeneous acoustic signal. There were no signs of malignancy. There was another lesion with similar echogenicity in ultrasound in the central part of the right breast, toward the chest wall. US BI-RADS right outer and central 3.

### Mammography

As expected, the glandular tissue was extremely dense (ACR type 4). There was a questionable round density between the outer quadrants of the right breast, possibly corresponding to the palpable lump. Mammography depicted no calcifications and no architectural distortion. BI-RADS right 1.

### MR Mammography

Corresponding to palpation and ultrasound findings, MRI showed a hypervascularized round, well-defined lesion with a high T2 signal between the outer quadrants of the right breast. Another lesion with comparable pre- and postcontrast signal characteristics was visible in the central part of the right breast close to the chest wall. However, this lesion had intermediate signal in T2-weighted imaging.

**MRI Artifact Category:** 2
**MRI Density Type:** 1

| MRM score | Right breast, outer quadrants | Points | Right breast, central region | Points |
|---|---|---|---|---|
| **Shape** | round | 0 | round | 0 |
| **Border** | well-defined | 0 | well-defined | 0 |
| **CM Distribution** | inhomogeneous | 1 | inhomogeneous | 1 |
| **Initial Signal Intensity Increase** | strong | 2 | strong | 2 |
| **Post-initial Signal Intensity Character** | plateau | 1 | plateau | 1 |
| **MRI score (points)** | | **4** | | **4** |
| **MRI BI-RADS** | | **4** | | **4** |

### → Preliminary Diagnosis

Bifocal fibroadenoma of the right breast (myxoid?), adenoma.

### → Differential Diagnosis

Carcinoma (medullary?)–very unlikely.

| BI-RADS Categorization | | |
|---|---|---|
| Clinical Findings | right 3 | left 1 |
| Ultrasound | right 3 | left 1 |
| Mammography | right 1 | left 1 |
| MR Mammography | right 4 | left 1 |
| **BI-RADS Total** | **right 4** | **left 1** |

**Procedure**

US-guided percutaneous core biopsy of the palpable mass for histological analysis was recommended. However, at the patient's request, and in view of the discomfort caused by the lump in the right breast, an open biopsy of both lesions in the right breast was performed without preoperative core biopsy.

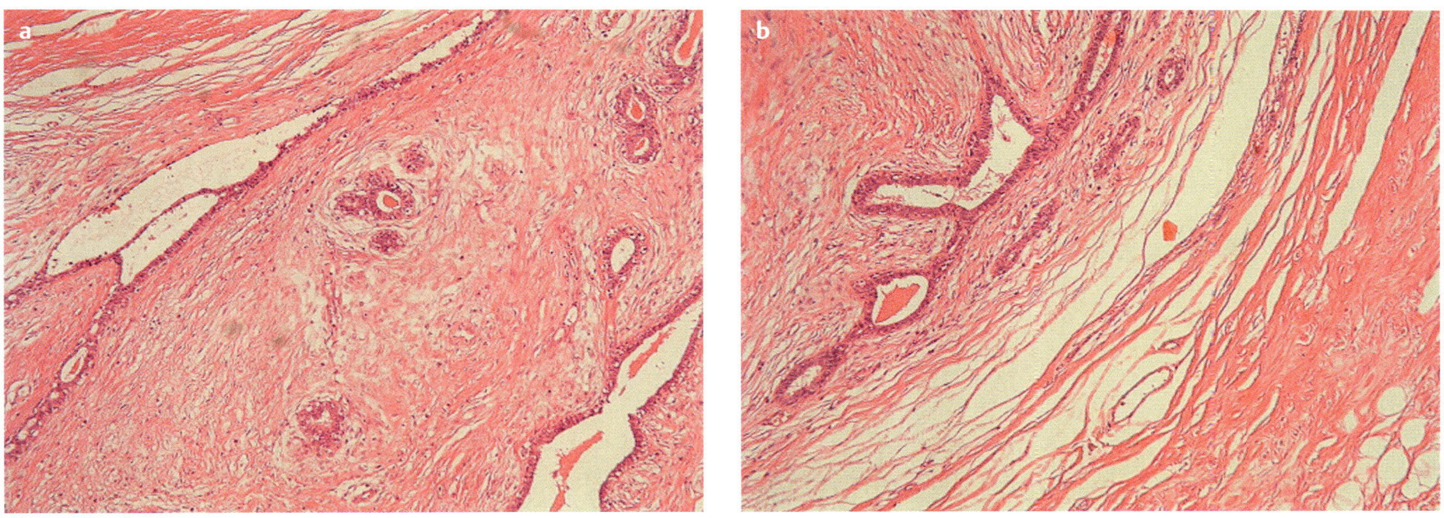

Fig. 44.**9 a, b** Specimens from both lesions in the right breast. Histologically typical fibroadenomas.

## Histology

20 mm and 22 mm fibroadenomas in the right breast.

Myxoid fibroadenoma (bifocal) in the right breast

## Treatment

Excisional biopsy.

Myxoid fibroadenoma is the most common breast tumor in younger women.

**Indication:** Screening.
**History:** Unremarkable.
**Risk profile:** No increased risk.
**Age:** 58 years.

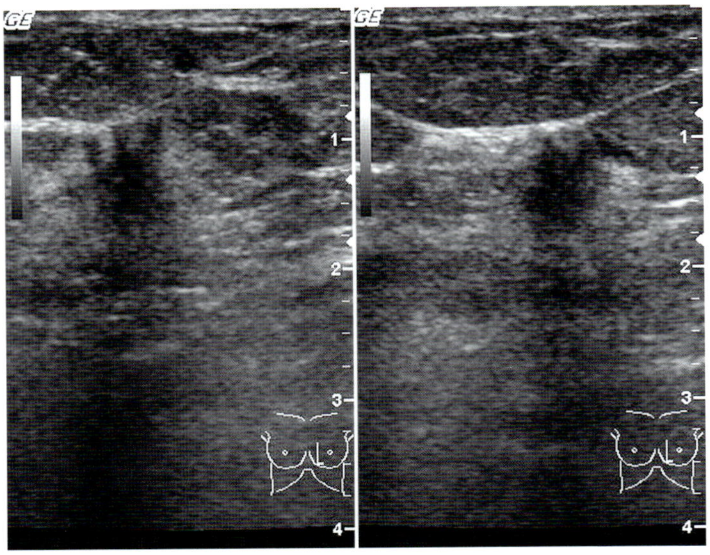


Fig. 45.**1** Ultrasound.

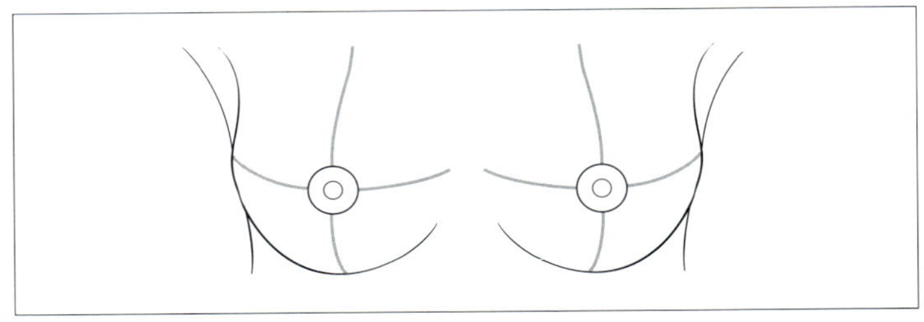

**Clinical Findings**

No suspect findings.

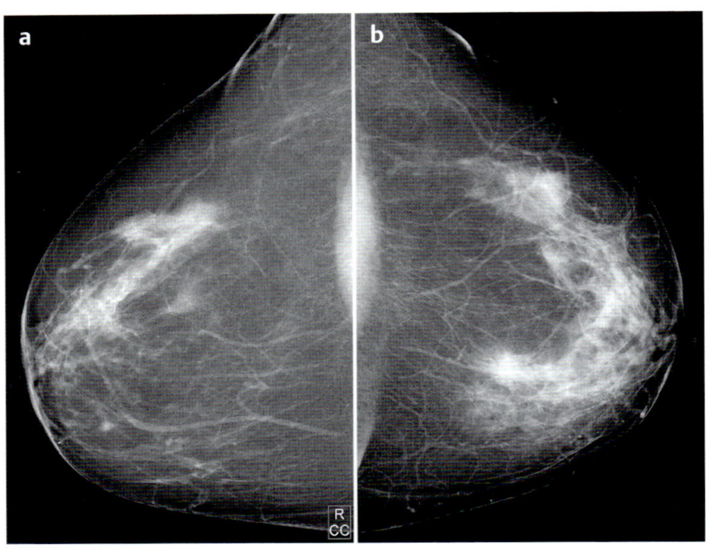


Fig. 45.**2 a, b** Digital mammography, CC view.

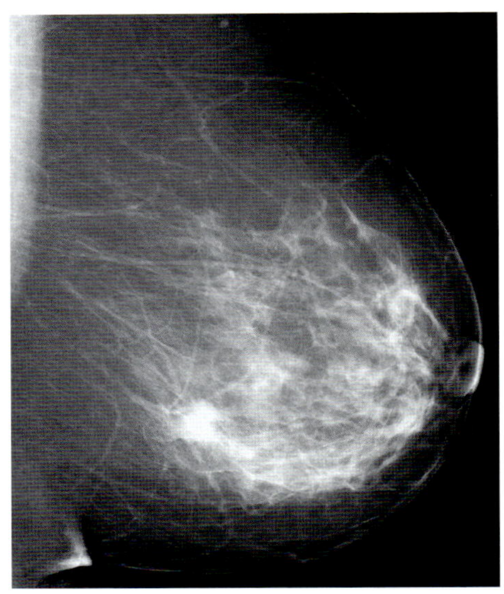

Fig. 45.**4** Digital mammography, left breast. ML view.

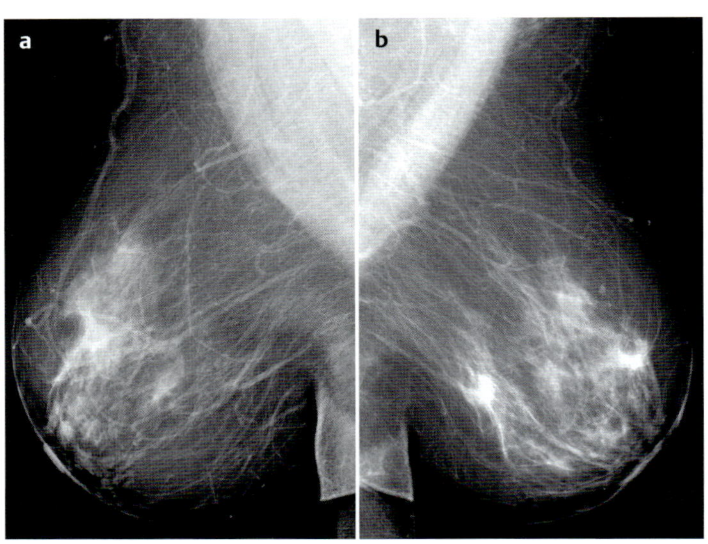


Fig. 45.**3 a, b** Digital mammography, MLO view.

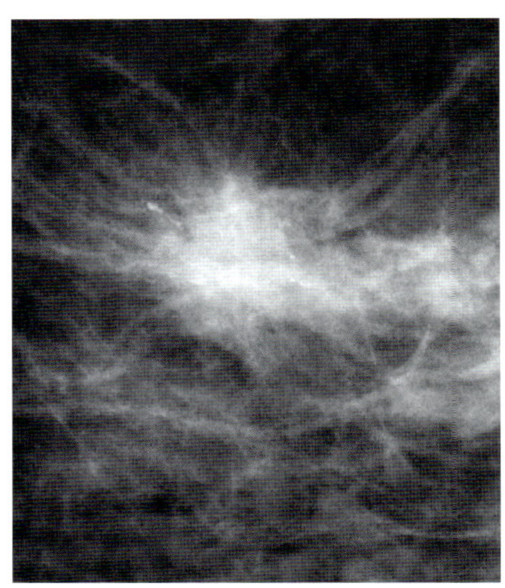

Fig. 45.**5** Magnification view, left breast (CC).

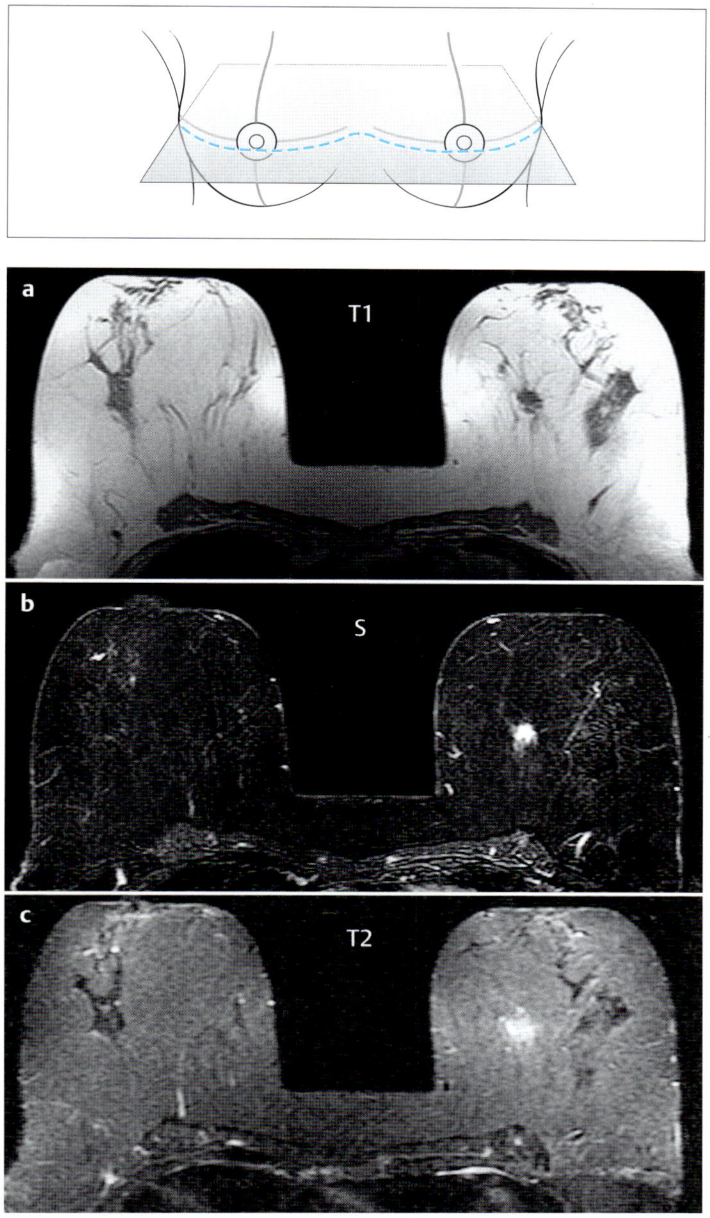


Fig. 45.**6 a – c** Contrast-enhanced MRI of the breasts.

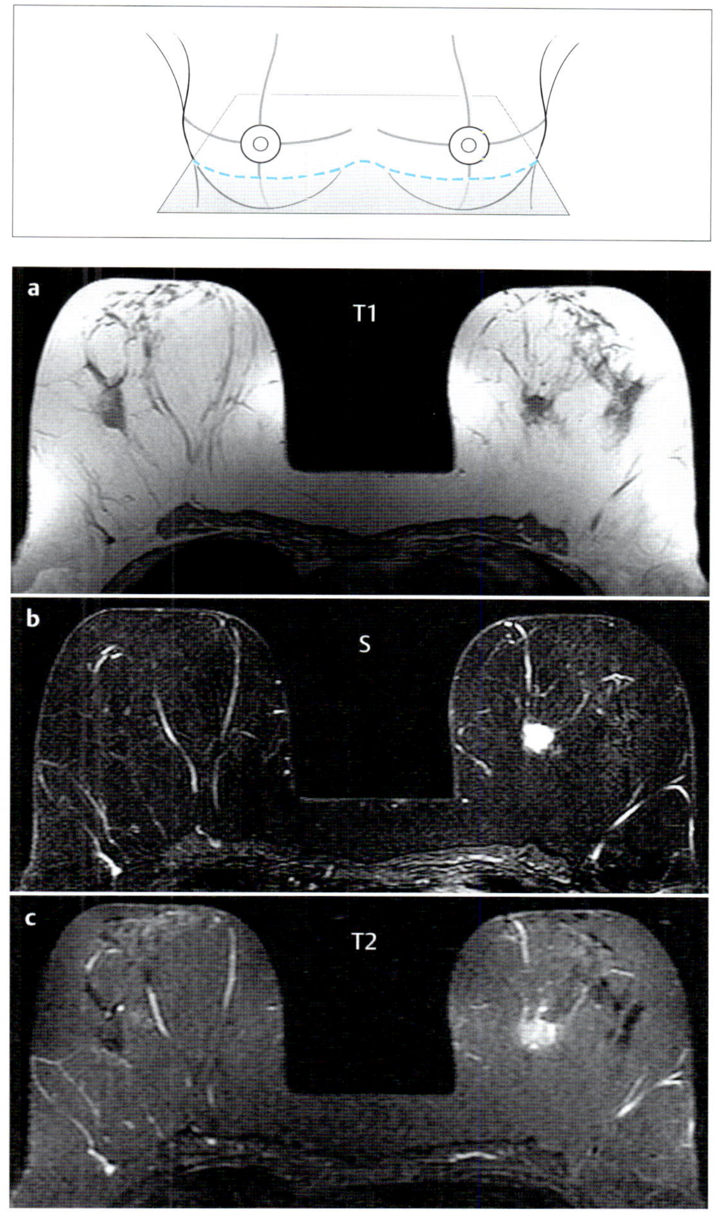


Fig. 45.**7 a – c** Contrast-enhanced MRI of the breasts.

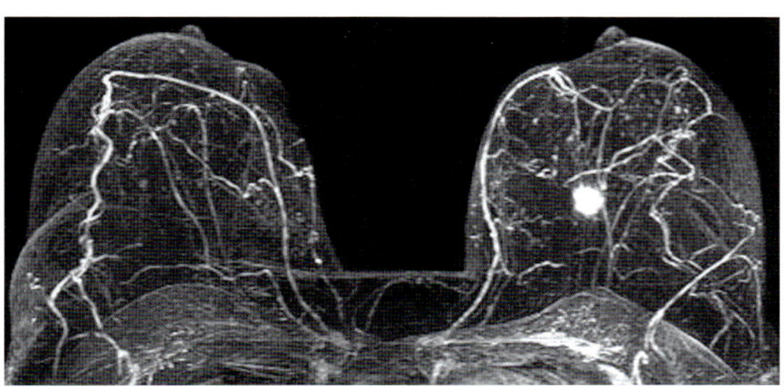

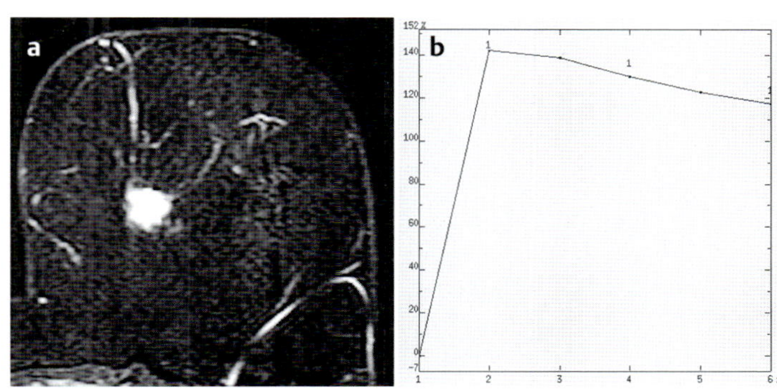


Fig. 45.**9 a, b** Signal-to-time curve.

Please characterize ultrasound, mammography, and MRI findings.
What is your preliminary diagnosis?
What are your next steps?

This case demonstrates the imaging studies of an asymptomatic woman.

### Ultrasound

Ultrasound showed an irregular hypoechoic lesion (diameter 1 cm) with distal shadowing and architectural distortion in the lower inner quadrant of the left breast. US BI-RADS 5.

### Mammography

The parenchyma was bilaterally symmetric with fibroglandular texture, ACR type 2. A hyperdense, lobulated mass of 1 cm diameter with spiculation and predominantly monomorphous microcalcifications was visible in the left lower inner quadrant. Mammograms showed no architectural distortion (BI-RADS right 1/left 5). PGMI: CC view P; MLO view G (inframammary fold).

### MR Mammography

MRI demonstrated a partially lobulated, partially spiculated, homogeneously enhancing mass in the lower inner quadrant of the left breast with a diameter of 1 cm. This mass had an initial signal increase of 115% and postinitial washout as well as increased signal in T2-weighted imaging.

**MRI Artifact Category:** 1
**MRI Density Type:** 1

| MRM score | Finding | Points |
|---|---|---|
| **Shape** | round | 0 |
| **Border** | spiculated | 1 |
| **CM Distribution** | inhomogenous | 1 |
| **Initial Signal Intensity Increase** | strong | 2 |
| **Post-initial Signal Intensity Character** | wash-out | 2 |
| **MRI score (points)** | | **6** |
| **MRI BI-RADS** | | **5** |

### → Preliminary Diagnosis

Carcinoma.

| BI-RADS Categorization | | |
|---|---|---|
| Clinical Findings | right 1 | left 1 |
| Ultrasound | right 1 | left 5 |
| Mammography | right 1 | left 5 |
| MR Mammography | right 1 | left 5 |
| **BI-RADS Total** | **right 1** | **left 5** |

### Procedure

Ultrasound guided core biopsy of the lesion in the left breast for histological analysis.

### Histology

Lobular invasive carcinoma.

### Further procedure

Resection of tumor after preoperative hook-wire localization (Fig. 45.**10 a, b**). Perioperative specimen radiography to verify complete excision of tumor (Fig. 45.**11**).

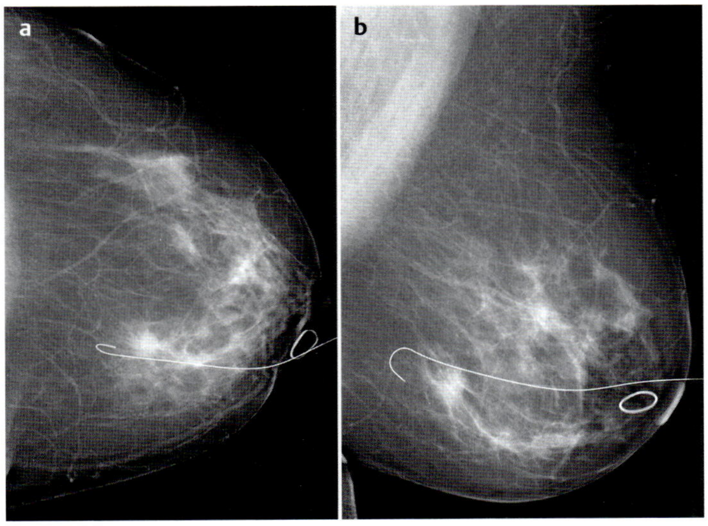


Fig. 45.**10 a, b** Hook-wire localization seen in mammography.

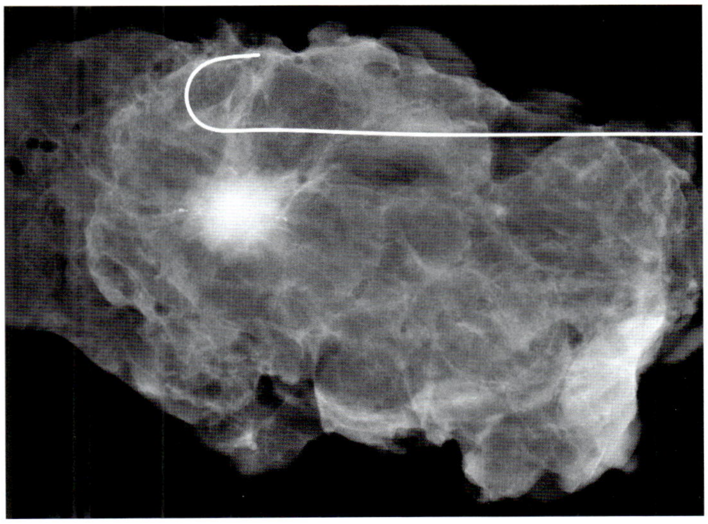

Fig. 45.**11** Specimen radiography.

### Histology

Lobular invasive breast carcinoma with a diameter of 12 mm. Axillary lymph node status normal.

ILC pT1c, pN0, G2.

### Treatment

Breast conservation therapy of the left breast.

This case is a good example of the classic carcinoma discovered through screening, with suspicious changes in all three imaging modalities.

**Indication:** Screening.
**History:** Unremarkable.
**Risk profile:** No increased risk.
**Age:** 53 years.

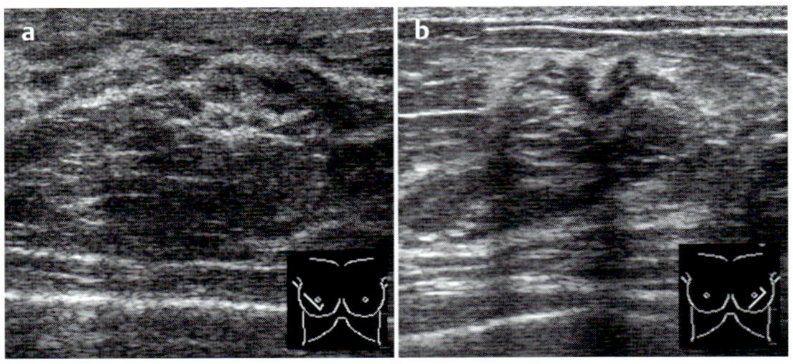


Fig. 46.1 **a, b** Sonography of both breasts.

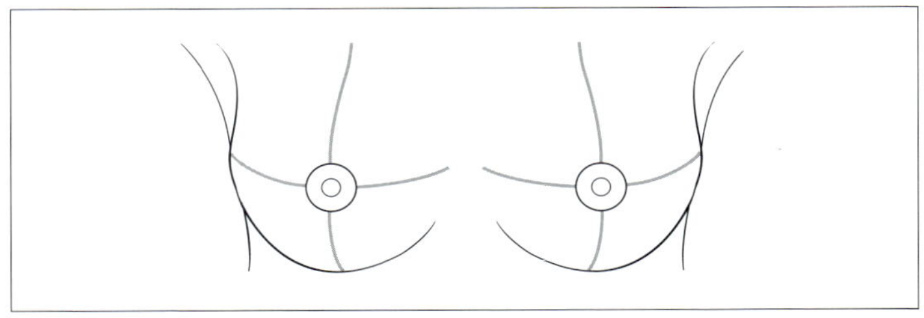

## Clinical Findings

Normal.

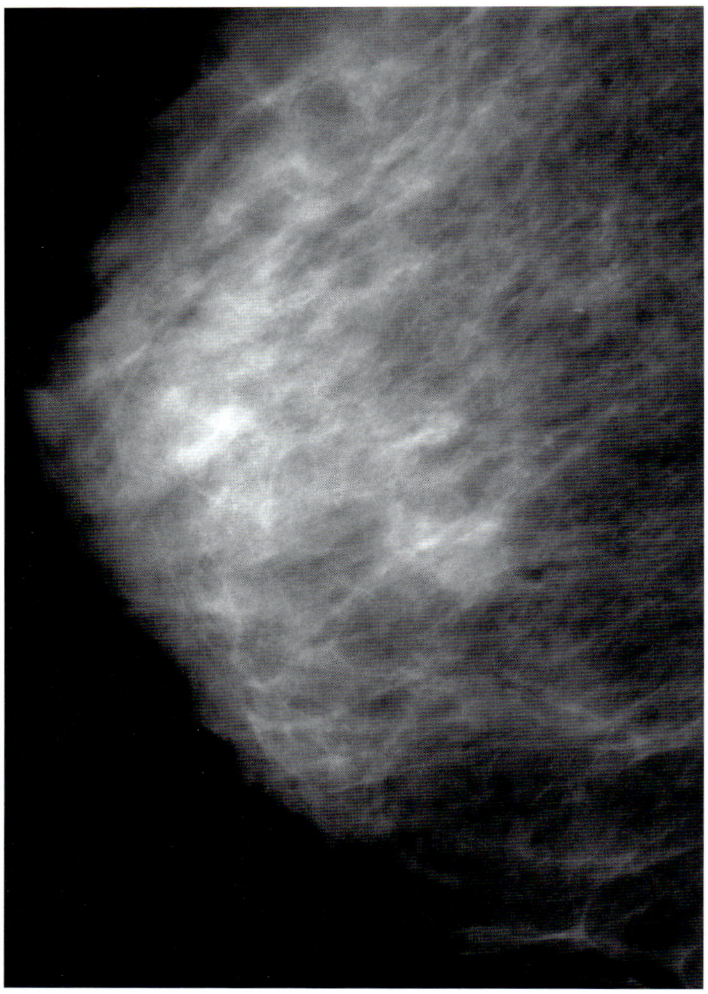

Fig. 46.**2** Digital mammography. Magnification view of right breast.

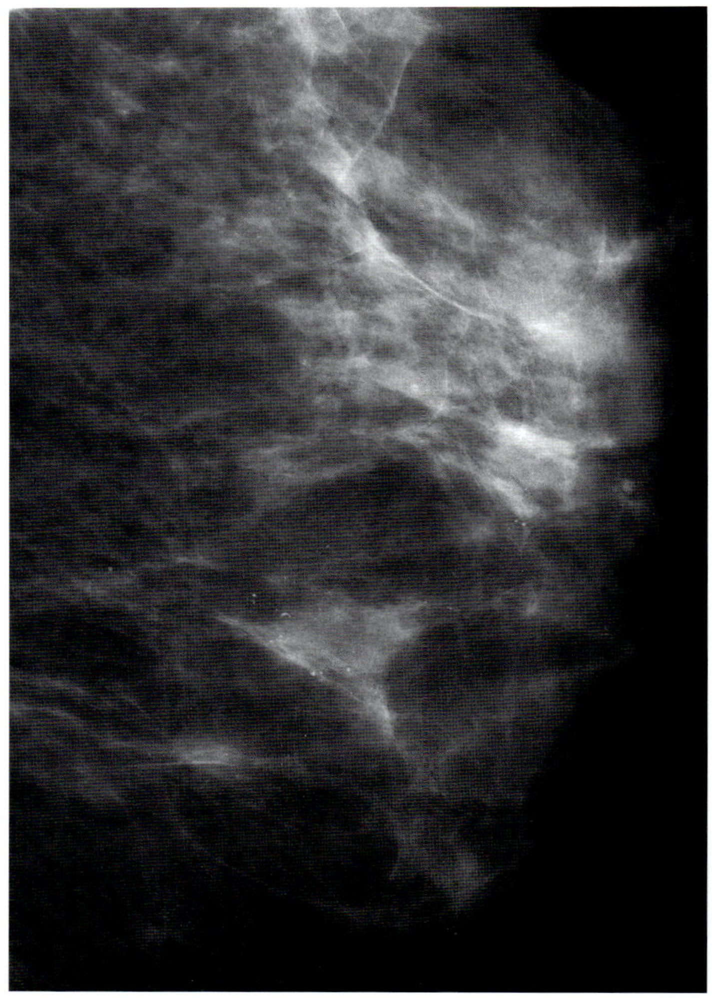

Fig. 46.**3** Digital mammography. Magnif cation view of left breast.

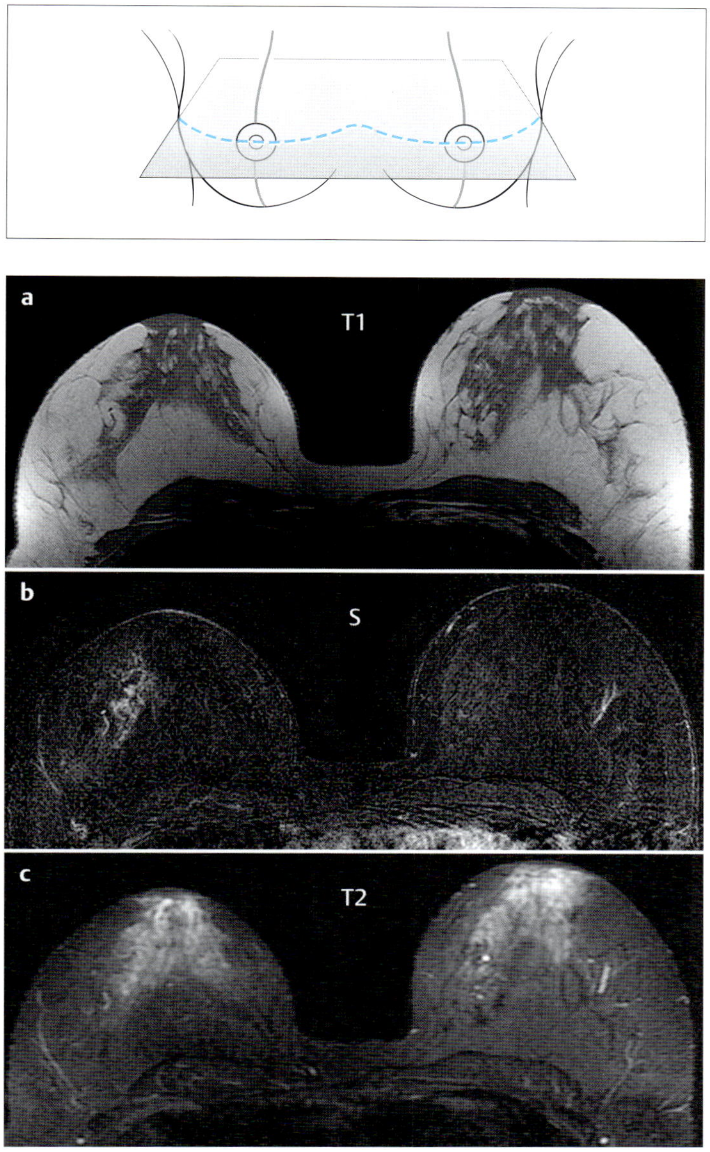


Fig. 46.**4 a–c** Contrast-enhanced MRI of the breasts.

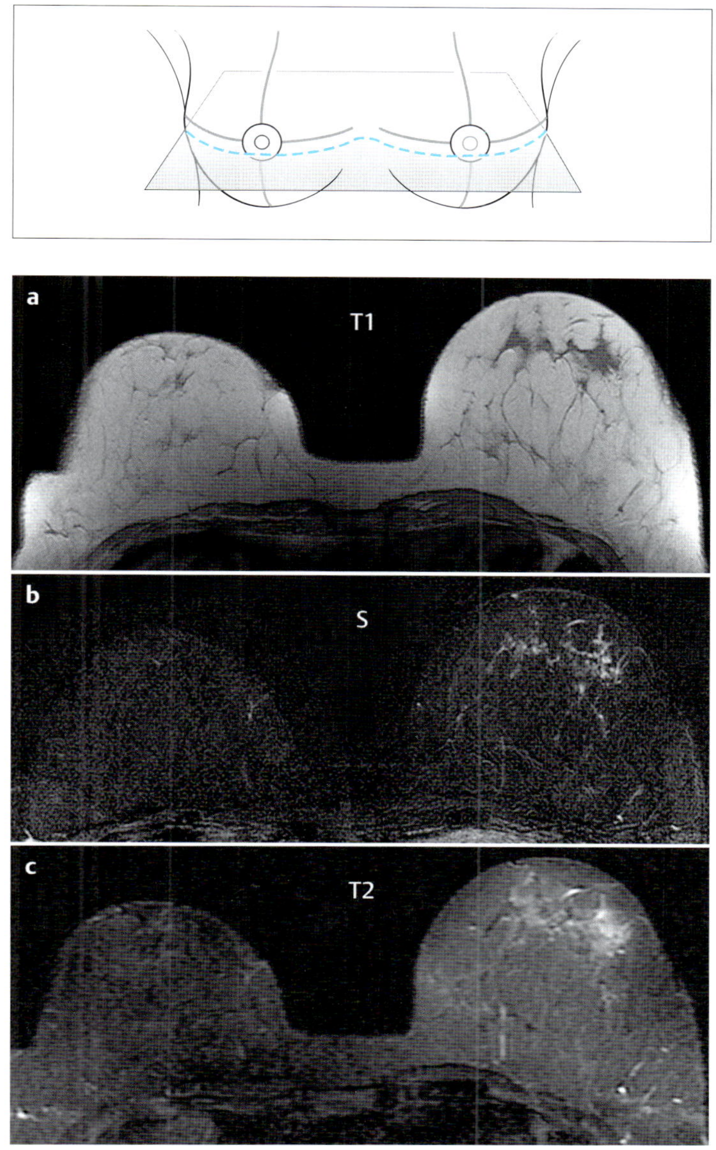


Fig. 46.**5 a–c** Contrast-enhanced MRI of the breasts.

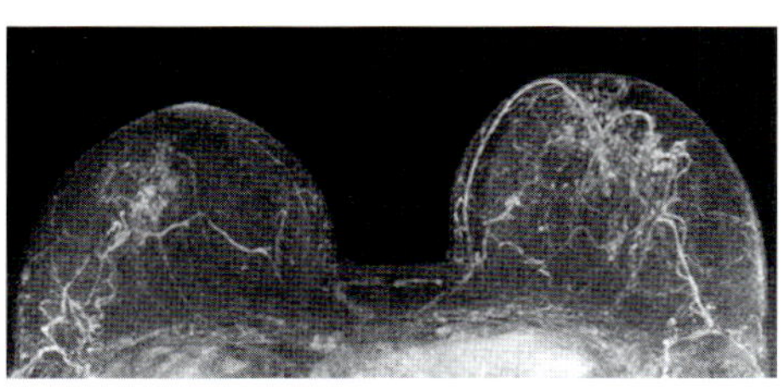

Fig. 46.**6** Contrast-enhanced MR mammography. Maximum intensity projection.

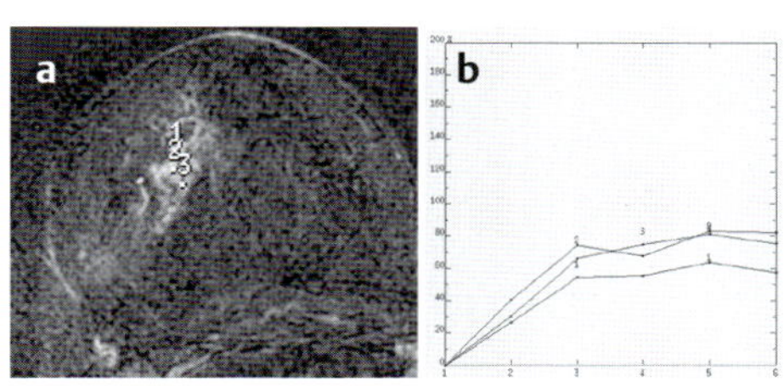


Fig. 46.**7 a, b** Signal-to-time curves.

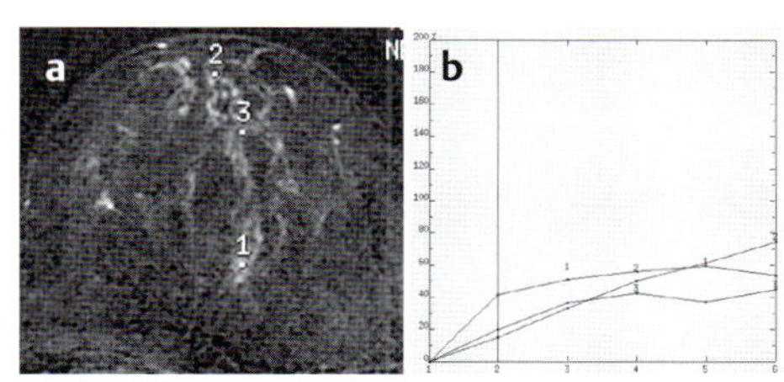


Fig. 46.**8 a, b** Signal-to-time curves (MR slice below the slice seen in Fig. 46.**5 b**).

**?**

Please characterize ultrasound, mammography, and MRI findings.
What is your preliminary diagnosis?
What are your next steps?

This case demonstrates the diagnostic imaging and additional investigations for an asymptomatic woman.

### Ultrasound

Images showed ectatic milk ducts in the lower outer quadrant of the left breast compared to the corresponding area in the right breast. Otherwise findings were sonographically normal. US BI-RADS right 1/left 3.

### Mammography

Mammograms demonstrated inhomogeneous dense parenchyma, ACR type 3. Comparison of the magnification views showed asymmetry of the glandular tissue accompanied by architectural distortion and retraction phenomenon in the left breast. There were diffuse polymorphous microcalcifications (predominantly round, some linear and curved), in the left breast, but no V-or Y-shaped calcifications. Some monomorphous calcifications were visible in the right breast. No masses or hyperdensities. BI-RADS right 3/left 4.

### MR Mammography

MRI showed dendritic enhancement in both lower quadrants of the left breast, but no circumscribed mass. Signal–time analysis is not particularly useful under such conditions, but in any case was unremarkable in the present examination. There was also a dendritic enhancing area in the right breast with a nonsuspect signal curve.

**MRI Artifact Category:** 1
**MRI Density Type:** 1

| MRM score | Finding right | Points | Finding left | Points |
|---|---|---|---|---|
| **Shape** | dendritic | 1 | dendritic | 1 |
| **Border** | ill-defined | 1 | ill-defined | 1 |
| **CM Distribution** | homogenous | 0 | homogeneous | 0 |
| **Initial Signal Intensity Increase** | low | 0 | moderate | 1 |
| **Post-initial Signal Intensity Character** | continuous | 0 | continuous | 0 |
| **MRI score (points)** | | **2** | | **3** |
| **MRI BI-RADS** | | **2** | | **3** |

### → Differential Diagnosis

Adenosis, DCIS.

| BI-RADS Categorization | | |
|---|---|---|
| Clinical Findings | right 1 | left 1 |
| Ultrasound | right 1 | left 3 |
| Mammography | right 3 | left 4 |
| MR Mammography | right 2 | left 3 |
| **BI-RADS Total** | **right 3** | **left 4** |

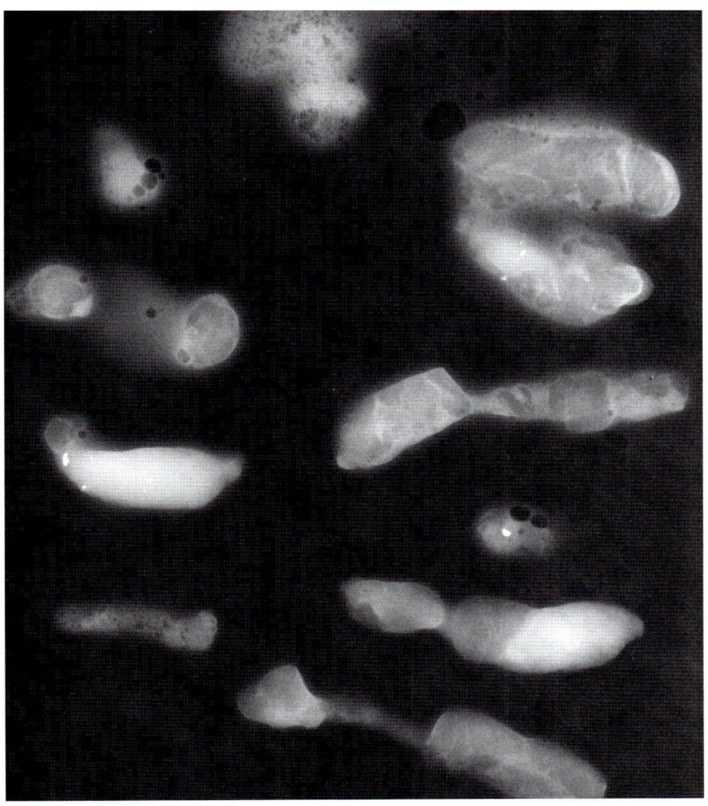

Fig. 46.**9** Radiography of the specimens from biopsy of the left breast.

**Procedure**

Histological evaluation of the microcalcifications in the left breast with stereotactic vacuum biopsy. If these show malignancy, additional stereotactic vacuum biopsy of the calcifications in the right breast should be carried out.

**Histology of the left breast specimens**

Intraductal carcinoma.

**Histology of the right breast specimen**

Ductal hyperplasia.

## Histology

Left: DCIS
Right: Ductal hyperplasia

## Treatment

Mastectomy of the left breast due to extensive DCIS; reduction surgery on the right breast.

In cases with dendritic enhancement in MRI, evaluation of dynamic criteria is often of secondary importance. Morphological criteria are more relevant for diagnosis in these circumstances.

**Indication:** Screening.
**History:** Unremarkable.
**Risk profile:** No increased risk.
**Age:** 47 years.

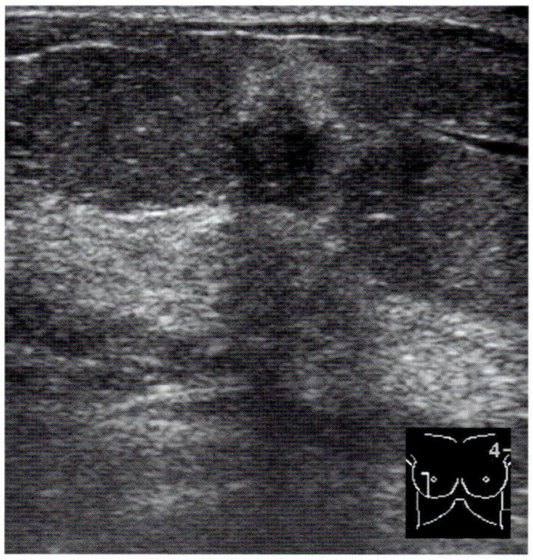

Fig. 47.**1** Sonography.

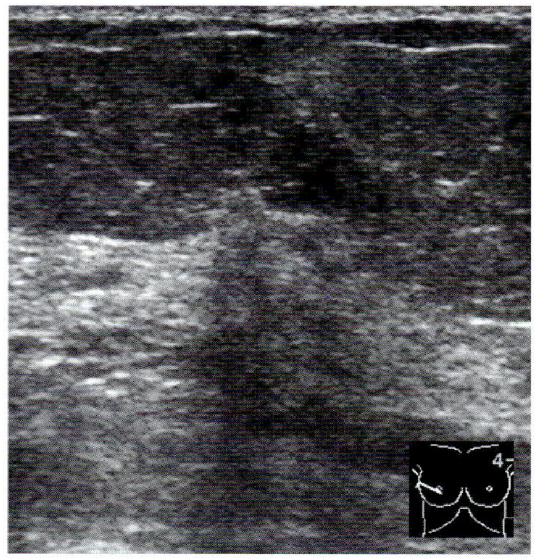

Fig. 47.**2** Sonography.

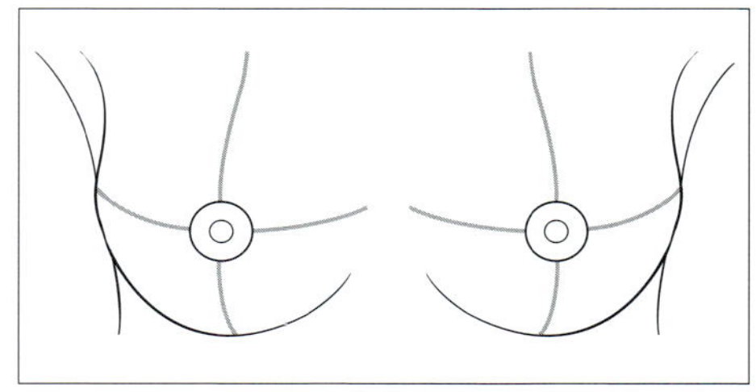

## Clinical Findings

Normal.

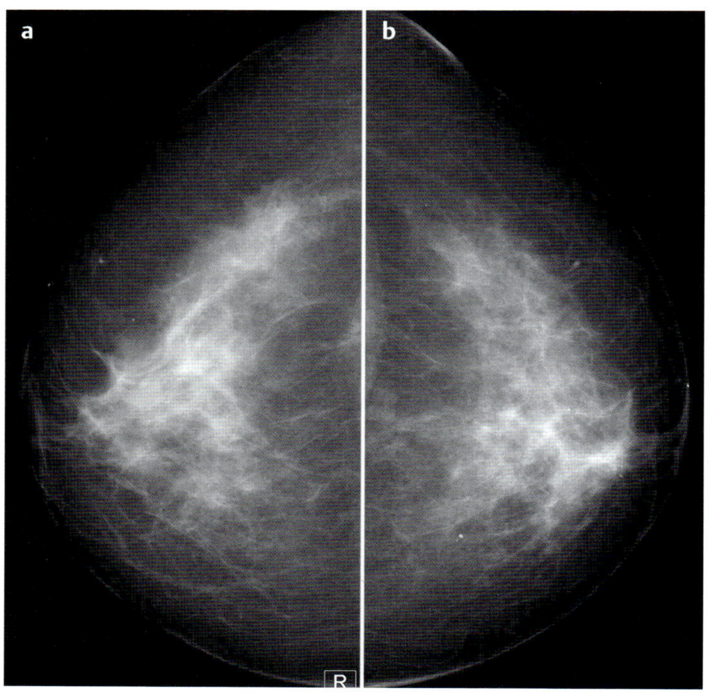


Fig. 47.**3 a, b** Digital mammography, CC view.

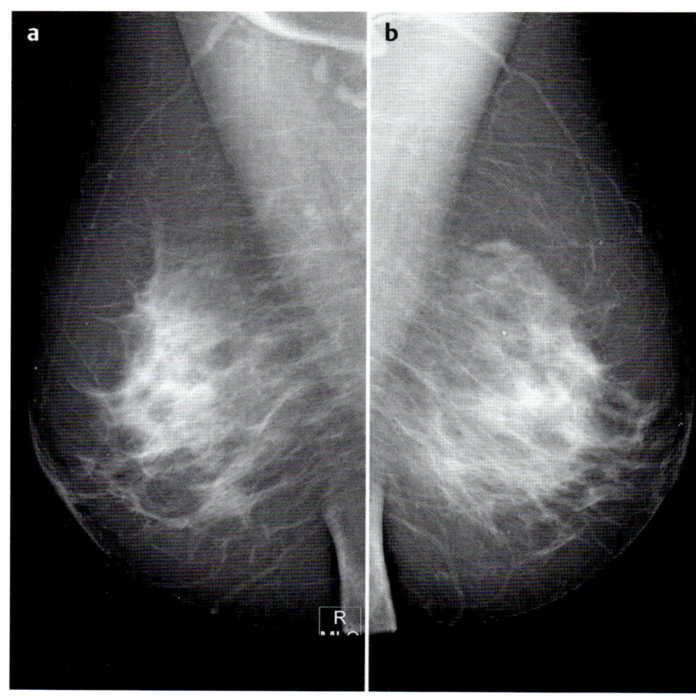


Fig. 47.**4 a, b** Digital mammography, MLO view.

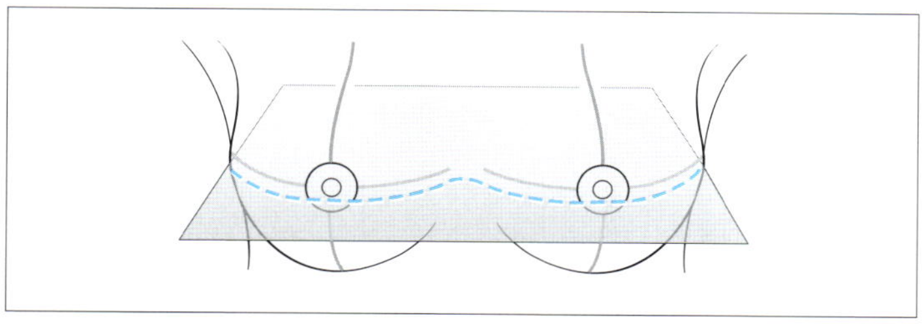

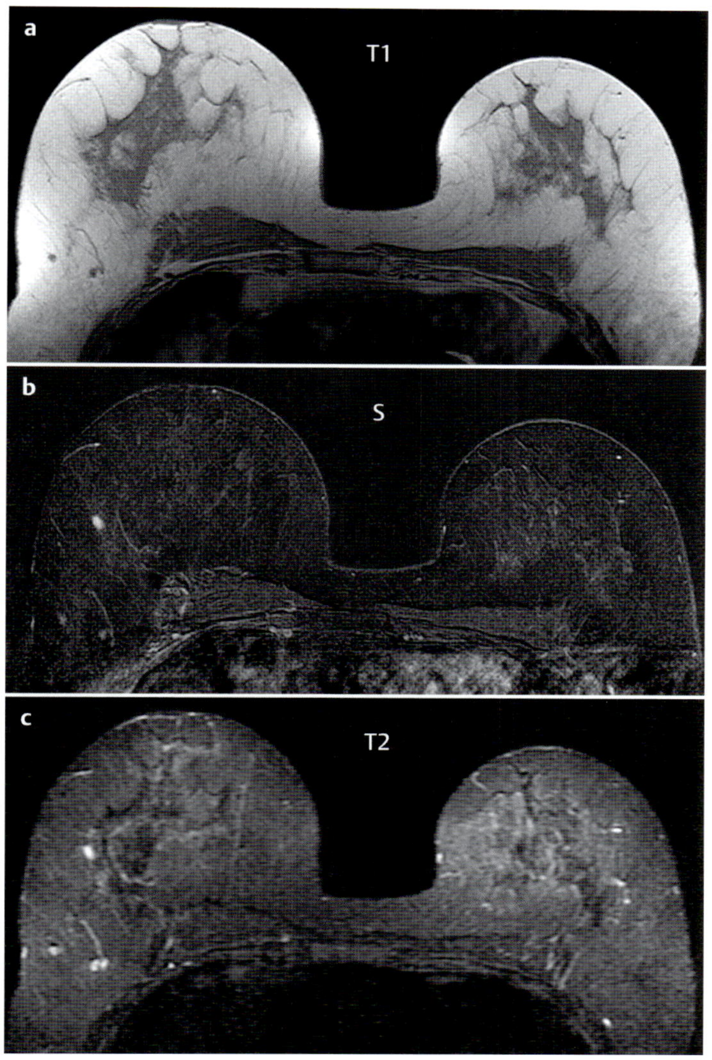


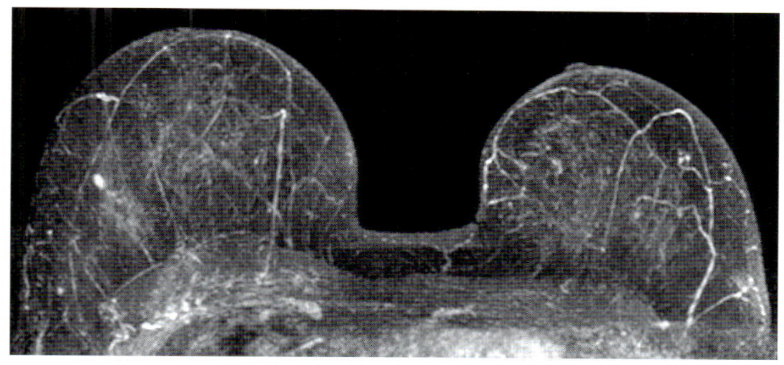

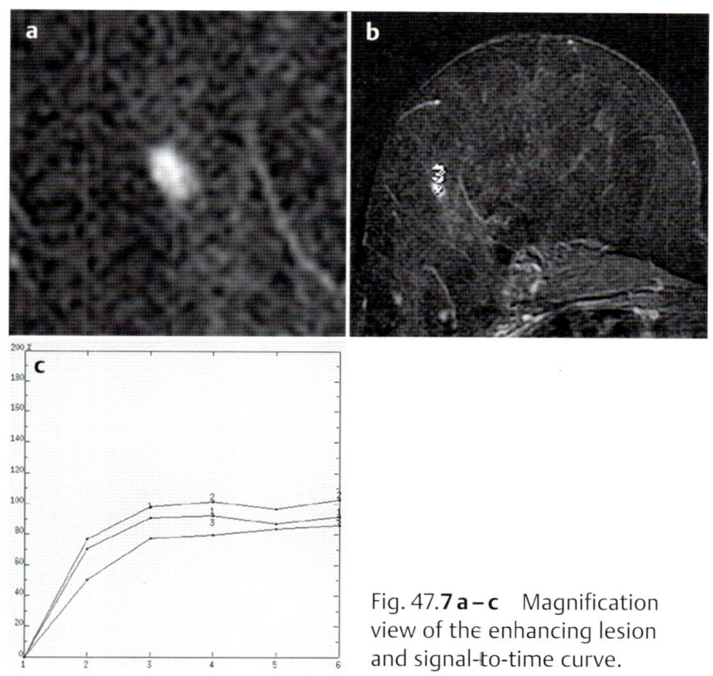


Fig. 47.5 **a – c** Contrast-enhanced MRI of the breasts.

Fig. 47.7 **a – c** Magnification view of the enhancing lesion and signal-to-time curve.

Please characterize ultrasound, mammography, and MRI findings.
What is your preliminary diagnosis?
What are your next steps?

This case presents the complete breast imaging diagnostics used in screening.

### Ultrasound

There was a hypoechoic lesion with ill-defined borders in the right breast lateral to the areola, with moderate acoustic shadowing behind the lesion. However, ultrasound did not show definitive signs of malignancy. US BI-RADS right lateral 4.

### Mammography

Mammograms showed inhomogeneous dense parenchyma, ACR type 3. Consistent with the ultrasound finding, in the CC view there was an impression of slight asymmetry in the lateral glandular tissue, with possible hyperdensity within the parenchyma. However, there were no clear signs of malignancy. Otherwise, no unusual findings. There were no architectural distortions and no calcifications were visible (BI-RADS right 3/left 1). PGMI: CC view P; MLO view G (skin fold, inframammary fold).

### MR Mammography

MRI depicted a single oval hypervascularized lesion measuring 7 mm in the lateral part of the right breast, clearly corresponding to the finding in ultrasound. This lesion had a high signal in T2-weighted imaging. MR imaging showed no other abnormalities.

**MRI Artifact Category:** 1
**MRI Density Type:** 1

| MRM score | Finding | Points |
|---|---|---|
| **Shape** | oval | 0 |
| **Border** | well-defined | 0 |
| **CM Distribution** | inhomogenous (septa?) | 1 |
| **Initial Signal Intensity Increase** | moderate | 1 |
| **Post-initial Signal Intensity Character** | plateau | 1 |
| **MRI score (points)** | | **3** |
| **MRI BI-RADS** | | **3** |

### → Preliminary Diagnosis

Fibroadenoma.

### → Differential Diagnosis

Adenoma, papilloma, carcinoma.

| BI-RADS Categorization | | |
|---|---|---|
| Clinical Findings | right 1 | left 1 |
| Ultrasound | right 4 | left 1 |
| Mammography | right 3 | left 1 |
| MR Mammography | right 3 | left 1 |
| **BI-RADS Total** | **right 3** | **left 1** |

### Procedure

Histological analysis of the lesion in the right breast after US-guided percutaneous core biopsy.

### Histology of the right breast (5 specimens)

Fat necrosis.

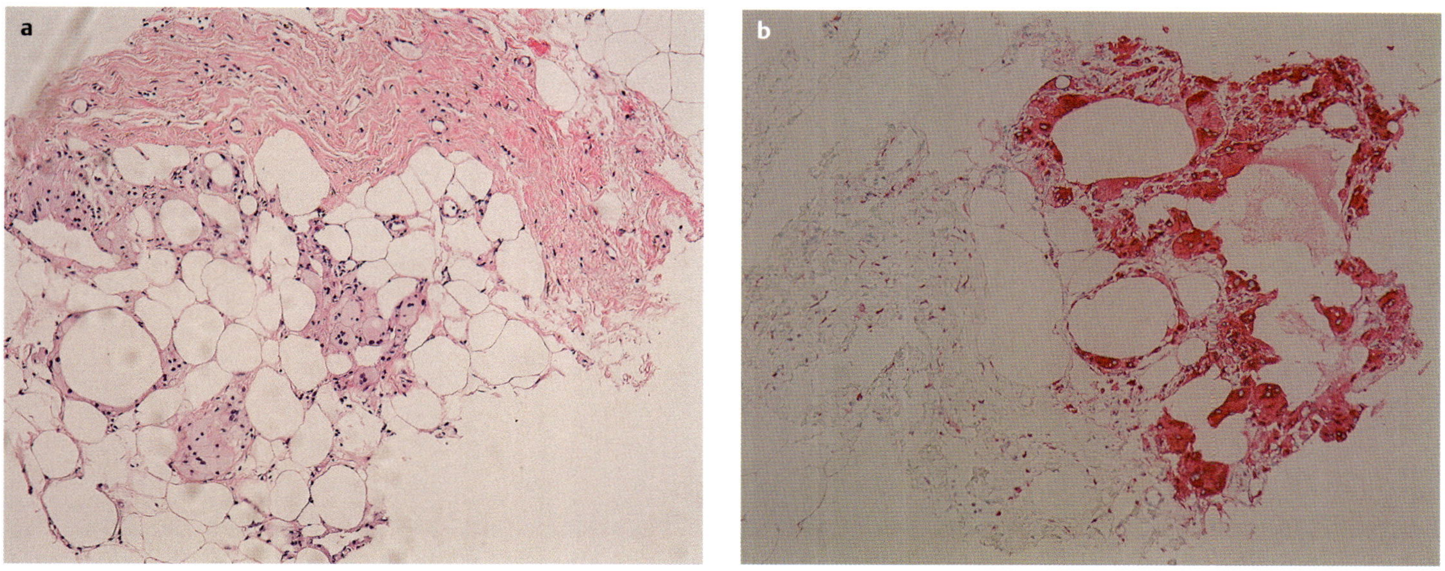


Fig. 47.**8 a, b** Macrohistology of a representative specimen showing fat necrosis.

## Histology

Fat necrosis.

## Treatment

Follow-up ultrasound examination after 6 months; MRI after 6 months if required.

Fat necroses can give rise to false-positive findings in all imaging modalities.

**Indication:** Screening mammography.
**History:** Unremarkable.
**Risk profile:** No increased risk.
**Age:** 64 years.

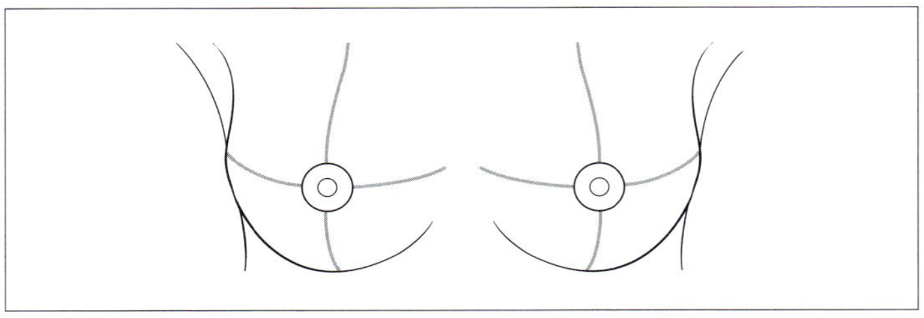

### Clinical Findings

Inspection and palpation unremarkable.

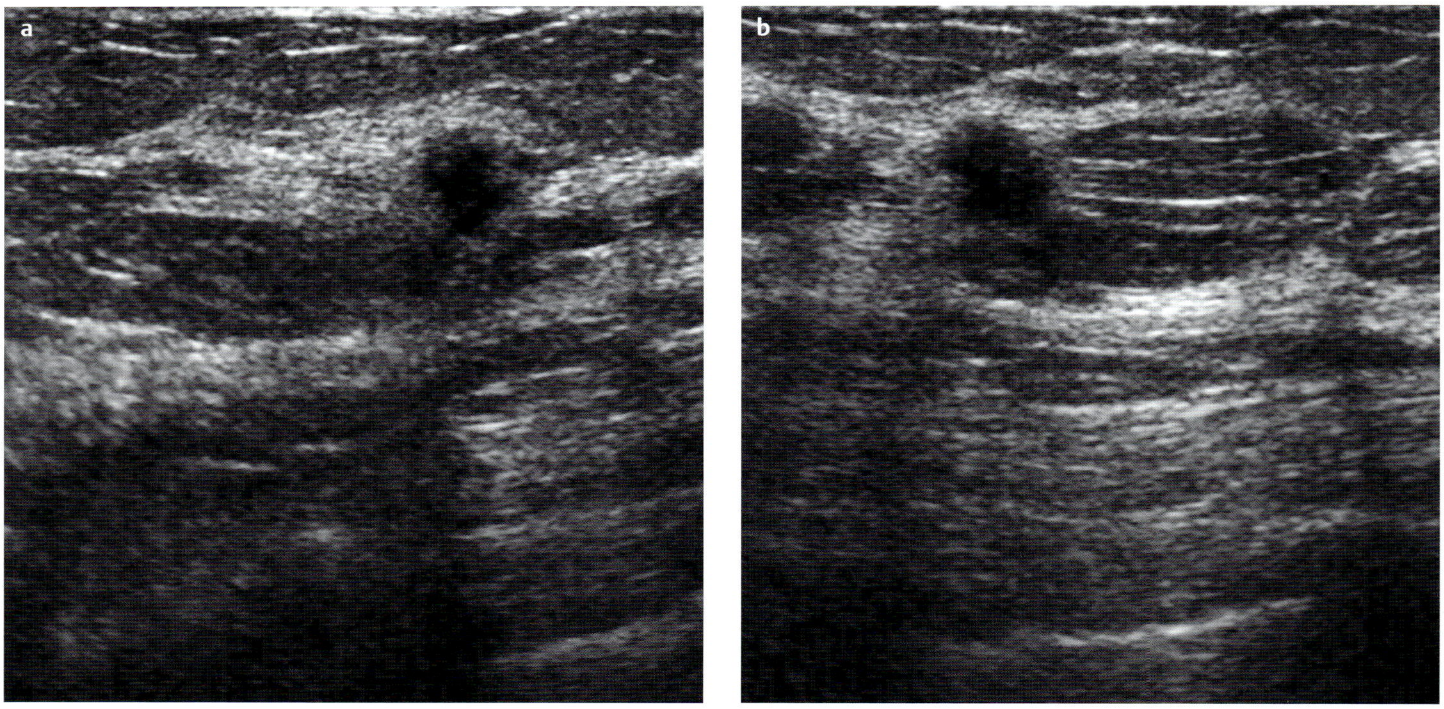

Fig. 48.**1 a, b** Ultrasound images of the central part of the right breast from two angles.

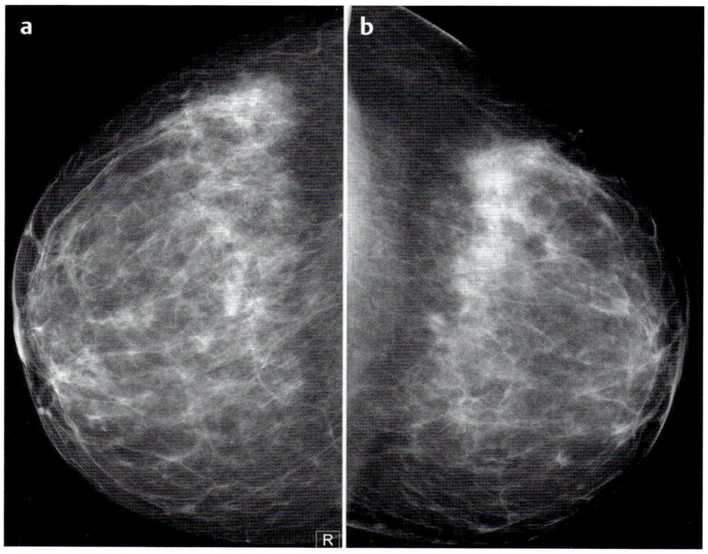


Fig. 48.**2 a, b** Digital mammography, CC view.

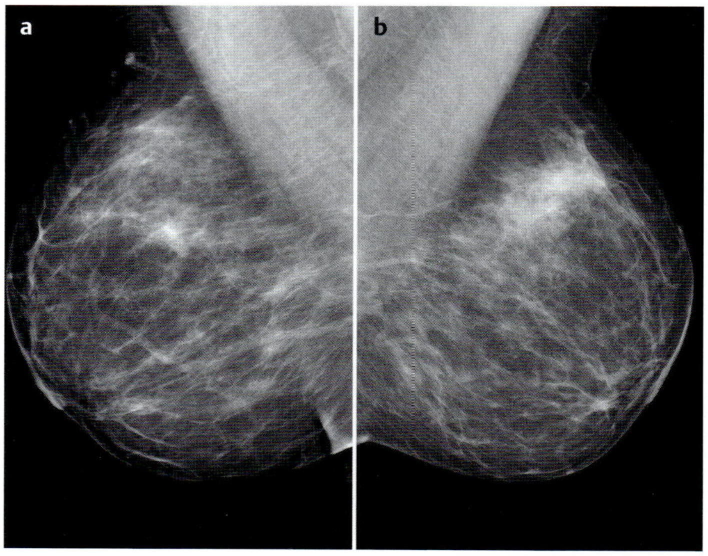

Fig. 48.**3 a, b** Digital mammography, MLO view.

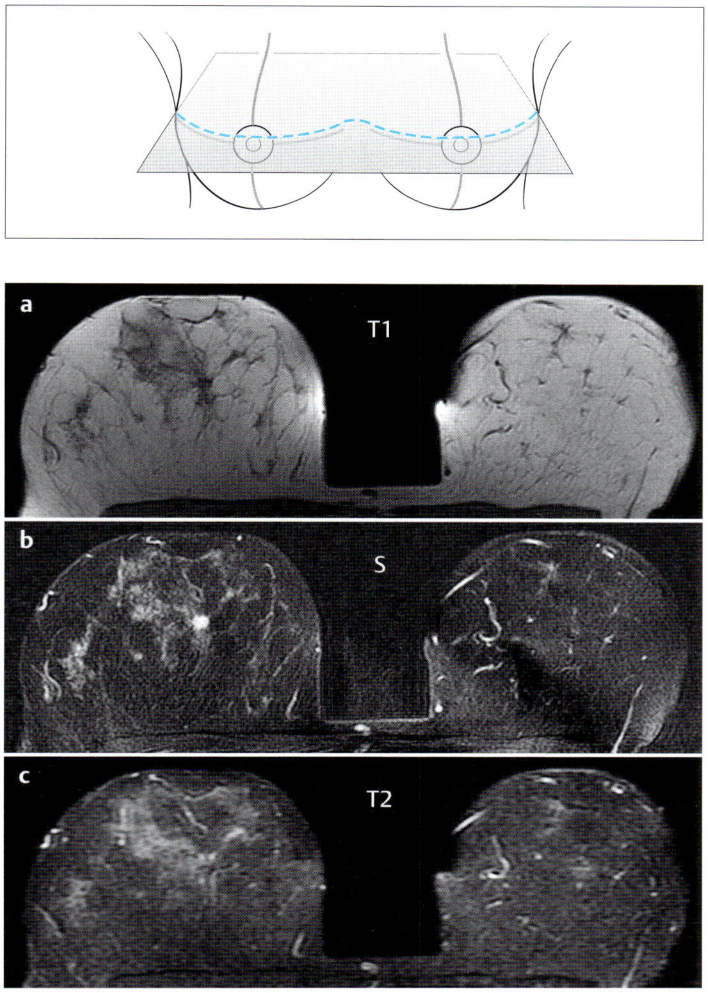


Fig. 48.**4 a – c** Contrast-enhanced MRI of the breasts.

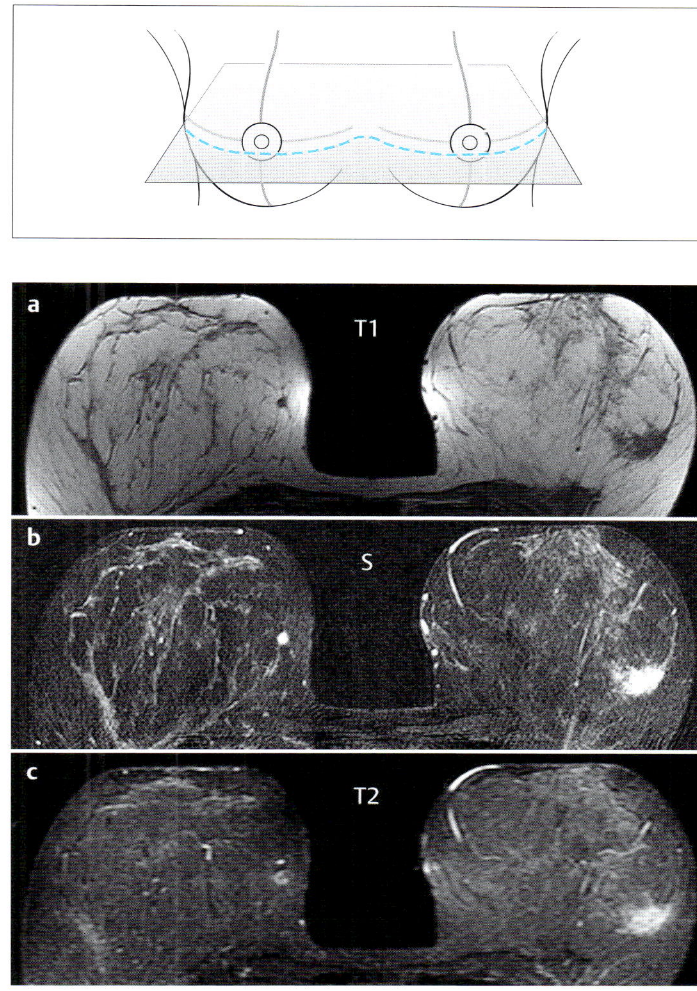


Fig. 48.**5 a – c** Contrast-enhanced MRI of the breasts.

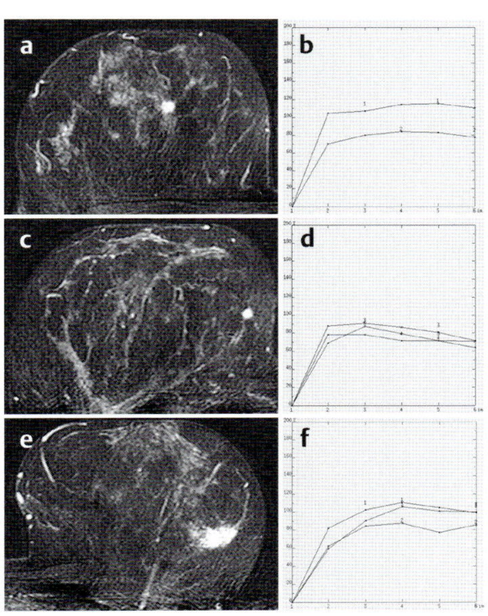


Fig. 48.**6 a – f** Signal-to-time curves.

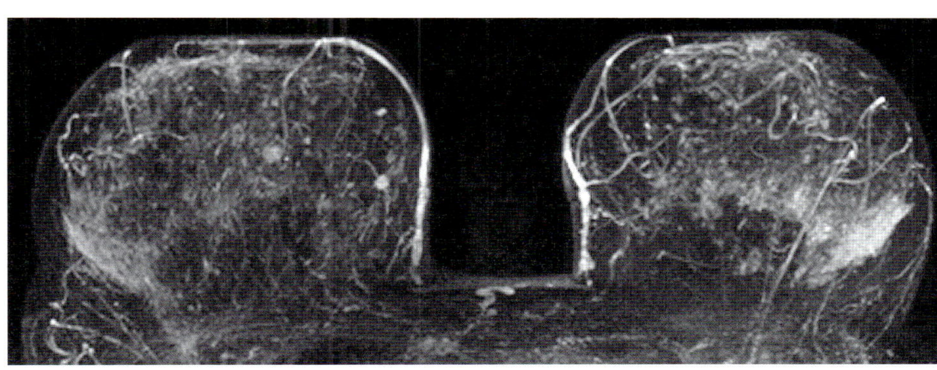

Fig. 48.**7** Contrast-enhanced MR mammography. Maximum intensity projection.

?

Please characterize ultrasound, mammography, and MRI findings.
What is your preliminary diagnosis?
What are your next steps?

This case shows the imaging studies of an asymptomatic woman.

### Ultrasound

In the right breast, ultrasound demonstrated a partially lobulated, hypoechoic lesion, measuring 9 mm, with echogenic margins. No architectural distortion. There were no further findings in ultrasound. US BI-RADS right 4/left 1.

### Mammography

The parenchyma was bilaterally almost completely symmetric and inhomogeneously dense, ACR type 3. Mammograms showed no suspicious findings. In particular, the area corresponding to the sonographic finding between the upper quadrants of the right breast showed no densities, no architectural distortions, and no calcifications. BI-RADS right 1/left 1. PGMI: CC view P; MLO view G (inframammary fold).

### MR Mammography

Between the upper quadrants of the right breast, MRI depicted a hypervascularized, irregular mass (diameter 1 cm) with intermediate signal in T2-weighted imaging. Initial signal increase was 110%, followed by a postinitial plateau (MRM score 4). Radial spiculations were clearly visible on precontrast images. MRI also showed another hypervascularized lesion measuring 8 mm in the lower inner quadrant of the right breast with centrally reduced and peripherally increased T2 signal. Initial signal increase was 90% with postinitial washout (MRM score 3). There was also regional enhancement in the lower outer quadrant of the left breast with an initial signal increase of 100%, postinitial plateau, and increased signal in T2-weighted imaging.

**MRI Artifact Category:** 1
**MRI Density Type:** 2

| MRM score | Right breast, central region | Points | Right breast, lower inner quadrant | Points | Left breast, lower quadrants | Points |
|---|---|---|---|---|---|---|
| **Shape** | round | 0 | round | 0 | irregular | 1 |
| **Border** | spiculated | 1 | well-defined | 0 | ill-defined | 1 |
| **CM Distribution** | homogenous | 0 | homogenous | 0 | homogenous | 0 |
| **Initial Signal Intensity Increase** | strong | 2 | moderate | 1 | moderate | 1 |
| **Post-initial Signal Intensity Character** | plateau | 1 | wash-out | 2 | plateau | 1 |
| **MRI score (points)** | | **4** | | **3** | | **4** |
| **MRI BI-RADS** | | **4** | | **3** | | **4** |

### → Differential Diagnosis

Right: Multicentric carcinoma, bifocal fibroadenoma.

Left: Adenosis, diffuse carcinoma.

| BI-RADS Categorization | | |
|---|---|---|
| Clinical Findings | right 1 | left 1 |
| Ultrasound | right 4 | left 1 |
| Mammography | right 1 | left 1 |
| MR Mammography | right 4 (multicentric) | left 4 |
| **BI-RADS Total** | **right 4** | **left 4** |

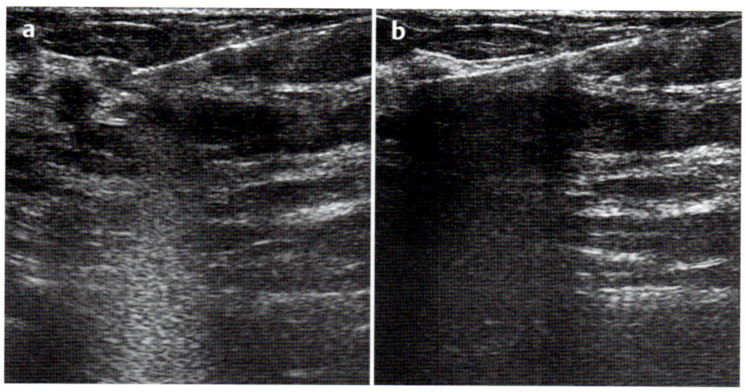


Fig. 48.**8 a, b** US-guided core biopsy of the central lesion in the right breast. Pre-fire and post-fire documentation.

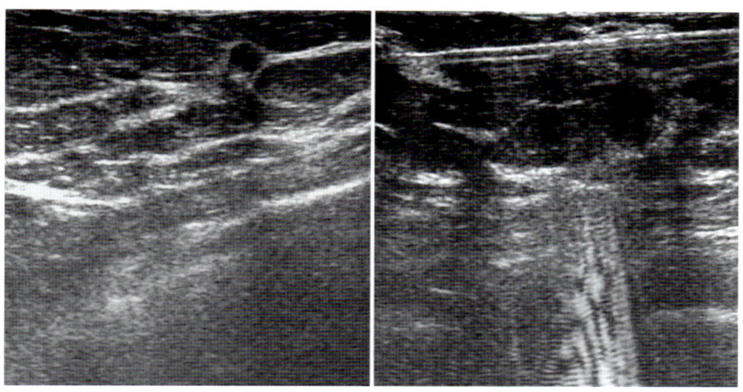

Fig. 48.**9** Ultrasound of the lower inner quadrant of the right breast.
Fig. 48.**10** US-guided core biopsy of the second lesion in the right breast.

### Procedure

Histopathological analysis of the lesion between the upper quadrants of the right breast by US-guided percutaneous core biopsy.

### Histopathology of the right breast

Invasive ductal carcinoma between the upper quadrants of the right breast.

### What about the second lesion seen in MRI in the right breast?

A targeted sonographic re-examination detected a hypoechoic lesion of diameter 4 mm with echogenic margins. Here US-guided core biopsy was also performed (Figs. 48.**9** and 48.**10**).

### Histopathology of the second lesion (lower inner quadrant of right breast)

Invasive ductal carcinoma.

### Regional enhancement in the left breast (MRI BI-RADS 4)

Because there were no findings in ultrasound and mammography consistent with this enhancing area, no biopsy was performed here. A follow-up was carried out after 6 months. This follow-up did not reproduce the enhancement in this area.

## Histology

Invasive ductal carcinomas of the right breast with a diameter of 8 mm and 7 mm. Lymph node status normal.

IDC (multicentric) pT1b, pN0, G2

## Treatment

Mastectomy of the right breast.

Where MR mammography results in additional findings, it is often worthwhile repeating sonographic examination, targeting the area of the known lesions.

**Indication:** Screening.
**History:** Unremarkable.
**Risk profile:** No increased risk.
**Age:** 59 years.

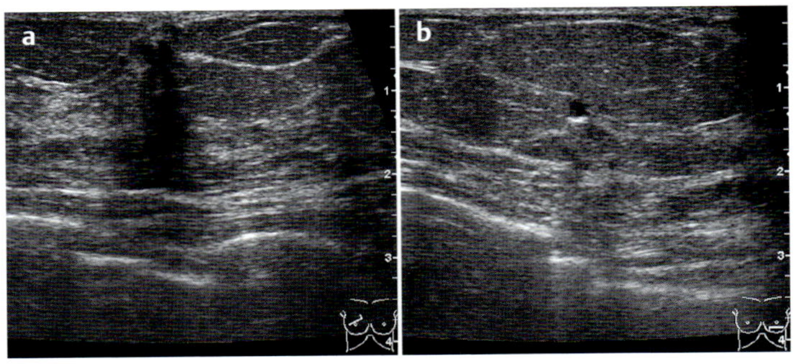


Fig. 49.**1 a, b** Ultrasound.

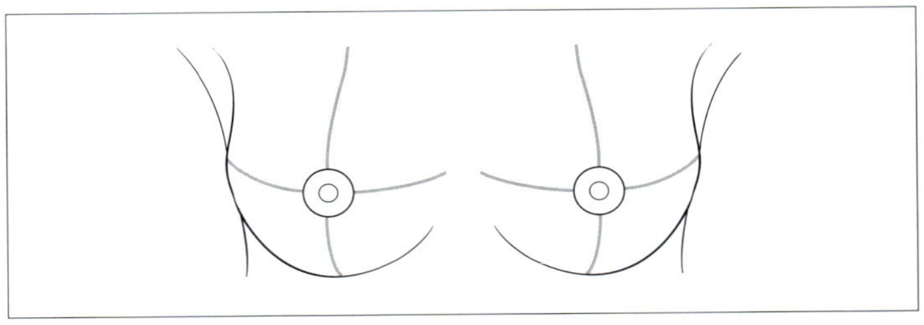

**Clinical Findings**

Normal findings on inspection and palpation.

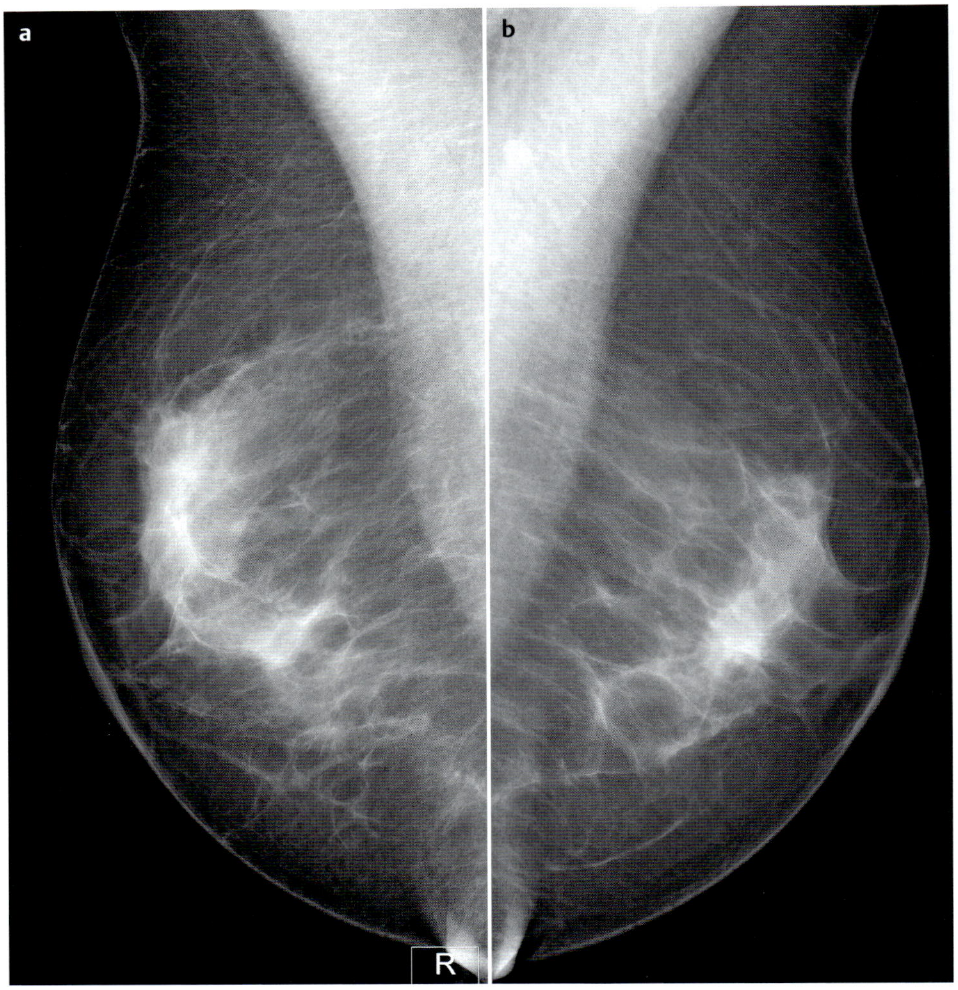


Fig. 49.**2 a, b** Digital mammography, MLO view.

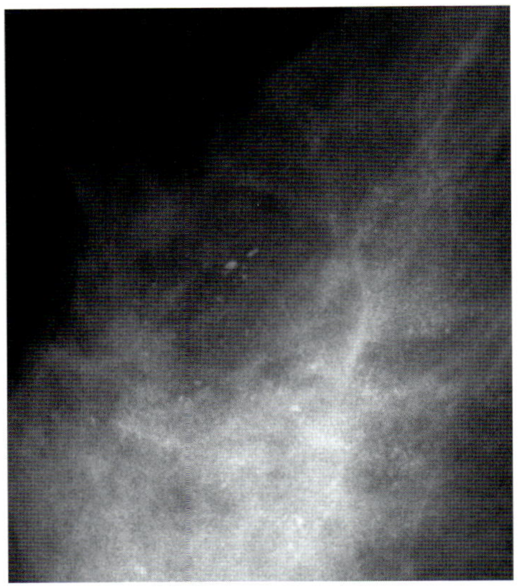

Fig. 49.**3** Magnification view of the upper quadrants of the right breast.

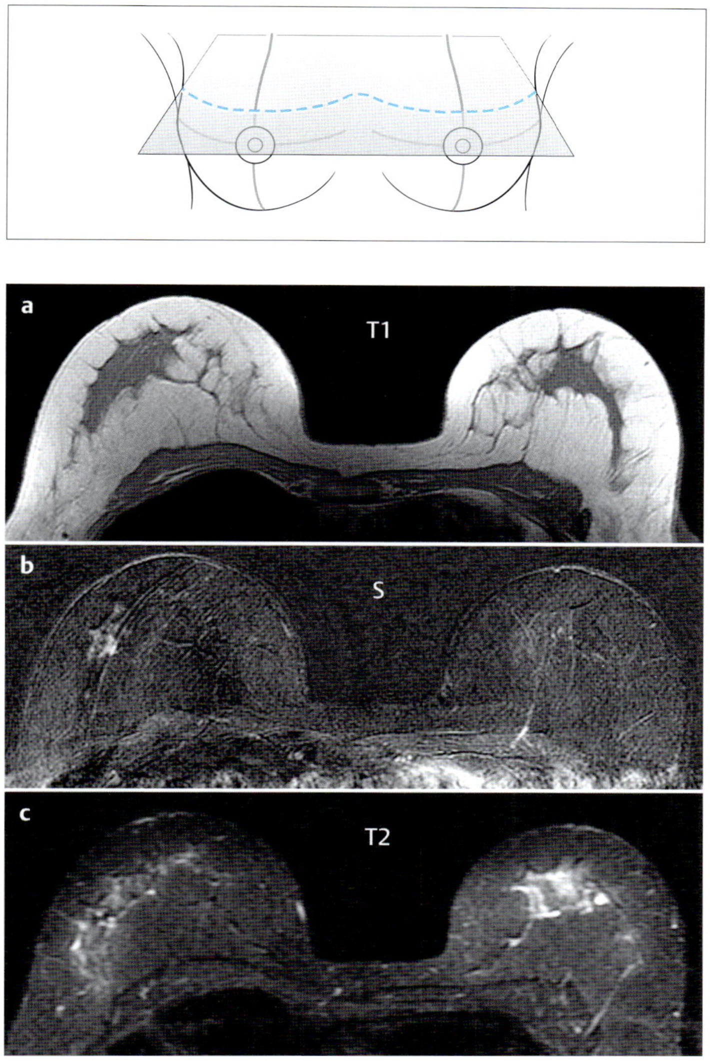


Fig. 49.**4 a–c** Contrast-enhanced MR mammography.

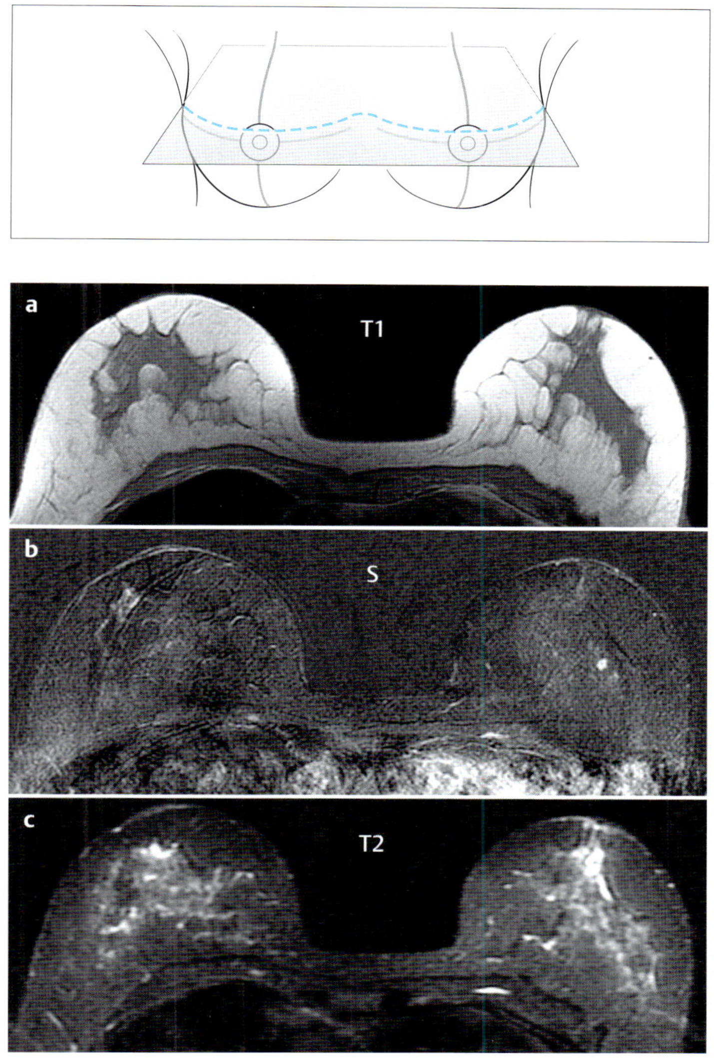


Fig. 49.**5 a–c** Contrast-enhanced MR mammography.

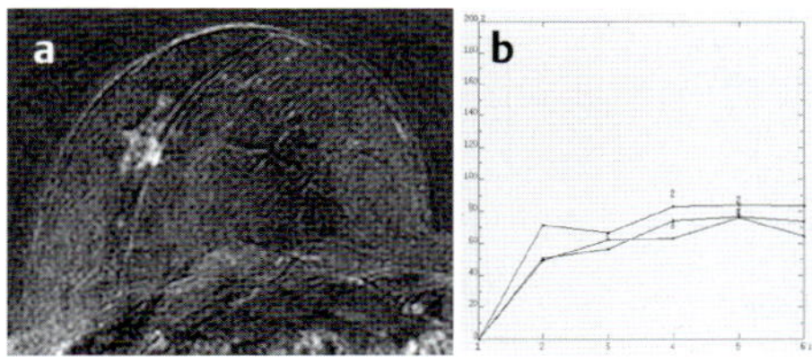


Fig. 49.**6 a, b** Signal-to-time curve.

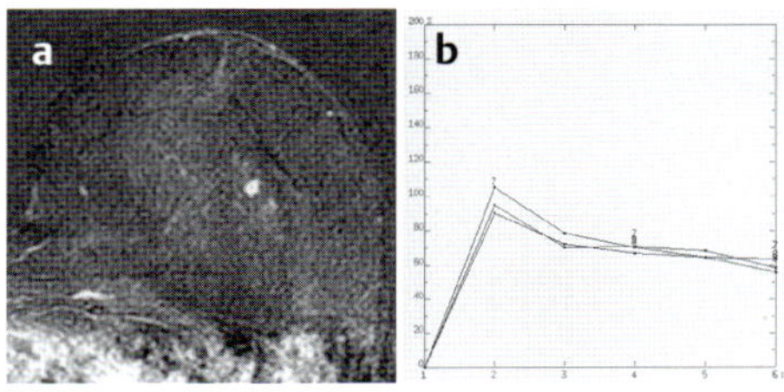


Fig. 49.**7 a, b** Signal-to-time curve.

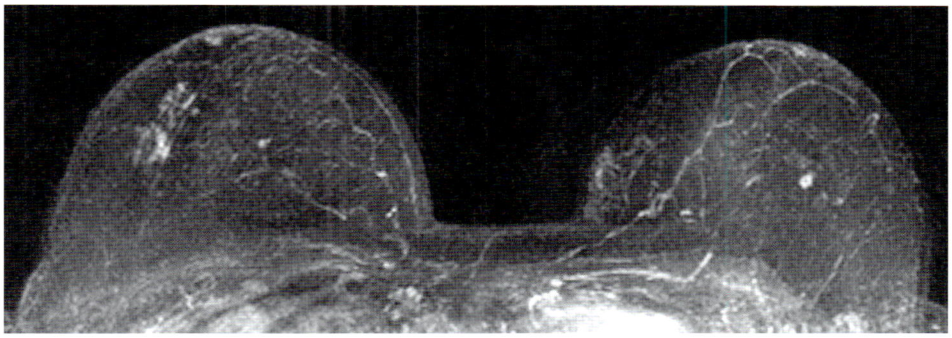

Fig. 49.**8** Contrast-enhanced MR mammography. Maximum intensity projection.

?

Please characterize ultrasound, mammography, and MRI findings.
What is your preliminary diagnosis?
What are your next steps?

This case demonstrates imaging in a screening situation.

### Ultrasound

Ultrasound showed a small hypoechoic area in the upper outer quadrant of the right breast. There was a possible unspecific lesion centrally located in the left breast. US BI-RADS right 3/left 2.

### Mammography

Mammography showed asymmetric, partially inhomogeneously dense parenchyma, ACR type 3. In the outer quadrants of the right breast, clustered, mainly monomorphous microcalcifications (round and oval) were visible. There were no masses, densities, or architectural distortions. BI-RADS right 4/left 1.

### MR Mammography

Segmentally distributed dendritic enhancements with nonspecific signal curves were visible in MRI, corresponding to the microcalcifications seen in mammograms. In addition, in the center of the left breast there was a well-defined lesion measuring 8 mm with ring enhancement and reduced signal in T2-weighted imaging.

**MRI Artifact Category:** 2
**MRI Density Type:** 1

| MRM score | Right | Points | Left | Points |
|---|---|---|---|---|
| **Shape** | dendritic | 1 | round | 0 |
| **Border** | ill-defined | 1 | well-defined | 0 |
| **CM Distribution** | homogenous | 0 | ring | 2 |
| **Initial Signal Intensity Increase** | moderate | 1 | strong | 2 |
| **Post-initial Signal Intensity Character** | continuous | 0 | wash-out | 2 |
| **MRI score (points)** | | **3** | | **6** |
| **MRI BI-RADS** | | **3** | | **5** |

### → Preliminary Diagnosis

Right: DCIS, diffuse carcinoma.
Left: Carcinoma

### → Differential Diagnosis

Right: Adenosis, focal inflammation.
Left: Fibroadenoma, papilloma, focal adenosis.

| BI-RADS Categorization | | |
|---|---|---|
| Clinical Findings | right 1 | left 1 |
| Ultrasound | right 3 | left 2 |
| Mammography | right 4 | left 1 |
| MR Mammography | right 3 | left 5 |
| **BI-RADS Total** | **right 4** | **left 5** |

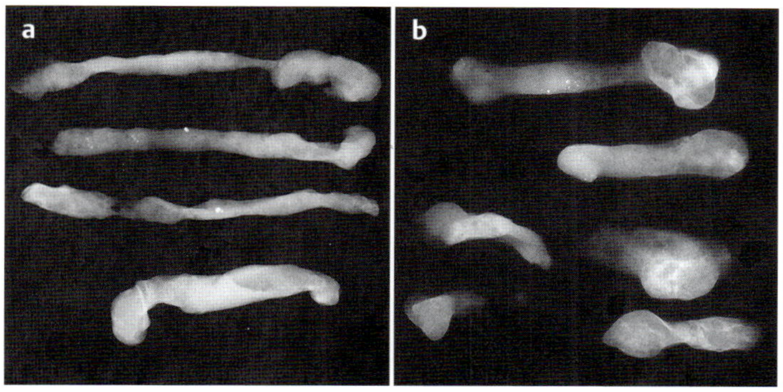


Fig. 49.**9 a, b** Radiogram of histological specimens from the right breast.

**Procedure (according to guidelines)**

Histopathological analysis of the calcifications in the right breast after stereotactic vacuum biopsy.
Histopathological analysis of the lesion in the left breast after MR-guided vacuum biopsy.

**Histopathology of the right breast**

Invasive lobular carcinoma.

**What about the second lesion seen in MRI (in the left breast)?**

Since an operation to remove the carcinoma from the right breast was already indicated, the lesion in the left breast was also excised following MR-guided hook-wire localization. Preoperative biopsy was therefore not performed.

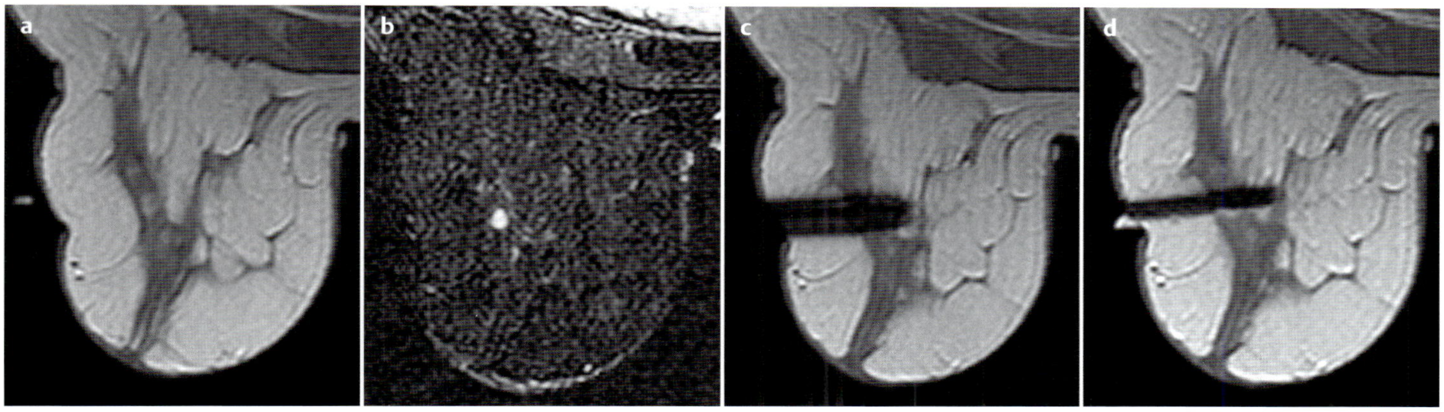


Fig. 49.**10 a – d** MR-guided preoperative hook-wire localization of the lesion in the left breast. Findings after contrast administration (**a**) and in subtraction image (**b**). Correct placement of the needle (**c**) and of the hook wire (**d**).

## Histology

Right: ILC pT2, pN0, G2
Left: Focal sclerosing adenosis

## Treatment

Mastectomy of the right breast, excisional biopsy of the lesion in left breast.

Invasive lobular carcinomas of the breast are not usually accompanied by microcalcifications.

**Indication:** Cutaneous changes in lower outer quadrant of the right breast.
**History:** Excisional biopsy of bilateral fibroadenomas 7 years previously.
**Risk profile:** Breast cancer in mother and grandmother.
**Age:** 50 years.

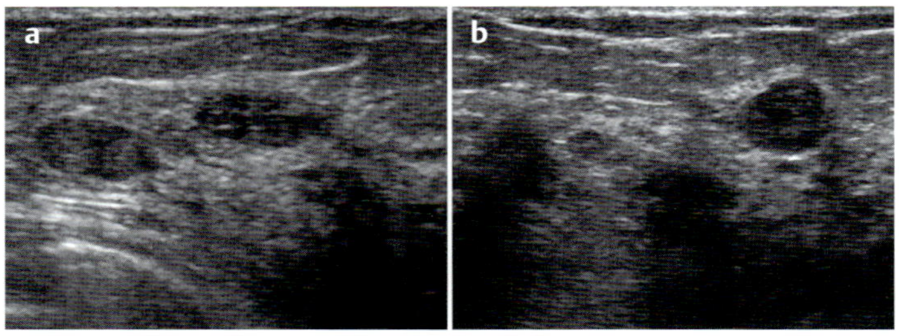

Fig. 50.**1 a, b** Ultrasound of the left breast, lower outer quadrant.

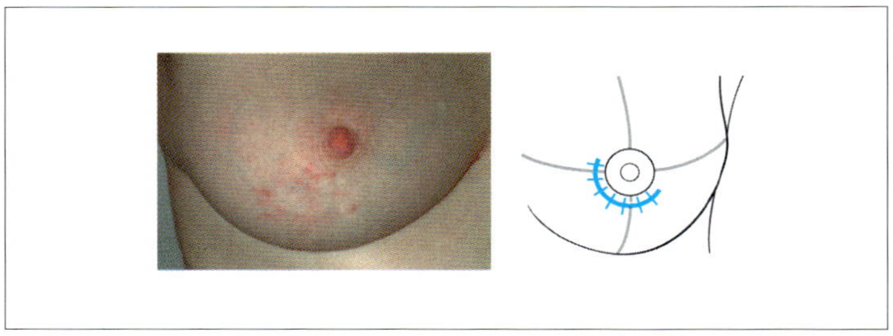

**Palpation**

Nodular parenchymal texture. No circumscribed resistance.

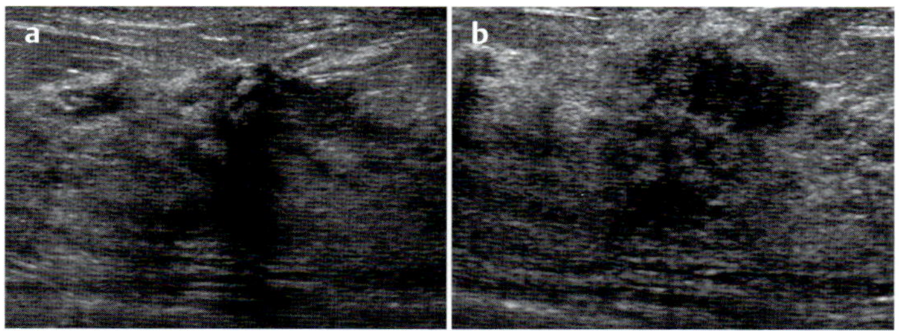

Fig. 50.**2 a, b** Ultrasound of the right breast, lower outer quadrant.

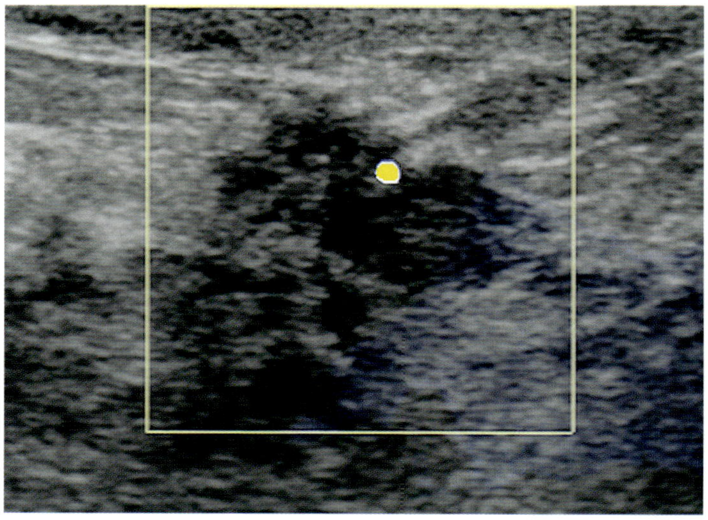

Fig. 50.**3** Color-coded Doppler sonography of the right breast, outer quadrants.

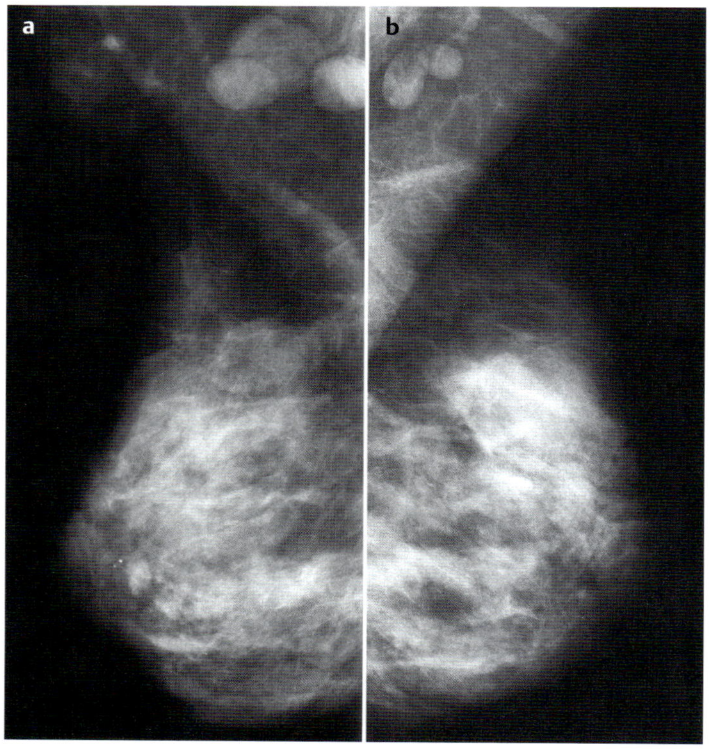

Fig. 50.**4 a, b** Conventional mammography, MLO view [imaging not performed by authors].

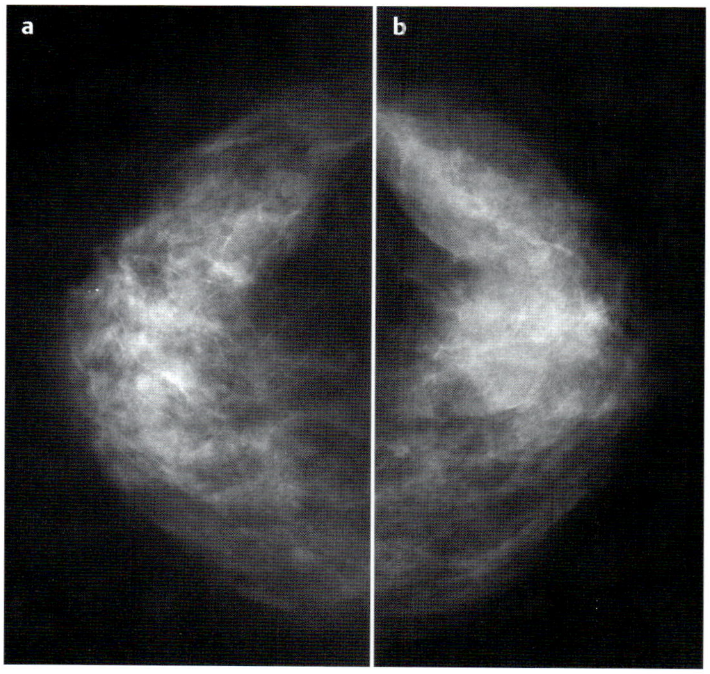

Fig. 50.**5 a, b** Conventional mammog-aphy, CC view [imaging not performed by authors].

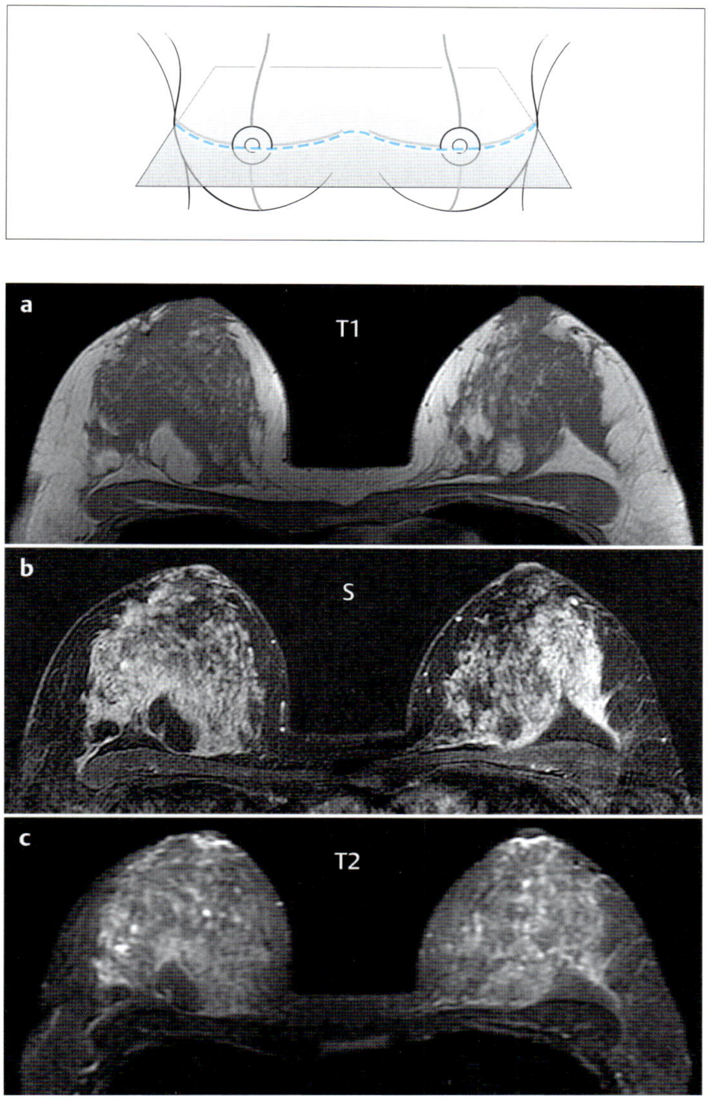


Fig. 50.**6 a–c** Contrast-enhanced MR mammography.

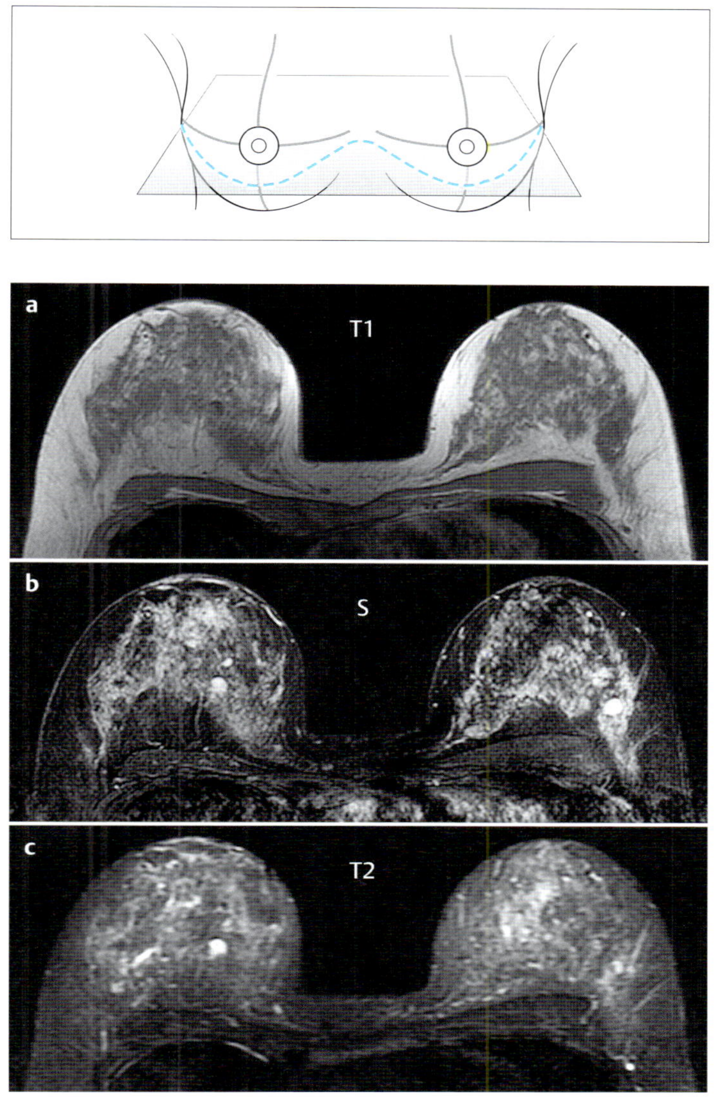


Fig. 50.**7 a–c** Contrast-enhanced MR mammography.

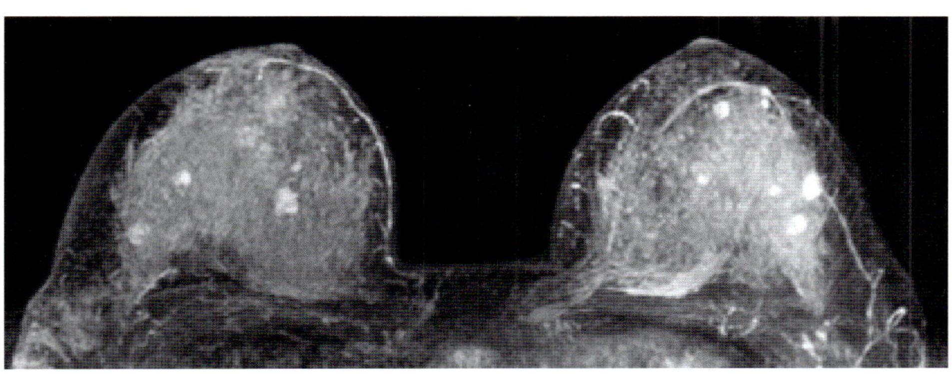

Fig. 50.**8** Contrast-enhanced MR mammography. Maximum intensity projection.

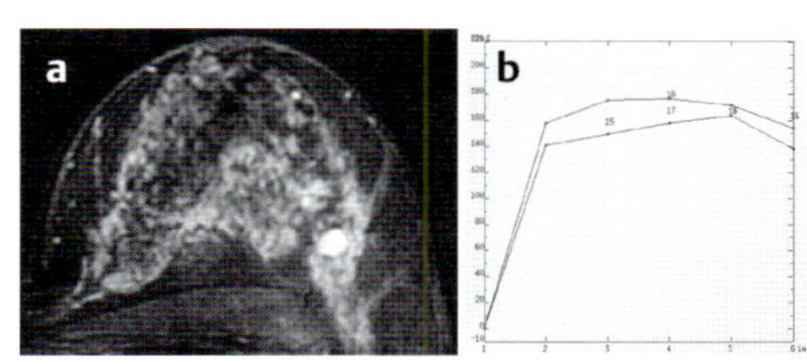


Fig. 50.**9 a, b** Signal-to-time curves.

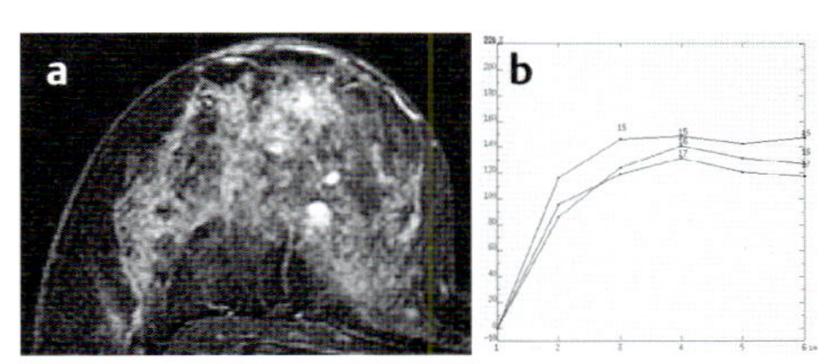


Fig. 50.**10 a, b** Signal-to-time curves.

?

Please characterize ultrasound, mammography, and MRI findings.
What is your preliminary diagnosis?
What are your next steps?

This case shows the imaging studies of a symptomatic woman with cutaneous changes of the lower outer quadrant of the right breast and a positive family history of breast cancer.

### Ultrasound

This method showed multiple, well-defined, hypoechoic lesions (maximum diameter 1.5 cm) with indeterminate distal echo pattern in the left breast. There were no signs of malignancy. In the lower outer quadrant of the right breast–in the area of the cutaneous changes–ultrasound detected a hypoechoic, microlobulated lesion without evident echogenic margins, but with partial distal shadowing and hyperperfusion of the lesion. Furthermore, ultrasound showed multiple compressible hypoechoic foci in both breasts. US BI-RADS right 4/left 2.

### Mammography

Mammograms showed bilaterally symmetric, extremely dense tissue, ACR type 4. There were isodense, well-defined lesions measuring up to 1.5 cm in both breasts. However, there was no circumscribed lesion in the lower outer quadrant of the right breast. There were no suspicious microcalcifications. Mammography showed enlarged axillary lymph nodes bilaterally. BI-RADS right 3/left 3. PGMI CC view P; MLO view M (pectoralis muscle does not reach the nipple line; inframammary fold not correctly depicted).

### MR Mammography

MRI demonstrated marked enhancement of the entire parenchyma of both breasts. There were no circumscribed findings corresponding to the cutaneous changes in the lower outer quadrant of the right breast. Pre-contrast images also showed no notable changes. However, MRI depicted multiple, well-defined, lobulated, hypervascularized lesions (maximum diameter 1.5 cm) in the upper inner, and lower outer quadrants of the left breast, and in the lower inner quadrant of the right breast. These lesions had initial signal increase of 180%, postinitial plateaus and increased signal in T2-weighted imaging.

**MRI Artifact Category:** 1
**MRI Density Type:** 4

| MRM score | Right breast, lower inner quadrant | Points | Left breast, upper inner and lower outer quadrants | Points |
|---|---|---|---|---|
| **Shape** | round/oval | 0 | round/oval | 0 |
| **Border** | well-defined | 0 | well-defined | 0 |
| **CM Distribution** | homogenous | 0 | homogenous | 0 |
| **Initial Signal Intensity Increase** | strong | 2 | strong | 2 |
| **Post-initial Signal Intensity Character** | plateau | 1 | plateau | 1 |
| **MRI score (points)** | | **3** | | **3** |
| **MRI BI-RADS** | | **3** | | **3** |

### → Differential Diagnosis

Bilateral fibroadenomas. Ambiguous skin changes in the lower outer quadrant of the right breast with indeterminate mammography and MRM results, but highly suspicious findings in ultrasound. Diffuse carcinoma? Inflammatory carcinoma?

| BI-RADS Categorization | | |
|---|---|---|
| Clinical Findings | right 4 | left 1 |
| Ultrasound | right 4 | left 2 |
| Mammography | right 3 | left 3 |
| MR Mammography | right 3 | left 3 |
| **BI-RADS Total** | **right 4** | **left 3** |

### Procedure

Histopathological evaluation of the sonographic findings after US-guided core biopsy. In case of benign histology, additional skin biopsy and/or referral to a dermatologist is recommended.

### Histology of the specimen

Invasive ductal carcinoma.

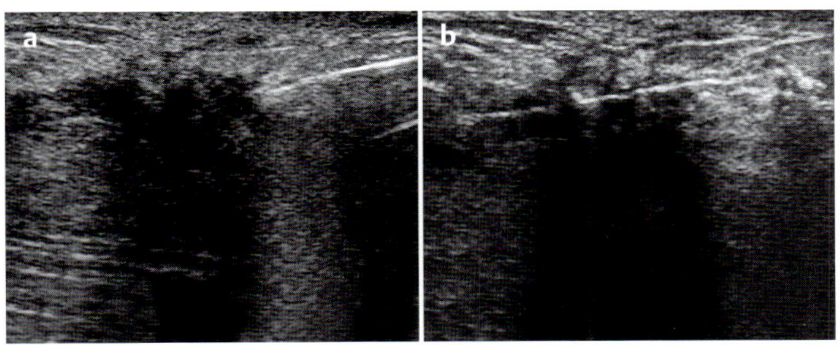


Fig. 50.**11 a, b** US-guided core biopsy (pre-fire and post-fire documentation).

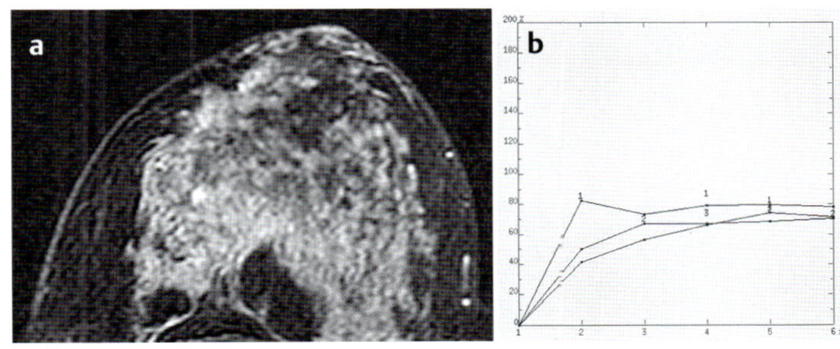


Fig. 50.**13 a, b** Signal-to-time curves in the outer quadrants of the right breast.

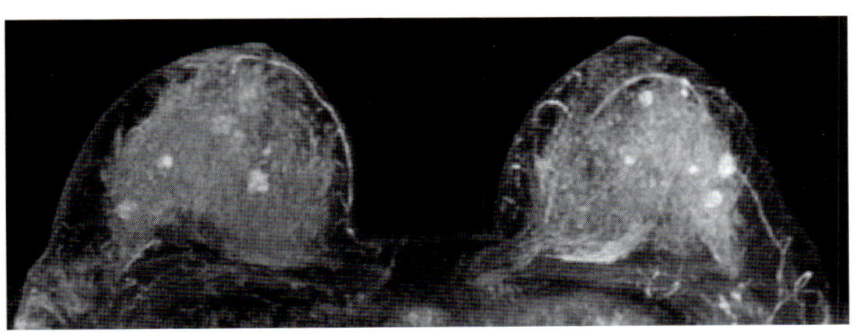

Fig. 50.**12** Maximum intensity projection of the earliest subtraction.

## Histology

Extended invasive ductal carcinoma of the right breast with skin infiltration.

IDC pT4 (cutaneous infiltration), pN1, G2.

## Treatment

Mastectomy of the right breast.

In cases of very high contrast uptake throughout the parenchyma in MRM (MRI density type 4) as well as extremely dense glandular tissue in mammography (ACR type 4), the diagnostic value of these modalities is very limited. Luckily this situation is very rare! When it does happen, suspicious clinical findings must be clarified by ultrasound or percutaneous biopsy.

**Indication:** Screening.
**History:** Thoracotomy at the age of 1 year. Changes in scar texture.
**Risk profile:** No increased risk.
**Age:** 45 years.

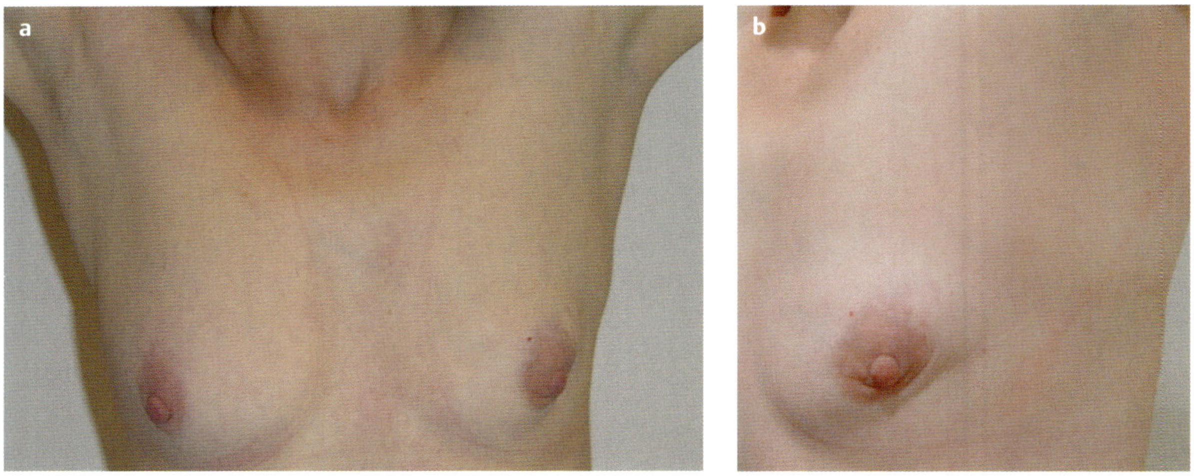


Fig. 51.**1 a, b** Clinical examination. The patient underwent thoracotomy in infancy for patent ductus arteriosus.

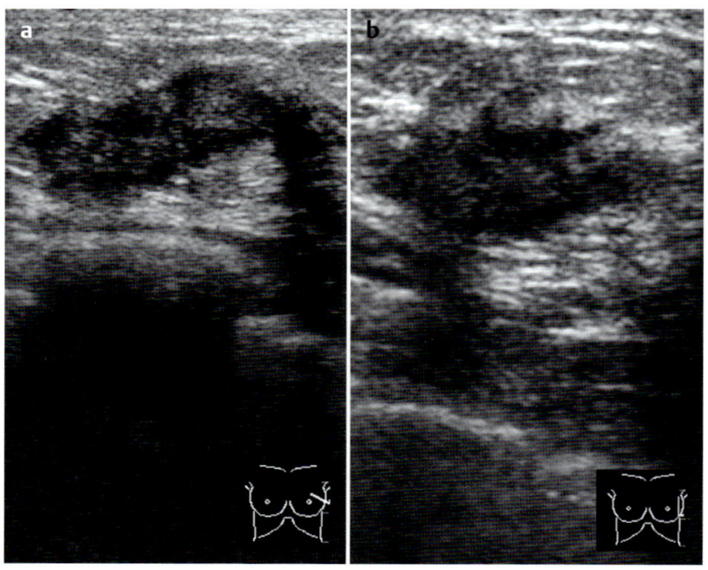


Fig. 51.**2 a, b** Sonography.

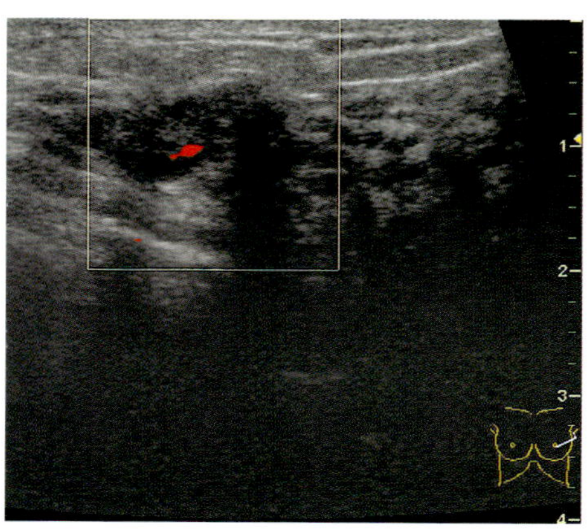


Fig. 51.**3** Color-coded Doppler sonography.

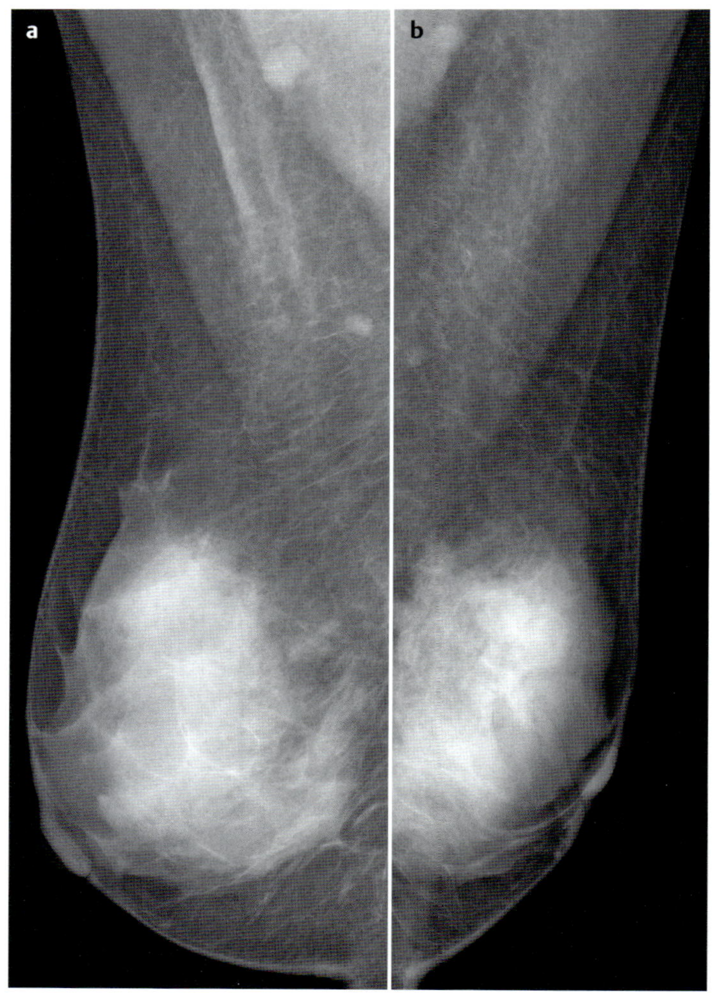


Fig. 51.**4 a, b** Digital mammography, MLO view.

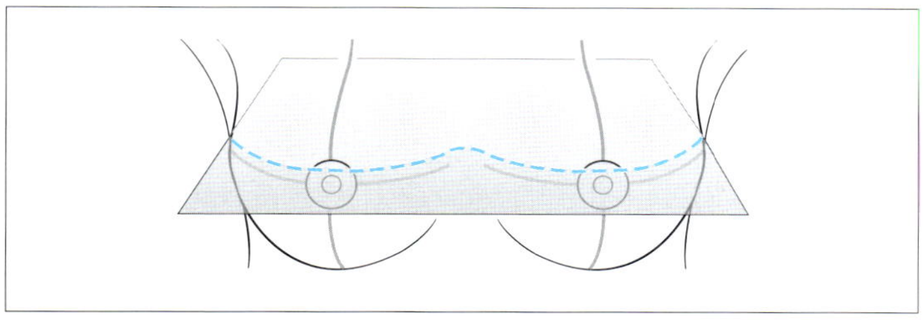

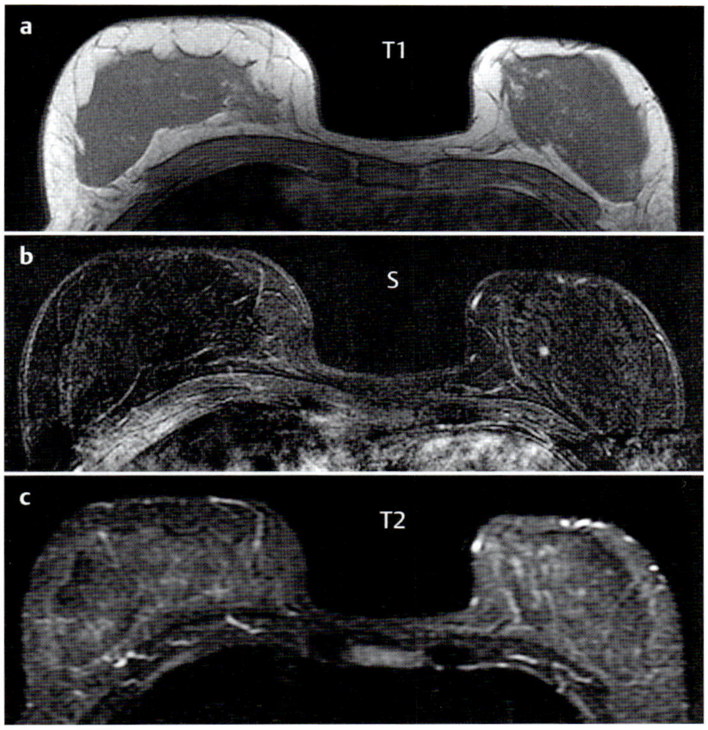


Fig. 51.5 a–c Contrast-enhanced MRI of the breasts.

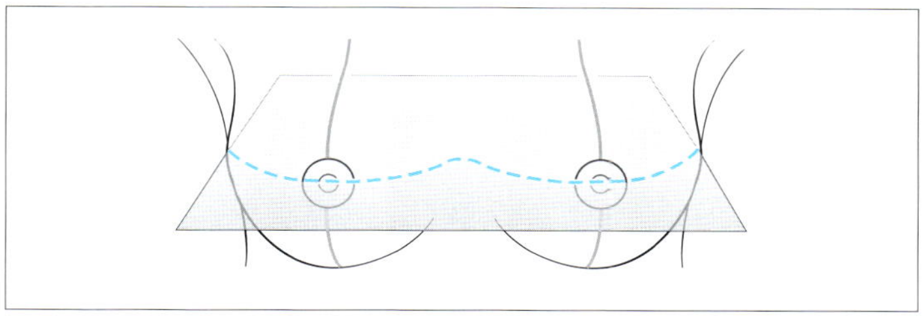

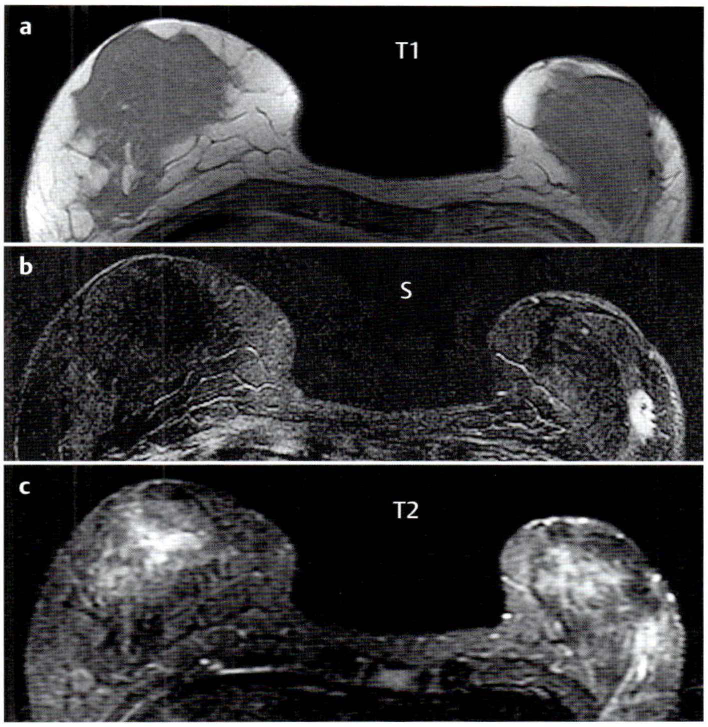


Fig. 51.6 a–c Contrast-enhanced MRI of the breasts.

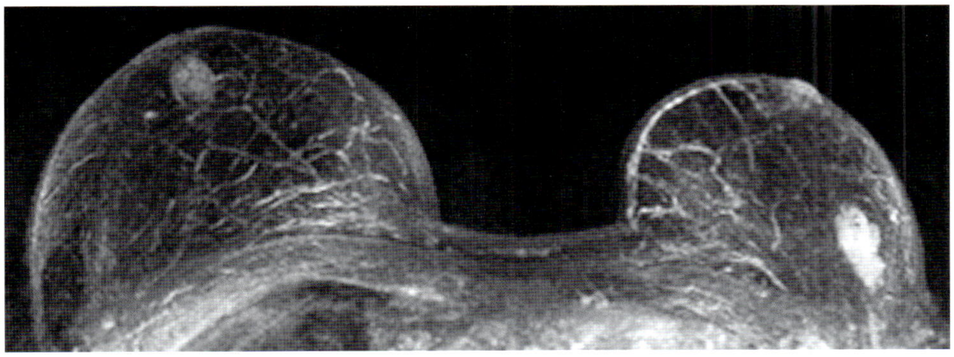

Fig. 51.7 Contrast-enhanced MR mammography. Maximum intensity projection.

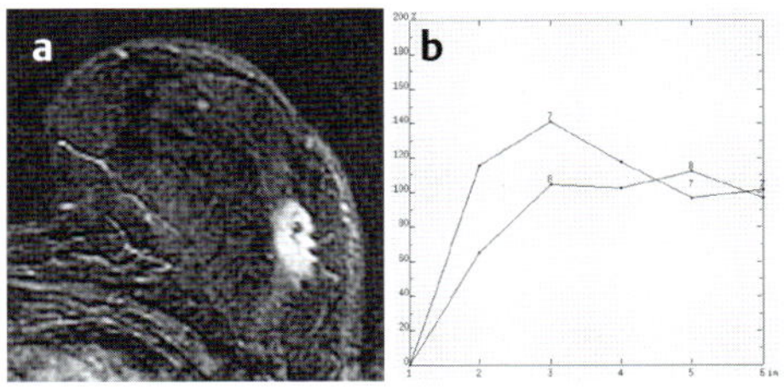


Fig. 51.8 a, b Signal-to-time curves.

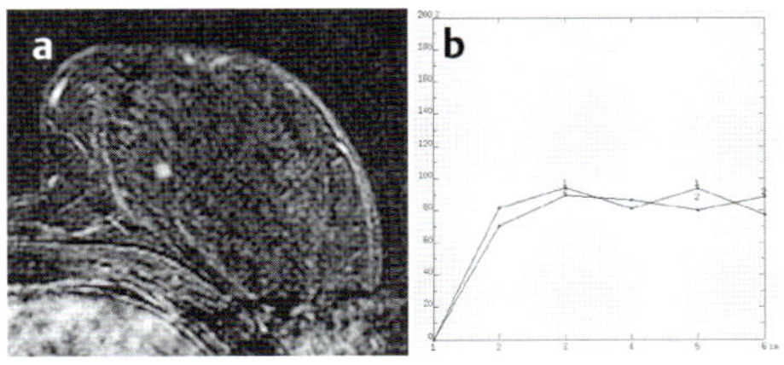


Fig. 51.9 a, b Signal-to-time curves.

?

Please characterize ultrasound, mammography, and MRI findings.
What is your preliminary diagnosis?
What are your next steps?

At the time screening was performed, the patient had experienced changes in the scar from a thoracotomy she underwent as an infant for patent ductus arteriosus.

### Ultrasound

Ultrasound showed an irregular hypoechoic lesion (diameter 16 mm) between the outer quadrants of the left breast with distal shadowing. Doppler sonography showed increased vascularization. US BI-RADS left 4.

### Mammography

The glandular texture was in part very dense, ACR type 4. Postoperative architectural distortion of the left breast was seen on mammograms, with no circumscribed lesions. BI-RADS right 1/ left 3. PGMI : MLO view P (despite extensive distortion by scar).

### MR Mammography

Between the outer quadrants of the left breast, MRI demonstrated a spiculated, ill-defined mass (diameter 18 mm) with ring enhancement, high initial signal increase, and postinitial wash-out as well as intermediate signal in T2-weighted imaging. 3 cm medial and 2 cm cranial from this lesion there was a second lesion (diameter 5 mm) which showed homogeneous enhancement and moderate initial signal increase, postinitial plateau, and reduced signal in T2-weighted imaging.

**MRI Artifact Category:** 2
**MRI Density Type:** 1

| MRM score | Left breast, between outer quadrants | Points | Left breast, central region | Points |
|---|---|---|---|---|
| **Shape** | irregular | 1 | round | 0 |
| **Border** | spiculated | 1 | well-defined | 0 |
| **CM Distribution** | ring | 2 | homogenous | 0 |
| **Initial Signal Intensity Increase** | strong | 2 | moderate | 1 |
| **Post-initial Signal Intensity Character** | wash-out | 2 | plateau | 1 |
| **MRI score (points)** | | **8** | | **2** |
| **MRI BI-RADS** | | **5** | | **2** |

### → Differential Diagnosis

Carcinoma, adenosis, focal inflammation.

| BI-RADS Categorization | | |
|---|---|---|
| Clinical Findings | right 1 | left 3 |
| Ultrasound | right 1 | left 4 |
| Mammography | right 1 | left 3 |
| MR Mammography | right 1 | left 5 |
| **BI-RADS Total** | **right 1** | **left 5** |

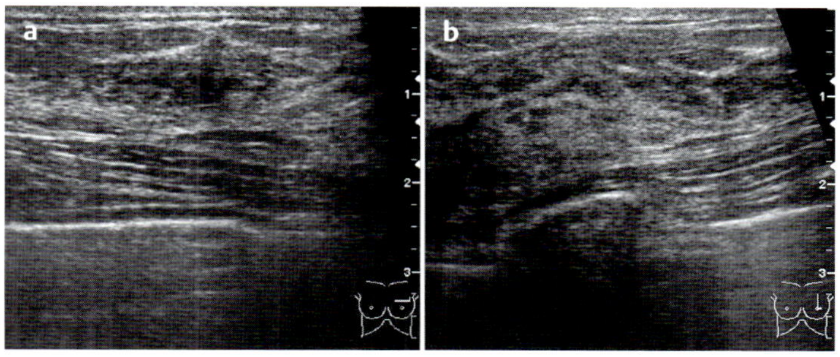

Fig. 51.**10 a, b** Sonography of the central region of the left breast showed no findings consistent with the second lesion seen in MRI.

### Procedure

Ultrasound-guided histopathological investigation of the lesion between the outer quadrants of the left breast.

### Histology

Invasive lobular carcinoma.

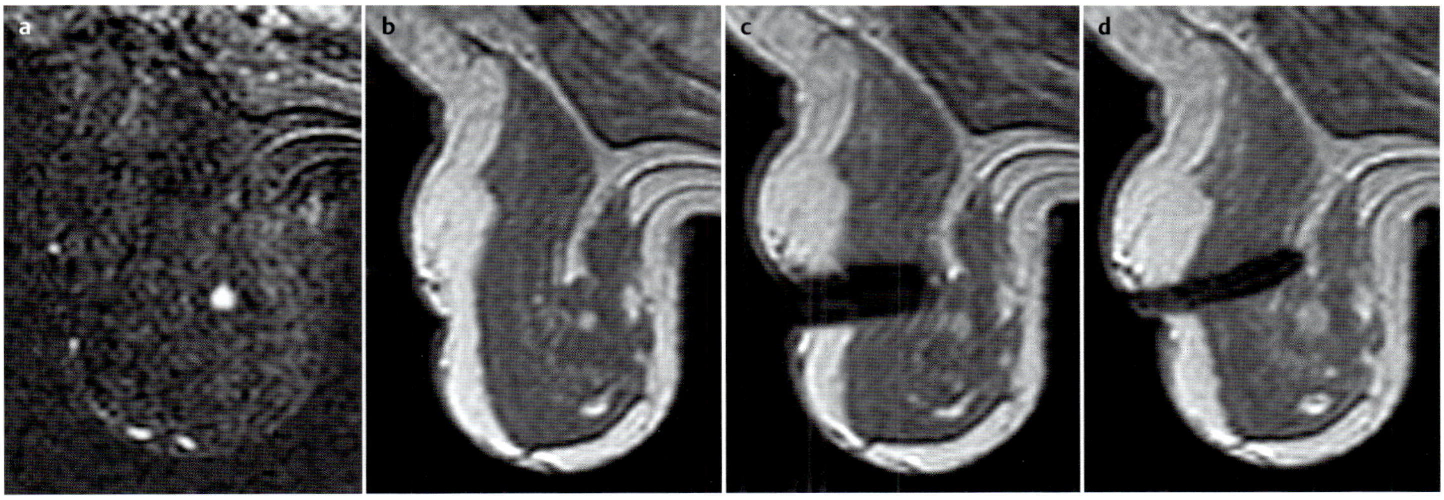

Fig. 51.**11 a – d** Preoperative MR-guided hook-wire localization of the central lesion in the left breast. Precontrast anc subtraction image are presented as well as documentation of the wire in position. Deviation of the hook-wire toward the chest wall due to the high density of the parenchyma can be seen.

### Histology

Invasive lobular carcinoma between the outer quadrants of the left breast. The second lesion, in the center of the left breast, was an adenosis.

ILC pT1c, pN0, G2.

### Treatment

Breast conservation therapy of the left breast.

Invasive lobular carcinomas will often become clinically manifest only at an advanced stage. In this case ultrasound findings pointed toward malignancy. In spite of the low MRM score for the second ipsilateral lesion, this too shculd be marked and analyzed. Malignant findings here would indicate multicentricity and therefore mastectomy.

**Indication:** Monitoring following earlier breast cancer.
**History:** Breast conservation therapy of left breast 4 years previously, relapse 2 years previously.
**Risk profile:** Increased by earlier incidence of breast cancer.
**Age:** 49 years.

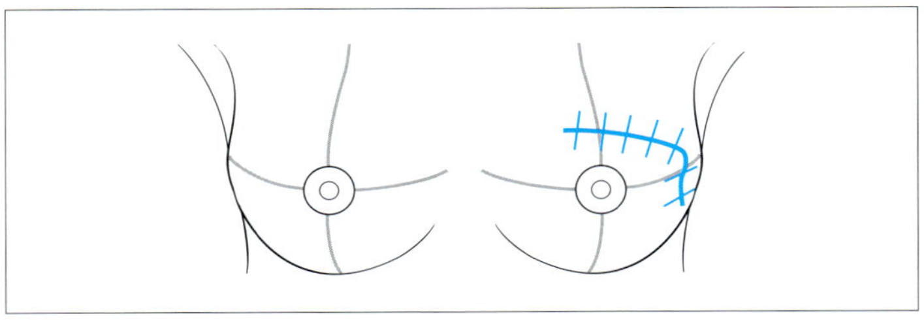

### Clinical Findings

Changes in the left breast due to treatment. Unremarkable scar. No other unusual findings.

### Ultrasound (not shown)

Changes in the left breast due to treatment. No abnormalities.

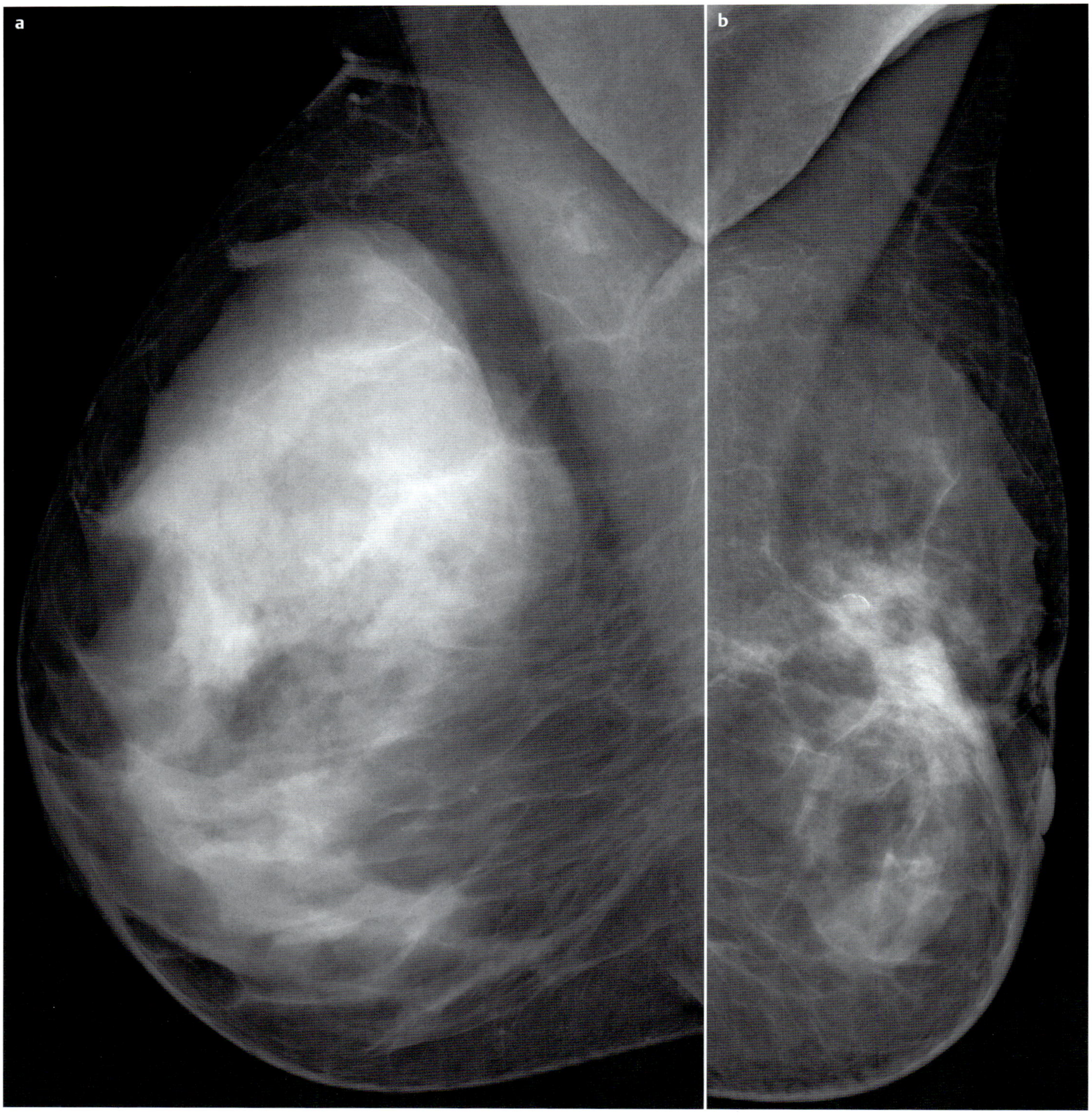


Fig. 52.**1 a, b** Digital mammography, MLO view.

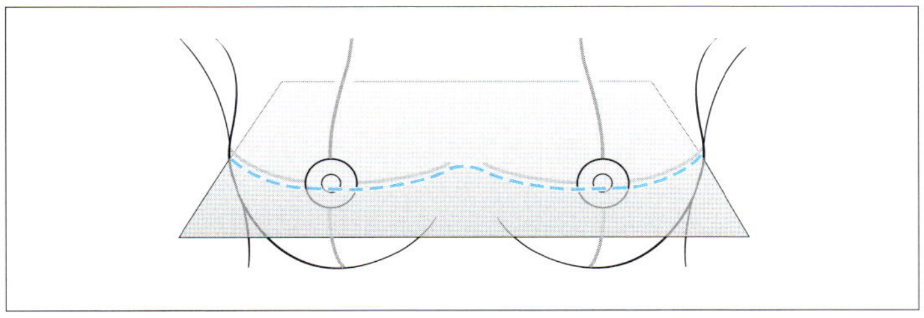

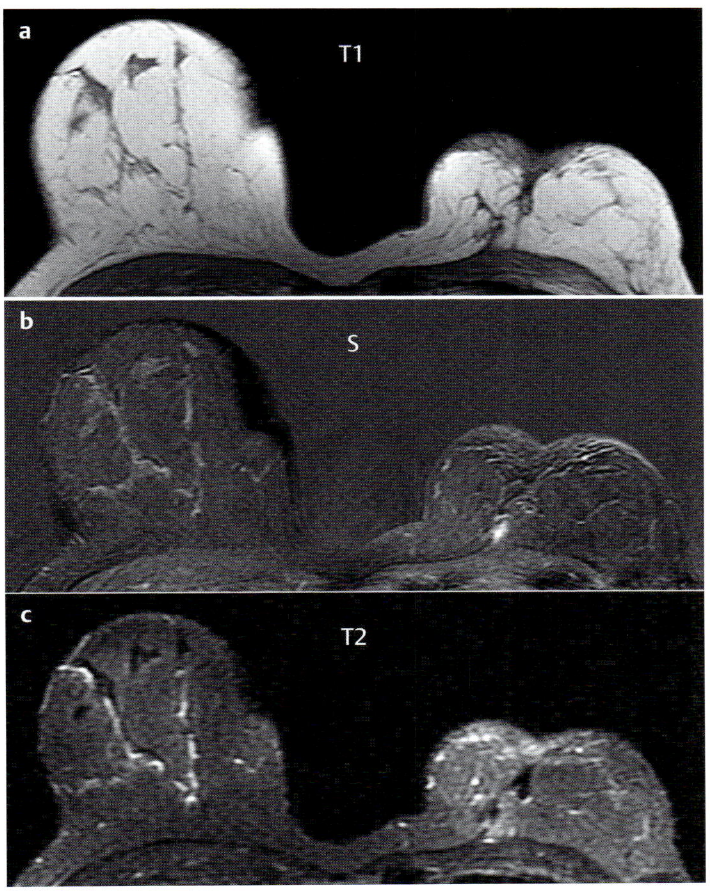


Fig. 52.**2 a–c** Contrast-enhanced MRI of the breasts.

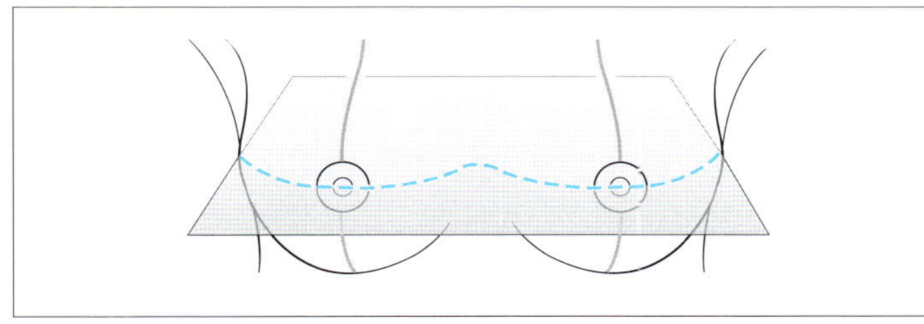

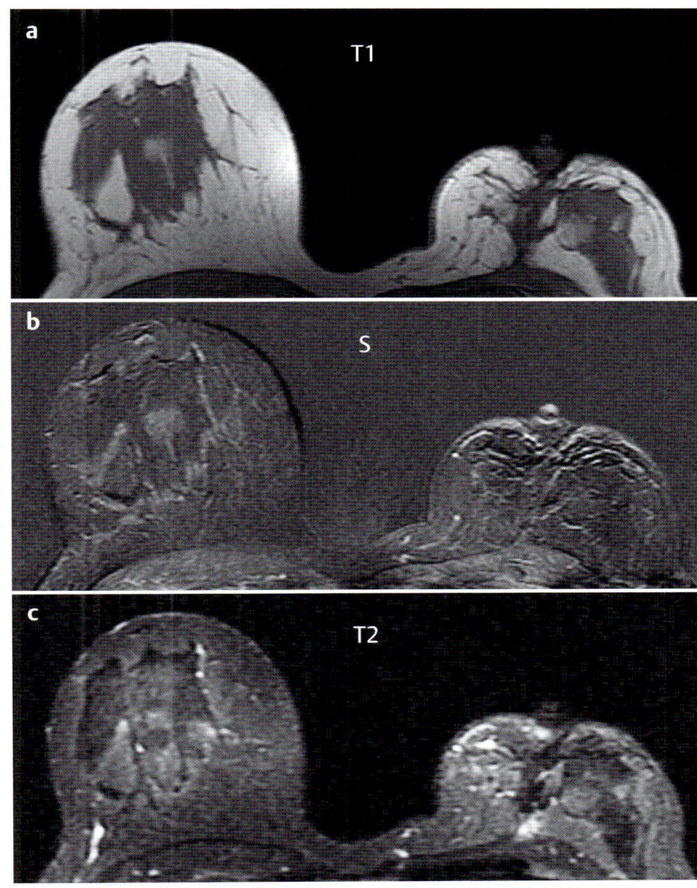


Fig. 52.**3 a–c** Contrast-enhanced MRI of the breasts.

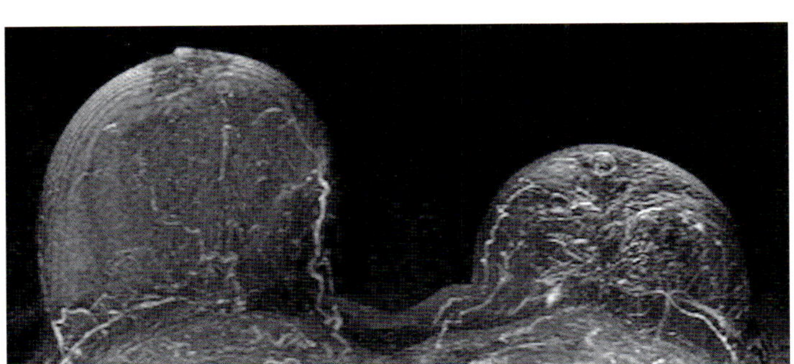

Fig. 52.**4** Contrast-enhanced MR mammography. Maximum intensity projection.

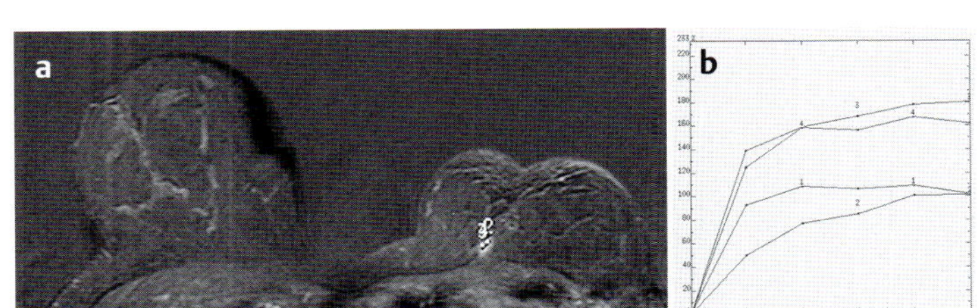


Fig. 52.**5 a, b** Signal-to-time curves.

?

Please characterize mammography and MRI findings.
What is your preliminary diagnosis?
What are your next steps?

These are the imaging studies of a patient being monitored after breast conservation therapy. The patient's risk profile is considered to be high because she did not undergo mastectomy even after suffering a relapse.

### Ultrasound

In the left breast, the only changes observed were related to the earlier treatment for breast cancer. Ultrasound did not show any echo patterns consistent with the enhancement seen in MRI. US BI-RADS right 1/left 2.

### Mammography

Mammograms showed an extremely dense parenchymal pattern, ACR type 4. Under these limiting conditions, there were no suspicious findings in the right breast. The left breast showed treatment-induced changes including marked architectural distortions, extending from behind the nipple to the chest wall. There were no signs of lesions or tumor recurrence. Mammograms depicted no microcalcifications. (BI-RADS right 1/left 3) PGMI classification was omitted due to earlier breast conservation therapy of the left breast.

### MR Mammography

MRI depicted a linear enhancement close to the chest wall in the imaging slice directly inferior to the nipple. The signal curve in this region showed a strong initial increase of about 100% and a postinitial plateau. The MRI slice directly through the nipple line was normal.

The patient's history of previous carcinoma and breast conservation therapy, and no mastectomy after tumor relapse, meant that the probability of the linear enhancement seen in MRI representing tumor recurrence was high.

**MRI Artifact Category:** 2
**MRI Density Type:** 1

| MRM score | Finding | Points |
|---|---|---|
| **Shape** | linear | 1 |
| **Border** | ill-defined | 1 |
| **CM Distribution** | homogenous | 0 |
| **Initial Signal Intensity Increase** | strong | 2 |
| **Post-initial Signal Intensity Character** | plateau | 1 |
| **MRI score (points)** | | **5** |
| **MRI BI-RADS** | | **4** |

### → Differential Diagnostic Considerations

Tumor recurrence, focal mastitis, fat necrosis.

| BI-RADS Categorization | | |
|---|---|---|
| Clinical Findings | right 1 | left 1 |
| Ultrasound | right 1 | left 1 |
| Mammography | right 1 | left 3 |
| MR Mammography | right 1 | left 4 |
| **BI-RADS Total** | **right 1** | **left 4** |

### Procedure

MR-guided percutaneous biopsy of the circumscribed enhancement near the chest wall in the left breast.
However, the patient declined this intervention and instead follow-up MR mammography was performed 6 months later.

### Follow-up MRI after 6 months

The previously seen linear enhancement in the left breast close to the chest wall was not reproduced to the same extent (Fig. 52.**6**).

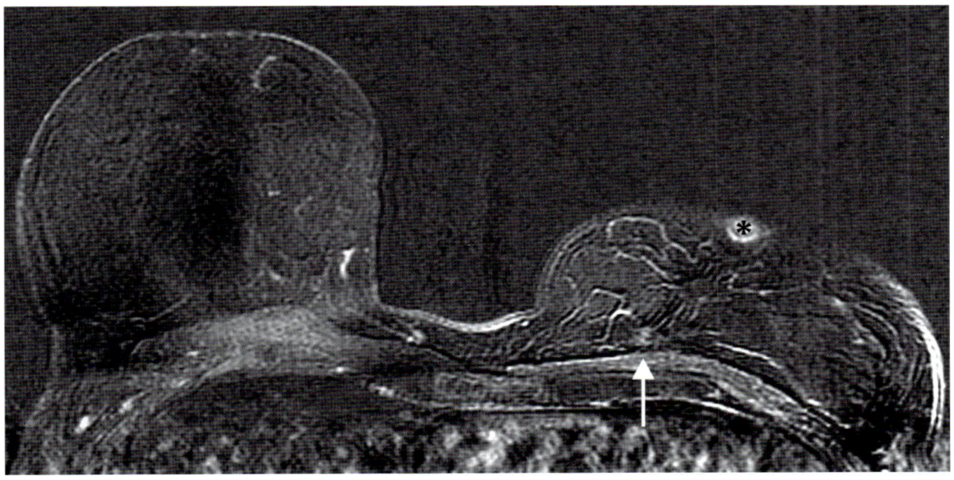


Fig. 52.**6** Single-slice subtraction image from the follow-up MRI six months later showing residual contrast uptake (arrow). Enhancement of the nipple (asterisk).

## Diagnosis (without histological verification)

Focal inflammation after surgery (breast conservation therapy, intervention after relapse).

## Treatment

None.

## Follow-up

Further monitoring at regular intervals (* see comment).

* After breast conservation therapy, monitoring is recommended at the following intervals:
Mammography of the ipsilateral breast at intervals of 6 months for 3 years.
Mammography of the contralateral breast at intervals of 12 months for 3 years.
Bilateral mammography yearly after 3 years.

**Indication:** Screening.
**History:** Unremarkable.
**Risk profile:** No increased risk.
**Age:** 52 years.

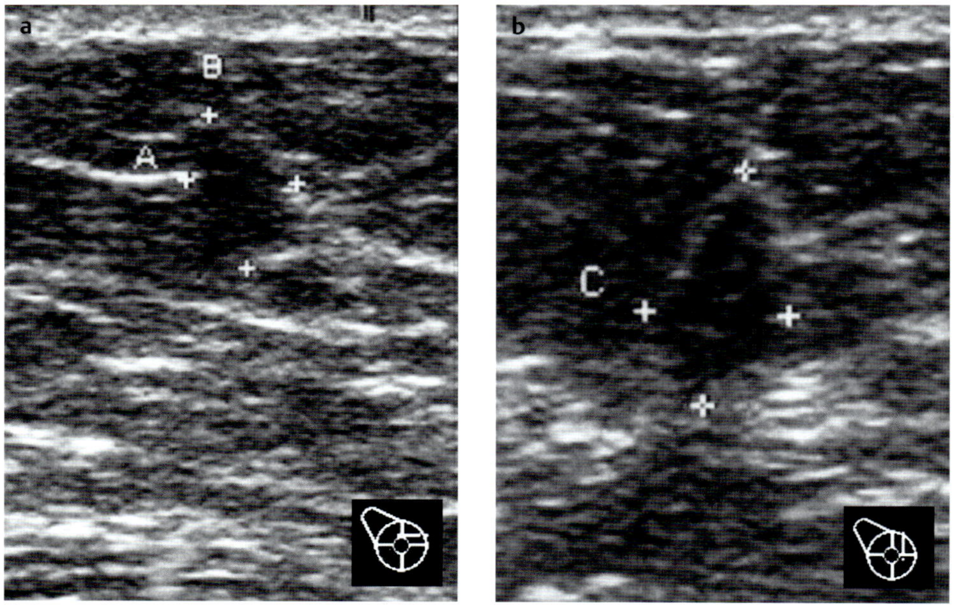


Fig. 53.**1 a, b** Ultrasound images of outer quadrants of the right breast [imaging not performed by authors].

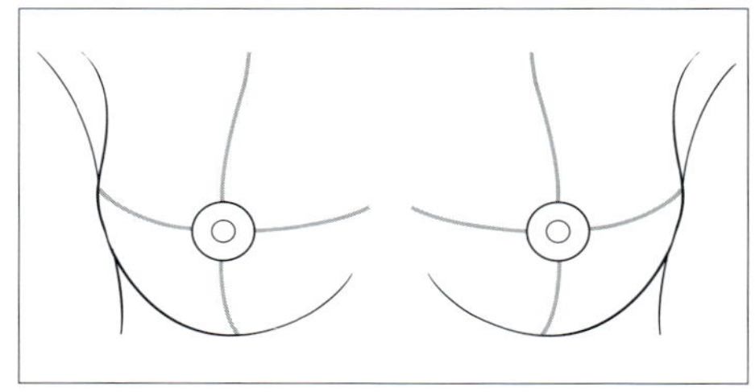

### Clinical Findings

Nodular parenchymal texture. No circumscribed findings.

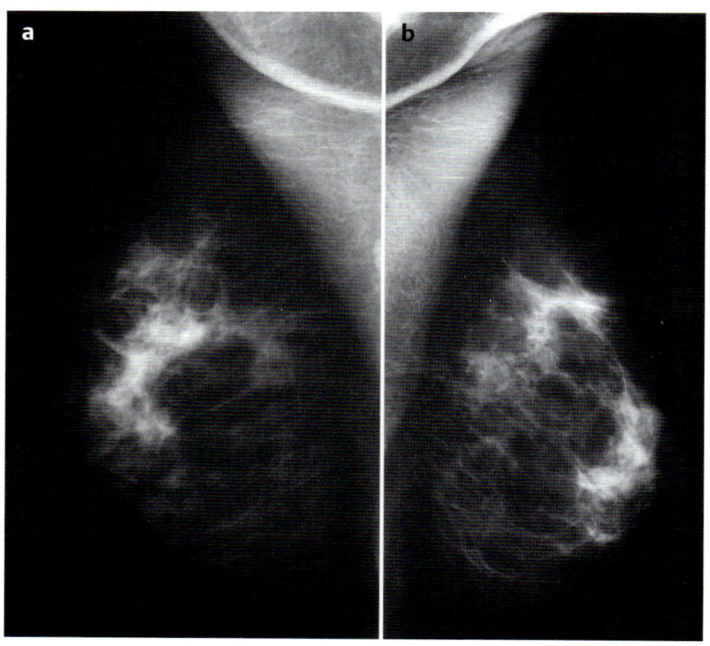


Fig. 53.**2 a, b** Conventional mammography, MLO view [imaging not performed by authors].

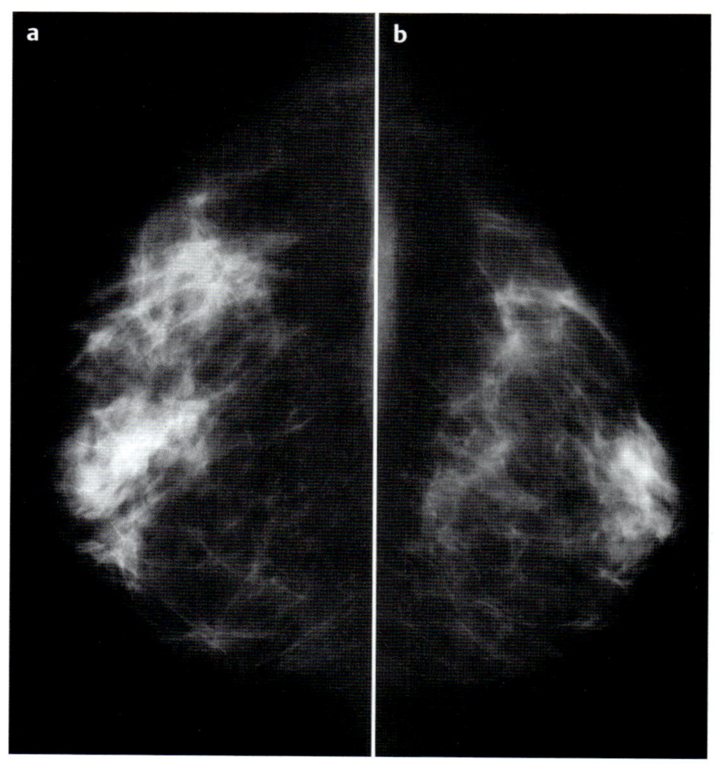


Fig. 53.**3 a, b** Conventional mammography, CC view [imaging not performed by authors].

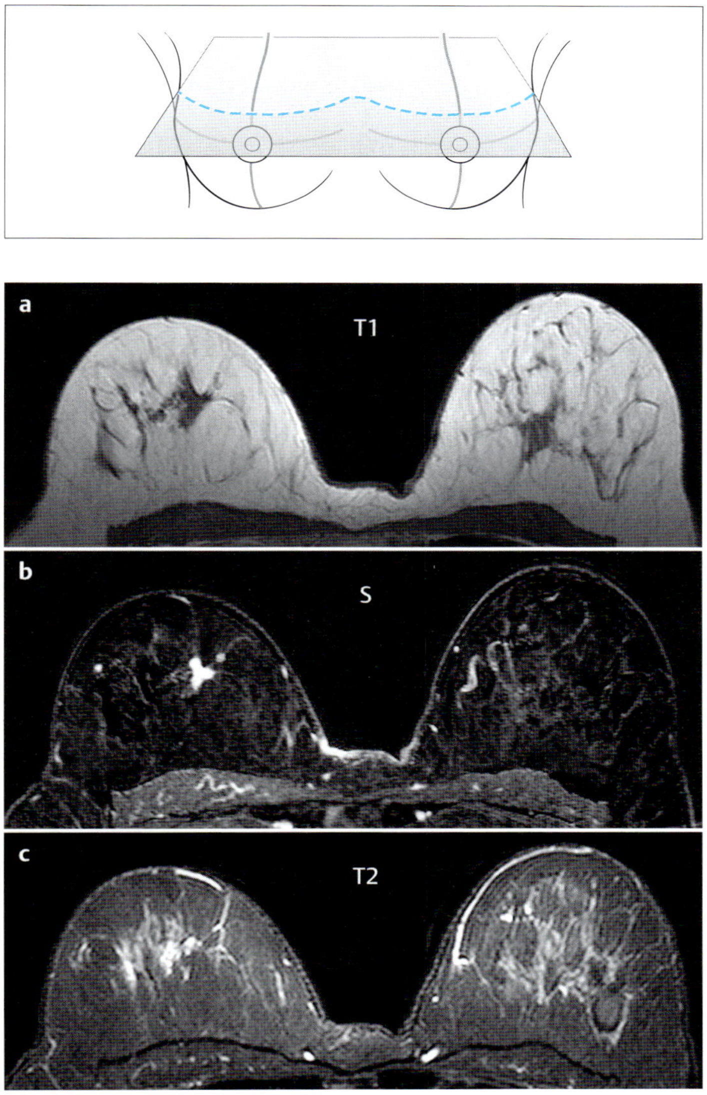


Fig. 53.**4 a – c** Contrast-enhanced MRI of the breasts.

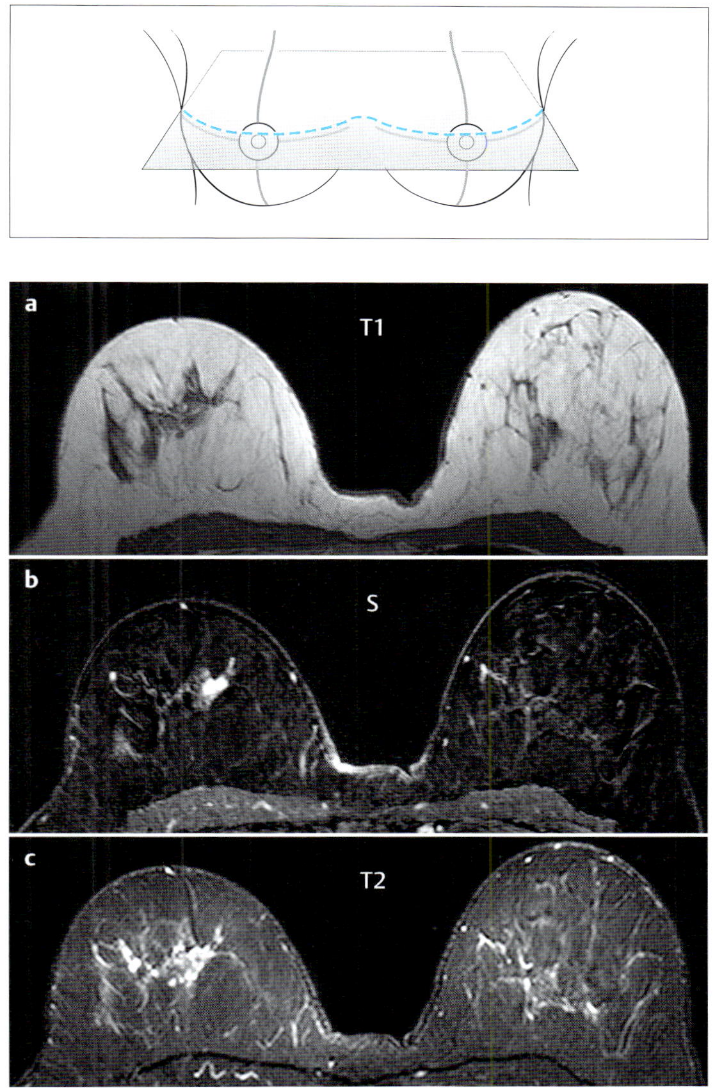


Fig. 53.**5 a – c** Contrast-enhanced MRI of the breasts.

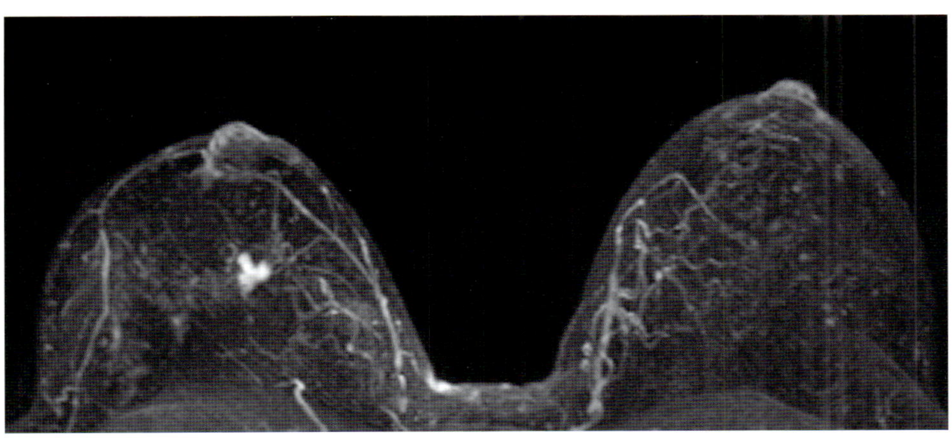

Fig. 53.**6** Contrast-enhanced MR mammography. Maximum intensity projection.

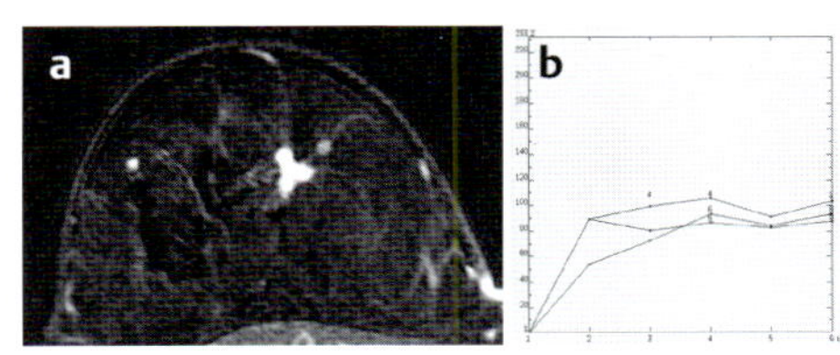


Fig. 53.**7 a, b** Signal-to-time curves.

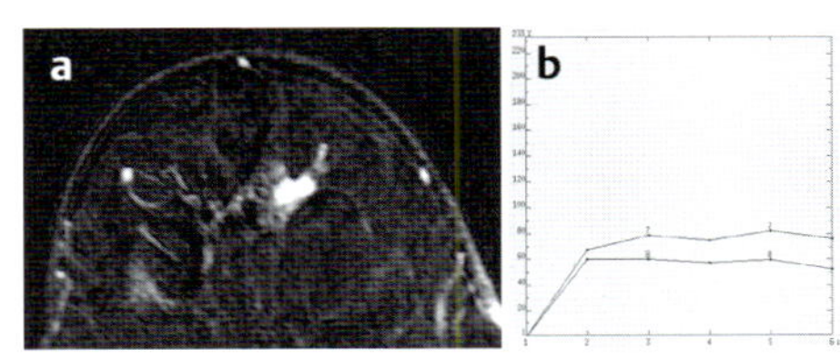


Fig. 53.**8 a, b** Signal-to-time curves.

?

Please characterize ultrasound, mammography, and MRI findings.
What is your preliminary diagnosis?
What are your next steps?

The images presented were taken during a screening examination of an asymptomatic woman.

### Ultrasound

Ultrasound demonstrated a hypoechoic lesion 8 mm in diameter with indeterminate distal echo pattern between the upper quadrants of the right breast. There were also signs of slight architectural distortion. Otherwise, acoustic texture was normal. US BI-RADS right 4/left 1.

### Mammography

Mammograms showed partially inhomogeneous dense parenchyma, ACR type 3. In the upper part of the right breast (MLO view) there was a hyperdensity and the resulting asymmetry was visible when both breasts were compared. There were no suspicious masses and no microcalcifications. BI-RADS right 3/left 1. PGMI: CC view P; MLO view G (bilateral axillary skin folds).

Additional imaging in a third view (LM) and a magnification mammography of the right breast were also performed (Fig. 53.**9 a, b, c**).

### MR Mammography (imaging performed elsewhere)

Between the upper quadrants of the right breast, a single partially ill-defined, partially spiculated mass with homogeneous enhancement was demonstrated. It showed moderate initial signal increase and a postinitial plateau, and had a slightly increased signal in T2-weighted imaging. The lesion diameter was 15 mm.

**MRI Artifact Category:** 2
**MRI Density Type:** 1

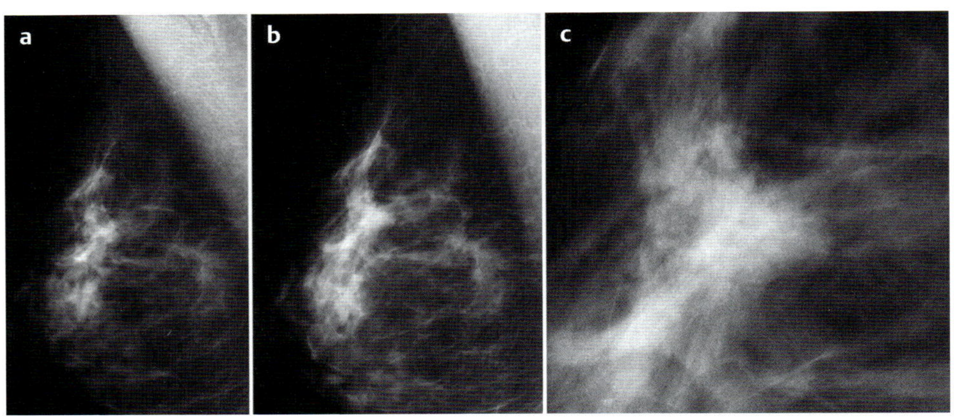


Fig. 53.**9 a – c** Analogue mammography (LM view), magnification view and enlarged image of the right breast [imaging not performed by authors].

| MRM score | Finding | Points |
|---|---|---|
| **Shape** | irregular | 1 |
| **Border** | spiculated | 1 |
| **CM Distribution** | inhomogenous | 1 |
| **Initial Signal Intensity Increase** | moderate | 1 |
| **Post-initial Signal Intensity Character** | plateau | 1 |
| **MRI score (points)** | | **4** |
| **MRI BI-RADS** | | **4** |

### → Differential Diagnosis

Radial scar, invasive carcinoma.

| BI-RADS Categorization | | |
|---|---|---|
| Clinical Findings | right 1 | left 1 |
| Ultrasound | right 4 | left 1 |
| Mammography | right 4 | left 1 |
| MR Mammography | right 4 | left 1 |
| **BI-RADS Total** | **right 4** | **left 1** |

### Procedure

Investigation of the lesion in the right breast by MR-guided vacuum biopsy.

### Histopathology of the core biopsy specimen

Tubular carcinoma.

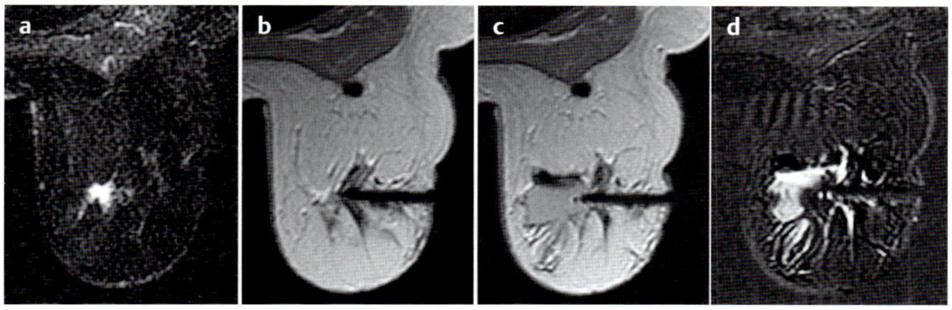


Fig. 53.**10 a – d** MR-guided core biopsy. The lesion in the right breast was reproducible. The coaxial needle is shown in position before the intervention. Precontrast and postcontrast images after removal of specimen are shown.

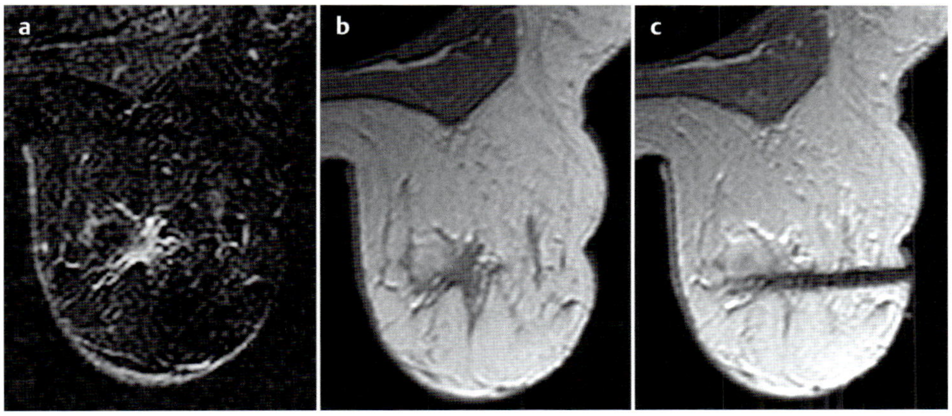


Fig. 53.**11 a – c** Preoperative MR-guided hook-wire localization before open biopsy.

## Histology

Tubular carcinoma.

TC pT1c pN0, G1.

## Treatment

Breast conservation therapy of the right breast.

Where standard mammography produces unclear findings, imaging in a third view (mediolateral or lateromedial) is useful. Based on the lateromedial imaging findings in this case, a stereotactic vacuum biopsy could have been an alternative next step.

**Indication:** Screening.
**History:** Unremarkable.
**Risk profile:** No increased risk.
**Age:** 44 years.

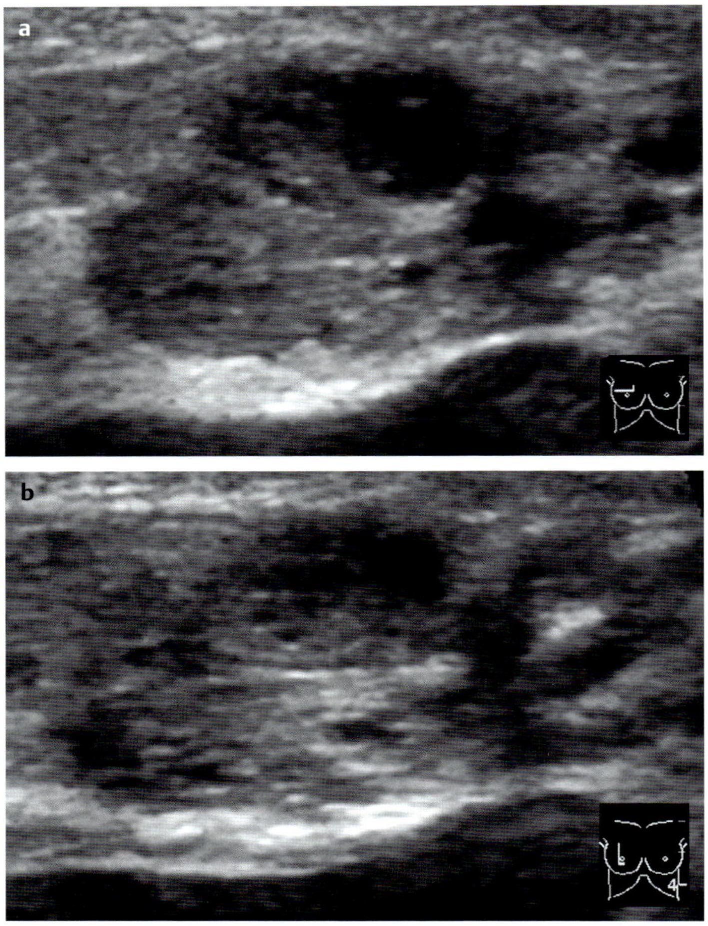

Fig. 54.**1 a, b** Ultrasound.

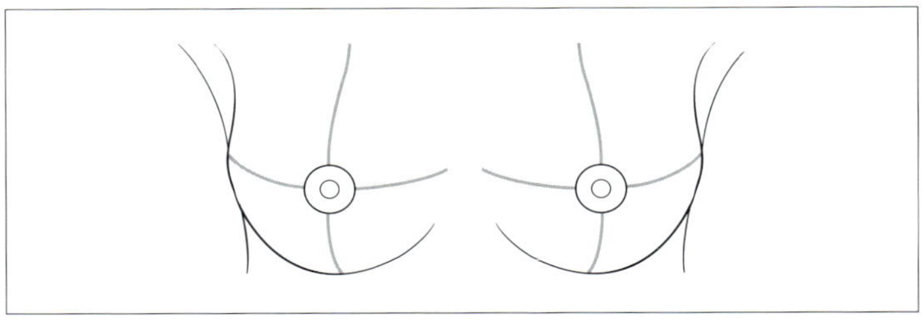

### Clinical Findings

Dense, nodular parenchyma, but no circumscribed lumps.

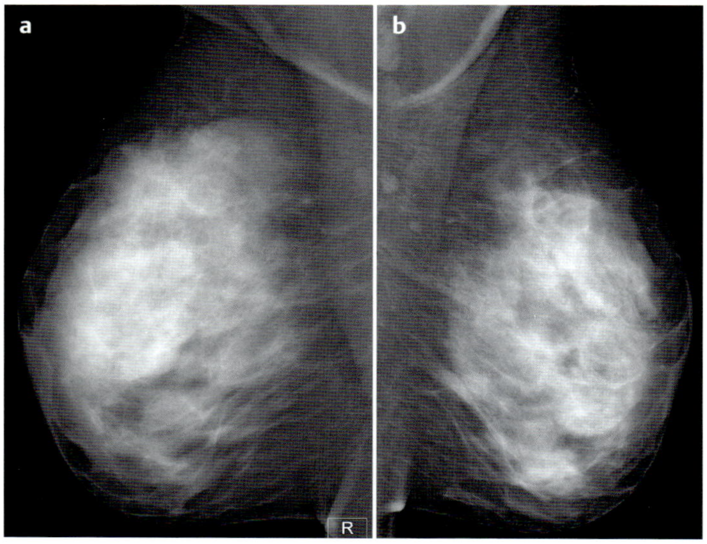

Fig. 54.**2 a, b** Digital mammography, MLO view.

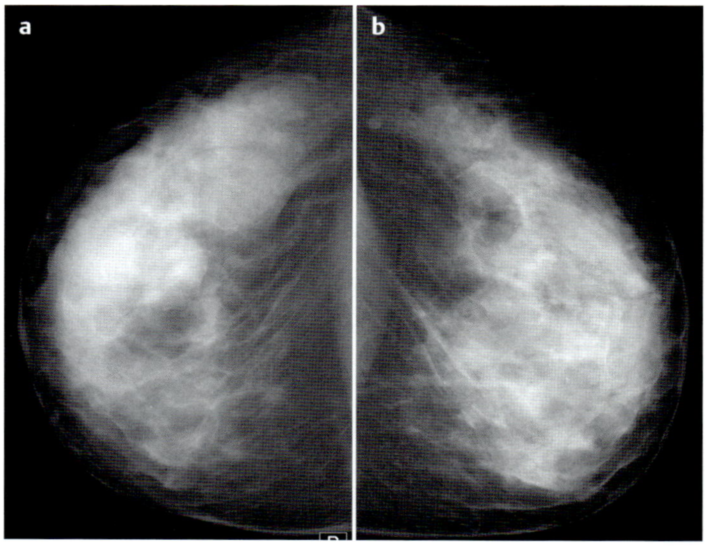

Fig. 54.**3 a, b** Digital mammography, CC view.

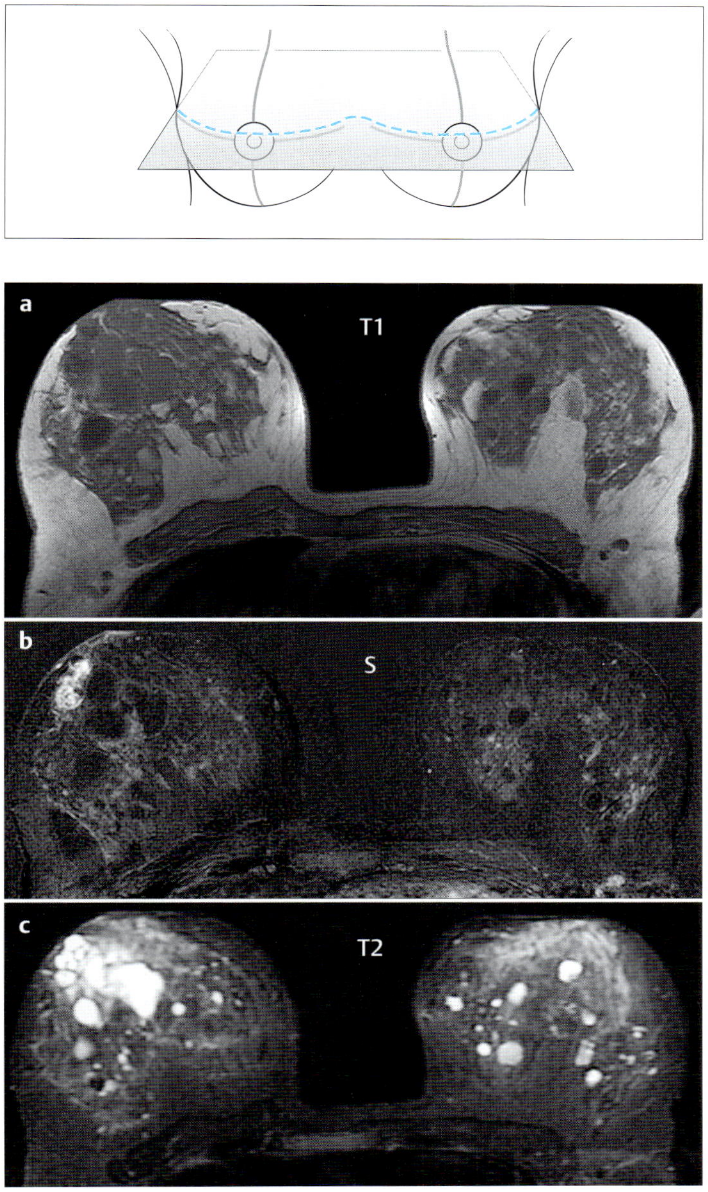


Fig. 54.**4 a – c** Contrast-enhanced MR mammography.

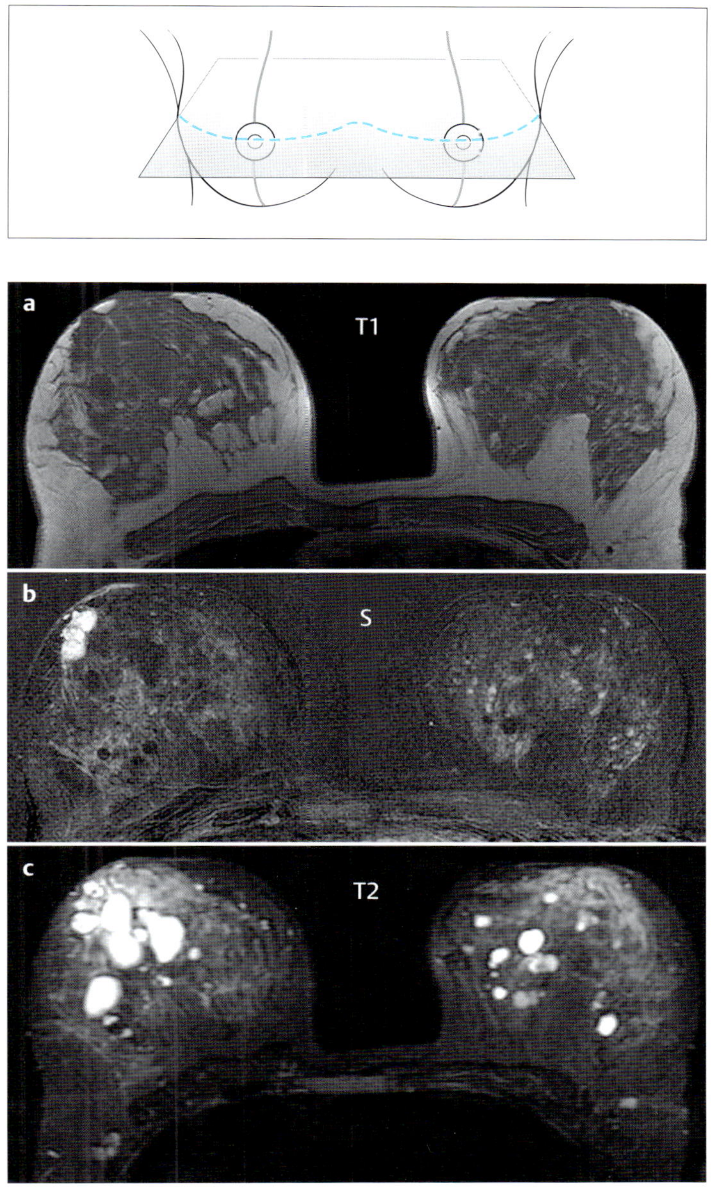


Fig. 54.**5 a – c** Contrast-enhanced MR mammography.

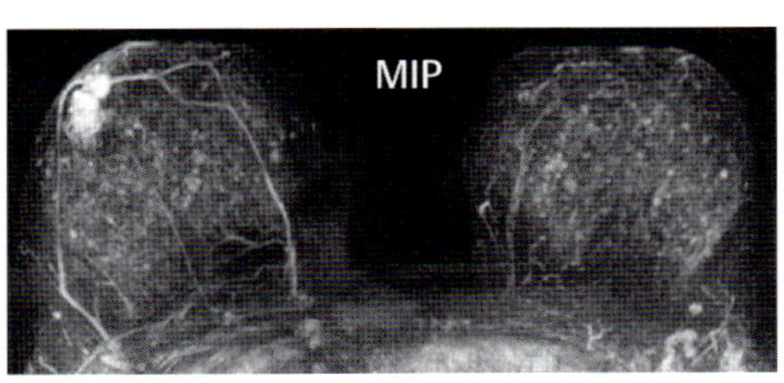


Fig. 54.**6** Contrast-enhanced MR mammography. Maximum intensity projection.

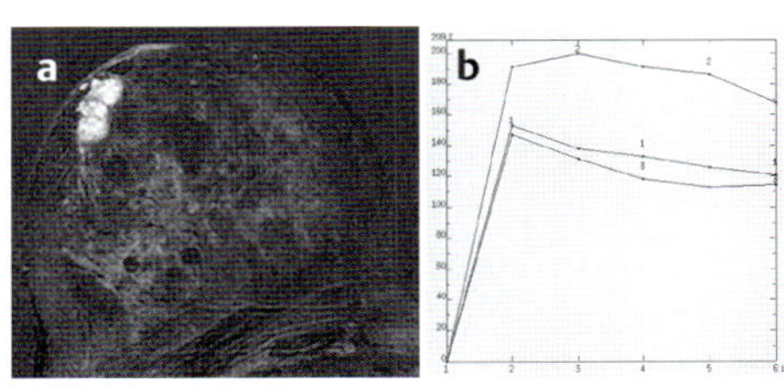


Fig. 54.**7 a, b** Signal-to-time curves.

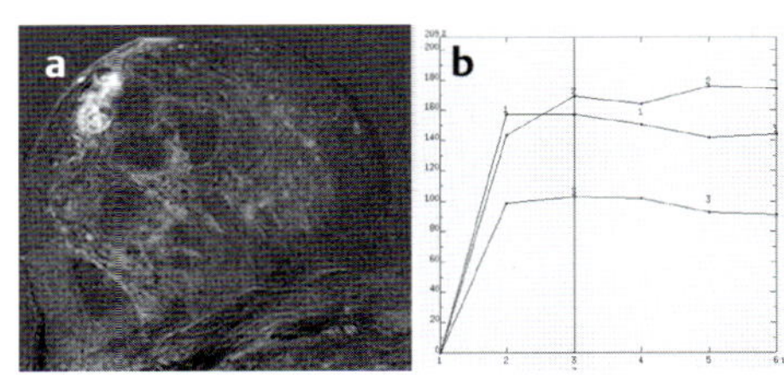


Fig. 54.**8 a, b** Signal-to-time curves.

?

Please characterize ultrasound, mammography, and MRI findings.
What is your preliminary diagnosis?
What are your next steps?

This case illustrates the imaging of an asymptomatic woman in a screening situation.

### Ultrasound

Ultrasound showed an inhomogeneous, partially hypoechoic lesion measuring 3 cm × 1.5 cm in the upper outer quadrant of the right breast. The distal echo pattern was indeterminate. Multiple cysts were also seen in both breasts. US BI-RADS right 3.

### Mammography

The parenchyma was bilaterally symmetric and extremely dense, ACR type 4. Under these limiting conditions, mammography showed no suspect densities or masses. No architectural distortion or calcifications. BI-RADS right 1/left 1. PGMI: CC view P; MLO view G (bilateral skin folds).

### MR Mammography

MRI depicted an inhomogeneous enhancing lesion 3 cm × 1.5 cm in size in the upper outer quadrant of the right breast, near the areola. This lesion had very high initial signal increase and postinitial washout. The signal in T2-weighted imaging was partially increased. There were multiple cysts of diameter up to 4 cm in both breasts.

**MRI Artifact Category:** 1
**MRI Density Type:** 2

| MRM score | Finding | Points |
|---|---|---|
| **Shape** | irregular | 1 |
| **Border** | well-defined | 0 |
| **CM Distribution** | inhomogeneous | 1 |
| **Initial Signal Intensity Increase** | strong | 2 |
| **Post-initial Signal Intensity Character** | wash-out | 2 |
| **MRI score (points)** | | **6** |
| **MRI BI-RADS** | | **5** |

### → Differential Diagnosis

Carcinoma, papilloma, fibroadenoma.

| BI-RADS Categorization | | |
|---|---|---|
| Clinical Findings | right 1 | left 1 |
| Ultrasound | right 3 | left 1 |
| Mammography | right 1 | left 1 |
| MR Mammography | right 5 | left 1 |
| **BI-RADS Total** | **right 5** | **left 1** |

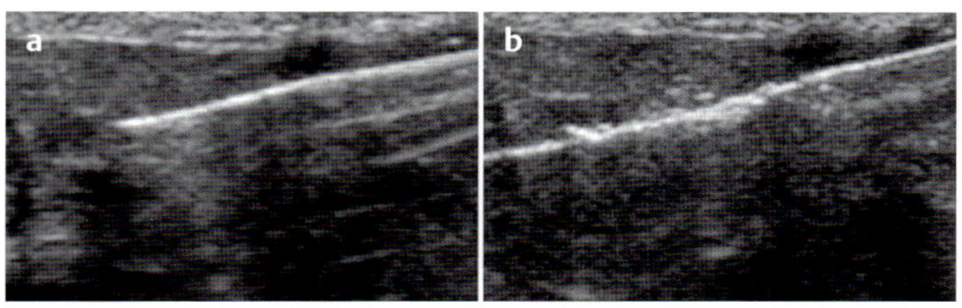

Fig. 54.**9 a, b** US-guided core biopsy (pre-fire, post-fire).

**Procedure**

Ultrasound-guided core biopsy of the right breast (Fig. 54.**9**).

**Histology**

Intraductal papilloma.

**Further Procedure**

Open biopsy of the papilloma.

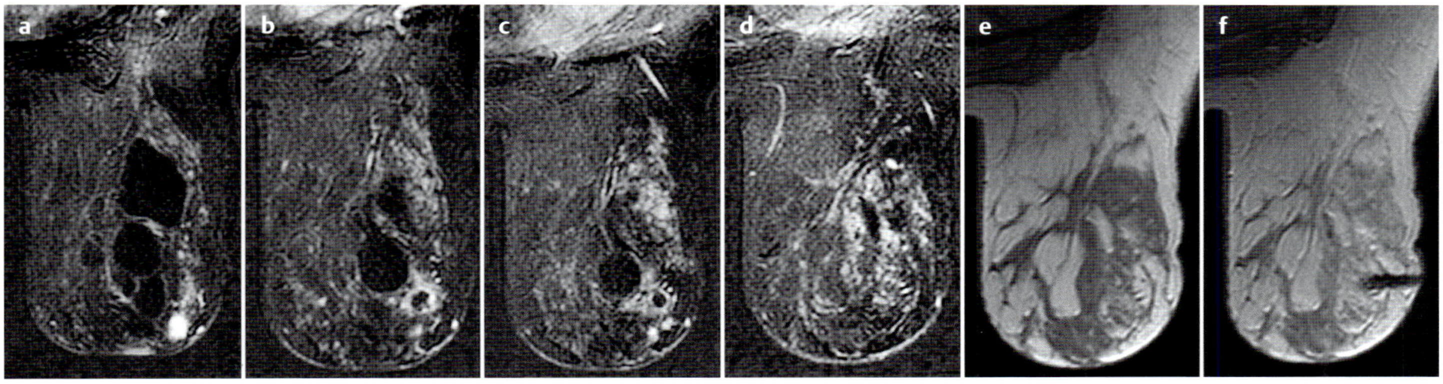

Fig. 54.**10 a–f** MR-guided localization to determine the precise extent of the tumor on the chest wall side. Consecutive subtraction images from the middle of the lesion to its caudal limit (**a–d**). Precontrast imaging of the tumor at its caudal border (**e**) and documentation of the correctly positioned hook-wire (**f**).

**Histology**

Multifocal minimally invasive papillary carcinoma.

IP pT1mic, pN0 (0/10), G2.

**Treatment**

Breast conservation therapy.

The risk of solitary intraductal papillomas becoming malignant is about 3–7%. In the case of multiple peripheral papillomas, the relative risk of breast cancer is 10–33%. For this reason, the resection of papillomas is recommended.

**Indication:** Screening before planned breast reduction surgery.
**History:** Unremarkable.
**Risk profile:** No increased risk.
**Age:** 60 years.

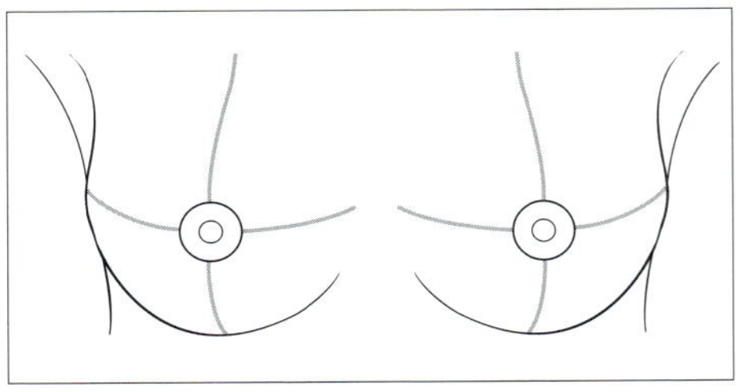

## Clinical Findings

Macromastia. No abnormalities.

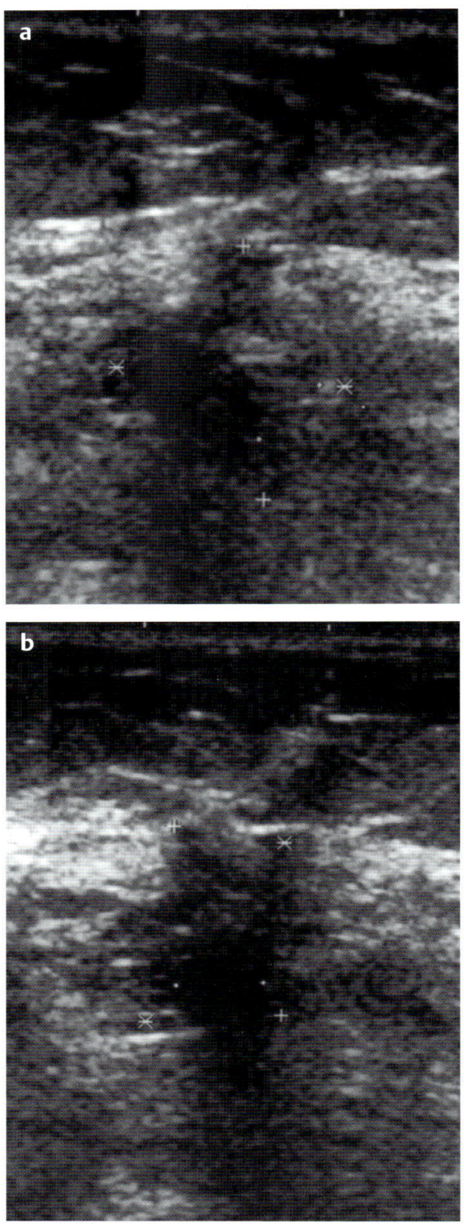

Fig. 55.**1 a, b** Ultrasound imaging between the upper quadrants of the right breast.

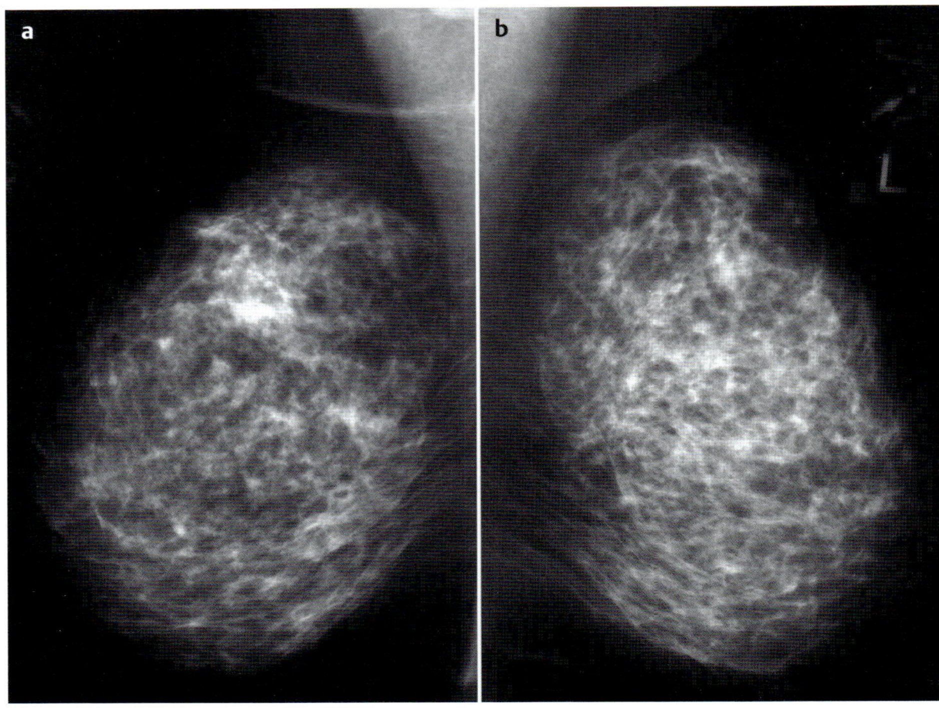

Fig. 55.**2 a, b** Conventional mammography, MLO view [imaging not performed by authors].

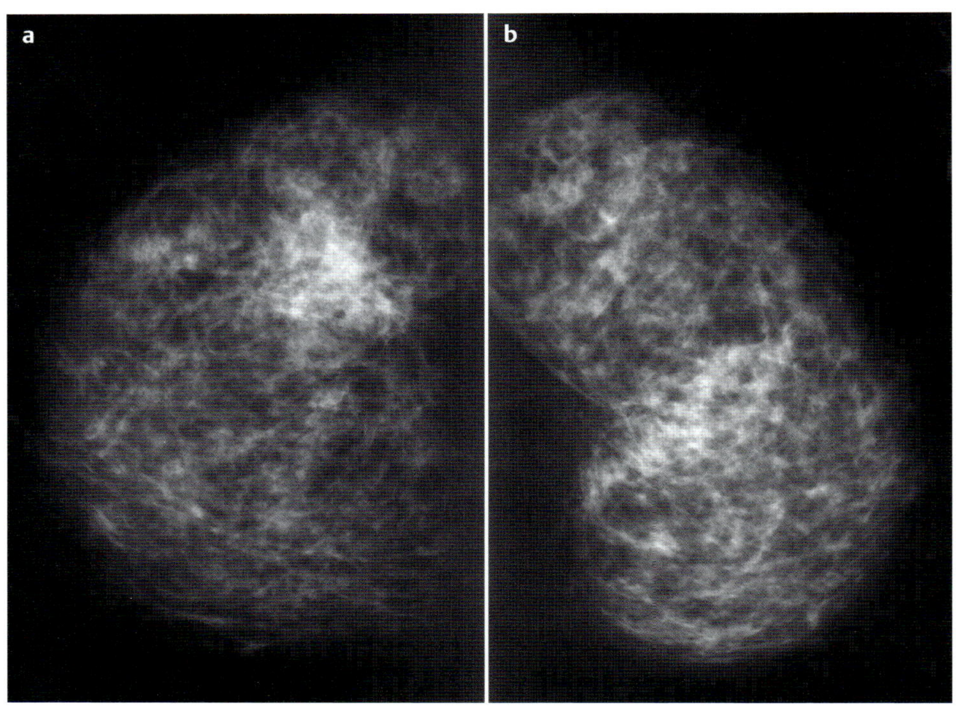

Fig. 55.**3 a, b** Conventional mammography, CC view [imaging not performed by authors].

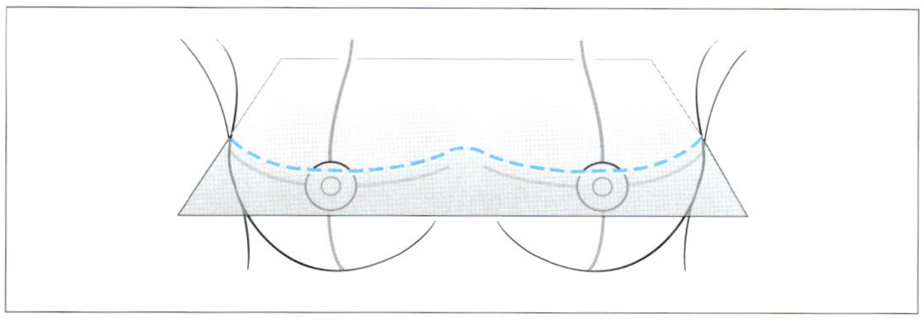

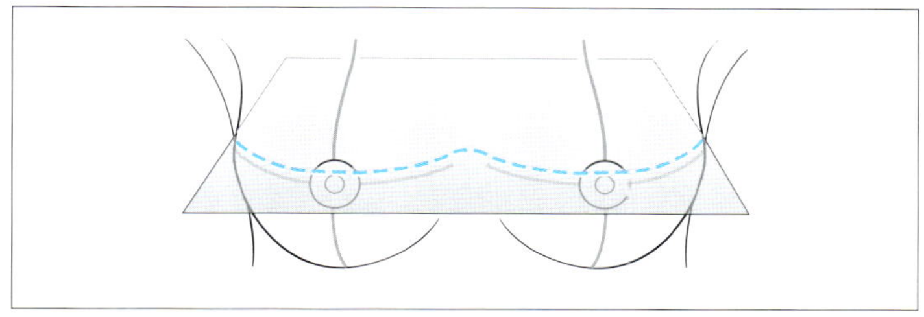

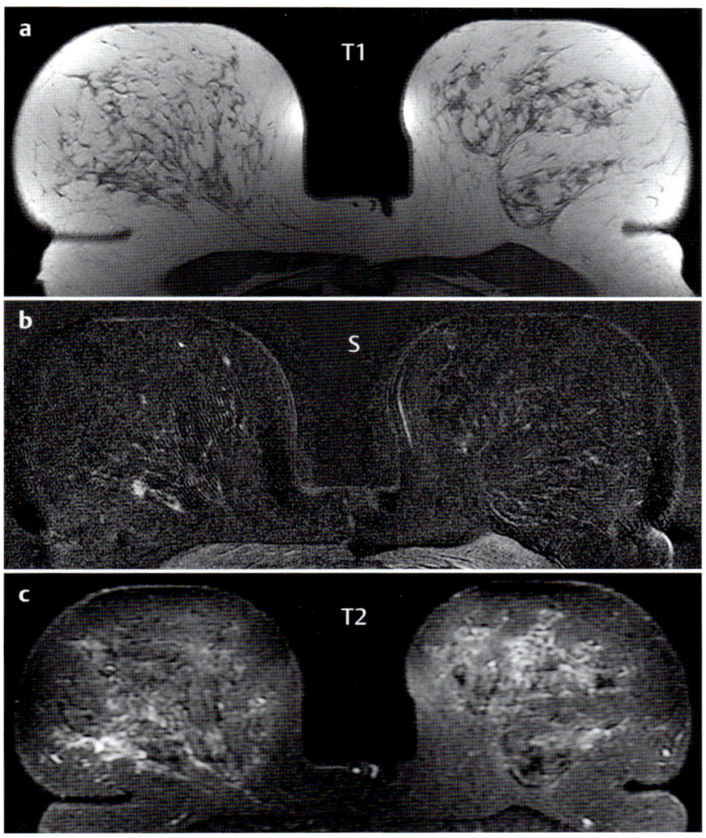


Fig. 55.**4 a – c** Contrast-enhanced MR mammography. Earliest subtraction.

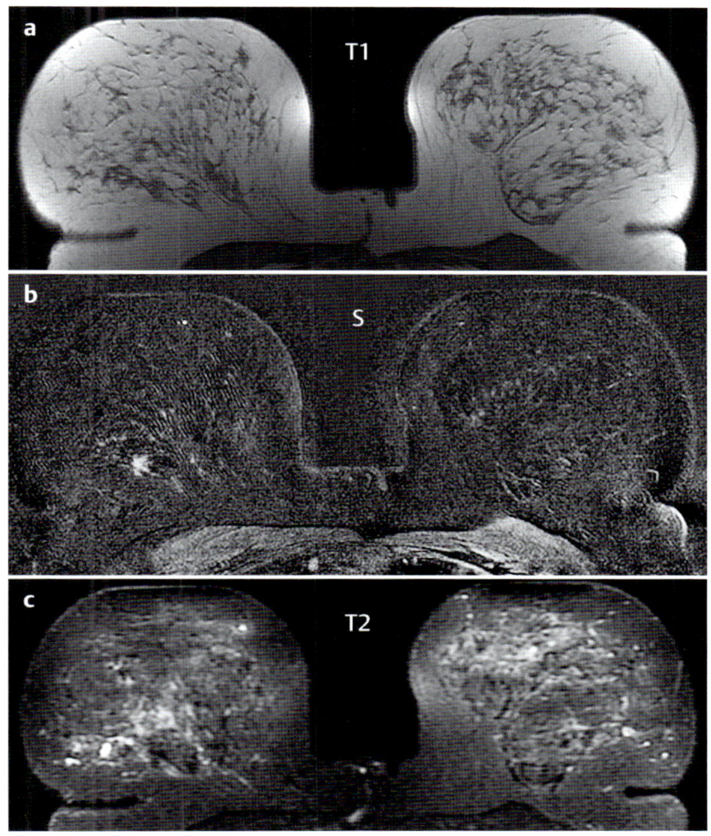


Fig. 55.**5 a – c** Contrast-enhanced MR mammography. Earliest subtraction.

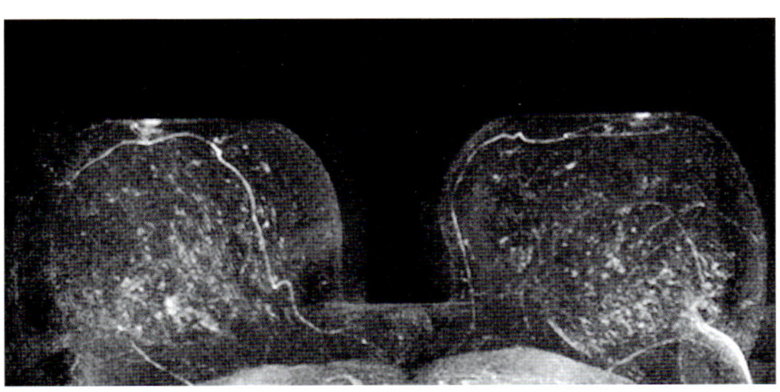

Fig. 55.**6** Contrast-enhanced MR mammography. Maximum intensity projection.

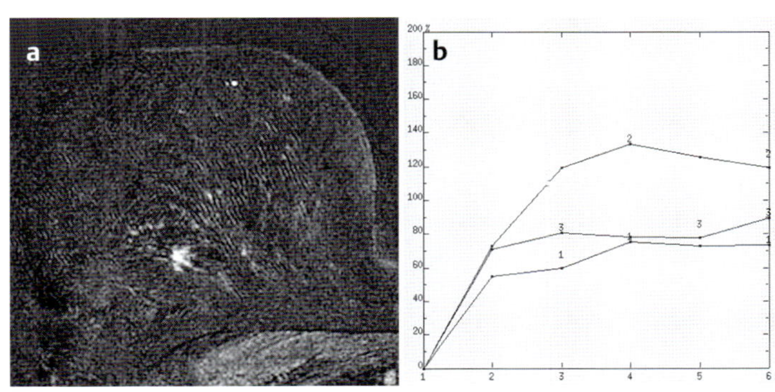


Fig. 55.**7 a, b** Signal-to-time curves.

Please characterize ultrasound, mammography, and MRI findings.
What is your preliminary diagnosis?
What are your next steps?

In view of the limited usefulness of mammography and sonography in this case, MR mammography was carried out on this patient in advance of planned bilateral reduction surgery.

### Ultrasound

Ultrasound showed inhomogeneous echogenicity of the breast parenchyma. No suspicious lesions were seen in the initial ultrasound images. However, once the results of MR mammography were known, the sonographic examination was repeated and a hypoechoic mass measuring 8 mm with distal echo shadowing was depicted between the upper quadrants of the right breast. No architectural distortion. US BI-RADS right 3/left 1.

### Mammography

Mammograms showed asymmetric, partially inhomogeneous dense parenchyma, ACR type 3. There were no suspicious findings and no microcalcifications. BI-RADS right 1/left 1. PGMI: CC view P; MLO view G (angle of pectoral muscle, inframammary fold).

### MR Mammography

A solitary, partially ill-defined, spiculated mass of 1.5 cm diameter with homogeneous enhancement was found between the upper quadrants of the right breast. Initial signal increase was 120% followed by a postinitial plateau. There was a partially reduced signal of this lesion in T2-weighted imaging. No other suspect findings.

**MRI Artifact Category:** 1
**MRI Density Type:** 2

| MRM score | Finding | Points |
|---|---|---|
| **Shape** | irregular | 1 |
| **Border** | spiculated | 1 |
| **CM Distribution** | homogeneous | 0 |
| **Initial Signal Intensity Increase** | strong | 2 |
| **Post-initial Signal Intensity Character** | plateau | 1 |
| **MRI score (points)** | | **5** |
| **MRI BI-RADS** | | **4** |

### → Differential Diagnosis

Focal adenosis, radial scar, carcinoma (tubular?).

| BI-RADS Categorization | | |
|---|---|---|
| Clinical Findings | right 1 | left 1 |
| Ultrasound | right 3 | left 1 |
| Mammography | right 1 | left 1 |
| MR Mammography | right 4 | left 1 |
| **BI-RADS Total** | **right 4** | **left 1** |

### Procedure

MR-guided vacuum biopsy. A US-guided biopsy could also be considered as an alternative. In the latter case, the correspondence between US and MRI findings must be very firmly established.

### Histology

Invasive lobular carcinoma.

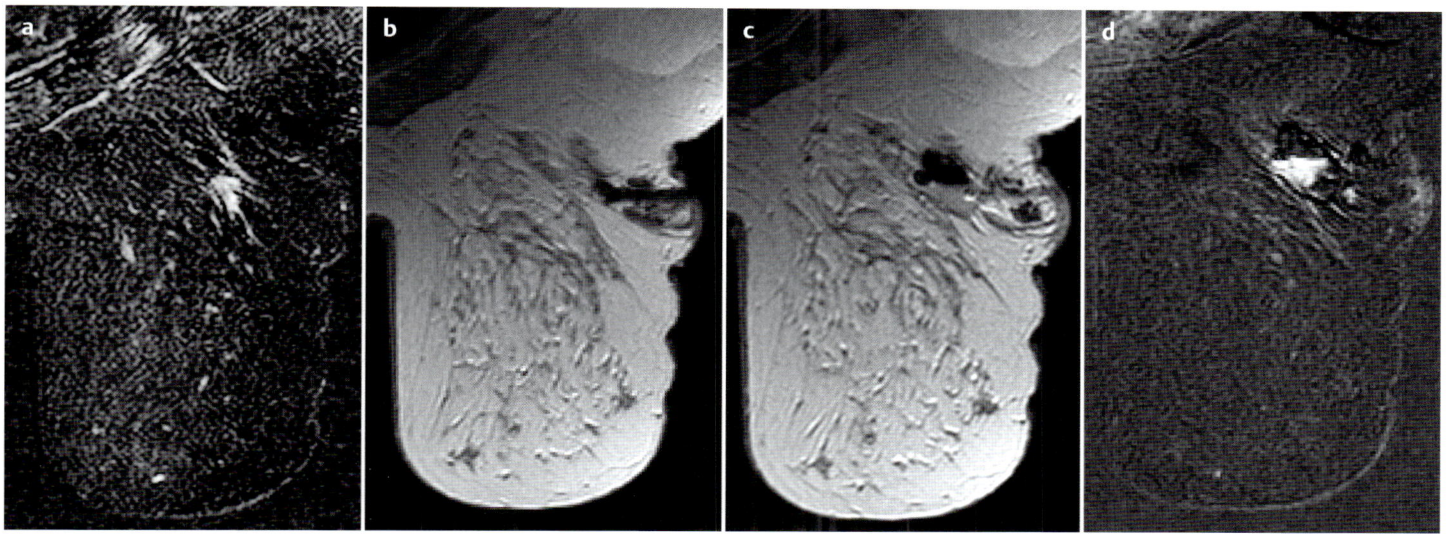

Fig. 55.**8 a – d** MR-guided vacuum biopsy.
**a** Subtraction image reproducing the suspicious finding.
**b** Documentation of coaxial needle.
**c** Area of resection after biopsy.
**d** Final documentation following further contrast administration, showing enhancement due to bleeding.

### Histology

Diffuse invasive lobular carcinoma.

ILC pT2 pN0, G1.

### Treatment

Breast conservation therapy of the right breast, and simultaneous bilateral reduction surgery.

When there is no correlation in sonography or mammography with suspect findings in MRI, further targeted ultrasound as well as alternative mammographic views should be obtained.

**Indication:** Inflammation of the left breast.
**History:** Unremarkable.
**Risk profile:** No increased risk.
**Age:** 73 years.

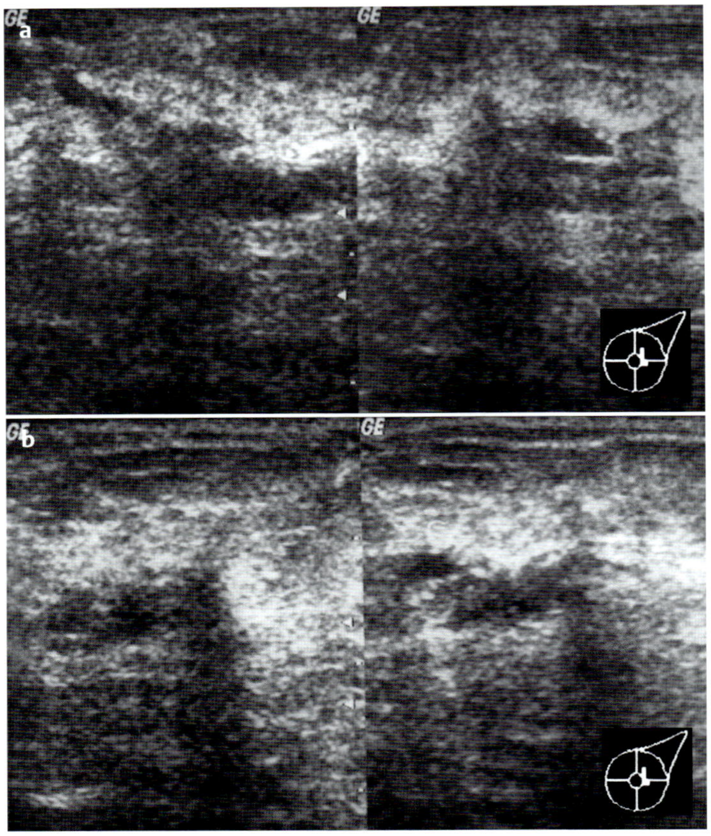

Fig. 56.1 **a, b** Ultrasound [imaging not performed by authors].

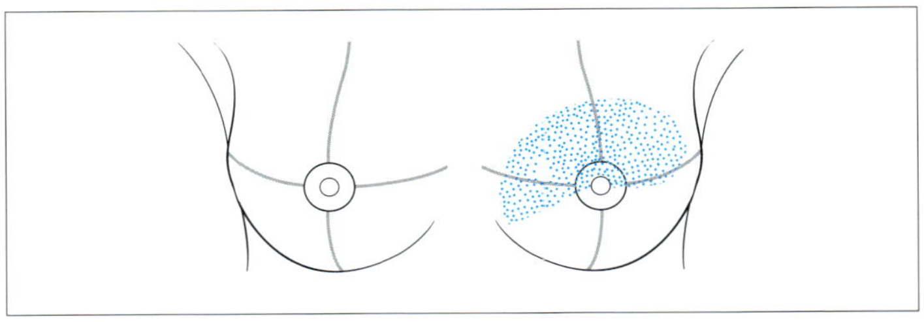

## Clinical Findings

Painful redness of both upper quadrants of the left breast. No resistance.

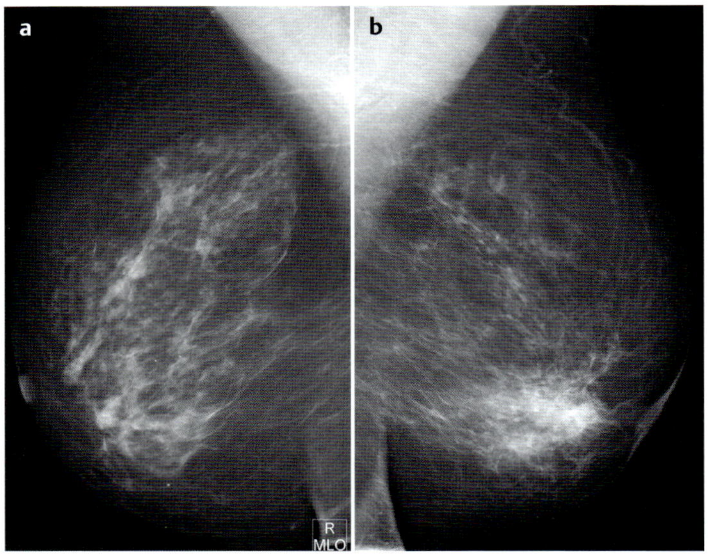


Fig. 56.2 **a, b** Digital mammography, MLO view [imaging not performed by authors].

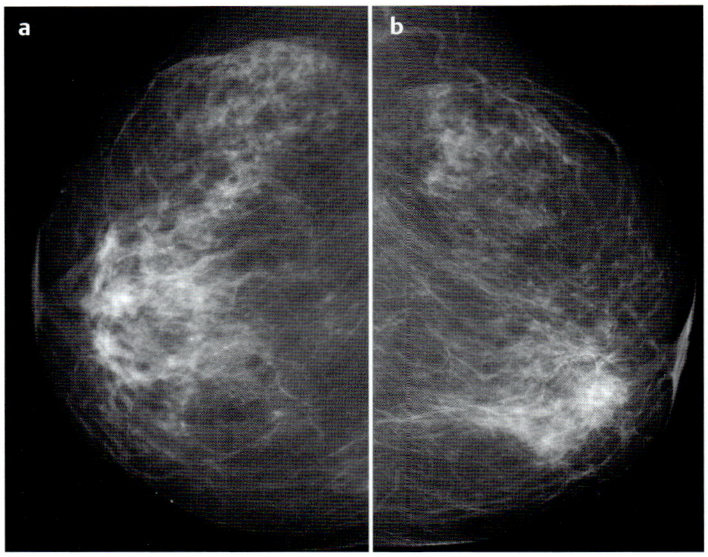


Fig. 56.3 **a, b** Digital mammography, CC view [imaging not performed by authors].

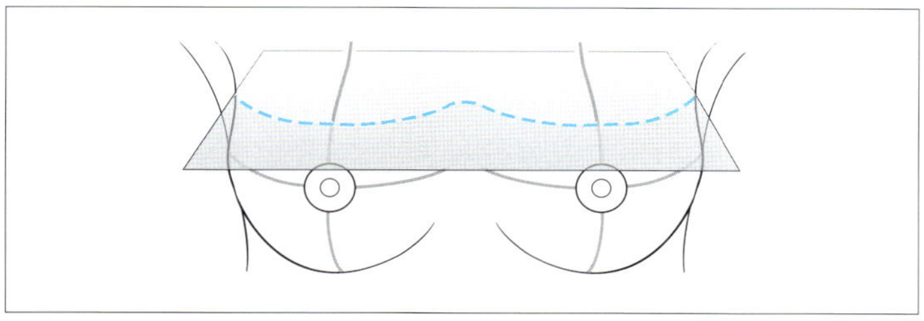

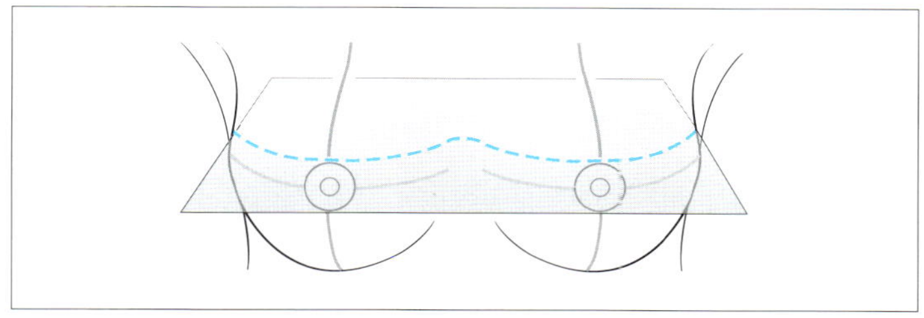

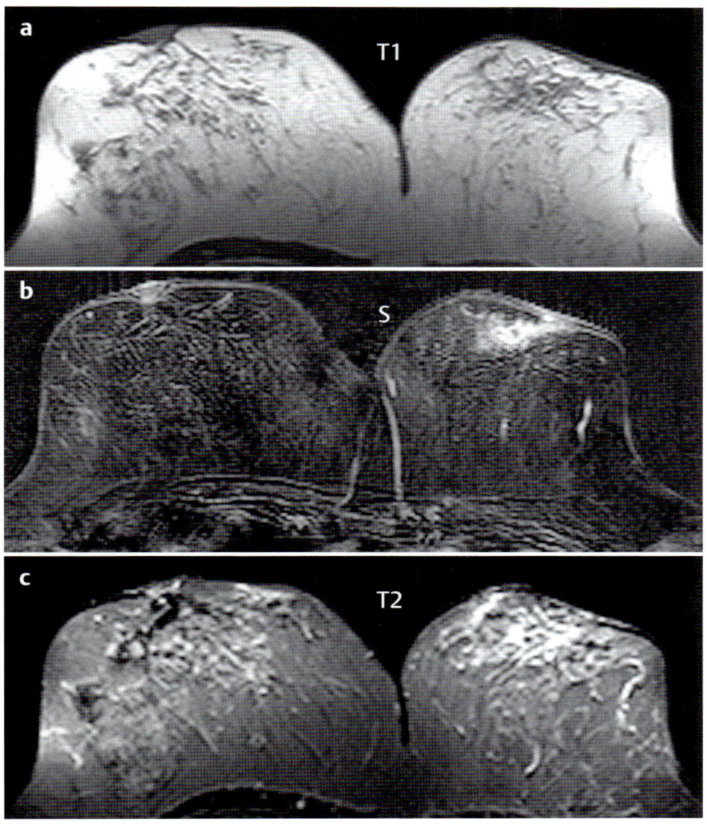


Fig. 56.**4 a–c** Contrast-enhanced MRI of the breasts.

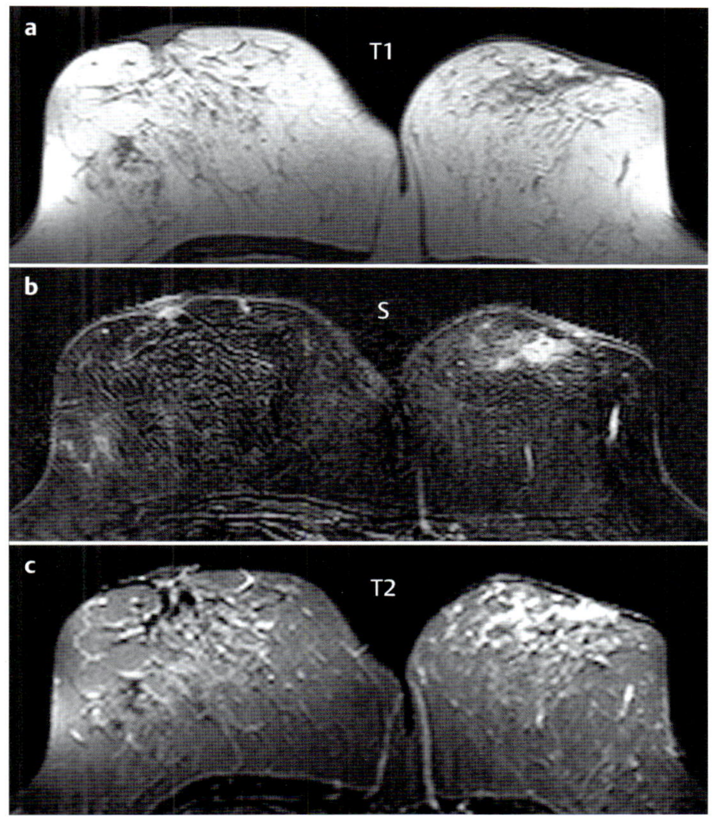


Fig. 56.**5 a–c** Contrast-enhanced MRI of the breasts.

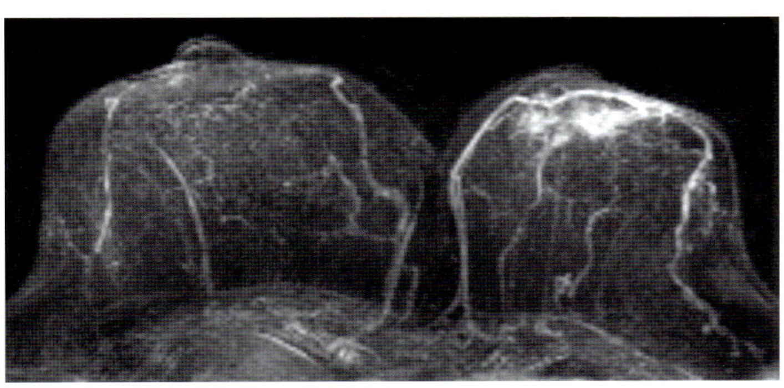

Fig. 56.**6** Contrast-enhanced MR mammography. Maximum intensity projection.

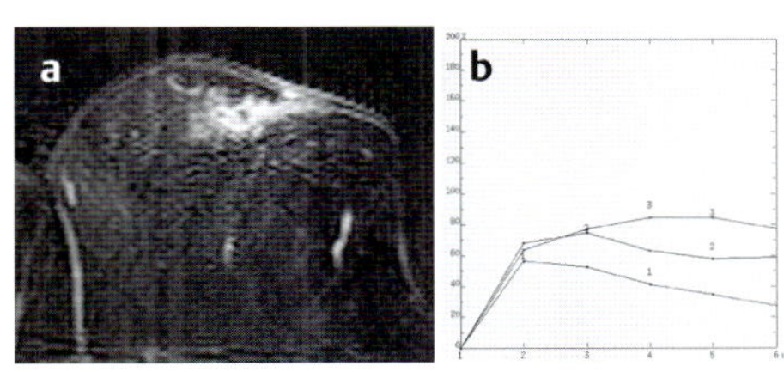


Fig. 56.**7 a, b** Signal-to-time curves.

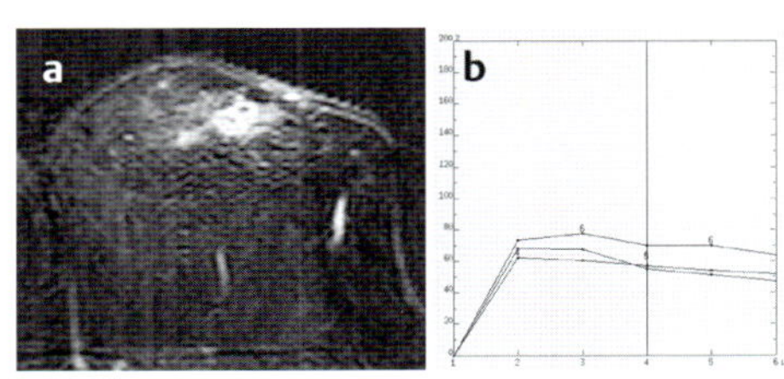


Fig. 56.**8 a, b** Signal-to-time curves.

?

Please characterize ultrasound, mammography, and MRI findings.
What is your preliminary diagnosis?
What are your next steps?

Imaging was carried out in this case to investigate inflammation of the left breast.

### Ultrasound

A linear hypoechoic region with distal shadowing was depicted in the upper quadrants of the left breast near the nipple. No circumscribed masses. US BI-RADS left 3.

### Mammography

The parenchyma had a fibroglandular texture, ACR type 2, and showed asymmetry in mammography with greater density of the left breast than the right. Mammograms showed no masses, no densities, and no microcalcifications. There was a possible thickening of the areolar region in the left breast when compared to the right (caution: digital images). BI-RADS right 1/left 3. PGMI: CC view P; MLO view M (right nipple not in profile, pectoral muscle).

### MR Mammography

An asymmetric enhancement was visible in the region above the left nipple, corresponding to the asymmetry depicted in mammography. It showed ring enhancement, an initial signal increase of 90%, and postinitial washout. Signal in T2-weighted imaging was increased.

**MRI Artifact Category:** 2
**MRI Density Type:** 1

| MRM score | Finding | Points |
|---|---|---|
| **Shape** | irregular | 1 |
| **Border** | ill-defined | 1 |
| **CM Distribution** | ring | 2 |
| **Initial Signal Intensity Increase** | moderate | 1 |
| **Post-initial Signal Intensity Character** | wash-out | 2 |
| **MRI score (points)** | | **7** |
| **MRI BI-RADS** | | **5** |

### → Differential Diagnosis

Inflammatory carcinoma, benign inflammation (e.g., nonpuerperal mastitis).

| BI-RADS Categorization | | |
|---|---|---|
| Clinical Findings | right 1 | left 4 |
| Ultrasound | right 1 | left 3 |
| Mammography | right 1 | left 3 |
| MR Mammography | right 1 | left 5 |
| **BI-RADS Total** | **right 1** | **left 5** |

**Procedure**

Antibiotic therapy (penicillin) for 10 days. Since this did not result in any improvement in the inflammation, open biopsy was performed to exclude the possibility of inflammatory carcinoma. MR mammography was performed for the purpose of preoperative staging of a potential carcinoma.

**Histopathology of the wedge biopsy**

Gout (Fig. 56.**9**).

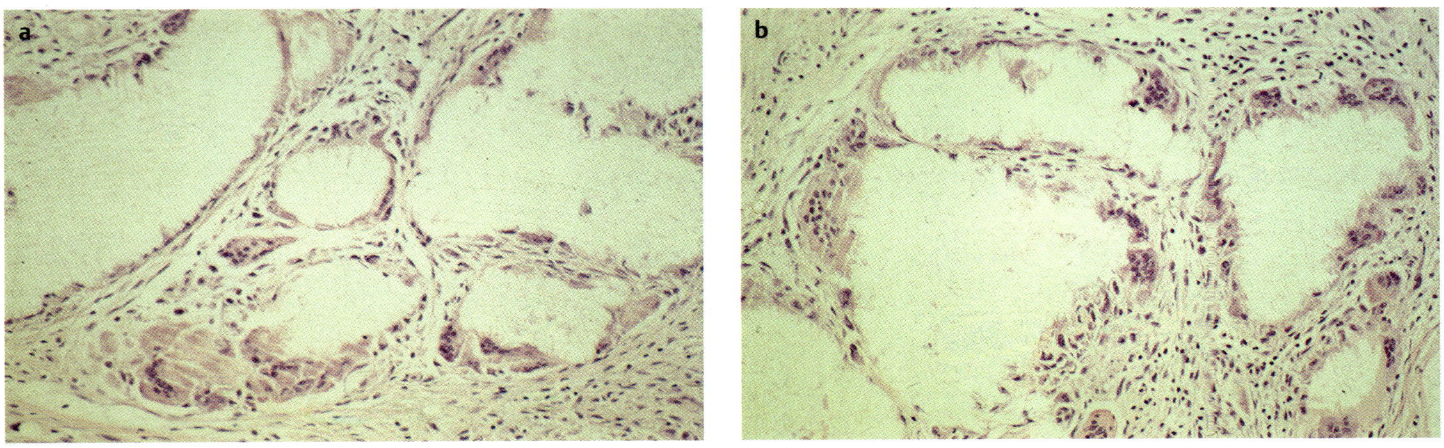


Fig. 56.**9 a, b** Histological step sections of the manifestation of gout in the breast.

## Histology

Gout.

## Treatment

Excisional biopsy.

Hyperuricemia in the breast is evidently possible, although extremely rare.
Also: MR mammography does not enable any differentiation between nonpuerperal mastitis and inflammatory breast cancer.

**Indication:** Mastodynia of the left breast.
**History:** Unremarkable.
**Risk profile:** No increased risk.
**Age:** 43 years.

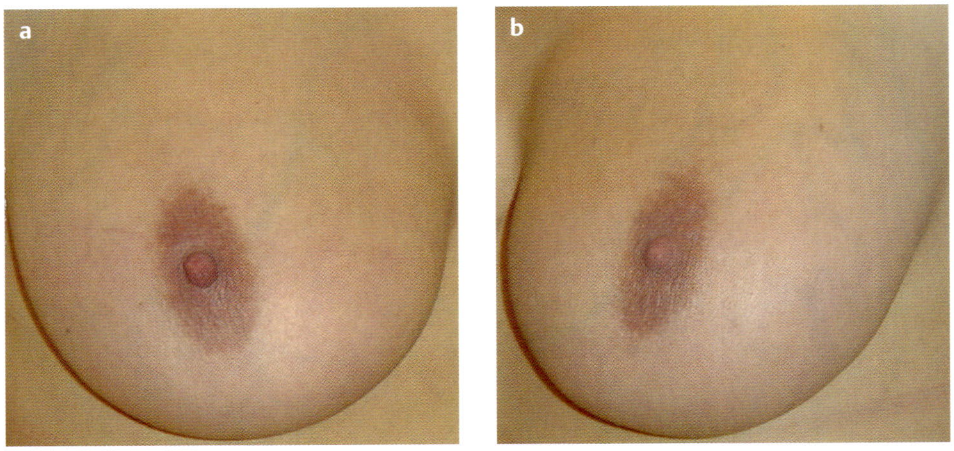

Fig. 57.**1 a, b** Clinical examination of the right (**a**) and left (**b**) breasts.

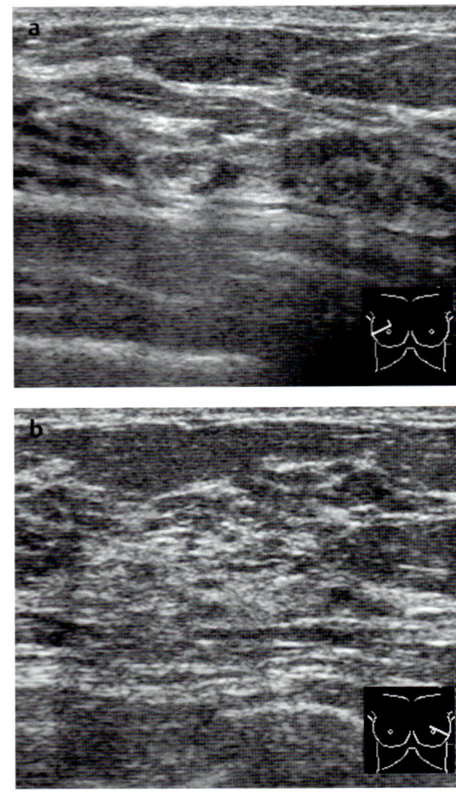

Fig. 57.**2 a, b** Sonography.

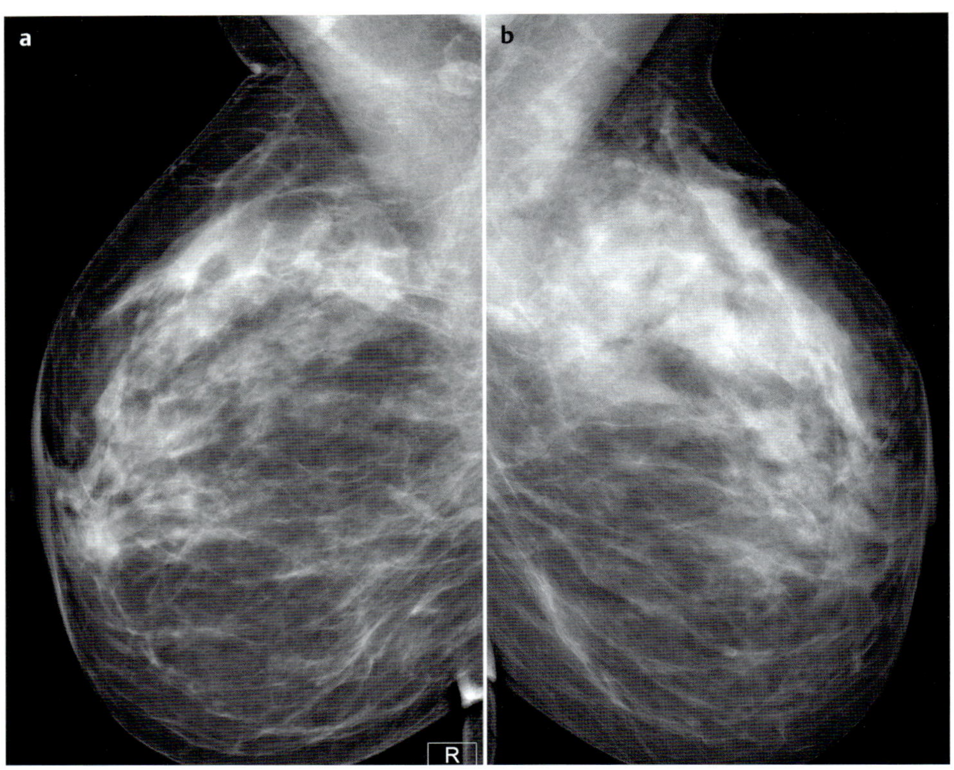

Fig. 57.**3 a, b** Digital mammography, MLO view.

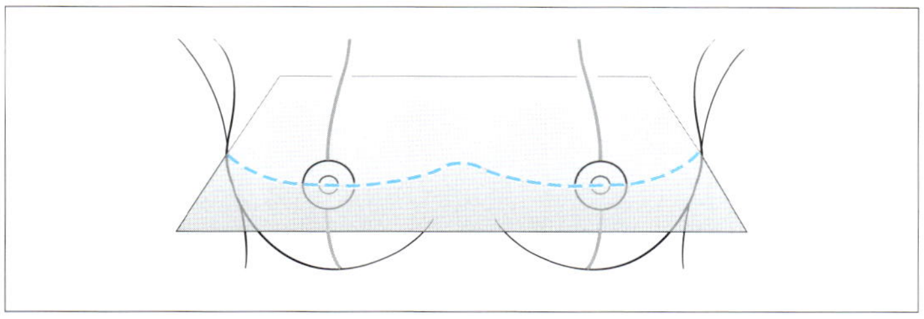

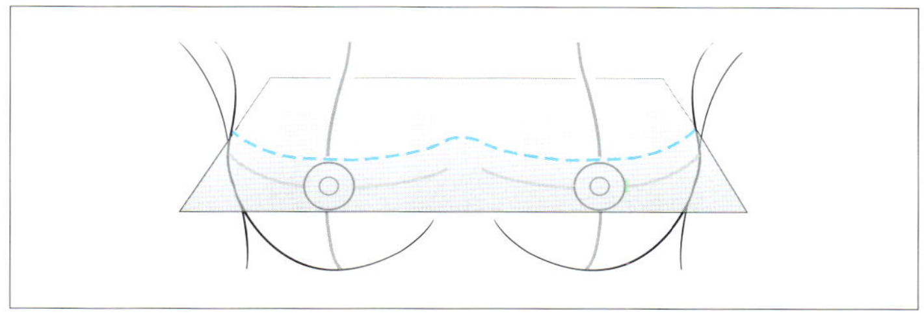

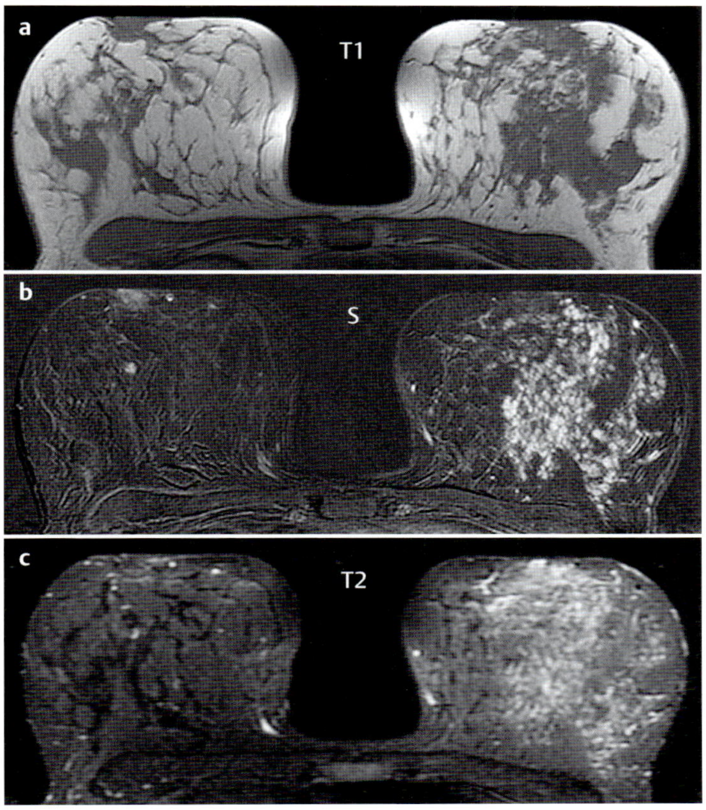


Fig. 57.4 **a – c** Contrast-enhanced MRI of the breasts.

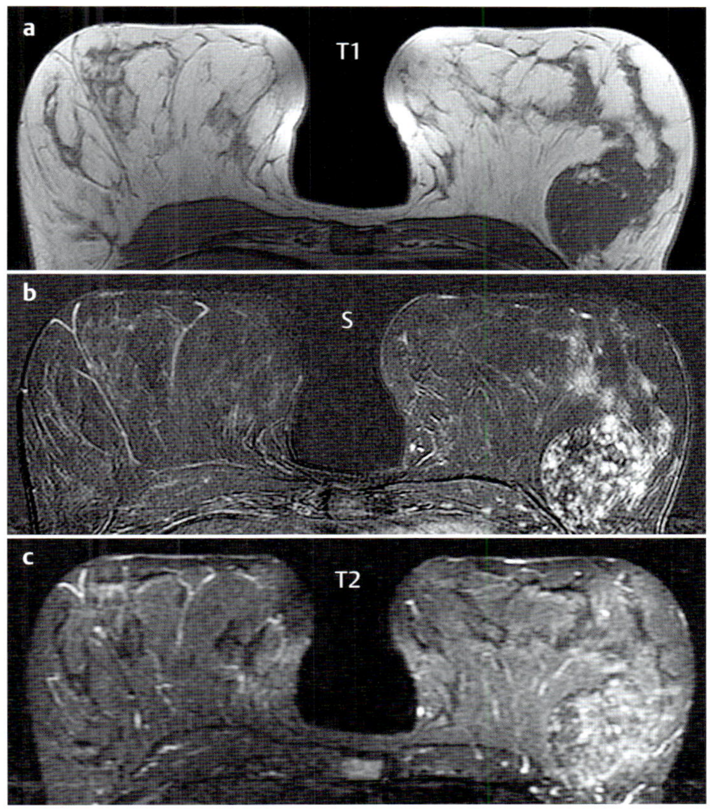


Fig. 57.5 **a – c** Contrast-enhanced MRI of the breasts.

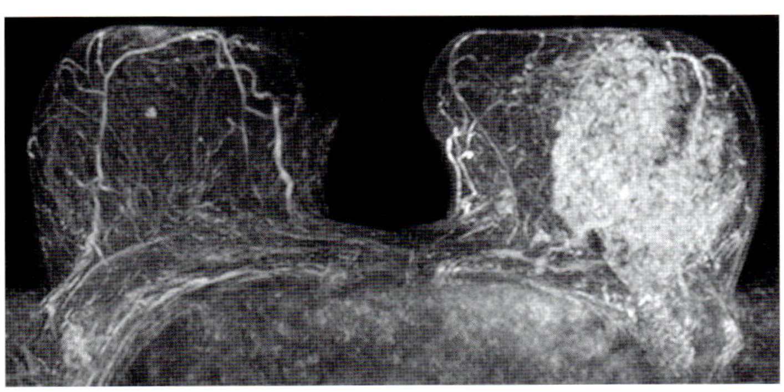

Fig. 57.6 Contrast-enhanced MR mammography. Maximum intensity projection.

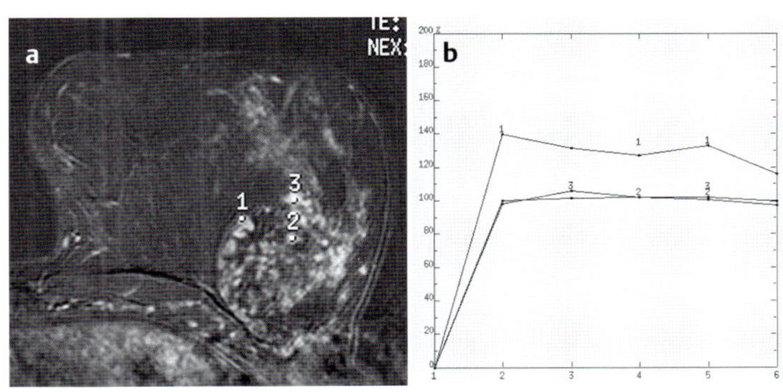


Fig. 57.7 **a, b** Signal-to-time curves.

?

Please characterize ultrasound, mammography, and MRI findings.
What is your preliminary diagnosis?
What are your next steps?

The imaging of a young woman with unilateral mastodynia is presented.

### Examination

The clinical aspect of both breasts was normal. No resistance in the area of the pain in the left breast.

### Ultrasound

Ultrasound demonstrated a marked difference between the echo textures of left and right breasts. There were no other abnormalities and no signs of malignancy. US BI-RADS right 1/left 1.

### Mammography

Mammography showed asymmetry of the parenchyma (right breast was inhomogenously dense, ACR type 3, left partially extremely dense, ACR type 4). No unusual findings. No densities or architectural distortion. No calcifications (BI-RADS right 1/left 2). PGMI: G (inframammary fold not correctly positioned).

### MR Mammography

As expected, the precontrast MRI showed asymmetry of the parenchymal structure (left > right). In the outer upper quadrant of the left breast there was a circumscribed, well-defined section of parenchyma. After contrast administration there was a marked difference between the enhancement pattern in each breast: the right breast demonstrated only a small, adenoma-like focal enhancement, whereas the left breast showed pronounced patchy enhancement throughout the parenchymal tissue as well as within the capsule-like circumscribed formation.

**MRI Artifact Category:** 2
**MRI Density Type:** 1

| MRM score | Finding | Points |
|---|---|---|
| **Shape** | round | 0 |
| **Border** | well-defined | 0 |
| **CM Distribution** | homogeneous | 0 |
| **Initial Signal Intensity Increase** | strong | 2 |
| **Post-initial Signal Intensity Character** | wash-out | 2 |
| **MRI score (points)** | | **4** |
| **MRI BI-RADS** | | **4** |

### → Differential Diagnostic Considerations

Right: Normal tissue with adenoma.
Left: Hamartoma (capsule-like area), adenosis, diffuse carcinoma.

| BI-RADS Categorization | | |
|---|---|---|
| Clinical Findings | right 1 | left 1 |
| Ultrasound | right 1 | left 1 |
| Mammography | right 1 | left 2 |
| MR Mammography | right 2 | left 4 |
| **BI-RADS Total** | **right 2** | **left 4** |

### Procedure

Histological investigation of the diffuse patchy enhancement seen in the left breast in MRI. Considering the homogeneity of the enhancement pattern, MR-guided vacuum biopsy was not required. Instead a US-guided representative "blind" biopsy was performed in three different regions of the left breast (upper outer quadrant, lateral to the nipple, and lower outer quadrant).

### Histology of the left breast

Mastopathy. Additionally, in one of the specimens a circumscribed region containing part of a "carcinoma lobulare in situ" was found. This carcinoma had minimal proliferative activity. There was no atypical ductal proliferation and no invasive lobular carcinoma. There was no suggestion of a ductal carcinoma in situ or an invasive carcinoma. These histology results were confirmed by supplementary immunohistochemical analysis.

### Further Procedure

A four-week trial of antihormonal therapy followed by repeat MR mammography. This repeat imaging showed no change in the findings of unilateral diffuse enhancement of the left breast (Fig. 57.**8**).

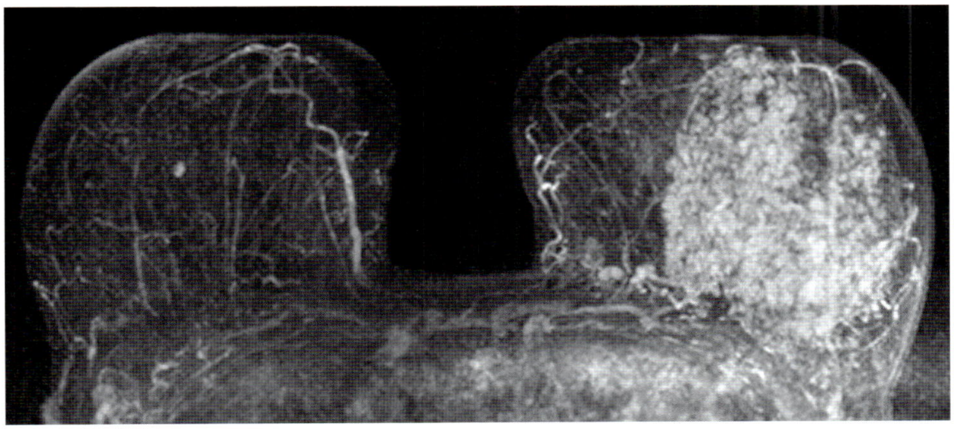

Fig. 57.**8** MR mammography with largely unchanged findings following four weeks of antihormonal therapy.

#### Further procedure

Although the histology revealed a CLIS in the core biopsy specimen, an open biopsy was avoided, because the blind biopsy results meant that a very extensive section of tissue from the outer quadrants of the left breast would be excised. In view of the unchanged enhancement of the left breast in MRI after 4 weeks of antihormonal therapy, close monitoring after a further 3, 6 and 12 months was recommended.

Borderline findings such as CLIS and/or ADH in the histopathological analysis of core biopsy specimens would usually necessitate open biopsy of the region from which the specimen was taken. In the present case this guideline was not followed, for the reasons indicated.

**Indication:** Monitoring post mastectomy.
**History:** Breast cancer and mastectomy of the right breast 23 years previously.
**Risk profile:** Increased by previous incidence of breast cancer.
**Age:** 73 years.

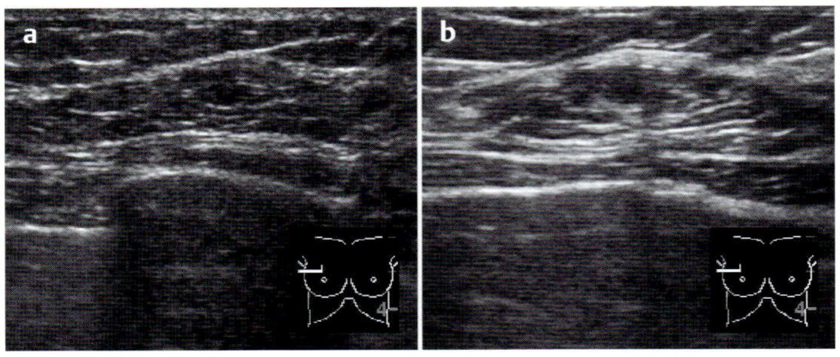


Fig. 58.**1 a, b** Ultrasound.

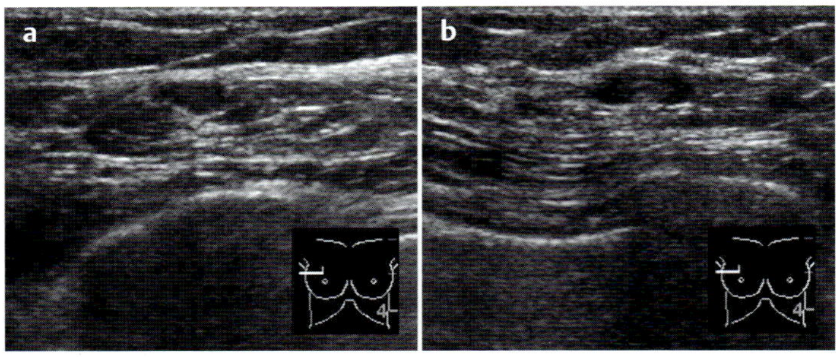


Fig. 58.**2 a, b** Ultrasound.

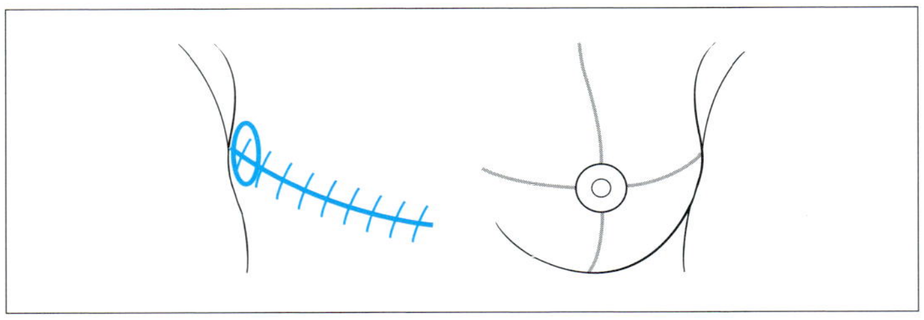

### Clinical Findings

Slight skin thickening in the axillary extension of the mastectomy scar. This was first noted by the patient after a mosquito bite 3 weeks before the examination.

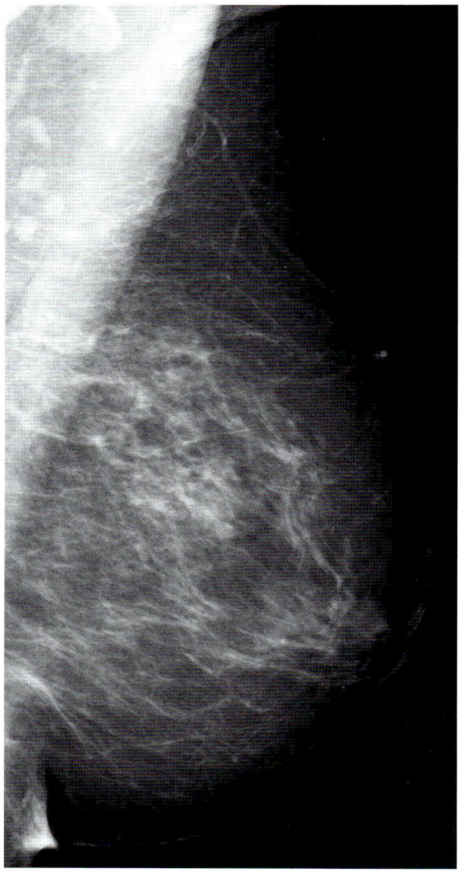

Fig. 58.**3** Digital mammography of the left breast, MLO view.

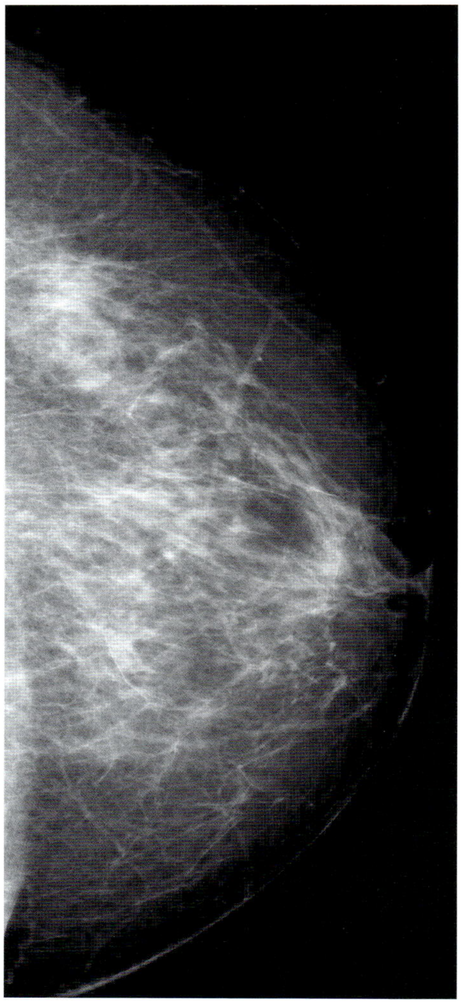

Fig. 58.**4** Digital mammography of the left breast, CC view.

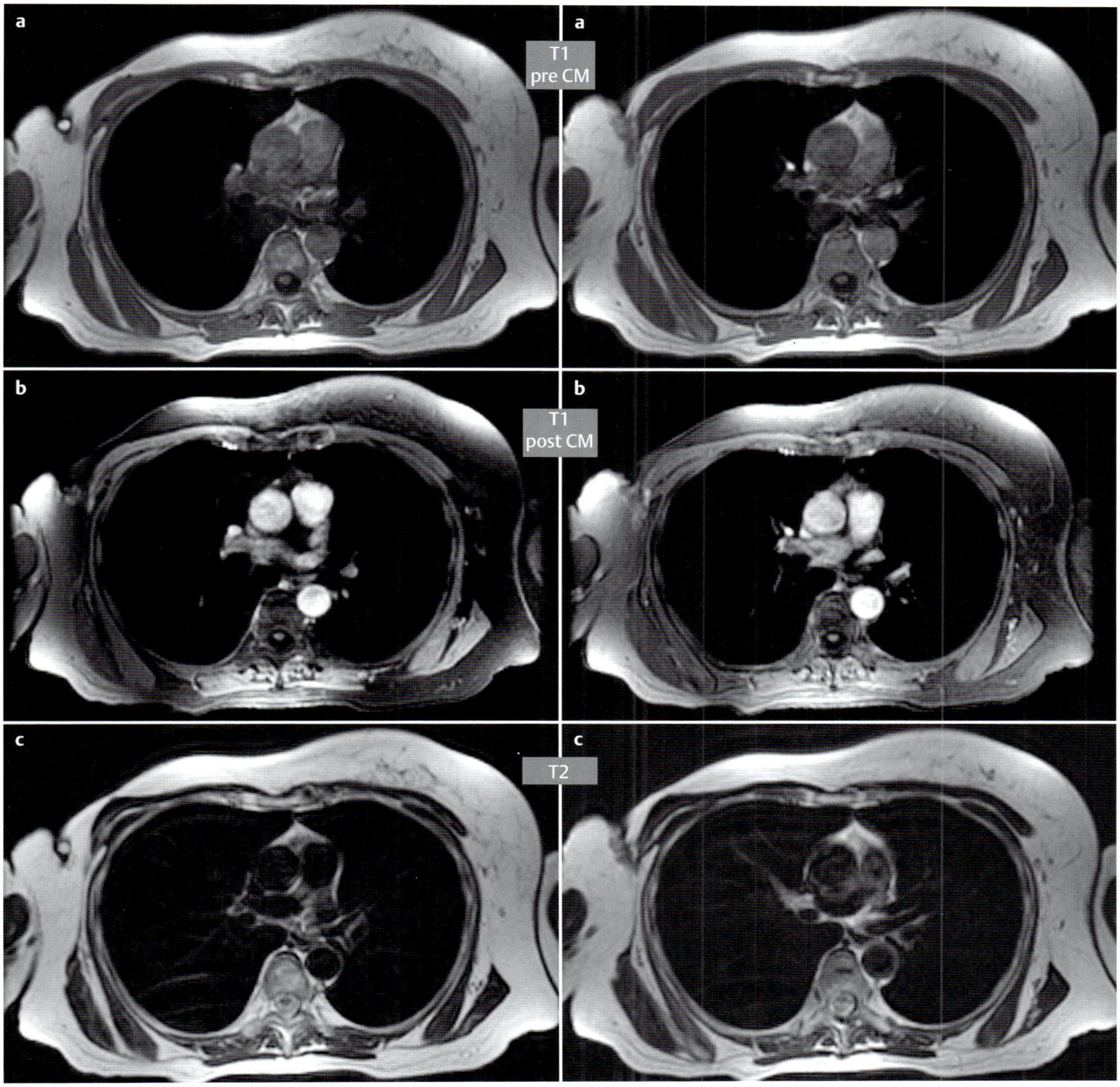


Fig. 58.5,6 MRI of the chest.

Please characterize ultrasound, mammography, and MRI findings.
What is your preliminary diagnosis?
What are your next steps?

This case demonstrates the follow-up of a woman 23 years after Halsted radical mastectomy for breast cancer. Clinically there is a slight, recently developed thickening in the axillary part of the scar.

### Ultrasound

There were no unusual sonographic findings within the scar. In the area around the axillary end of the scar there were two lymph nodes each with a diameter of 6 mm. US BI-RADS 1.

### Mammography

Mammograms showed that the parenchyma of the left breast was fibroglandular, ACR type 2. There were no masses, densities, or microcalcifications. After Halsted mastectomy a mammography of the residual breast tissue is not usually possible. BI-RADS left 1.

### MR Imaging

After marking of the slight axillary thickening with a nitro capsule, a subcutaneous enhancement was visible in this region. There were no further relevant findings. No additional information was supplied by T2-weighted images.

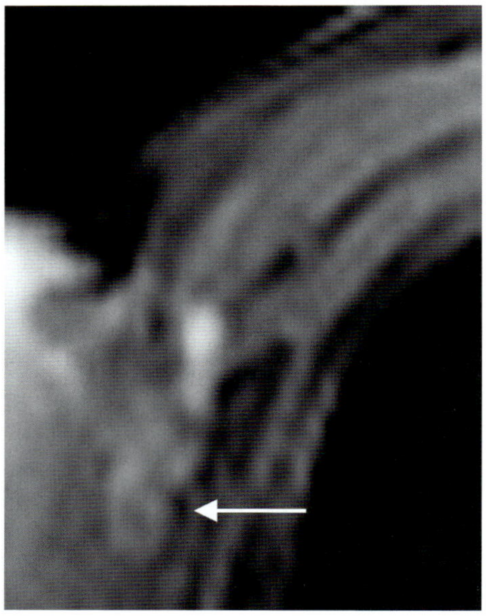

Fig. 58.**7** Enlarged post-contrast image of the MRI of the chest.

Analysis of the enhancing area using the Göttingen-Score is not useful in this case.
The general patterns observed following surgery and and healing are:

**Scar tissue does not show enhancement post-contrast.**

**Local tumor recurrence shows enhancement post-contrast.**

**Caution: Focal inflammation may lead to false positive findings!**

**MRI BI-RADS 4**

## → Preliminary Diagnosis

Late relapse.

## → Differential Diagnosis

Infection following mosquito bite (wishful thinking on the part of the patient?).

| **BI-RADS Categorization** | | |
|---|---|---|
| Clinical Findings | right 4 | left 1 |
| Ultrasound | right 1 | left 1 |
| Mammography | right – | left 1 |
| MRI (Thorax) | right 4 | left 1 |
| **BI-RADS Total** | **right 4** | **left 1** |

### Procedure

A repeat examination after 4 weeks was recommended to the patient in order to differentiate between a subcutaneous infection caused by the mosquito bite and a possible local relapse. Taking the aesthetic aspect of the mastectomy scar into consideration, the patient opted for immediate open biopsy.

## Histology

Local relapse of a tubular carcinoma with 6 lymph node metastases.

## Treatment

Tumor resection.

Even 23 years after the primary manifestation of a carcinoma, local tumor relapse can occur.
When differentiating between a local relapse and a scar, MRI provides a Yin and Yang rule of thumb:
Local relapses enhance in MRI, scars do not.

**Indication:** Screening.
**History:** Unremarkable.
**Risk profile:** No increased risk.
**Age:** 43 years.

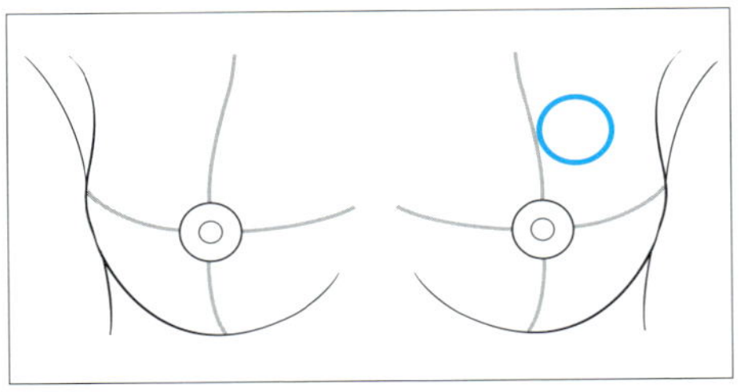

## Clinical Findings

Mobile resistance in the upper outer quadrant of the left breast.

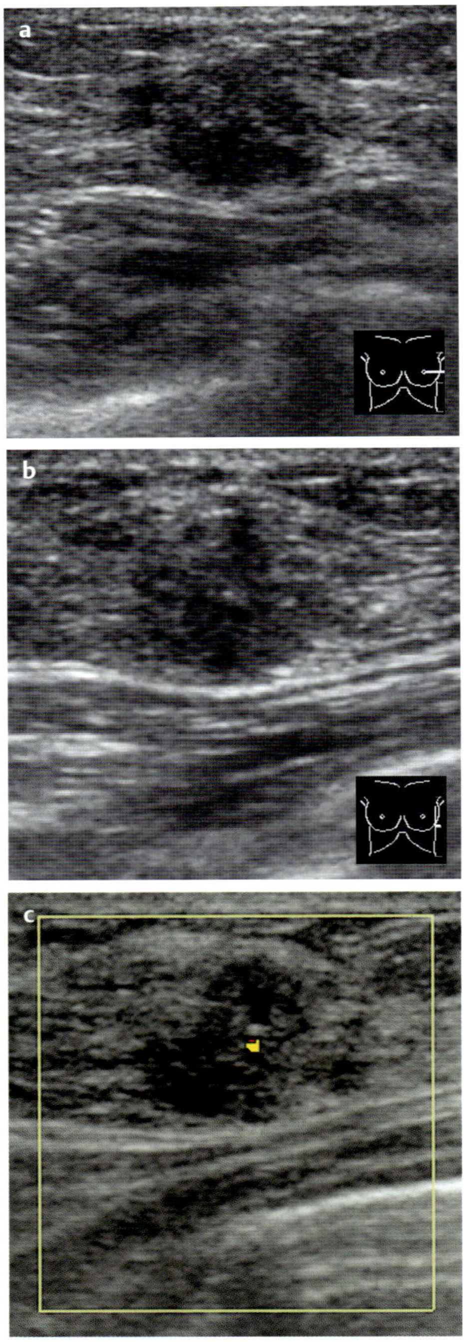

Fig. 59.**1 a–c** Conventional and color-coded Doppler sonography.

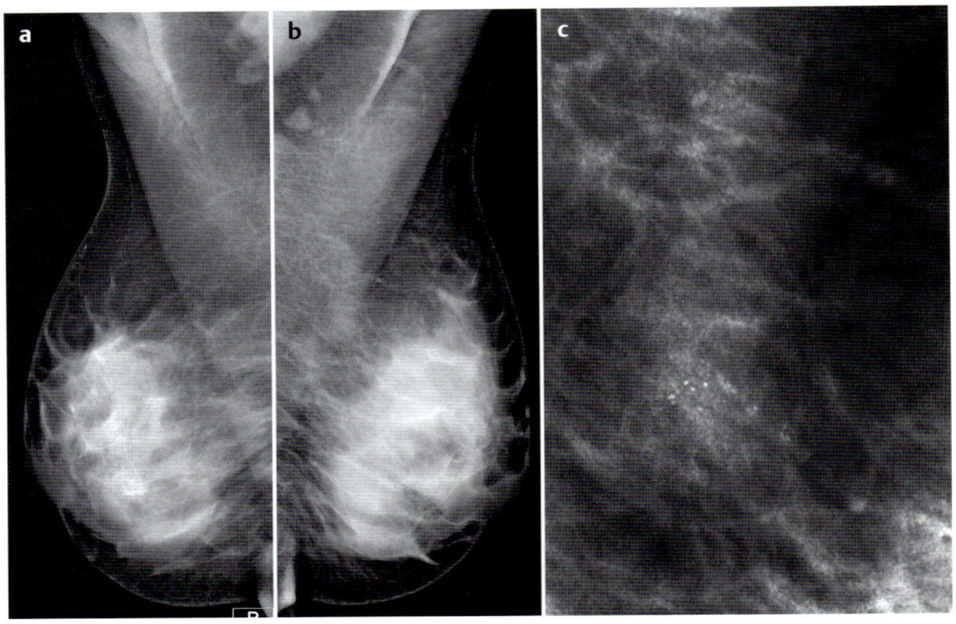

Fig. 59.**2 a–c** Digital mammography (MLO) with magnification view of the left breast.

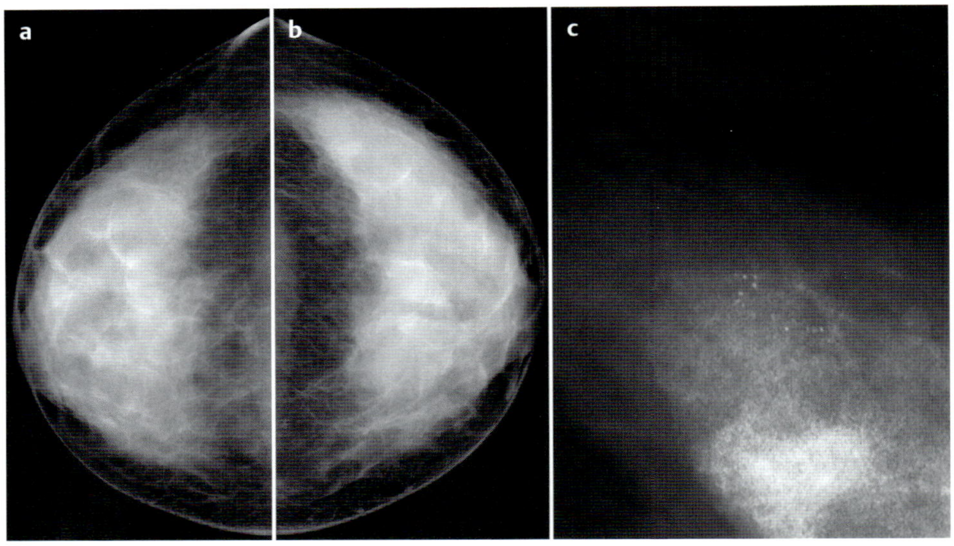

Fig. 59.**3 a–c** Digital mammography (CC) with magnification view of the left breast.

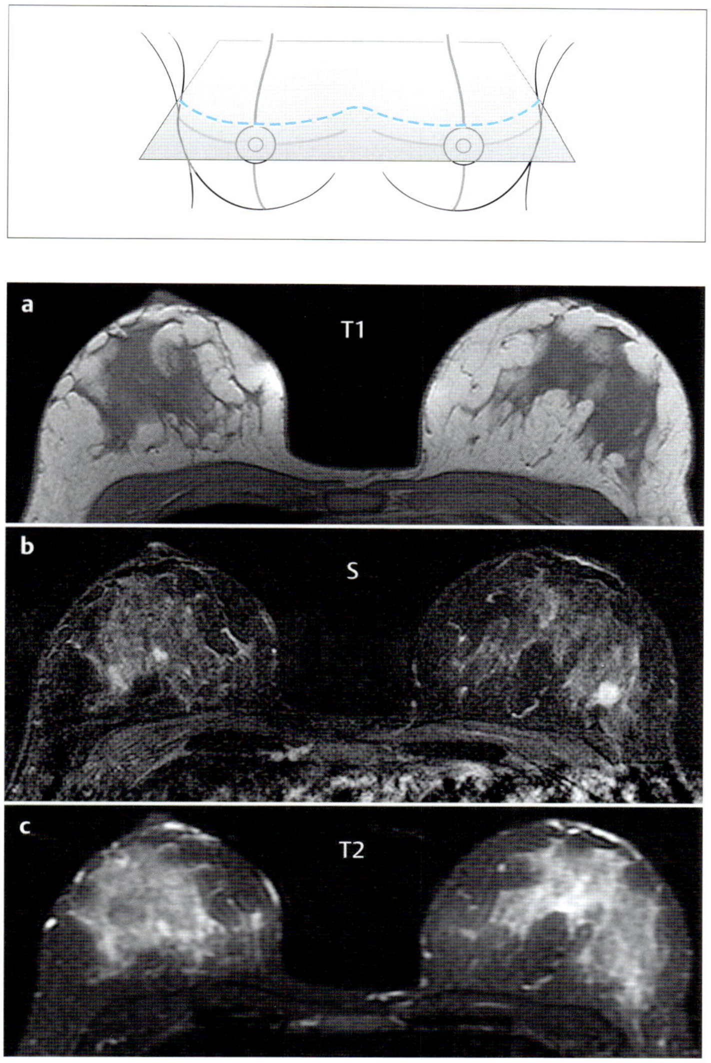


Fig. 59.**4 a – c** Contrast-enhanced MRI of the breasts.

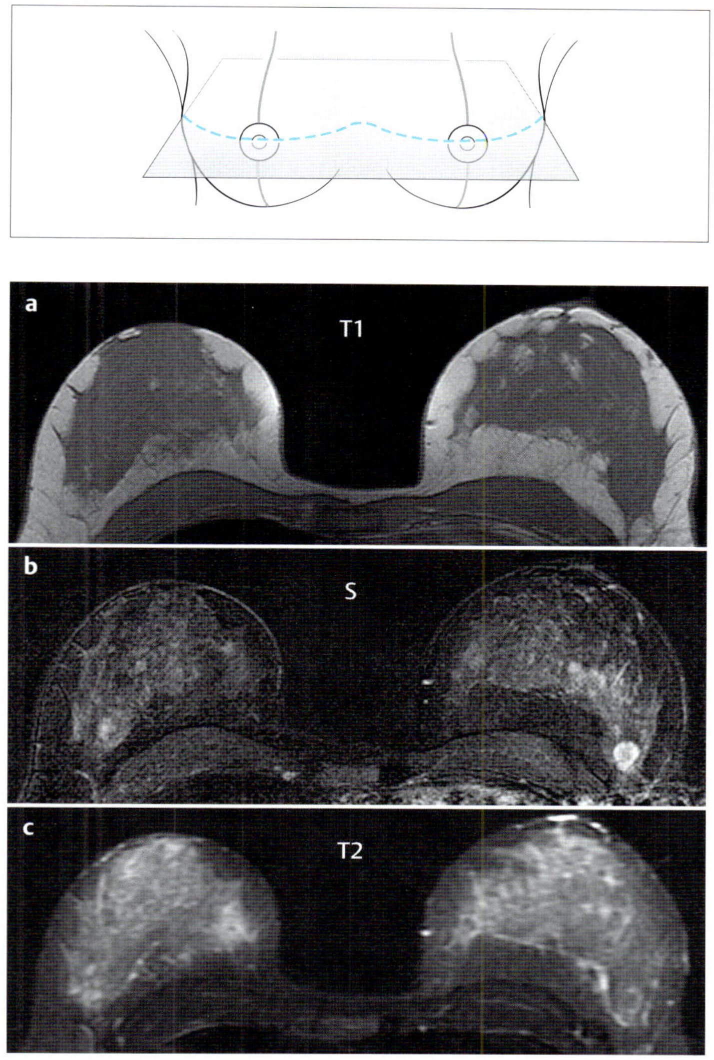


Fig. 59.**5 a – c** Contrast-enhanced MRI of the breasts.

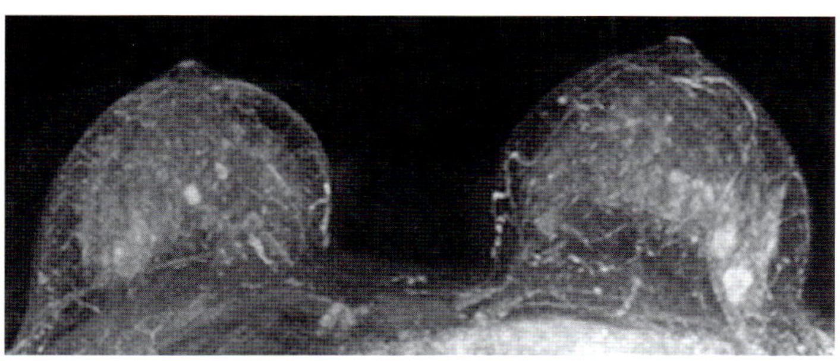

Fig. 59.**6** Contrast-enhanced MR mammography. Maximum intensity projection.

Please characterize ultrasound, mammography, and MRI findings.
What is your preliminary diagnosis?
What are your next steps?

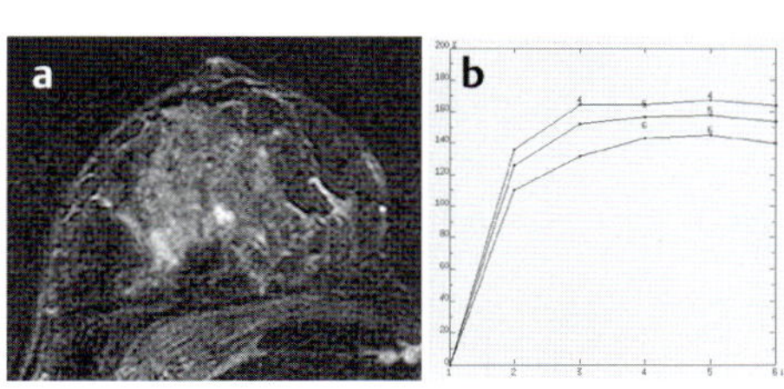


Fig. 59.**7 a, b** Signal-to-time curves.

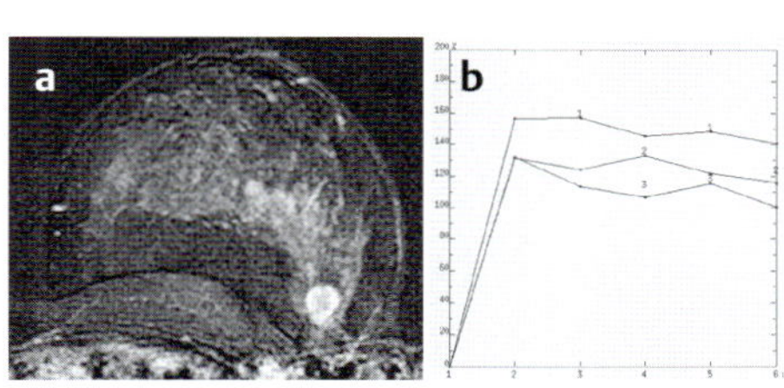


Fig. 59.**8 a, b** Signal-to-time curves.

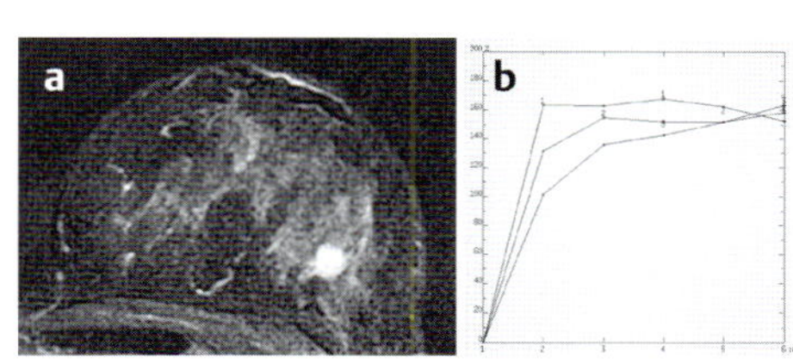


Fig. 59.**9 a, b** Signal-to-time curves.

The imaging of a woman presenting for screening is shown. The palpable resistance was first detected in the clinical examination.

### Ultrasound

Ultrasound demonstrated a lobulated, inhomogeneously hypoechoic lesion, 12 mm in diameter, without distal shadowing in the upper outer quadrant of the left breast. There was no evident architectural distortion. In the central part of the left breast, Doppler sonography showed signs of arterial hyperperfusion. US BI-RADS left 4.

### Mammography

There was symmetric extremely dense glandular tissue, ACR type 4, visible in mammography. No masses or densities could be identified. However, there was a cluster of predominantly monomorphous microcalcifications in the upper outer quadrant of the left breast. BI-RADS right 1/left 4. PGMI: CC view P; MLO view P.

### MR Mammography

MRI showed a diffuse, variegated contrast uptake throughout the parenchyma. In the upper outer quadrant of the left breast, a lesion of 13 mm diameter with ring enhancement, initial signal increase of 190%, and postinitial washout was visible. This lesion showed intermediate signal in T2-weighted imaging. There was another ill-defined lesion with inhomogeneous enhancement, initial signal increase of 160%, and postinitial plateau nearby. In the central parts of the right breast a lobulated septate lesion with a high water component in inversion recovery sequence was seen.

**MRI Artifact Category:** 1

**MRI Density Type:** 2

| MRM score | Left breast, between outer quadrants | Points | Left breast, upper outer quadrant | Points | Right breast, central region | Points |
|---|---|---|---|---|---|---|
| **Shape** | irregular | 1 | round | 0 | lobulated | 0 |
| **Border** | ill-defined | 1 | ill-defined | 1 | well-defined | 0 |
| **CM Distribution** | ring | 2 | ring | 2 | homogeneous | 0 |
| **Initial Signal Intensity Increase** | strong | 2 | strong | 2 | strong | 2 |
| **Post-initial Signal Intensity Character** | wash-out | 2 | plateau | 1 | plateau | 1 |
| **MRI score (points)** | | **8** | | **6** | | **3** |
| **MRI BI-RADS** | | **5** | | **5** | | **3** |

### → Preliminary Diagnosis

Left: Bifocal carcinoma.

Right: Fibroadenoma, adenosis, carcinoma.

| BI-RADS Categorization | | |
|---|---|---|
| Clinical Findings | right 1 | left 4 |
| Ultrasound | right 1 | left 4 |
| Mammography | right 1 | left 4 |
| MR Mammography | right 3 | left 5 |
| **BI-RADS Total** | **right 3** | **left 5** |

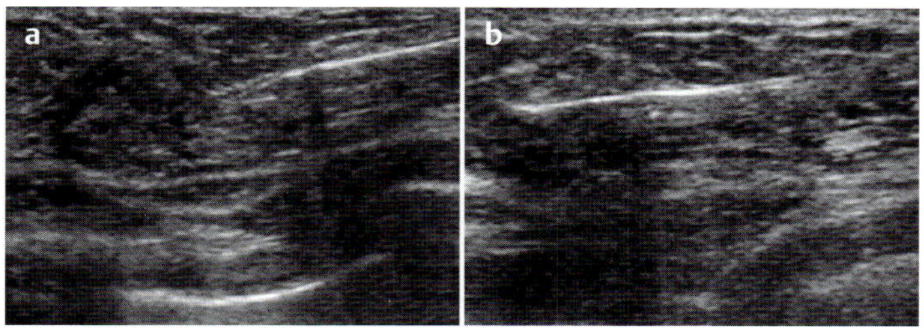


Fig. 59.**10 a, b** Core biopsy (pre-fire, post-fire).

### Further procedure

Open biopsy of left and right breasts following adequate localization of findings.

### Procedure

US-guided core biopsy and specimen radiography to obtain correlation of the lesion seen in ultrasound and the microcalcifications (Figs. 59.**10** and 59.**11**).

### Histology

Invasive ductal carcinoma.

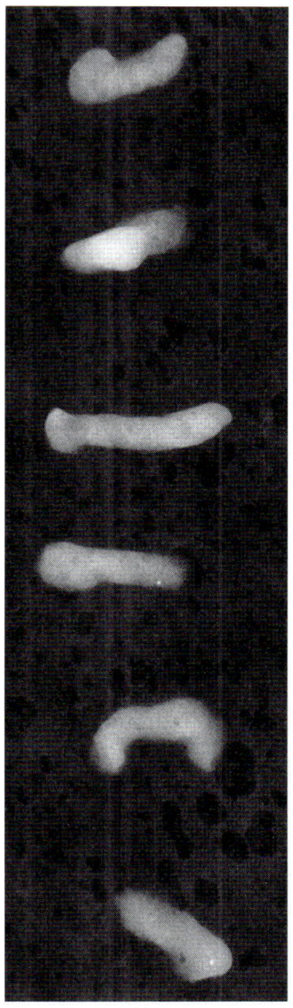

Fig. 59.**11** Specimen radiography with positive findings of microcalcifications.

### Histology

Left breast: Bifocal invasive ductal carcinoma (12 mm, 16 mm) with an extensive intraductal component.
Right breast: Lobular hyperplasia.

Left: IDC pT1c + EIC, pN1c (2/36), G2.
Right: LH.

### Treatment

Breast conservation therapy of the left breast; excisional biopsy of the right breast.

When microcalcifications are present, specimen radiography can confirm that the targeted tissue has in fact been excised.

**Indication:**. Suspicious ultrasound findings in the left breast in examination performed elsewhere.
**History:** Unremarkable.
**Risk profile:** No increased risk.
**Age:** 38 years.

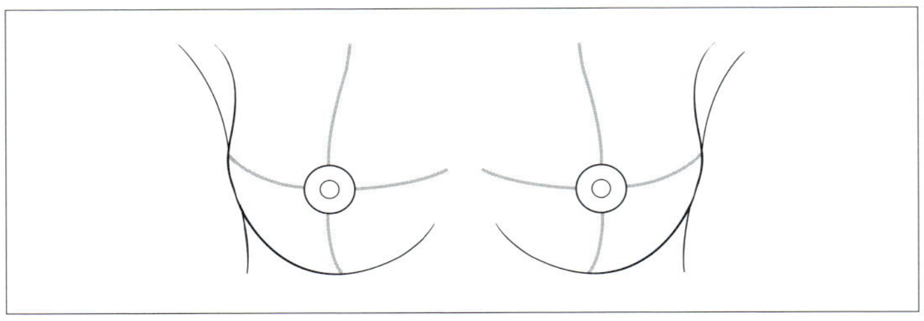

### Clinical Findings

Normal.

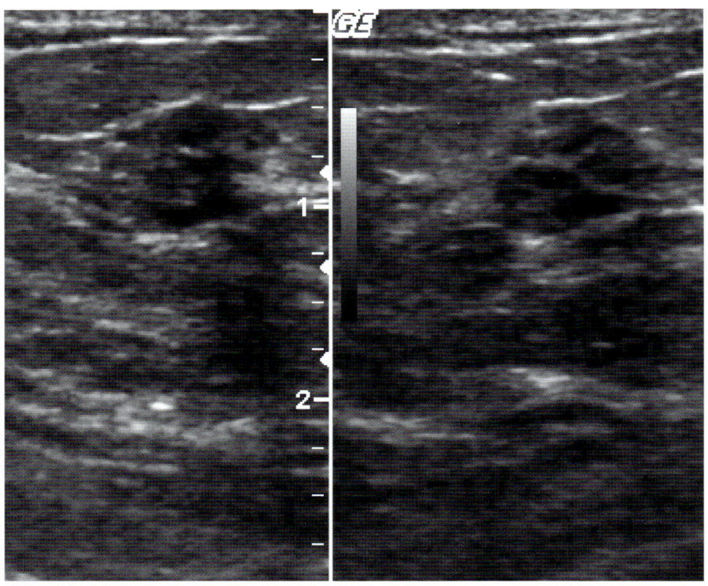


Fig. 60.**1** Ultrasound images from the center of the left breast.

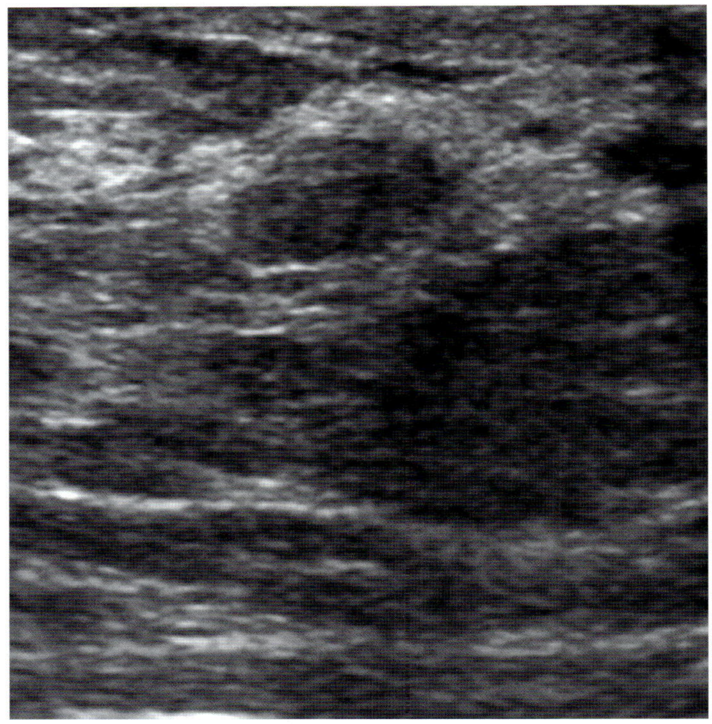

Fig. 60.**2** Ultrasound image from between the lower quadrants of the left breast.

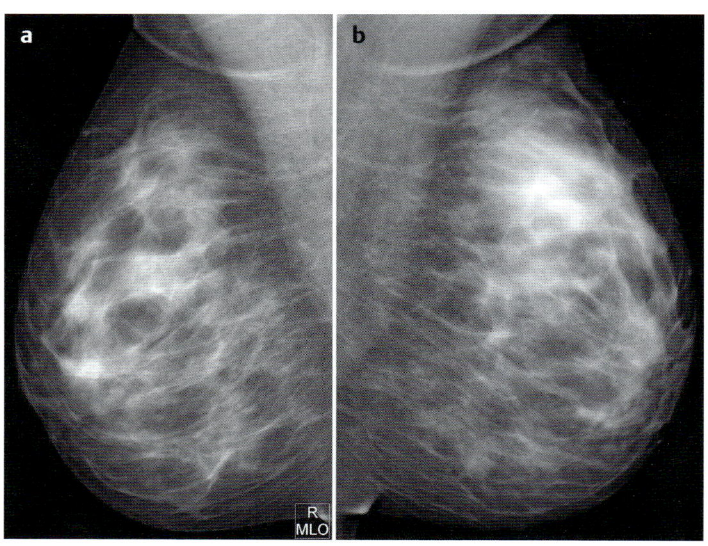


Fig. 60.**3 a, b** Digital mammography, MLO view.

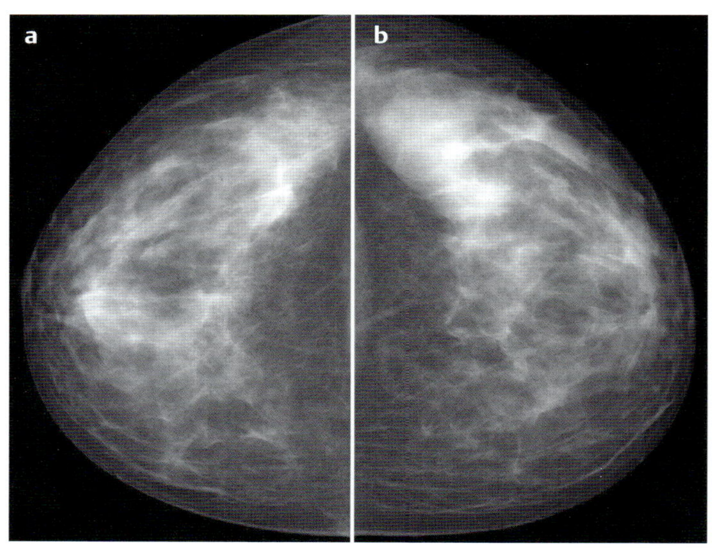


Fig. 60.**4 a, b** Digital mammography, CC view.

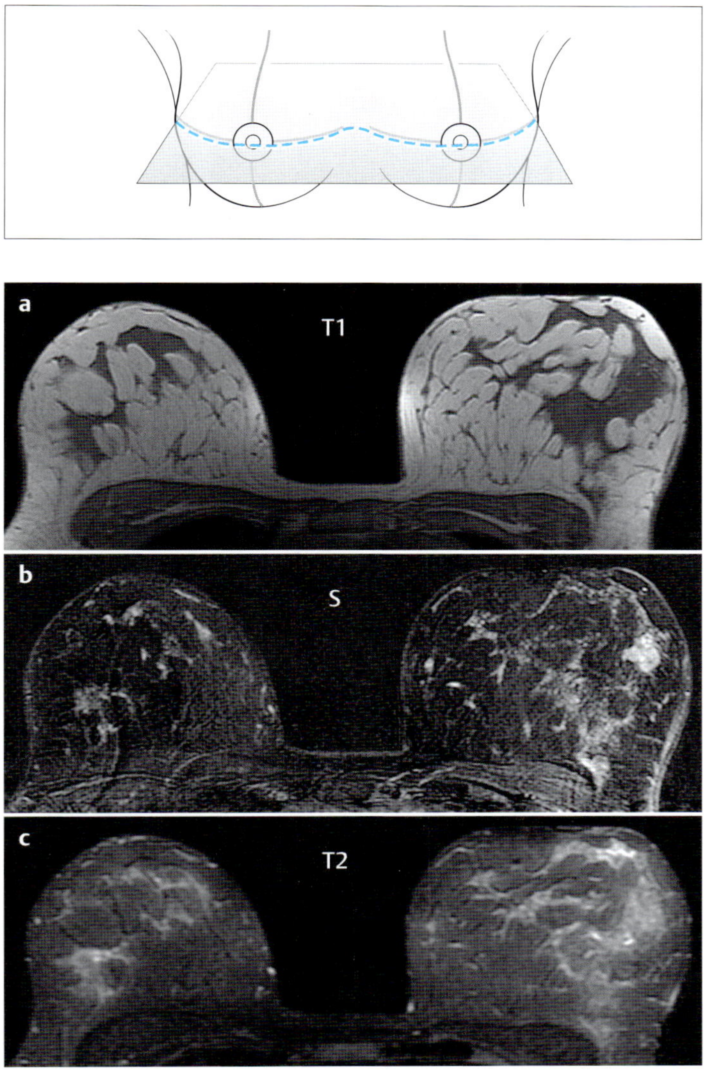


Fig. 60.5 a–c Contrast-enhanced MR mammography in fourth week of menstrual cycle.

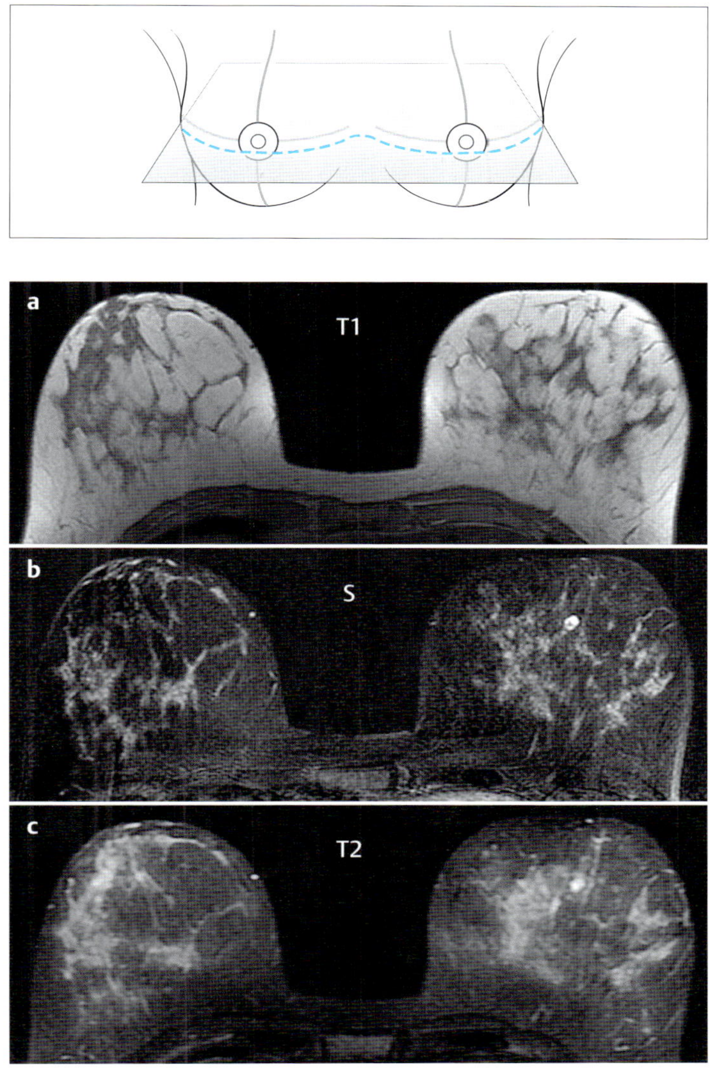


Fig. 60.6 a–c Contrast-enhanced MR mammography in fourth week of menstrual cycle.

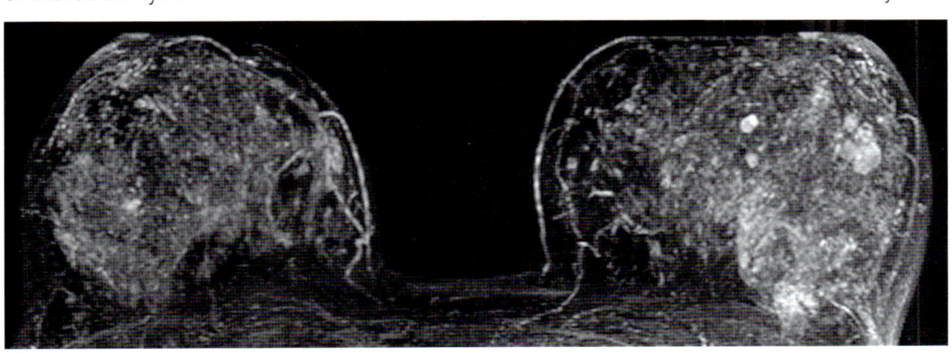

Fig. 60.7 Contrast-enhanced MR mammography. Maximum intensity projection.

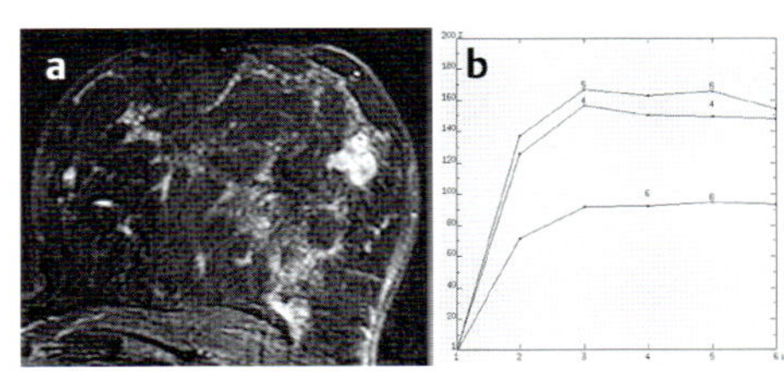


Fig. 60.8 a, b Signal-to-time curves.

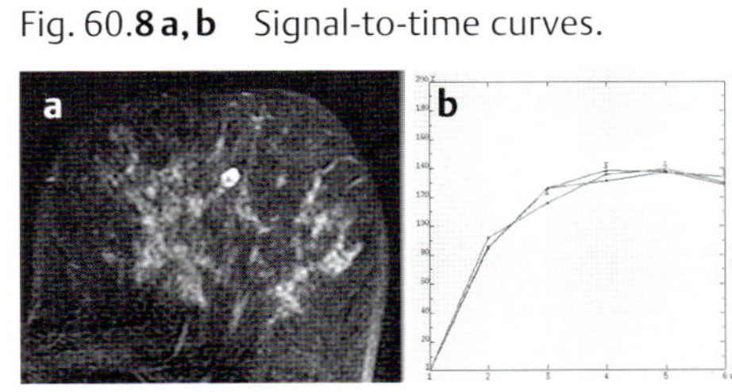


Fig. 60.9 a, b Signal-to-time curves.

?

Please characterize ultrasound, mammography, and MRI findings.
What is your preliminary diagnosis?
What are your next steps?

The diagnostic imaging presented was performed to investigate a suspicious finding in the left breast on sonograms performed elsewhere.

### Ultrasound

Ultrasound showed a lobulated, hypoechoic lesion 8 mm in diameter with indeterminate distal echo pattern between the outer quadrants of the left breast. There was another lobulated, hypoechoic lesion, 7 mm in diameter, with indeterminate distal echo pattern between the lower quadrants of the left breast. Ultrasound showed no architectural distortion. US BI-RADS left 3.

### Mammography

Mammograms demonstrated bilaterally symmetric, extremely dense parenchyma, ACR type 4. Particularly in the left breast there were no circumscribed findings, in the area of the ultrasound findings or elsewhere. Mammography showed no microcalcifications and no architectural distortion. BI-RADS right 1/left 1. PGMI: CC view P; MLO view P.

### MR Mammography

Strong contrast uptake was seen within the whole parenchyma, assessed as MRI density type 3. There was a well-defined, lobulated, septate lesion, 1.4 cm in diameter, between the outer quadrants of the left breast. The initial signal increase was 170% followed by a postinitial plateau. There was increased signal in T2-weighted imaging. Another well-defined, septate oval mass with elevated signal in T2-weighted imaging was visible between the lower quadrants of the left breast. Here the initial signal increase was 140% with a postinitial plateau.

**MRI Artifact Category:** 1
**MRI Density Type:** 3

| MRM score | Left breast, between outer quadrants | Points | Left breast, between lower quadrants | Points |
|---|---|---|---|---|
| **Shape** | lobulated | 0 | lobulated | 0 |
| **Border** | well-defined | 0 | well-defined | 0 |
| **CM Distribution** | ring | 2 | homogenous | 0 |
| **Initial Signal Intensity Increase** | strong | 2 | strong | 2 |
| **Post-initial Signal Intensity Character** | plateau | 1 | plateau | 1 |
| **MRI score (points)** | | **5** | | **3** |
| **MRI BI-RADS** | | **4** | | **3** |

### → Differential Diagnosis

Between outer quadrants: Carcinoma, fibroadenoma, papilloma, adenosis.
Between lower quadrants: Fibroadenoma, papilloma, carcinoma.

| BI-RADS Categorization | | |
|---|---|---|
| Clinical Findings | right 1 | left 1 |
| Ultrasound | right 1 | left 3 |
| Mammography | right 1 | left 1 |
| MR Mammography | right 1 | left 4 |
| **BI-RADS Total** | **right 1** | **left 4** |

### Procedure

Since the core biopsy indicated by guidelines was declined in this case, follow-up ultrasound (Fig. 60.**10**) and MRI after 6 months (Figs. 60.**11**–60.**14**), in an optimal stage of the menstrual cycle, was the procedure followed here.

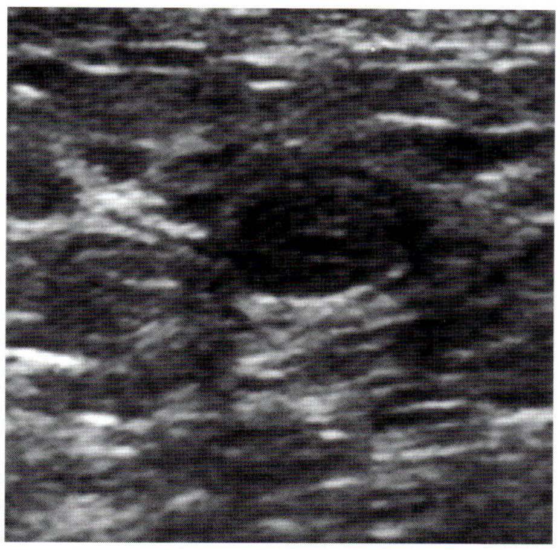

Fig. 60.**10** Follow-up ultrasound after six months between lower quadrants of the left breast.

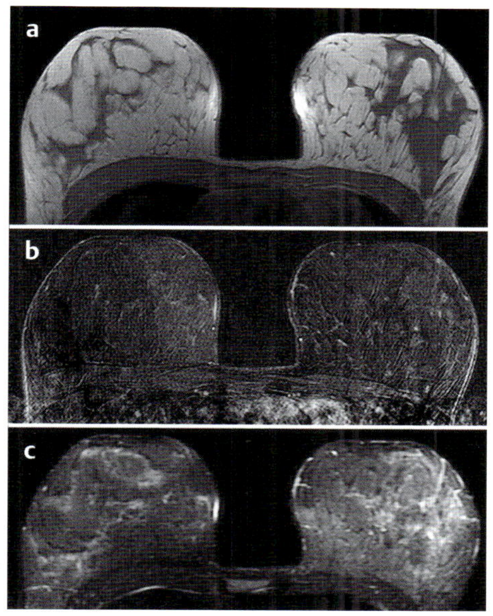

Fig. 60.**11 a–c** Contrast-enhanced MR mammography in second week of menstrual cycle.

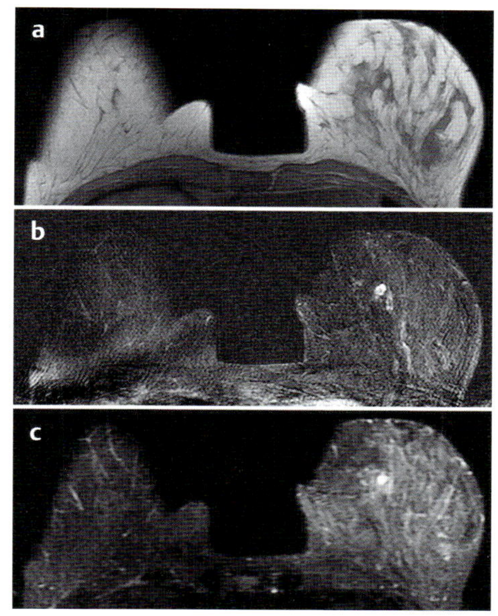

Fig. 60.**12 a–c** Contrast-enhanced MR mammography in second week of menstrual cycle.

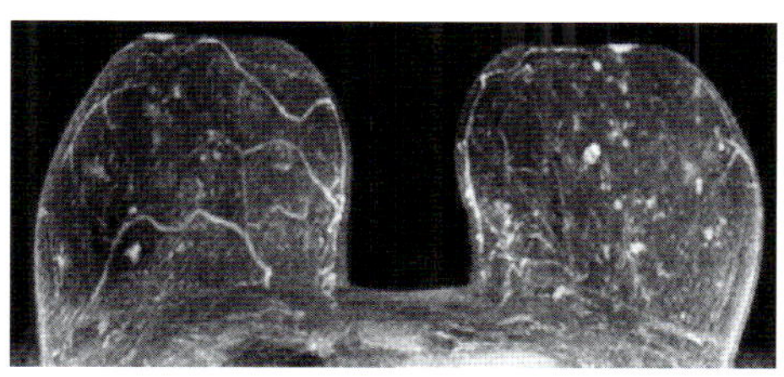

Fig. 60.**13** Contrast-enhanced MR mammography, in second week of menstrual cycle six months after first examination. Maximum intensity projection.

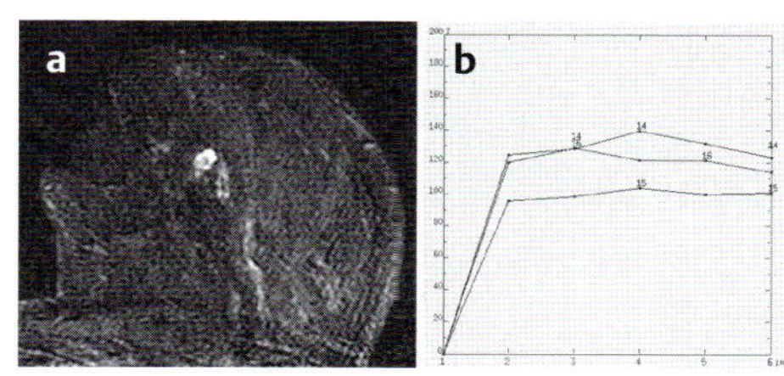

Fig. 60.**14 a, b** Signal-to-time curves.

## Diagnosis (without histopathological verification)

Myxoid fibroadenoma between lower quadrants. Hormone-induced “pseudo-lesion” between outer quadrants.

## Procedure

Screening.

Adenomas and fibroadenomas, as well as the glandular tissue, can display intraindividual variation in contrast enhancement.

**Indication:** Screening.
**History:** Unremarkable.
**Risk profile:** No increased risk.
**Age:** 65 years.

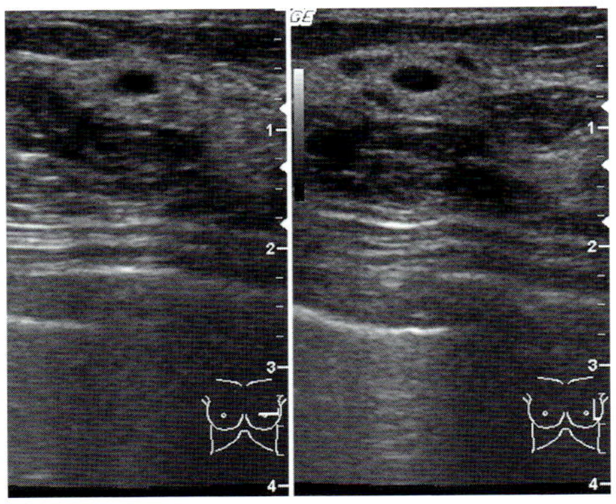

Fig. 61.**1** Ultrasound of the center of the left breast.

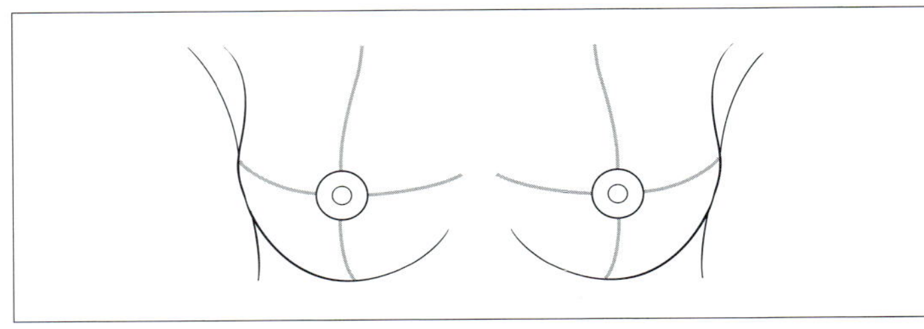

**Clinical Findings**

normal.

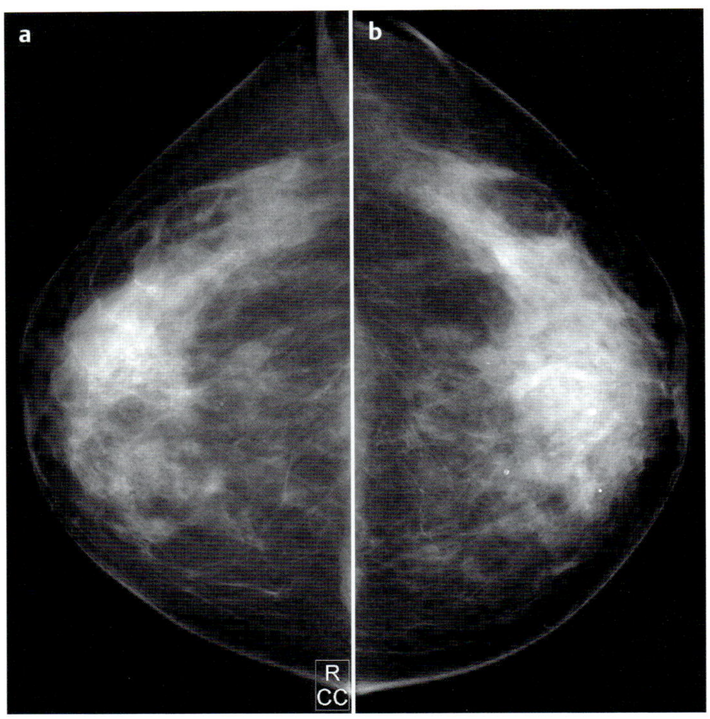


Fig. 61.**2 a, b** Digital mammography, CC view.

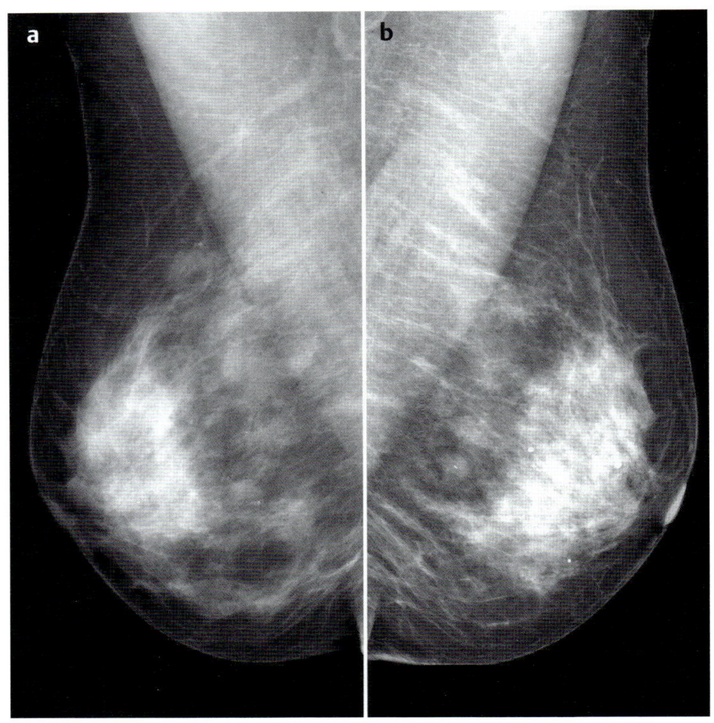


Fig. 61.**3 a, b** Digital mammography, MLO view.

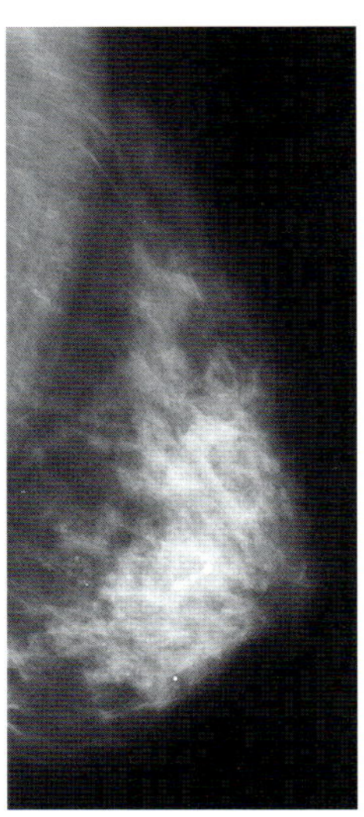

Fig. 61.**4** Conventional mammography two years earlier, MLO view [imaging not performed by authors].

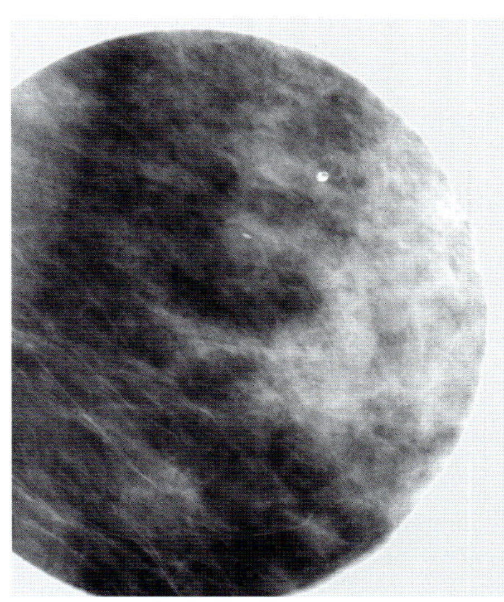

Fig. 61.**5** Spot compression of the left breast, MLO view.

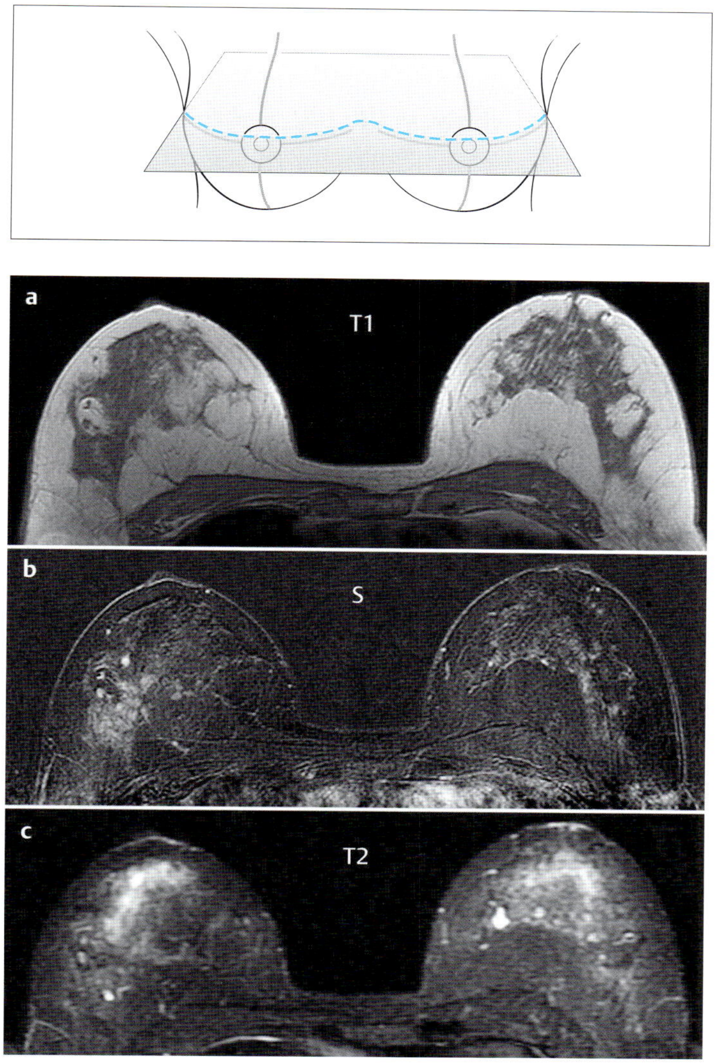


Fig. 61.**6 a – c** Contrast-enhanced MRI of the breasts.

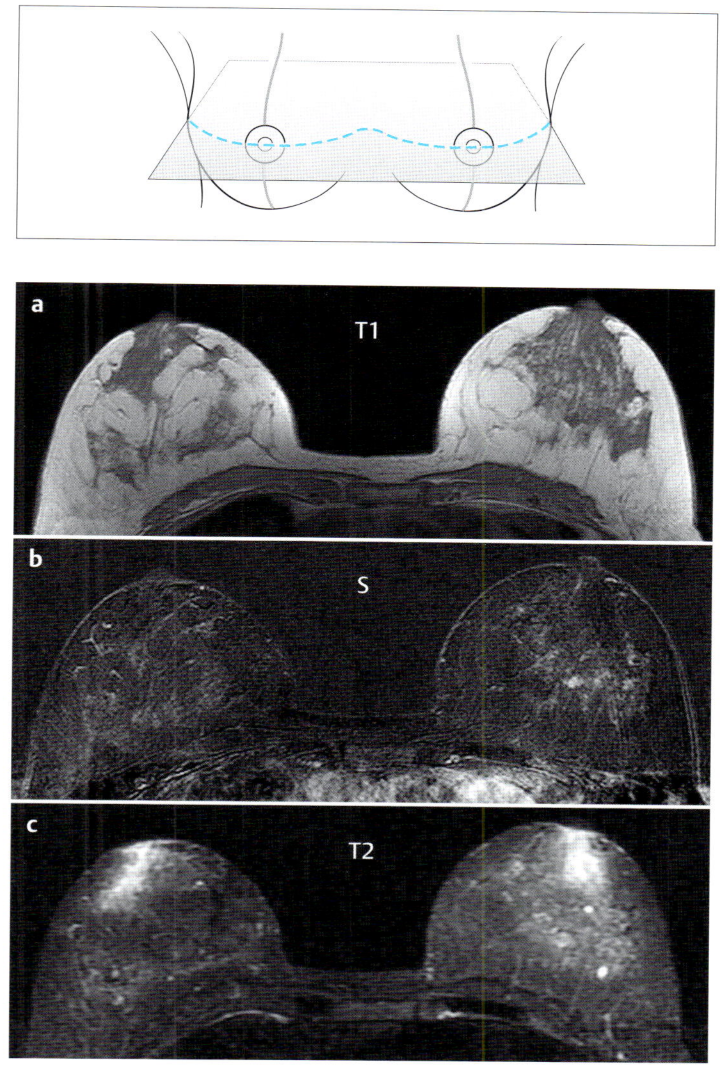


Fig. 61.**7 a – c** Contrast-enhanced MRI of the breasts.

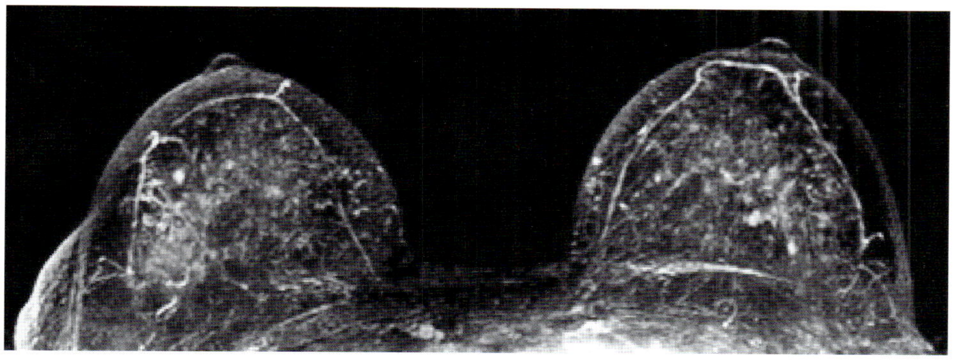

Fig. 61.**8** Contrast-enhanced MR mammography. Maximum intensity projection.

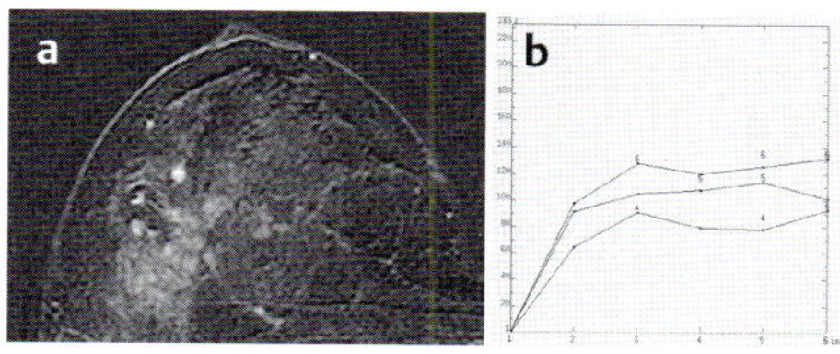


Fig. 61.**9 a, b** Signal-to-time curves, right breast.

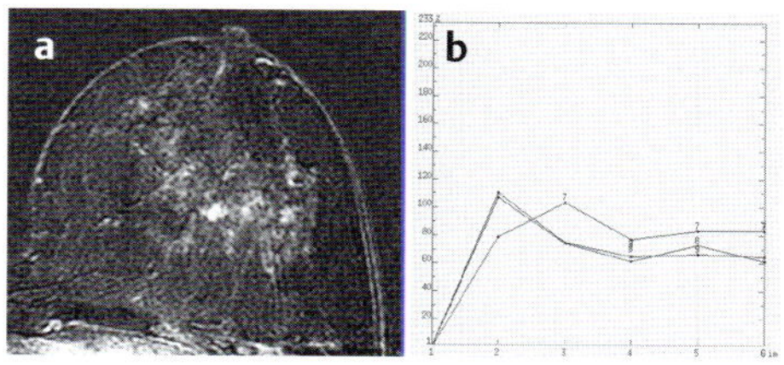


Fig. 61.**10 a, b** Signal-to-time curve, left breast.

**?**

Please characterize ultrasound, mammography, and MRI findings.
What is your preliminary diagnosis?
What are your next steps?

This is the imaging study of an asymptomatic woman.

## Ultrasound

There was a well-defined, hypoechoic lesion 3 mm in diameter with indeterminate distal echo pattern between the outer quadrants of the left breast. Ultrasound showed architectural distortion of the parenchyma by this lesion. US BI-RADS left 2.

## Mammography

Mammograms demonstrated inhomogeneously dense parenchyma, ACR type 3. In comparison with the mammography two years previously, there was a new, well-defined density (diameter 8 mm) in the prepectoral region of the left breast, accompanied by a small linear microcalcification also not depicted in the previous imaging. BI-RADS right 1/left 3.

## MR Mammography

Multiple cysts with maximum diameter of 1 cm were visible bilaterally. There was an ill-defined, homogeneously enhancing lesion of 8 mm diameter in the central part of the left breast with an initial signal increase of 110% and a postinitial washout as well as an intermediate signal in T2-weighted imaging. Another well-defined lesion of 6 mm diameter was visible between the outer quadrants of the right breast with homogeneous contrast uptake, an initial signal increase of 130%, and a postinitial plateau as well as an increased signal in T2-weighted imaging.

**MRI Artifact Category:** 1
**MRI Density Type:** 2

| MRM score | Right | Points | Left | Points |
|---|---|---|---|---|
| **Shape** | round | 0 | lobulated | 0 |
| **Border** | well-defined | 0 | ill-defined | 1 |
| **CM Distribution** | homogenous | 0 | homogeneous | 0 |
| **Initial Signal Intensity Increase** | strong | 2 | strong | 2 |
| **Post-initial Signal Intensity Character** | plateau | 1 | wash-out | 2 |
| **MRI score (points)** | | **3** | | **5** |
| **MRI BI-RADS** | | **3** | | **4** |

## → Differential Diagnosis

Right: Adenosis, fibroadenoma, papilloma.
Left: Adenosis, fibroadenoma, carcinoma, papilloma.

| BI-RADS Categorization | | |
|---|---|---|
| Clinical Findings | right 1 | left 1 |
| Ultrasound | right 1 | left 2 |
| Mammography | right 1 | left 3 |
| MR Mammography | right 3 | left 4 |
| **BI-RADS Total** | **right 3** | **left 4** |

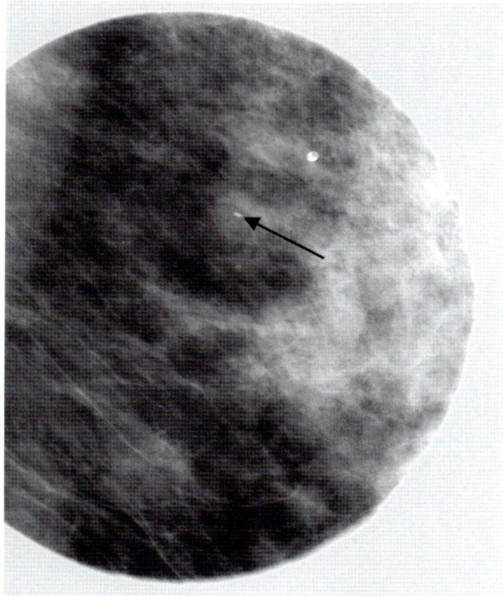

Fig. 61.**11** In comparison with images from the previous examination, a new lesion with microcalcifications (arrow) was visible.

**Procedure**

MR-guided vacuum core biopsy of the lesion in the central part of the left breast.

**Histology**

Adenosis.

## Histology

Adenosis.

## Treatment

None. Follow-up-MRI in 6 months.

In MRI, washout is rarely seen in benign changes of the breast, but can occasionally occur.

**Indication:** Further investigation of suspicious finding in sonography of the left breast.
**History:** Unremarkable.
**Risk profile:** No increased risk.
**Age:** 60 years.

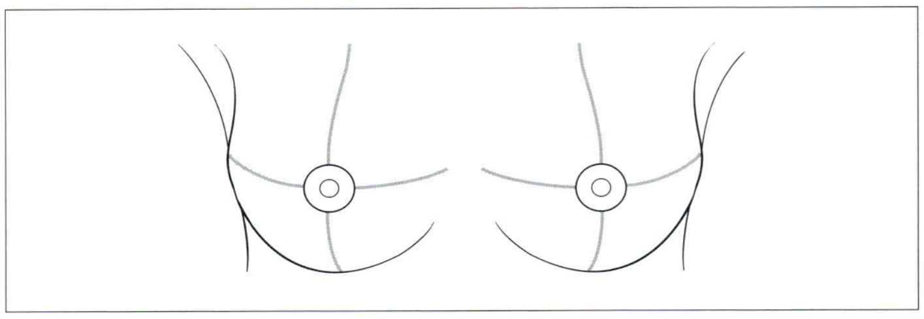

## Clinical Findings

No findings.

## Ultrasound (not shown)

No findings. The suspicious lesion detected in the left breast in sonography conducted elsewhere was not reproducible.

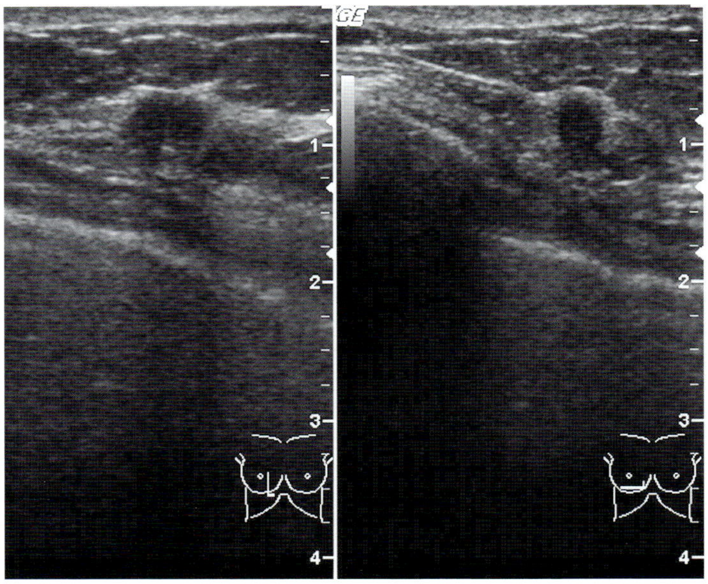

Fig. 62.3 Targeted repeat sonography in view of the MRI findings.

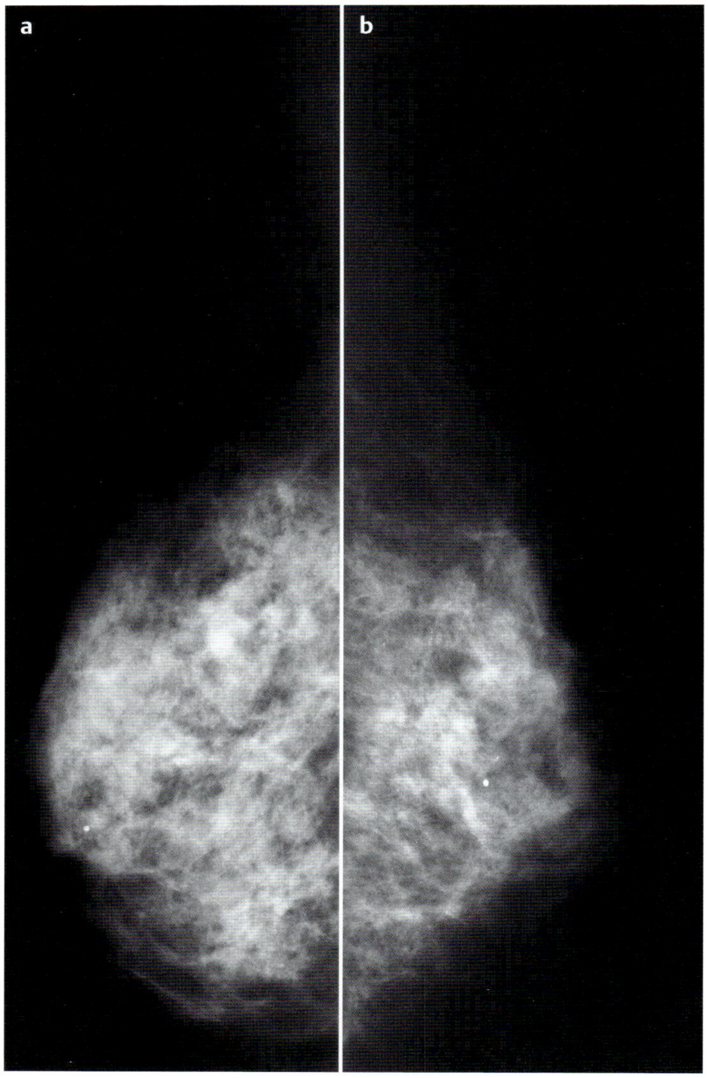

Fig. 62.1 **a, b** Conventional mammography, MLO view [imaging not performed by authors].

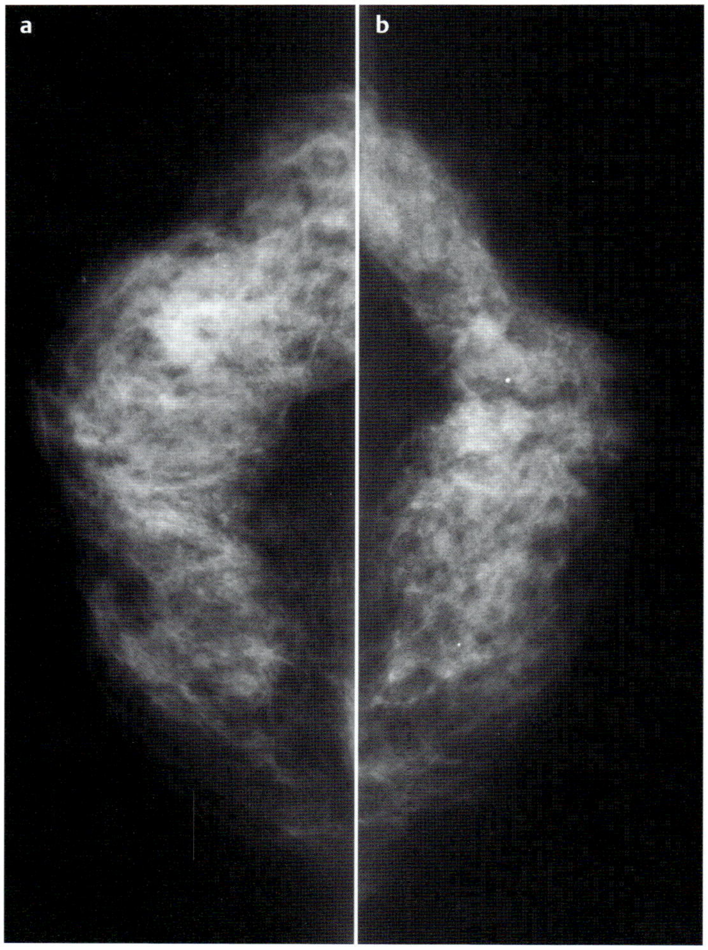

Fig. 62.2 **a, b** Conventional mammography, CC view [imaging not performed by authors].

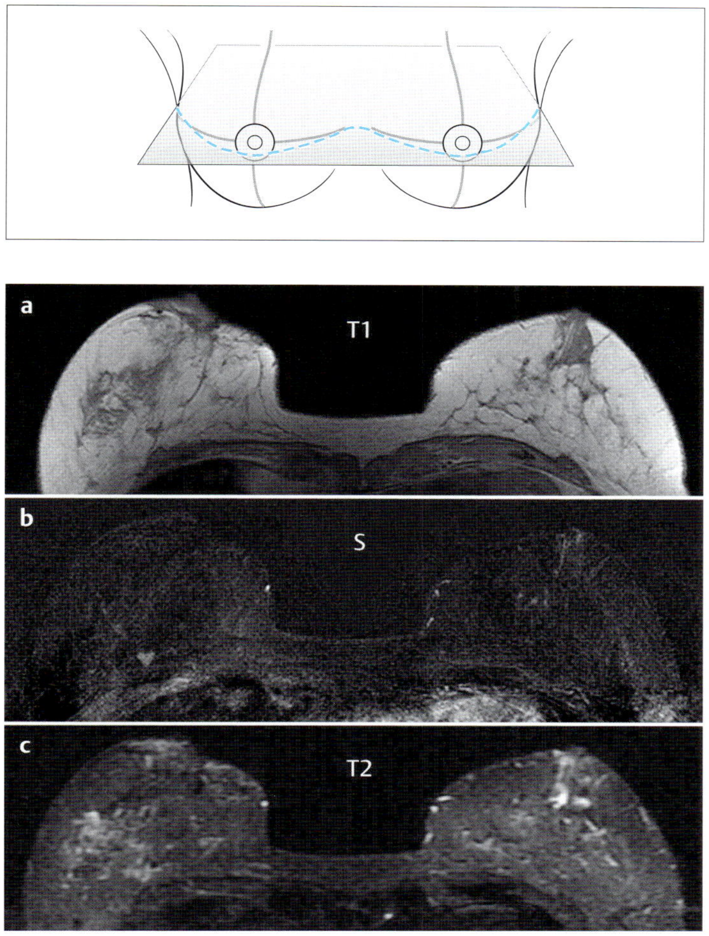


Fig. 62.**4 a – c** Contrast-enhanced MRI of the breasts.

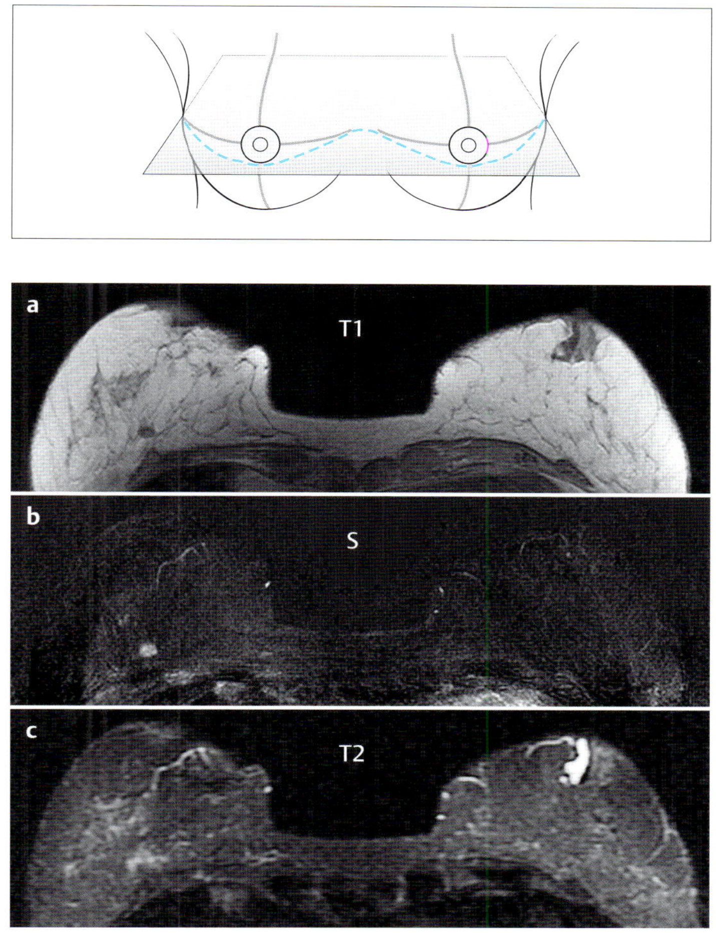


Fig. 62.**5 a – c** Contrast-enhanced MRI of the breasts.

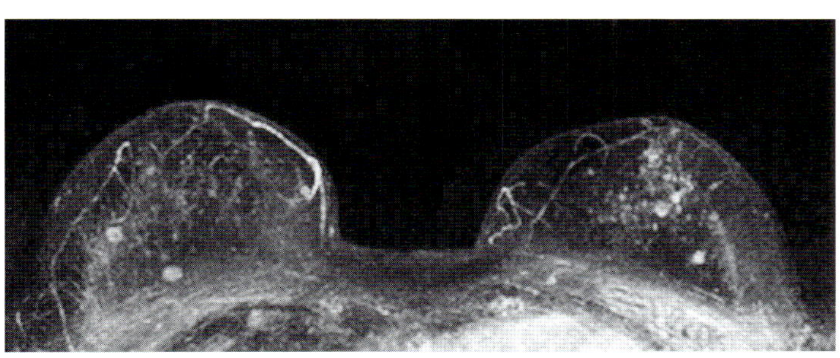

Fig. 62.**6** Contrast-enhanced MR mammography. Maximum intensity projection.

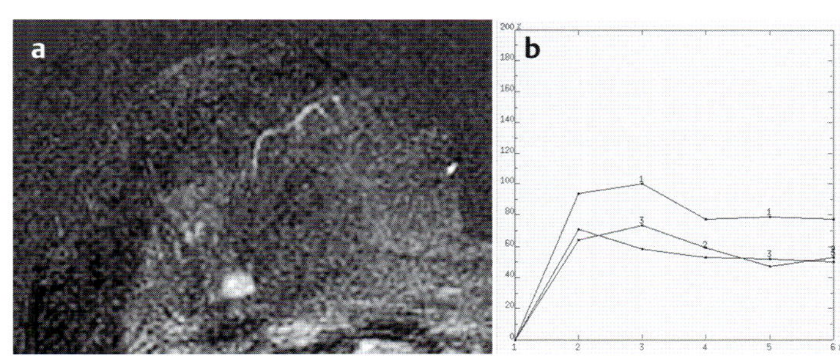

Fig. 62.**7 a, b** Signal-to-time curves.

?

Please characterize ultrasound, mammography, and MRI findings.
What is your preliminary diagnosis?
What are your next steps?

Diagnostic imaging was conducted in this case to investigate suspect findings in sonography of the left breast performed elsewhere on the asymptomatic patient.

### Ultrasound

Ultrasound showed inhomogeneous echogenicity of the tissue in both breasts with multiple hypoechoic, compressible lesions. The lesion between the upper quadrants of the left breast detected in a previous examination could not be reproduced. After MR mammography, further targeted sonography between the lower quadrants of the right breast showed a hypoechoic lesion (diameter 8 mm) with displacement of a Cooper's ligament. There was partial distal shadowing. No relevant architectural distortions. US BI-RADS 3.

### Mammography

The glandular tissue was bilaterally symmetric and extremely dense, ACR type 4. Under these limiting conditions–even retrospectively–no suspicious masses or densities were visible, particularly between the lower quadrants of the right breast. There were no microcalcifications suspect for malignancy. BI-RADS right 1/ left 1. PGMI: MLO view I (asymmetry, right pectoral muscle angle < 20°, left not depicted, inframammary fold incompletely depicted); CC view P.

### MR Mammography

MRI demonstrated a lobulated, ill-defined, inhomogeneously* enhancing mass, 8 mm in diameter, between the lower quadrants of the right breast. The lesion had marked initial signal increase and postinitial washout as well as reduced signal in T2-weighted imaging. There were no suspicious findings in the upper quadrants of the left breast. In maximum intensity projection, additional enhancing foci with no criteria of malignancy were visible. There was also a duct ectasia on the left side behind the nipple.

**MRI Artifact Category:** 1
**MRI Density Type:** 1

| MRM score | Finding | Points |
|---|---|---|
| **Shape** | lobulated | 0 |
| **Border** | ill-defined | 1 |
| **CM Distribution** | inhomogeneous | 1 |
| **Initial Signal Intensity Increase** | strong | 2 |
| **Post-initial Signal Intensity Character** | wash-out | 2 |
| **MRI score (points)** | | **6** |
| **MRI BI-RADS** | | **5** |

### → Differential Diagnosis

Right breast: Carcinoma (medullary?), adenosis, fibroadenoma, papilloma.

* Differentiation between inhomogeneity and internal septations was not possible.

| BI-RADS Categorization | | |
|---|---|---|
| Clinical Findings | right 1 | left 1 |
| Ultrasound | right 3 | left 1 |
| Mammography | right 1 | left 1 |
| MR Mammography | right 5 | left 1 |
| **BI-RADS Total** | **right 5** | **left 1** |

### Procedure

MR-guided vacuum biopsy (Fig. 62.**8**), since the correlation of the findings in MRI and in ultrasound was not firmly established.

### Histopathology

Invasive ductal carcinoma.

### Further procedure

Tumor excision following preoperative MR-guided localization.

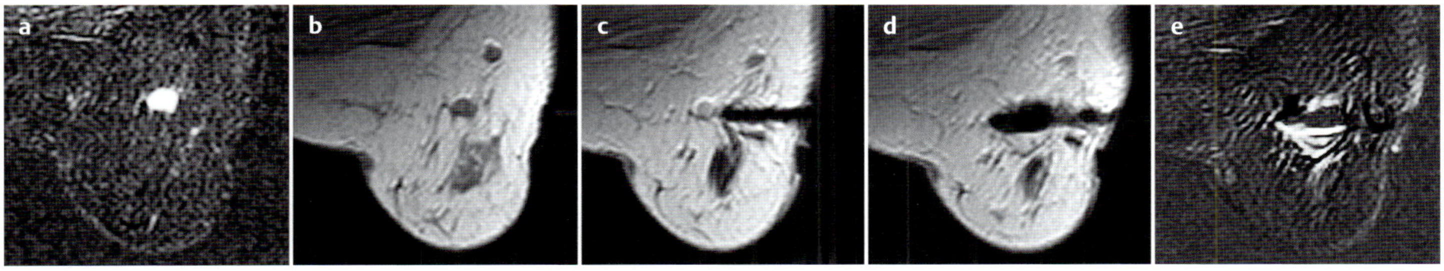


Fig. 62.**8 a – e** MR-guided vacuum biopsy of the right breast.

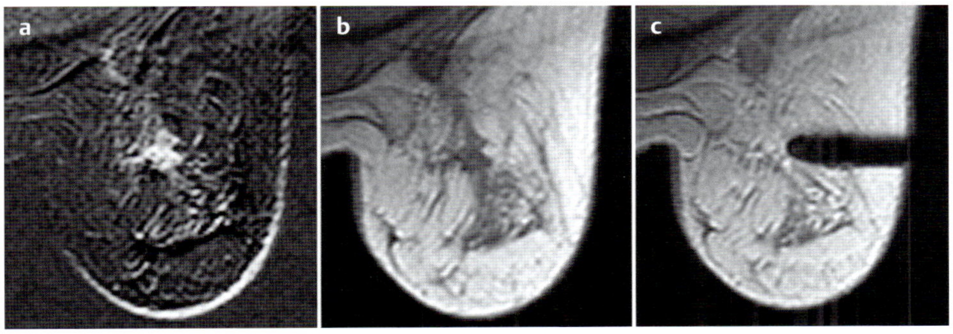


Fig. 62.**9 a – c** MR-guided localization of the lesion in the right breast.

### Diagnosis

IDC pT1b, pN0, G2

### Treatment

Breast conservation therapy of the right breast.

In extremely dense parenchyma (ACR type 4) up to 50 % of carcinomas are occult in mammography. Additional imaging modalities such as ultrasound or MR mammography are essential under these conditions.

**Indication:** Resistance in the upper outer quadrant of the left breast.
**History:** Unremarkable.
**Risk profile:** No increased risk.
**Age:** 49 years.

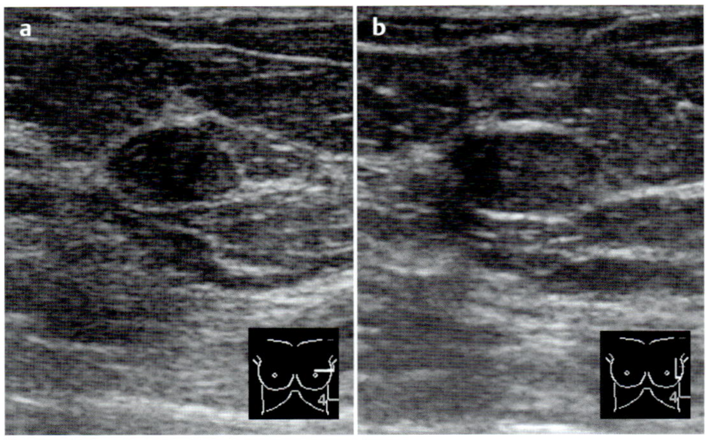


Fig. 63.**1 a, b** Ultrasound.

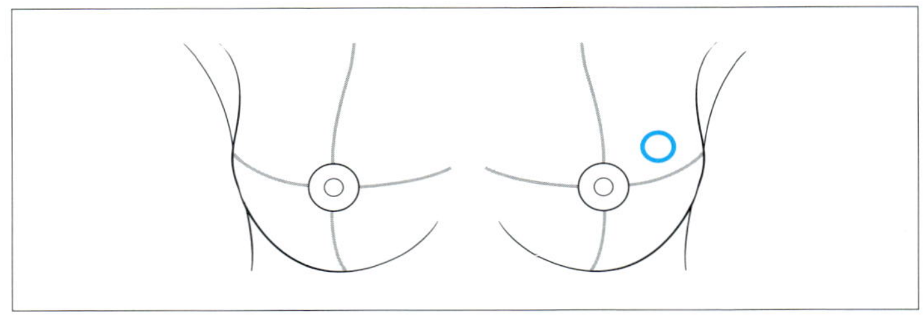

## Clinical Findings

Palpable, mobile mass 1 cm in diameter in the upper outer quadrant of the left breast.

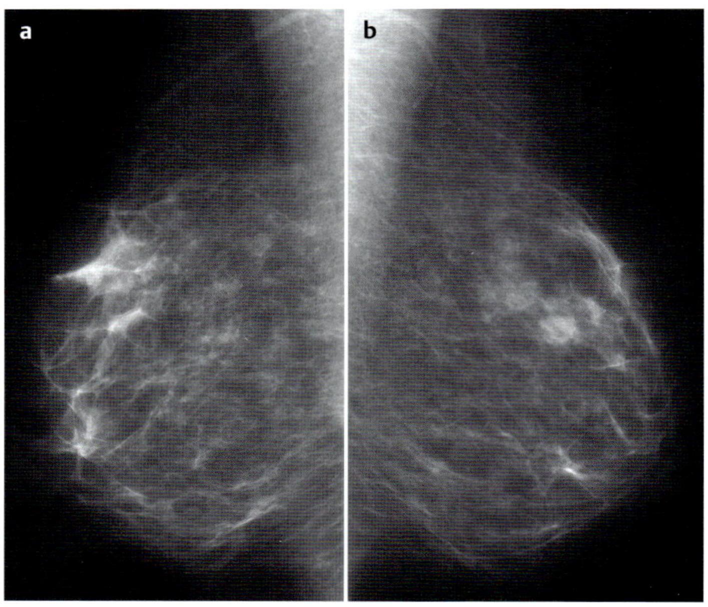


Fig. 63.**2 a, b** Conventional mammography, MLO view [imaging not performed by authors].

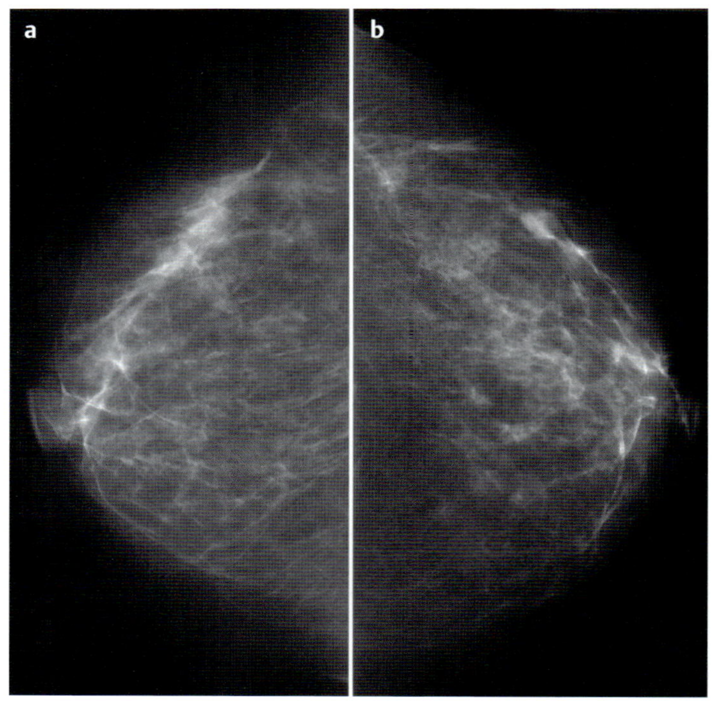


Fig. 63.**3 a, b** Conventional mammography, MLO view [imaging not performed by authors].

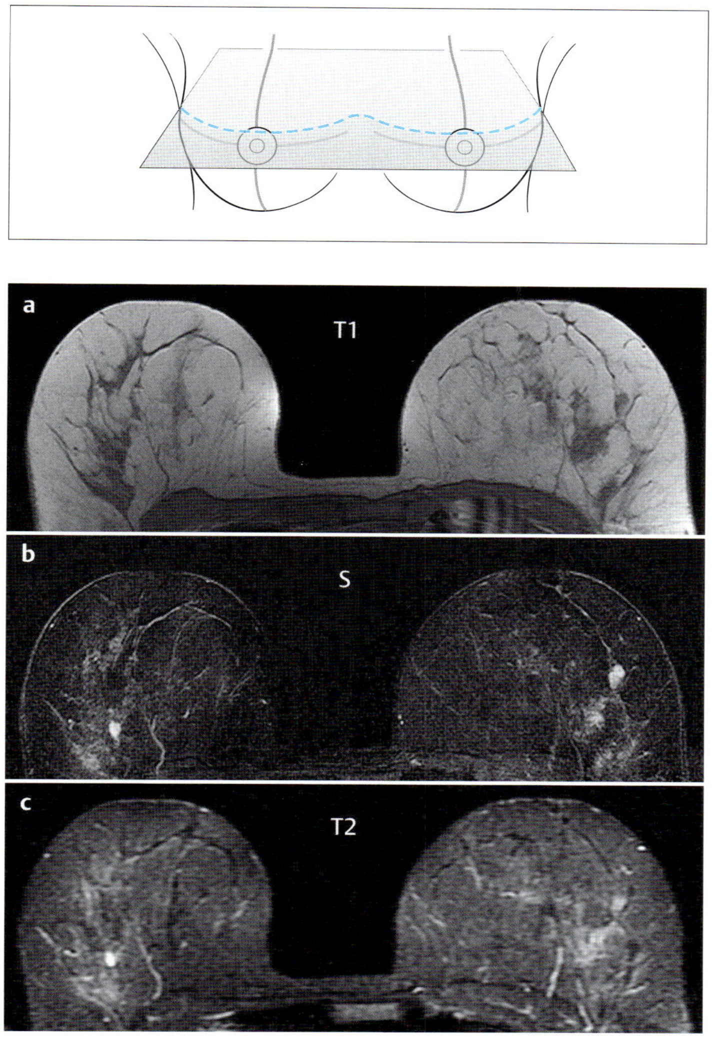


Fig. 63.**4 a–c** Contrast-enhanced MRI of the breasts.

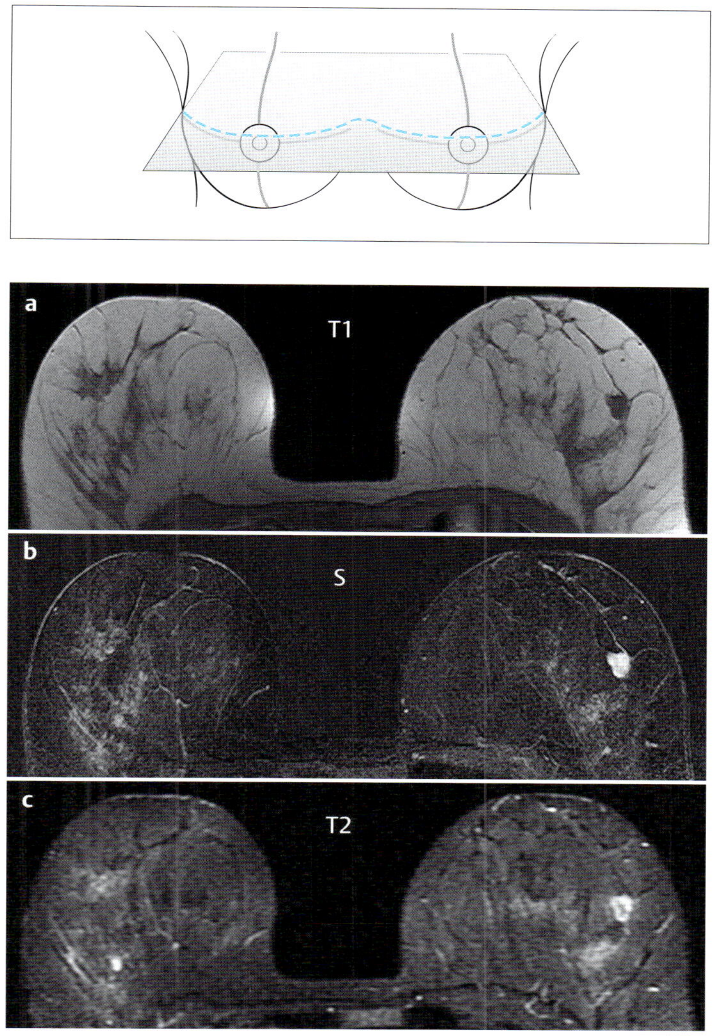


Fig. 63.**5 a–c** Contrast-enhanced MRI of the breasts.

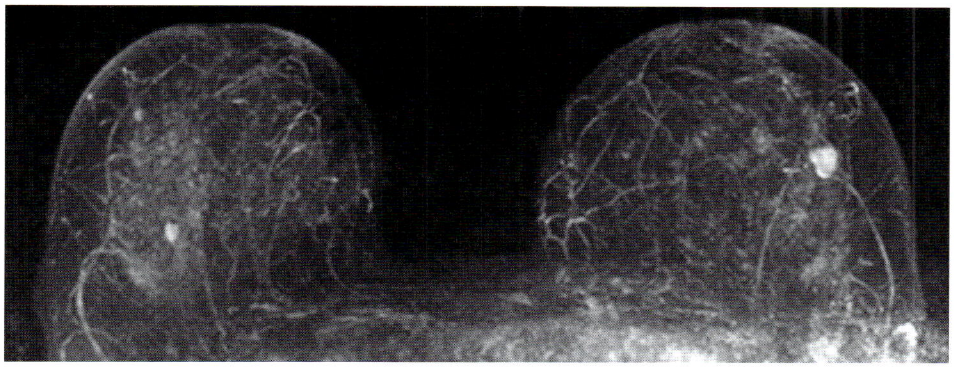

Fig. 63.**6** Contrast-enhanced MR mammography. Maximum intensity projection.

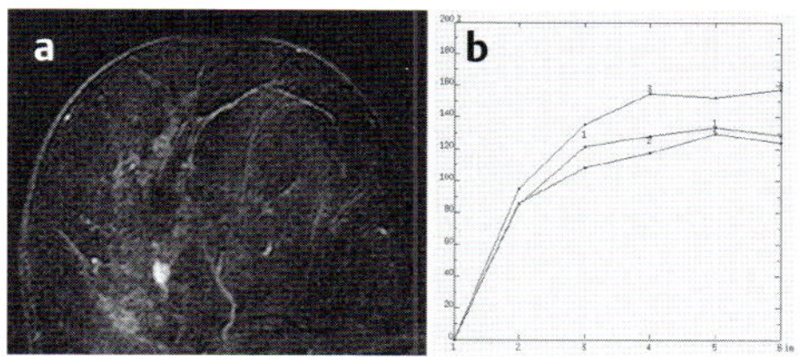


Fig. 63.**7 a, b** Signal-to-time curves.

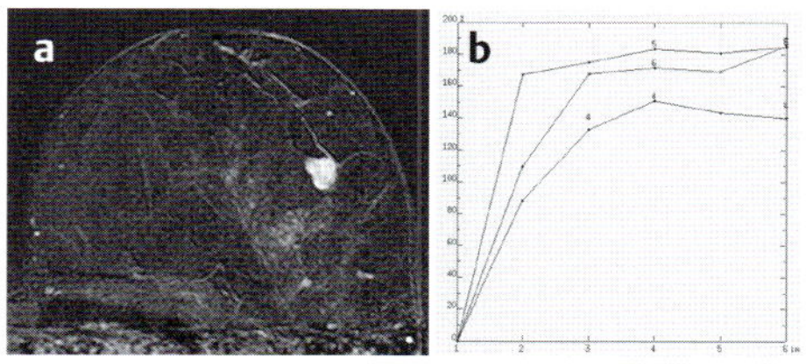


Fig. 63.**8 a, b** Signal-to-time curves.

?

Please characterize ultrasound, mammography, and MRI findings.
What is your preliminary diagnosis?
What are your next steps?

This case demonstrates the imaging studies of a symptomatic woman with a palpable mass measuring 1 cm in the upper outer quadrant of the left breast.

### Ultrasound

Lobulated, hypoechoic lesion in the upper outer quadrant of the left breast with indeterminate distal echo pattern. Orientation of the longer axis parallel to the skin. No architectural distortion. US BI-RADS 2.

### Mammography

The parenchyma was bilaterally symmetric and of fibroglandular texture, ACR type 2.
Mammography depicted an isodense, lobulated mass 1 cm in diameter between the outer quadrants of the left breast. In CC view this lesion was well defined; in MLO view it was partially superimposed. Imaging showed no microcalcifications and no architectural distortion. BI-RADS right 1/left 3. PGMI CC view M (nipple not in profile); MLO view M (angle of pectoralis muscle < 20°; inframammary fold not depicted).

### MR Mammography

There was a well-defined, lobulated, inhomogeneously enhancing mass (diameter 1 cm) between the outer quadrants of the left breast. Initial signal increase was 170%, followed by a postinitial plateau. This lesion showed an increased signal in T2-weighted imaging. There was another well-defined homogeneously enhancing oval lesion (diameter 6 mm) in the right breast. Here, the initial signal increase was 140% followed by a postinitial plateau. Signal in T2-weighted imaging was increased.

**MRI Artifact Category:** 1
**MRI Density Type:** 2

| MRM score | Right | Points | Left | Points |
|---|---|---|---|---|
| **Shape** | oval | 0 | lobulated | 0 |
| **Border** | well-defined | 0 | well-defined | 0 |
| **CM Distribution** | homogenous | 0 | inhomogeneous | 1 |
| **Initial Signal Intensity Increase** | strong | 2 | strong | 2 |
| **Post-initial Signal Intensity Character** | plateau | 1 | plateau | 1 |
| **MRI score (points)** | | **3** | | **4** |
| **MRI BI-RADS** | | **3** | | **4** |

### → Differential Diagnosis

Right: Fibroadenoma, papilloma, carcinoma (mucinous?).
Left: Carcinoma, fibroadenoma, papilloma.

| BI-RADS Categorization | | |
|---|---|---|
| Clinical Findings | right 1 | left 4 |
| Ultrasound | right 1 | left 2 |
| Mammography | right 1 | left 3 |
| MR Mammography | right 3 | left 4 |
| **BI-RADS Total** | **right 3** | **left 4** |

### Procedure

MRI follow-up of the lesion in the right breast after 6 months.
Histopathological analysis of the palpable resistance in the left breast with US-guided core biopsy.
In the MRI follow-up 6 months later, there were no changes in the findings in the right breast.

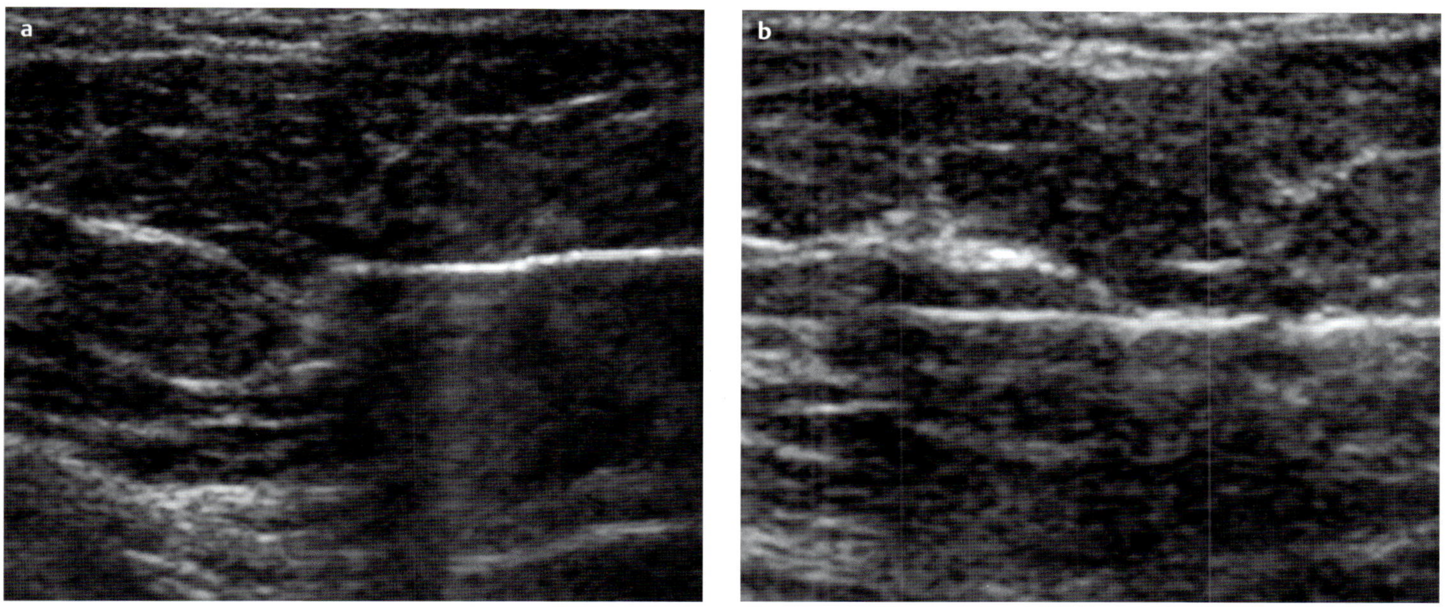


Fig. 63.**9 a, b** US-guided core biopsy. Pre-fire and post-fire images.

## Histology

Pericanalicular fibroadenoma of the left breast.
Fibroadenoma (no histological verification) of the right breast.

## Treatment

None. Screening at usual intervals.

Lesions categorized BI-RADS 4 must be investigated histopathologically. Percutaneous biopsy is the preferred method.

**Indication:** Monitoring after bilateral breast cancer.
**History:** Invasive lobular carcinoma of the left breast 5 years previously and ductal carcinoma in situ of the right breast 3 years previously. Bilateral breast conservation therapy and radiation therapy.
**Risk profile:** Increased by earlier bilateral cancer. **Age:** 52 years.

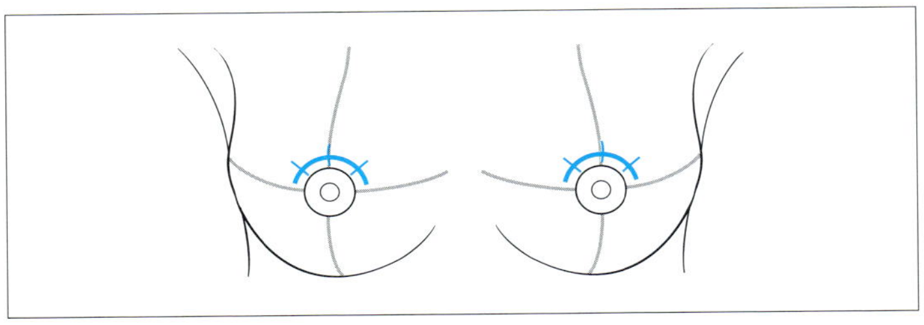

### Clinical Findings

Normal scarring of both breasts. No palpable findings.

### Ultrasound (not shown)

Bilateral lumpectomy scars; no other unusual findings.

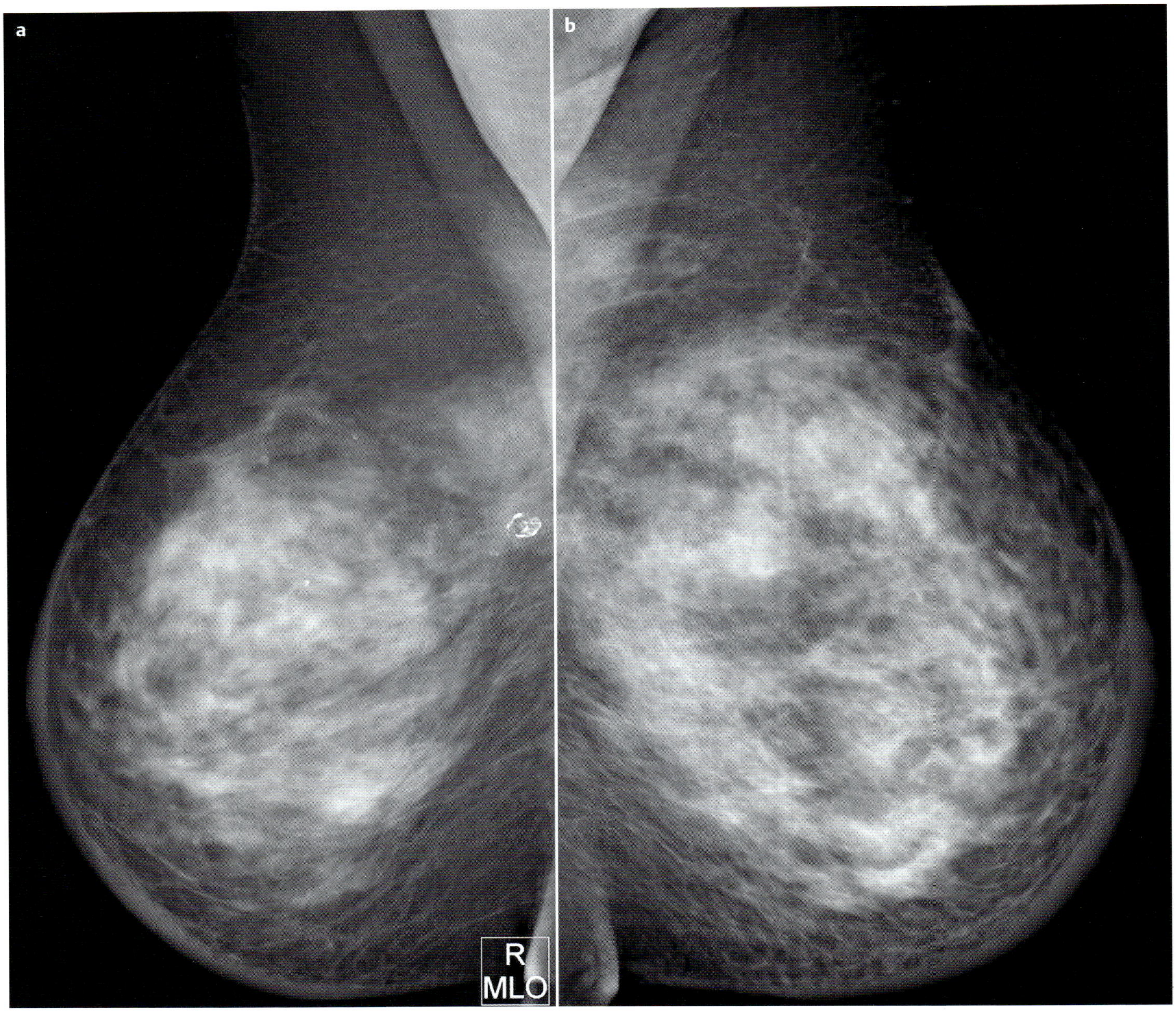


Fig. 64.**1 a, b** Digital mammography, MLO view.

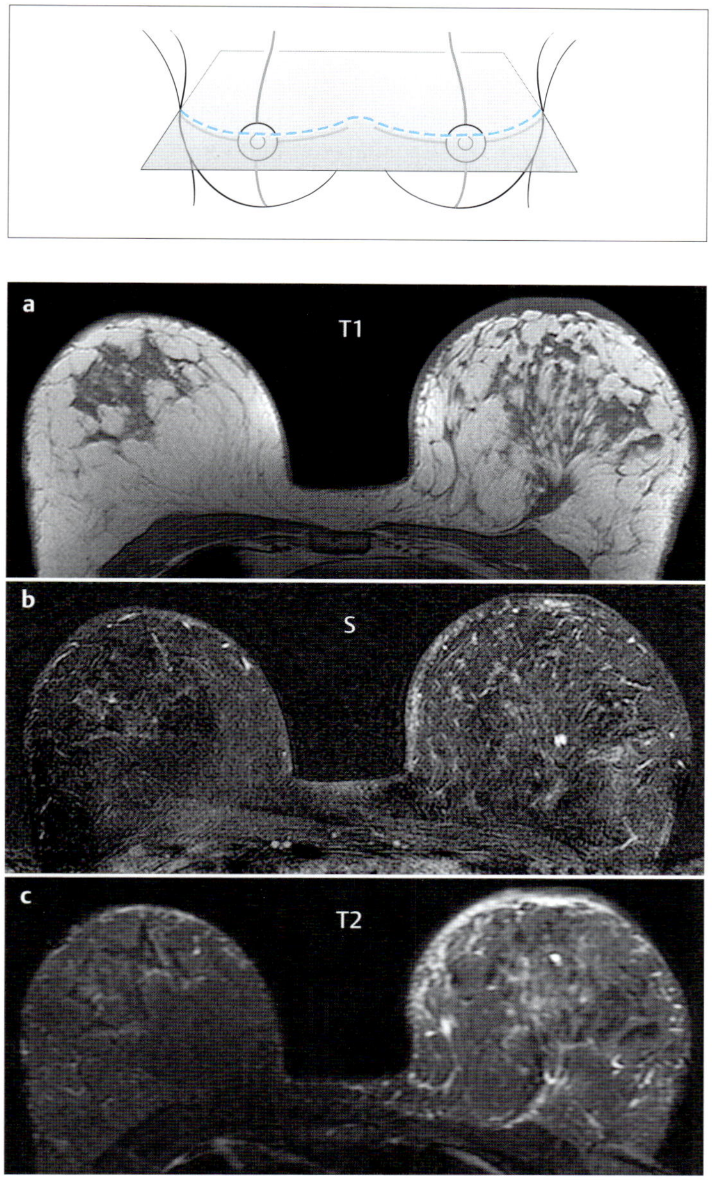


Fig. 64.**2 a, b** Contrast-enhanced MRI of the breasts.

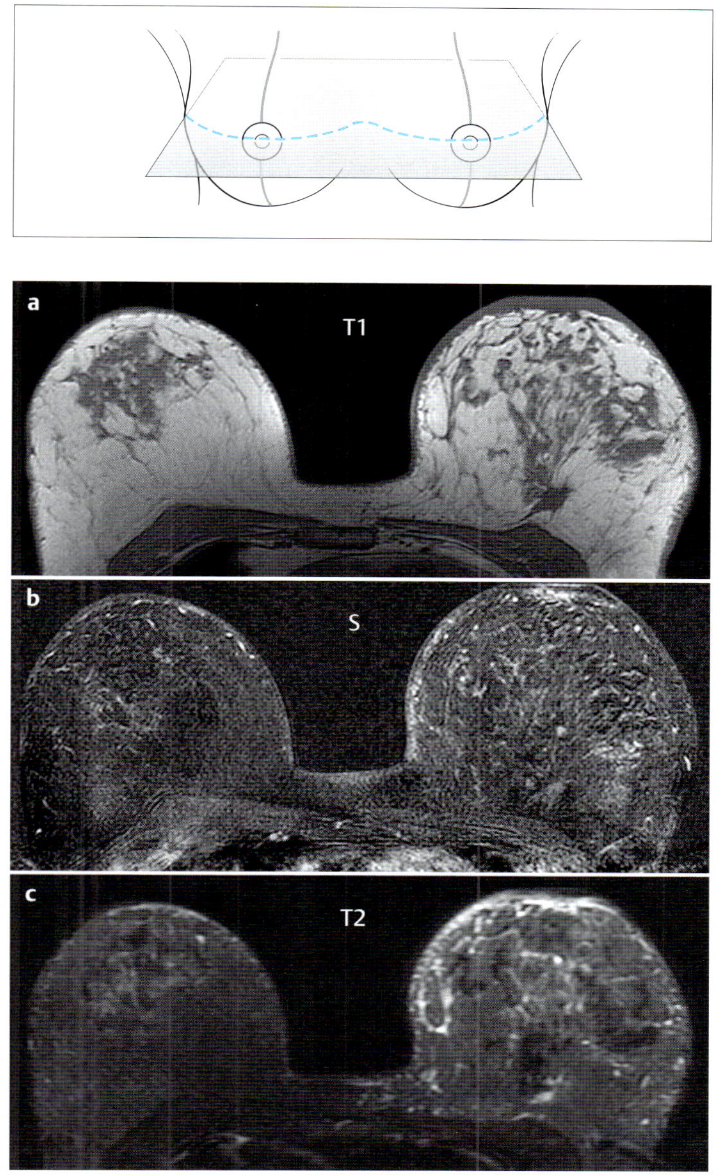


Fig. 64.**3 a, b** Contrast-enhanced MRI of the breasts.

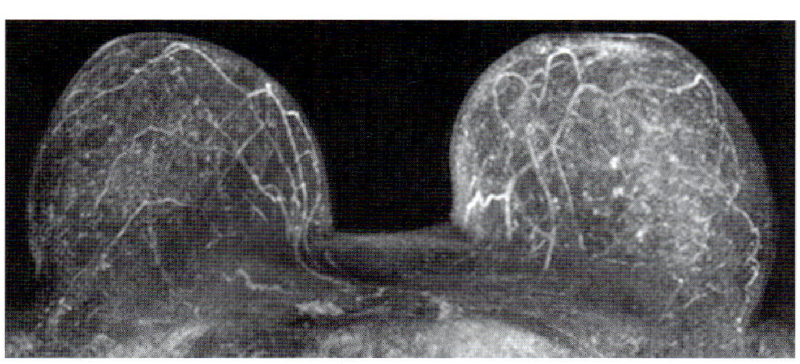

Fig. 64.**4 a, b** Contrast-enhanced MR mammography. Maximum intensity projection.

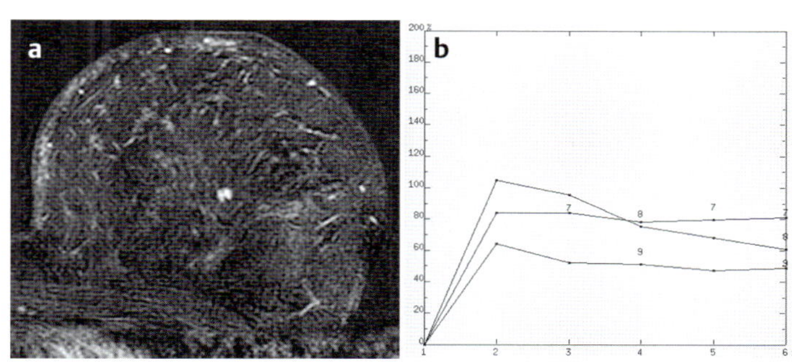


Fig. 64.**5 a, b** Signal-to-time curves.

?

Please characterize mammography and MRI findings.
What is your preliminary diagnosis?
What are your next steps?

This case presents the routine follow-up imaging of a 52-year-old woman after bilateral breast cancer 3 and 5 years previously.

### Ultrasound

Bilateral hypoechoic lumpectomy scars were visible. There were no suspicious findings. US BI-RADS right 2/left 2 (scars). (Not shown).

### Mammography

Mammograms showed bilaterally symmetric, inhomogeneously dense parenchyma, ACR type 3. Skin thickening due to previous treatment was visible around the circumference of both breasts, as well as postoperative architectural distortion in the upper quadrants of the right breast toward the chest wall. Here there were also eggshell-like calcifications, suggesting an oil cyst. There were no suspicious lesions or microcalcifications. BI-RADS right 2/ left 1. PGMI: MLO view G (inframammary fold).

### MR Mammography

T1-weighted MRI demonstrated a postoperative architectural distortion in the center of the left breast. Within this area there was an ill-defined lesion 6 mm in diameter that showed postcontrast hypervascularization, initial signal increase of 110%, postinitial washout, and reduced signal in T2-weighted imaging.

**MRI Artifact Category:** 1
**MRI Density Type:** 2

| MRM score | Finding left | Points |
|---|---|---|
| **Shape** | oval | 0 |
| **Border** | ill-defined | 1 |
| **CM Distribution** | homogeneous | 0 |
| **Initial Signal Intensity Increase** | strong | 2 |
| **Post-initial Signal Intensity Character** | wash-out | 2 |
| **MRI score (points)** | | **5** |
| **MRI BI-RADS** | | **4** |

### → Differential Diagnosis

Left breast: Focal infection, local tumor relapse, fibroadenoma, adenoma, papilloma.

| BI-RADS Categorization | | |
|---|---|---|
| Clinical Findings | right 2 | left 2 |
| Ultrasound | right 2 | left 2 |
| Mammography | right 2 | left 1 |
| MR Mammography | right 1 | left 4 |
| **BI-RADS Total** | **right 2** | **left 4** |

### Procedure

MR-guided vacuum biopsy.

### Histopathology

Invasive lobular carcinoma.

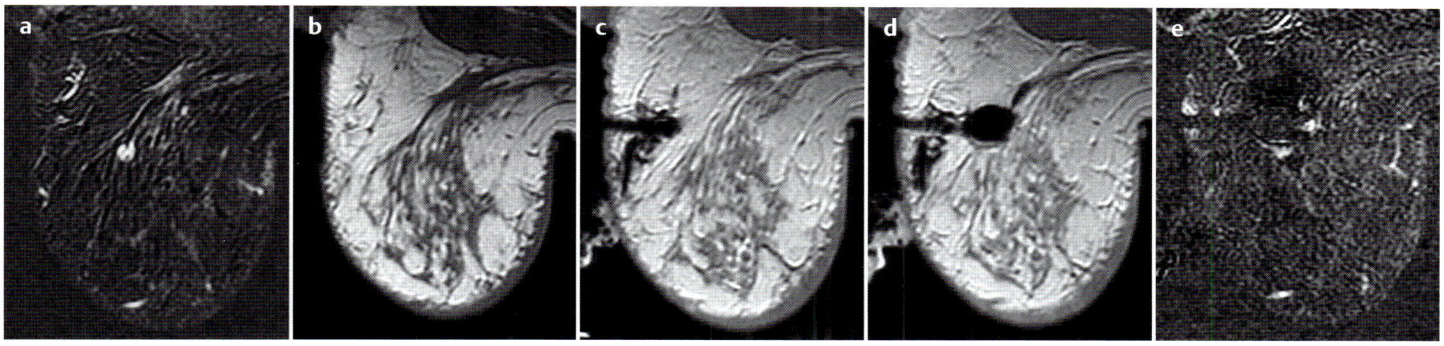

Fig. 64.**6 a – e** MR-guided vacuum biopsy.

### Histology

Local tumor recurrence of invasive lobular carcinoma (diameter 7 mm).

ILC pT1b, pN0, G2.

### Treatment

Mastectomy of the left breast.

In case of local tumor relapse after breast conservation therapy (BCT) and radiotherapy, BCT can no longer be considered as a treatment option.

**Indication:** Suspicious findings in ultrasound screening of the left breast performed elsewhere.
**History:** Unremarkable.
**Risk profile:** Breast cancer in a sister at the age of 44 years.
**Age:** 52 years.

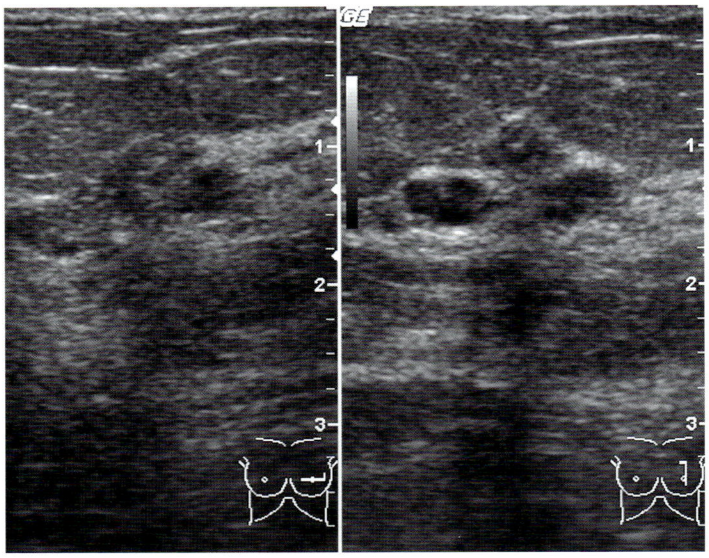


Fig. 65.**1** Ultrasound.

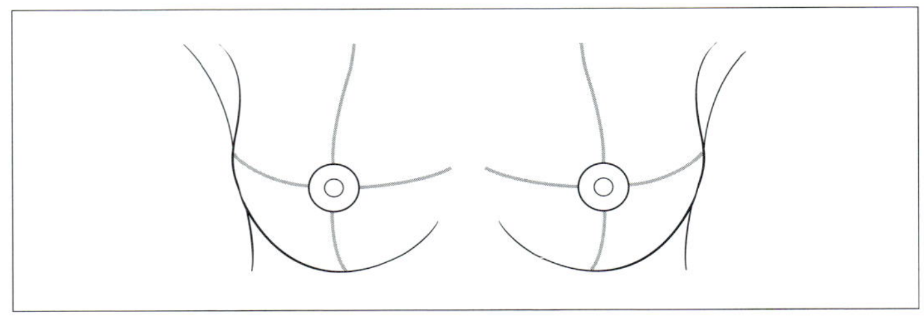

## Clinical Findings

No findings.

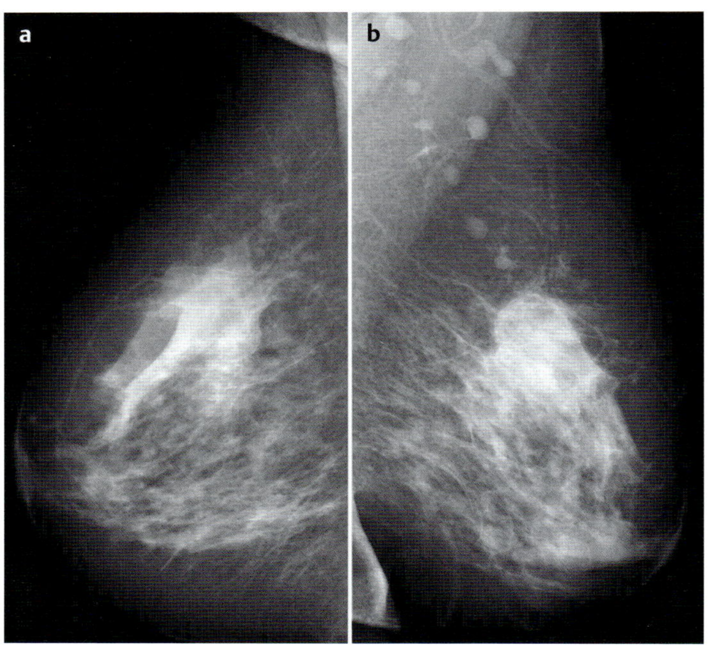


Fig. 65.**2 a, b** Digital mammography, MLO view [imaging not performed by authors].

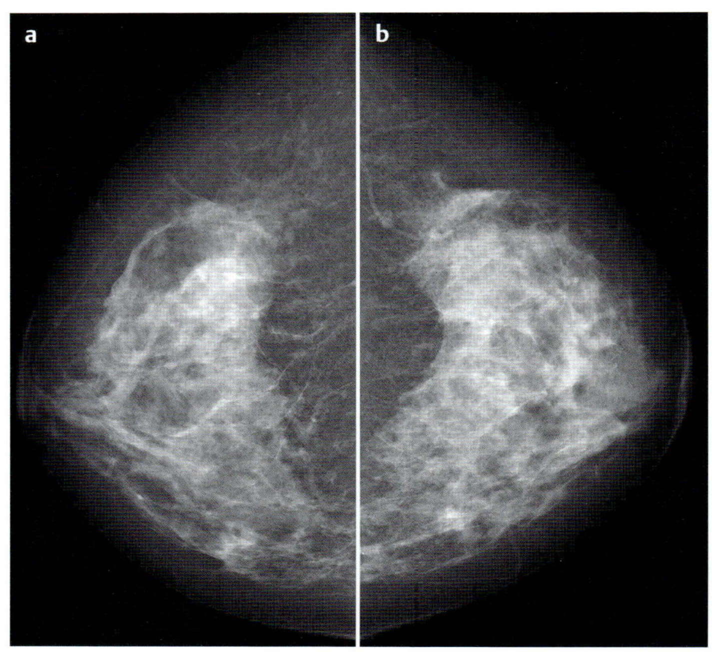


Fig. 65.**3 a, b** Digital mammography, CC view [imaging not performed by authors].

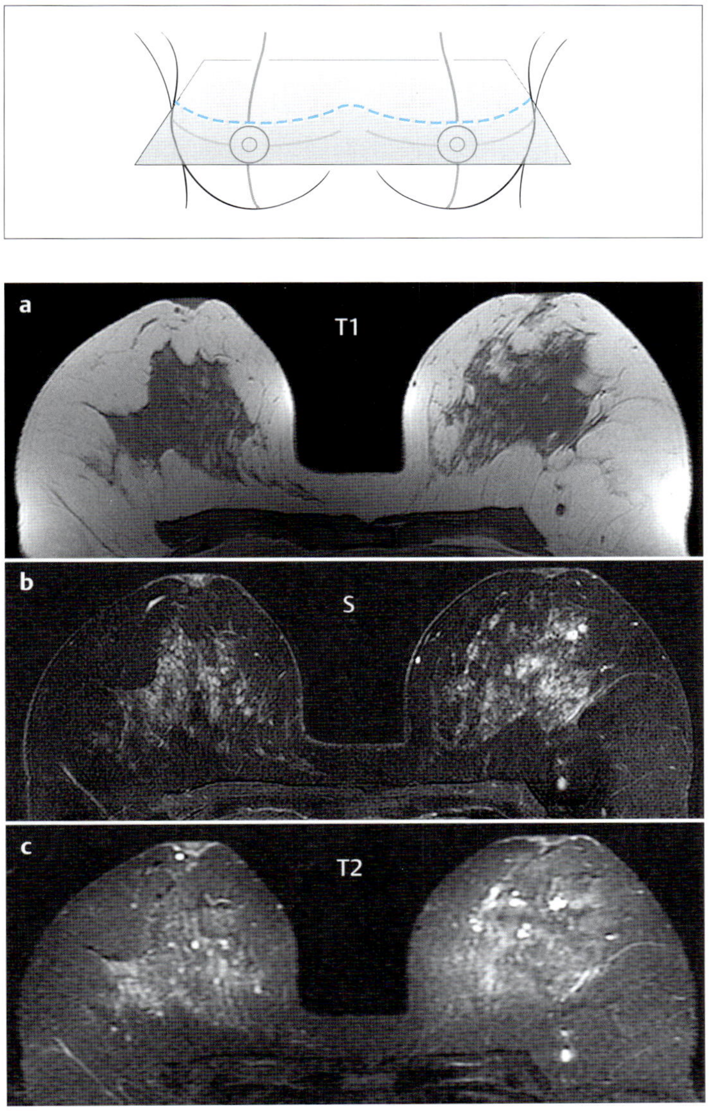


Fig. 65.**4 a–c** Contrast-enhanced MRI of the breasts.

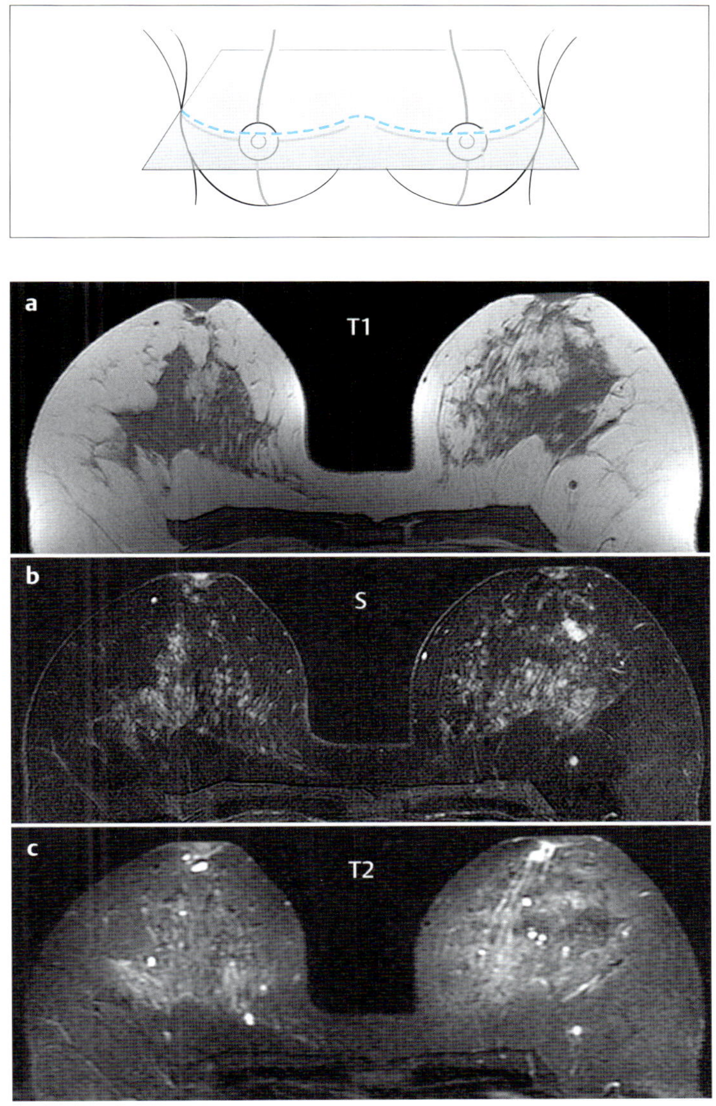


Fig. 65.**5 a–c** Contrast-enhanced MRI of the breasts.

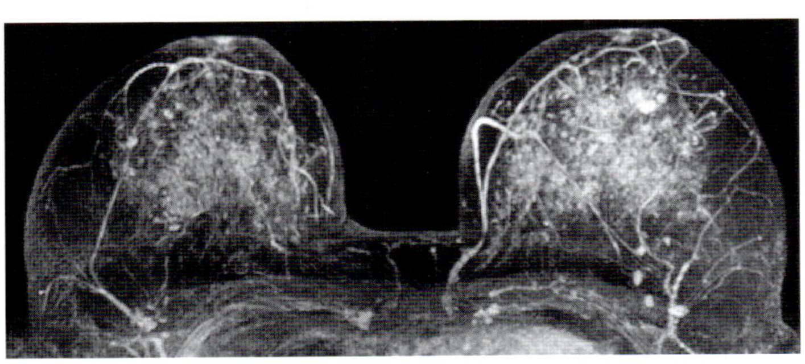

Fig. 65.**6** Contrast-enhanced MR mammography. Maximum intensity projection.

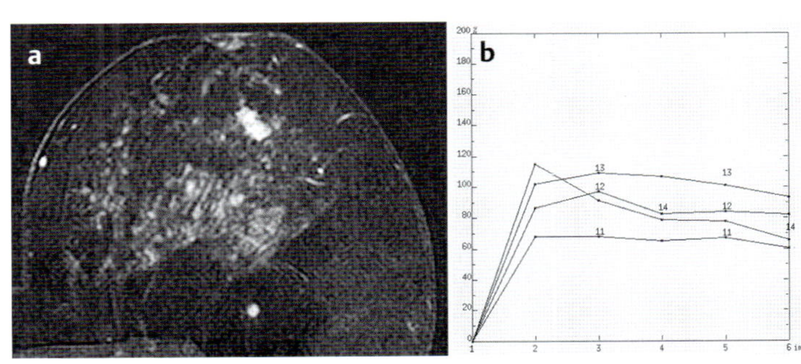


Fig. 65.**7 a, b** Signal-to-time curves.

?

Please characterize ultrasound, mammography, and MRI findings.
What is your preliminary diagnosis?
What are your next steps?

This case demonstrates supplementary imaging to investigate suspicious findings in an ultrasound examination performed elsewhere.

## Ultrasound

Ultrasound showed a cluster of round, hypoechogenic lesions with linear distal echo shadowing situated in the left breast behind the nipple. US BI-RADS 4.

## Mammography

Mammograms showed bilaterally symmetric, inhomogeneously dense parenchyma, ACR type 3. Particularly in the center of the left breast there were no suspicious lesions or densities. Images showed no suspicious microcalcifications and no architectural distortion. BI-RADS right 1/left 1. PGMI: MLO view I (right pectoralis muscle not depicted; inframammary fold not depicted, prominent abdominal skin fold); CC view M (medial parenchyma not fully visible).

## MR Mammography

A mass composed of three well-defined, oval, homogeneously enhancing components, each around 1 cm in diameter, was visible in the center of the left breast. It had initial signal increase of 150% and a postinitial washout. In T2-weighted imaging the section of the triple lesion nearest the nipple showed increased signal, while the two sections farther from the nipple had reduced signal. Maximum intensity projection showed a chain of lymph nodes within the breast.

**MRI Artifact Category:** 1
**MRI Density Type:** 3

| MRM score | Finding | Points |
|---|---|---|
| **Shape** | lobulated | 0 |
| **Border** | well-defined | 0 |
| **CM Distribution** | homogeneous | 0 |
| **Initial Signal Intensity Increase** | strong | 2 |
| **Post-initial Signal Intensity Character** | wash-out | 2 |
| **MRI score (points)** | | **4** |
| **MRI BI-RADS** | | **4** |

## → Differential Diagnosis

Left: Papilloma, fibroadenoma, adenoma, carcinoma.

| BI-RADS Categorization | | |
|---|---|---|
| Clinical Findings | right 1 | left 1 |
| Ultrasound | right 1 | left 4 |
| Mammography | right 1 | left 1 |
| MR Mammography | right 1 | left 4 |
| **BI-RADS Total** | **right 1** | **left 4** |

### Procedure

MR-guided vacuum biopsy was performed because ultrasound could not categorize the suspicious triple lesion seen in MR mammography.

### Histopathology

Focal sclerosing adenosis.

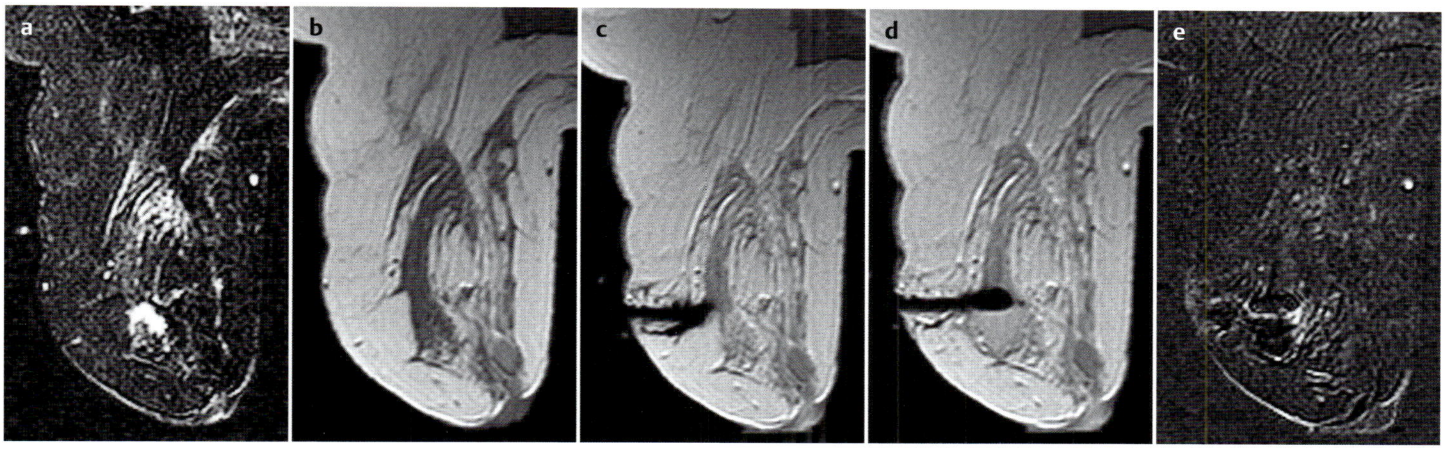


Fig. 65.**8 a – e** MR-guided vacuum biopsy of the left breast.

## Diagnosis

Sclerosing adenosis.

## Treatment

None. Follow-up examination after 6 months.

The differentiation of adenosis from carcinoma presents difficulties in all breast imaging modalities.

**Indication:** Recently discovered lump in the right breast.
**History:** Unremarkable.
**Risk profile:** Breast cancer in mother at the age of 47 years and in grandmother at the age of 62 years.
**Age:** 48 years.

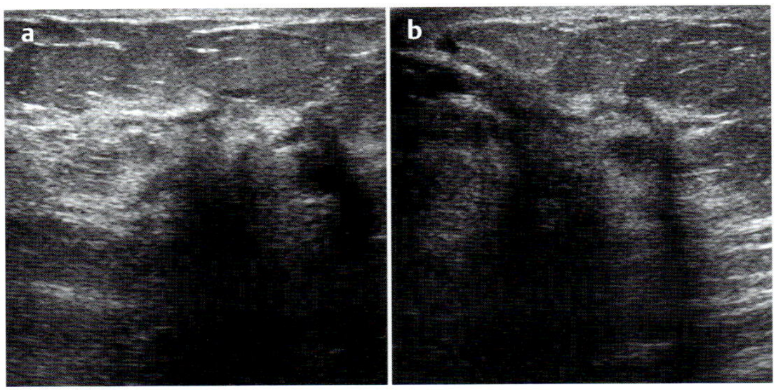


Fig. 66.**1 a, b** Ultrasound images from the area of the palpable mass.

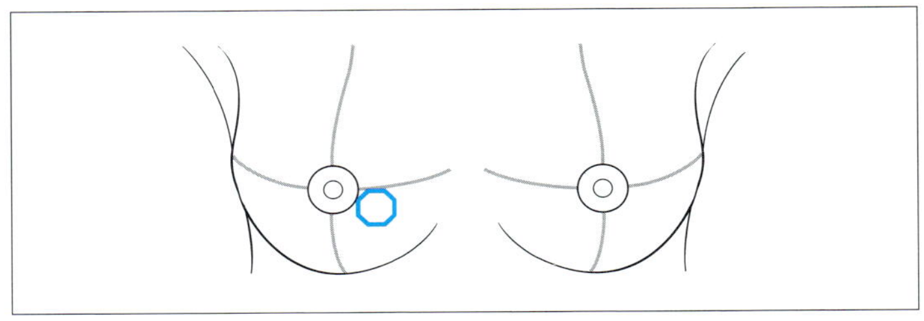

## Clinical Findings

Nodular parenchymal texture. Palpable mass in the deep tissue of the lower inner quadrant of the right breast.

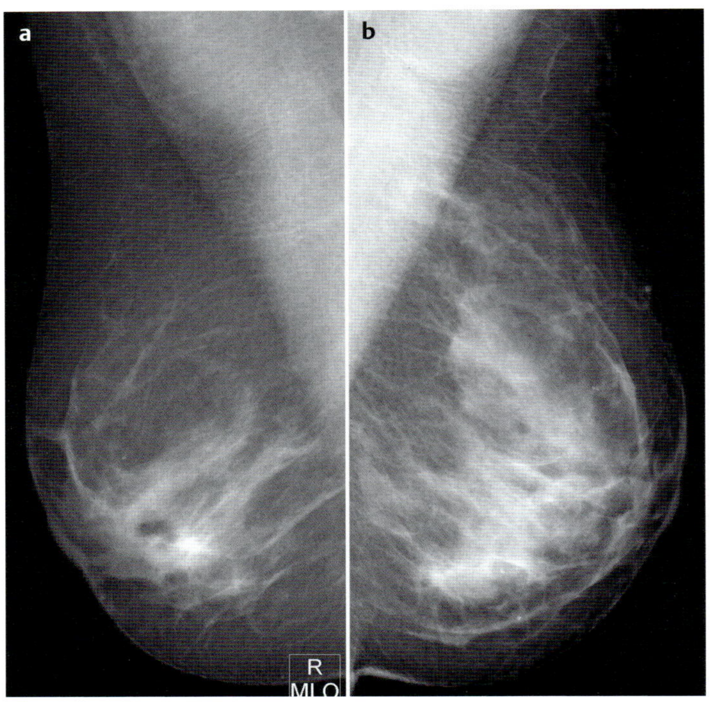


Fig. 66.**2 a, b** Digital mammography, MLO view.

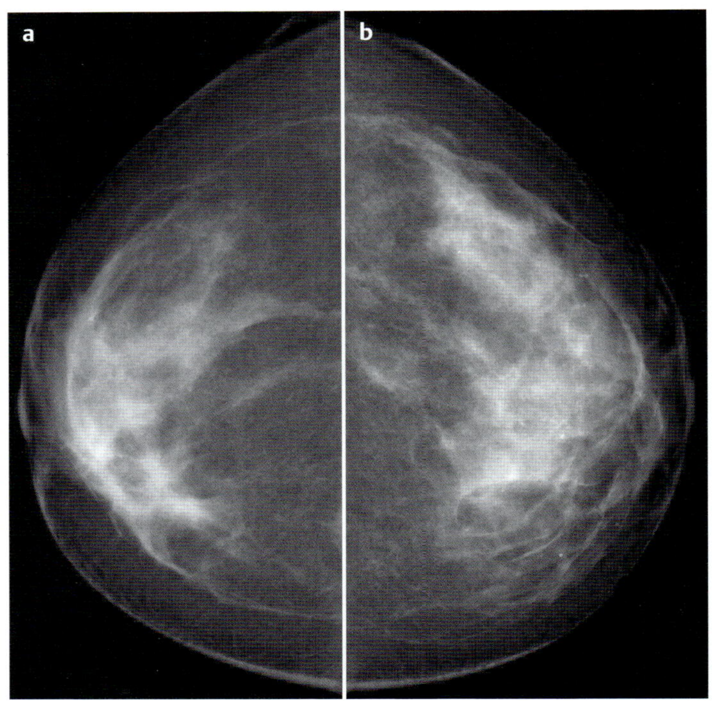


Fig. 66.**3 a, b** Digital mammography, CC view.

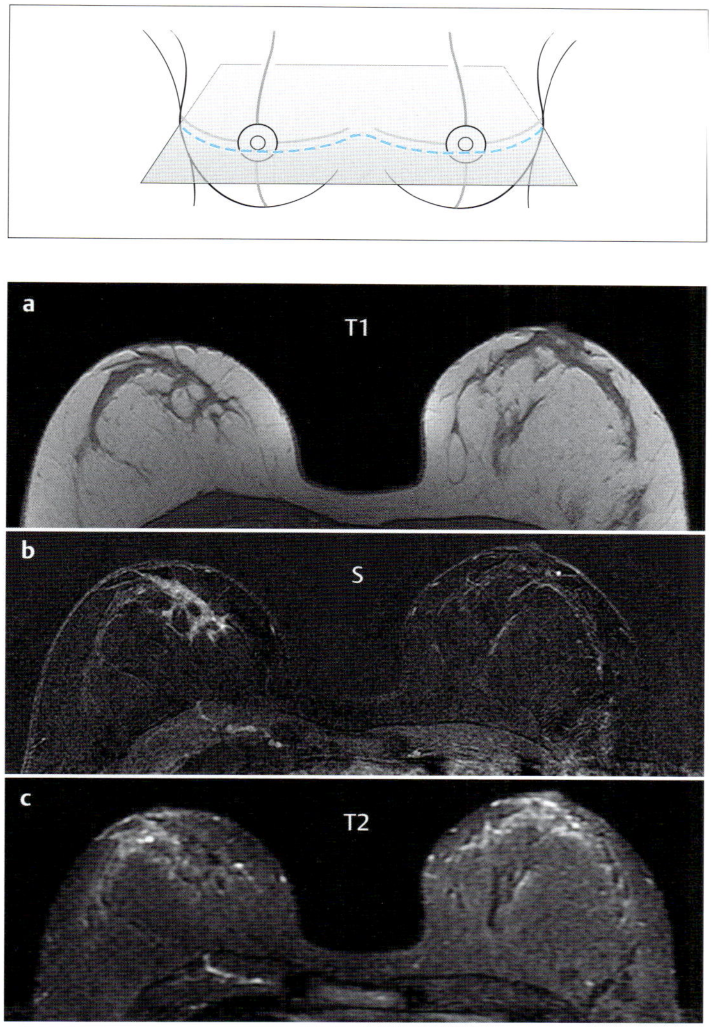


Fig. 66.**4 a – c** Contrast-enhanced MRI of the breasts.

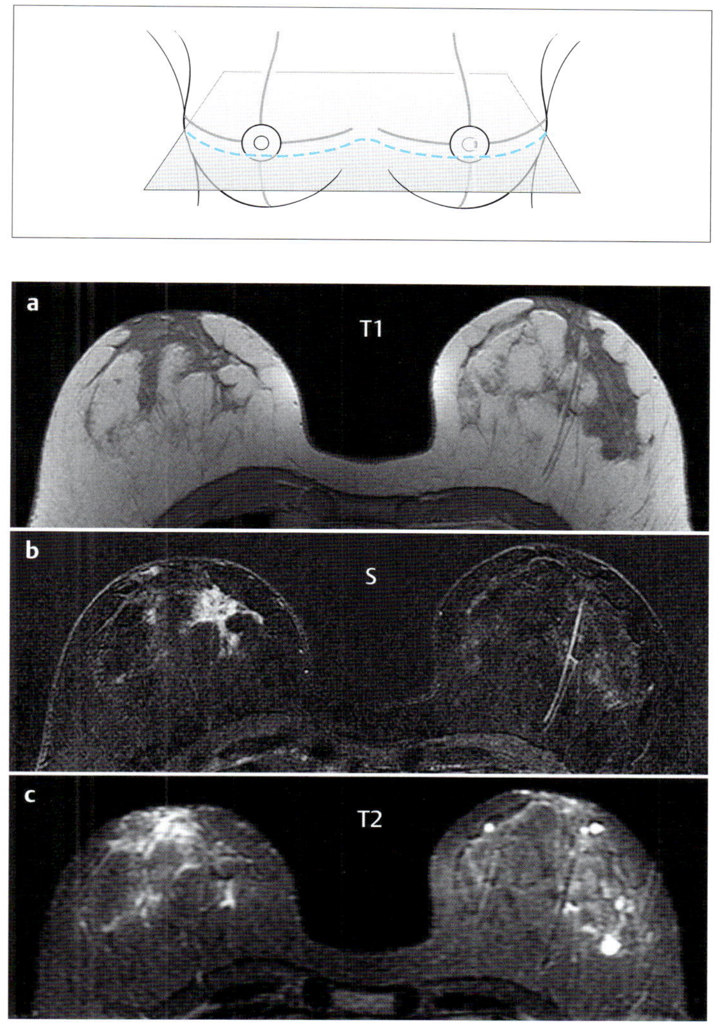


Fig. 66.**5 a – c** Contrast-enhanced MRI of the breasts.

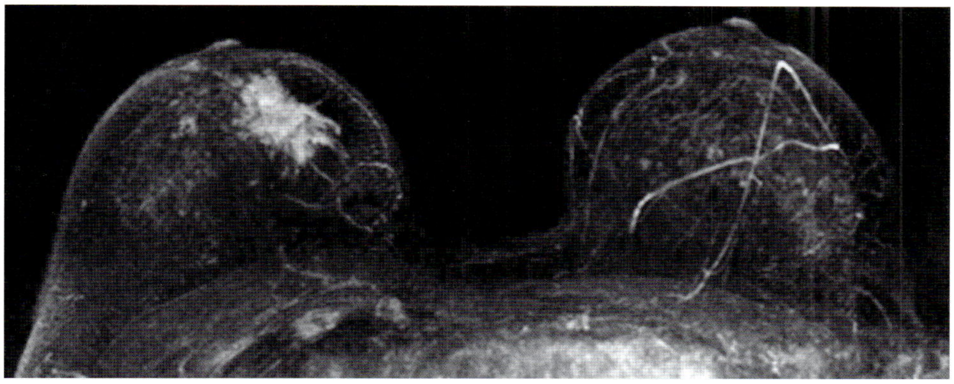

Fig. 66.**6** Contrast-enhanced MR mammography. Maximum intensity projection.

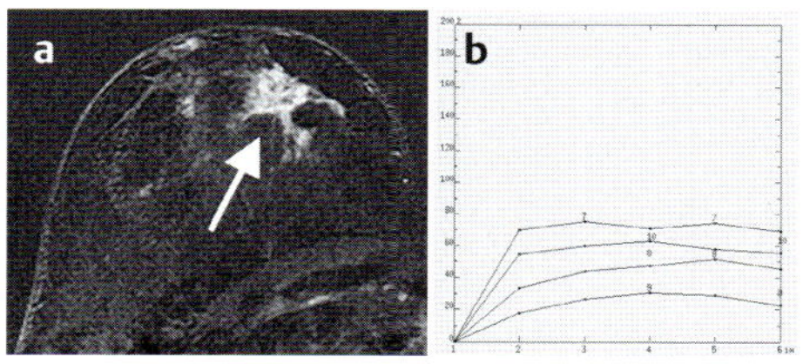


Fig. 66.**7 a, b** Signal-to-time curves of the lesion in the inner quadrants of the right breast (arrow).

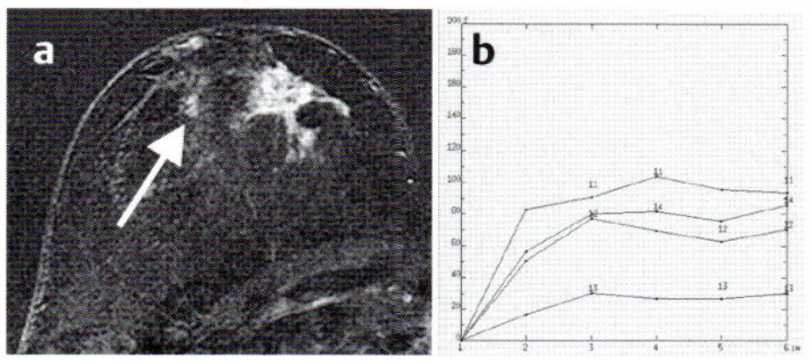


Fig. 66.**8 a, b** Signal-to-time curves of the lesion in the outer quadrants of the right breast (arrow).

?

Please characterize ultrasound, mammography, and MRI findings.
What is your preliminary diagnosis?
What are your next steps?

This case presents the imaging studies of a symptomatic woman. The resistance in the right breast had characteristics of a benign sclerotic gland but was the reason for further examination.

### Ultrasound

In the area of the palpable lump there was a corresponding dendritic, hypoechoic lesion with relatively indistinct echogenic margins and architectural distortion. US BI-RADS right 5.

### Mammography

There was an asymmetric inhomogeneous dense parenchyma ACR type 3, with greater density of the left breast. In the region of the palpable lump, in the lower inner quadrant of the left breast, vague architectural distortion (shrinking sign) was visible. There were no microcalcifications. BI-RADS right 4/left 1. PGMI: CC view P; MLO view G (inframammary fold).

### MR Mammography

Consistent with the palpable lump and the ultrasound findings, an irregular, inhomogeneously enhancing area 4 cm in diameter was depicted. This region had a moderate initial signal increase and a postinitial plateau as well as reduced signal in T2-weighted imaging. 2 cm lateral to this area there was an ill-defined mass (diameter 1 cm) with an initial signal increase of 90%, postinitial plateau, and reduced signal in T2-weighted imaging.
*Note:* An apparent ring enhancement between the inner quadrants of the right breast is actually due to fat contained in the lesion.

**MRI Artifact Category:** 1
**MRI Density Type:** 1

| MRM score | Right breast, inner quadrants | Points | Right breast, outer quadrants | Points |
|---|---|---|---|---|
| **Shape** | irregular | 1 | irregular | 1 |
| **Border** | ill-defined | 1 | ill-defined | 1 |
| **CM Distribution** | inhomogenous | 1 | homogeneous | 0 |
| **Initial Signal Intensity Increase** | moderate | 1 | moderate | 1 |
| **Post-initial Signal Intensity Character** | plateau | 1 | plateau | 1 |
| **MRI score (points)** | | **5** | | **4** |
| **MRI BI-RADS** | | **4** | | **4** |

## → Differential Diagnostic Considerations

In the present case, the change seen in the right breast (lipomatous region in MRI) is "non-mass" rather than circumscribed.

## → Preliminary Diagnosis

Diffuse tumor (lobular carcinoma? DCIS?); inflammatory condition.

| BI-RADS Categorization | | |
|---|---|---|
| Clinical Findings | right 4 | left 1 |
| Ultrasound | right 5 | left 1 |
| Mammography | right 4 | left 1 |
| MR Mammography | right 5 | left 1 |
| **BI-RADS Total** | **right 5** | **left 1** |

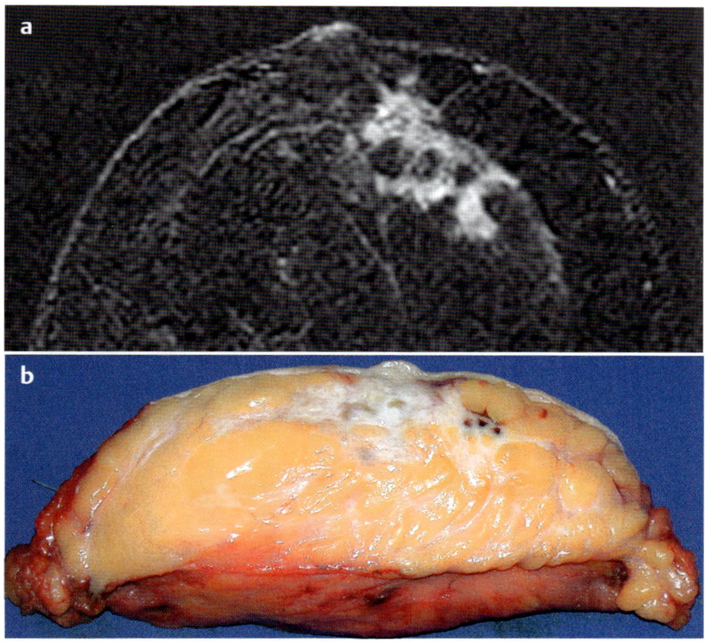


Fig. 66.**9 a, b** Documentation of correlation between MRI findings and macroscopic changes visible in the right breast after removal.

### Procedure

Histopathological analysis of the palpable mass, preferably by US-guided percutaneous core biopsy.

### Histology of the specimen

Invasive lobular carcinoma.

### Further procedure

At the patient's request and bearing in mind the size of the tumor between the inner quadrants of the right breast and the potential multicentricity, mastectomy was performed.

### Histology

Bifocal (45 mm and 9 mm) invasive lobular carcinomas in the right breast. Axillary lymph node status normal.

ILC pT 2, pN0, G2.

### Treatment

Mastectomy of the right breast.

In diffuse invasive lobular carcinoma the glandular tissue is replaced by tumor tissue. For this reason, there is no displacement and a shrinking of the glandular tissue is observed ("shrinking sign"). Fatty tissue remains intact.

**Indication:** Raised tumor marker level.
**History:** Breast conservation therapy and radiation therapy for a breast carcinoma 3 years previously (right breast).
**Risk profile:** Increased by earlier incidence of breast cancer.
**Age:** 64 years.

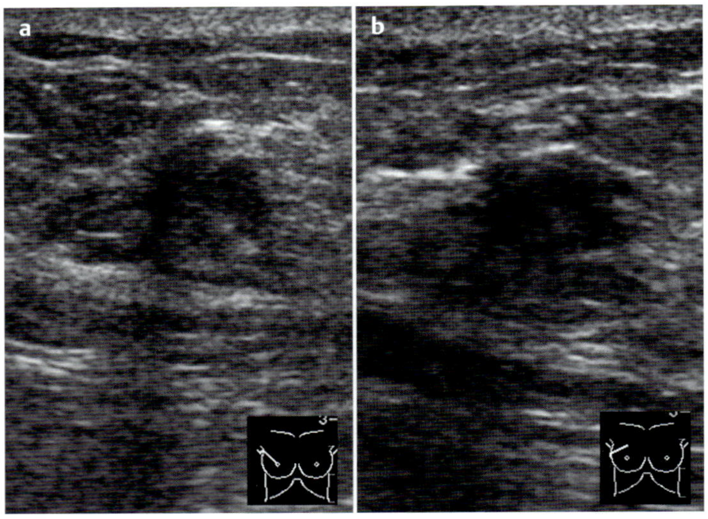

Fig. 67.**1 a, b** Ultrasound images from the area of the scar in the upper outer quadrant of the right breast.

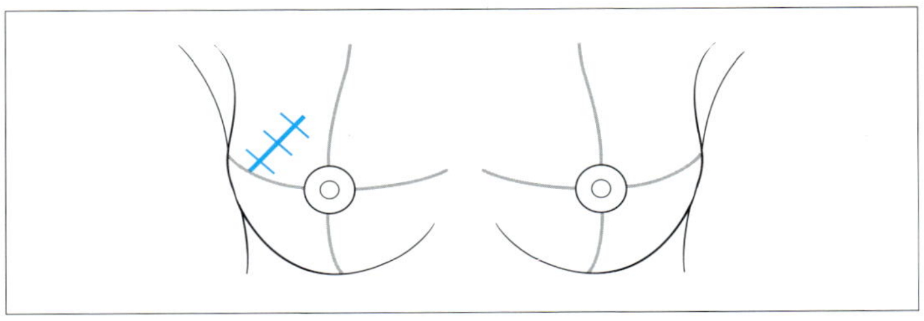

### Clinical Findings

Normal scar. No findings at palpation.

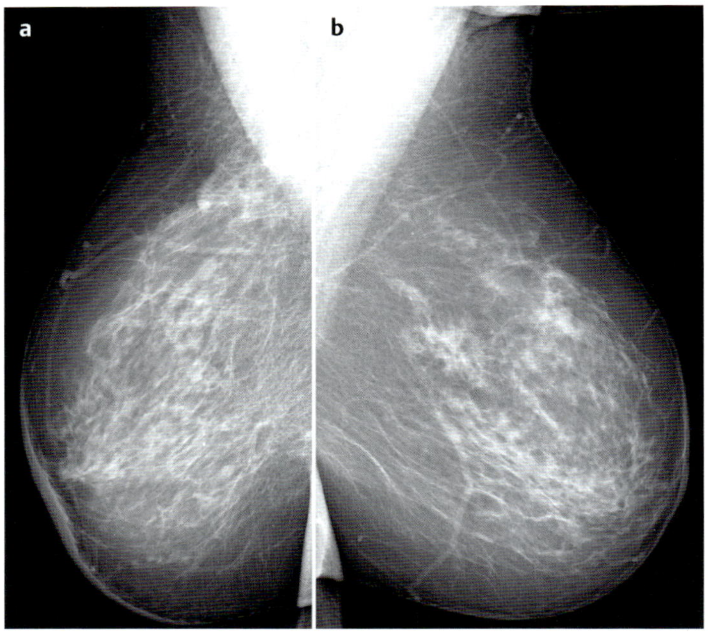

Fig. 67.**2 a, b** Digital mammography, MLO view.

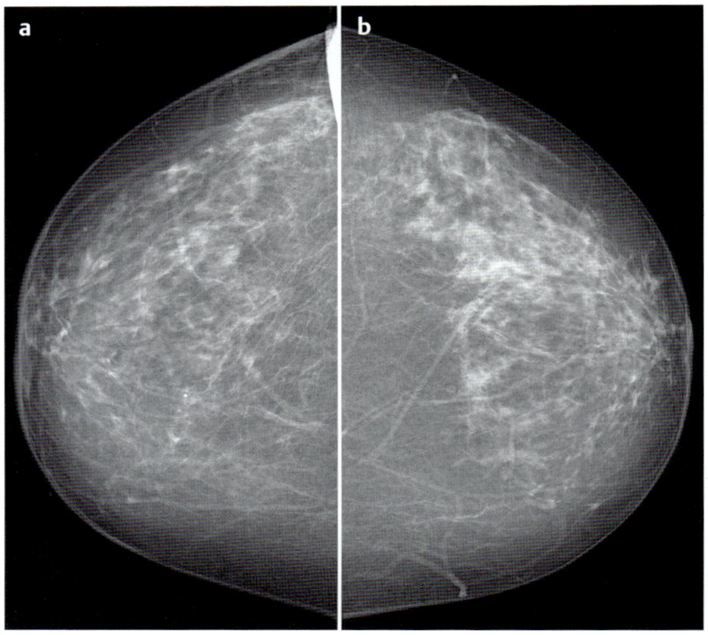

Fig. 67.**3 a, b** Digital mammography, CC view.

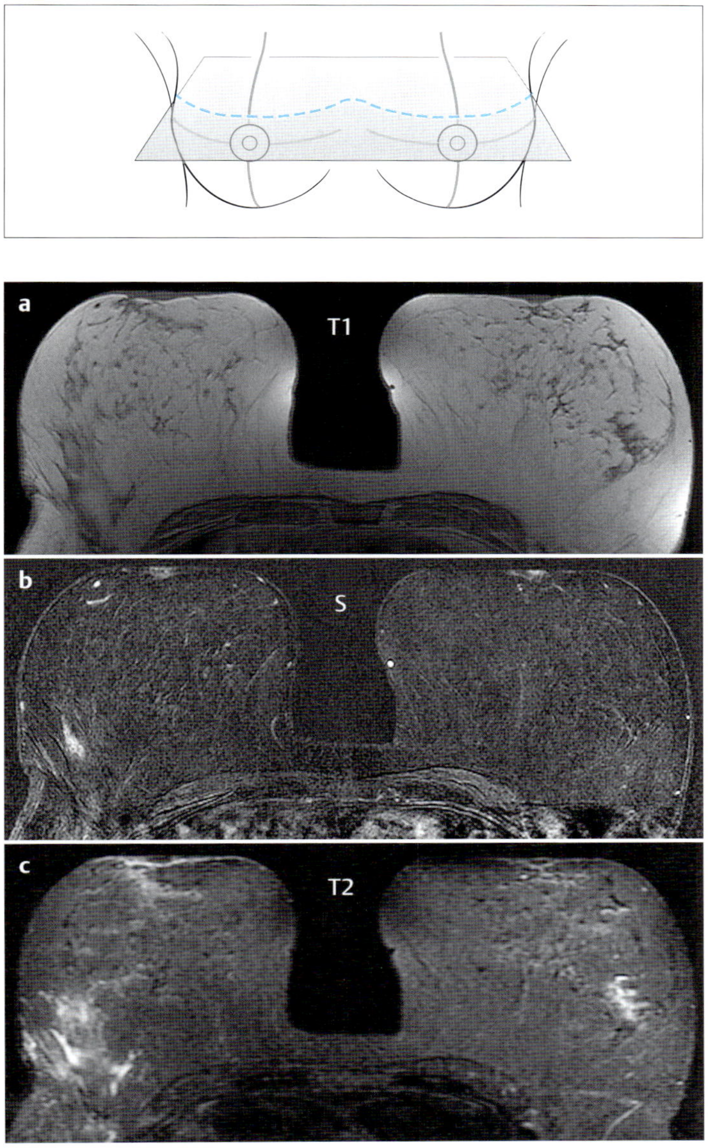


Fig. 67.**4 a – c** Contrast-enhanced MRI of the breasts.

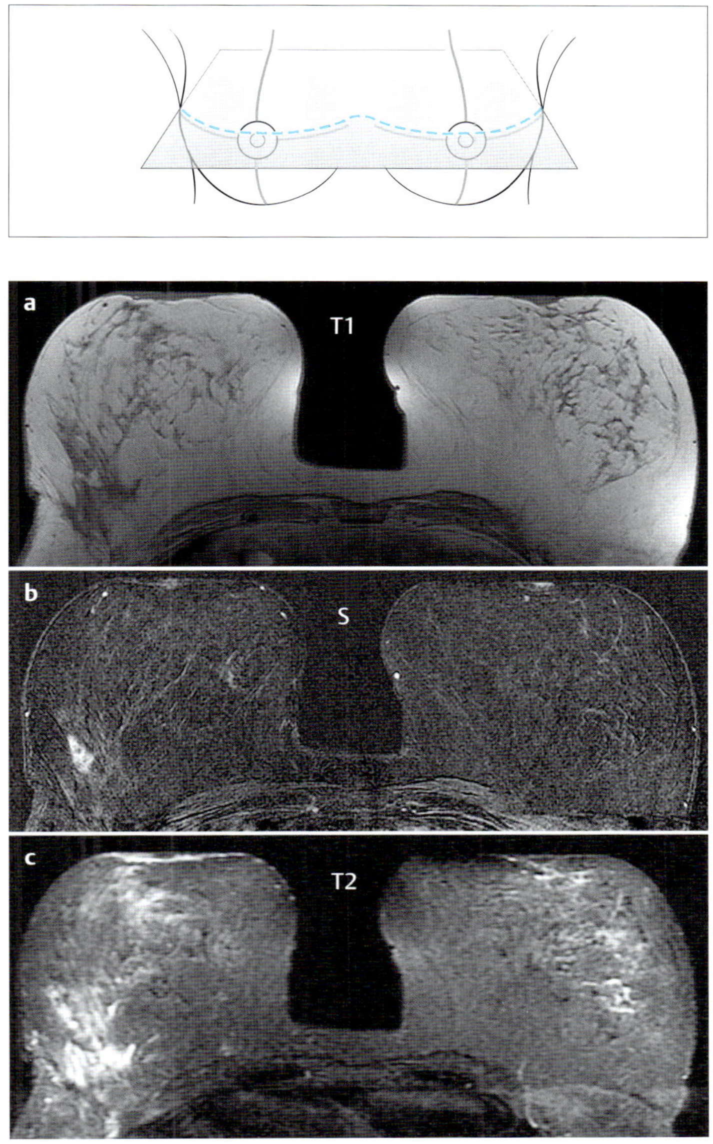


Fig. 67.**5 a – c** Contrast-enhanced MRI of the breasts.

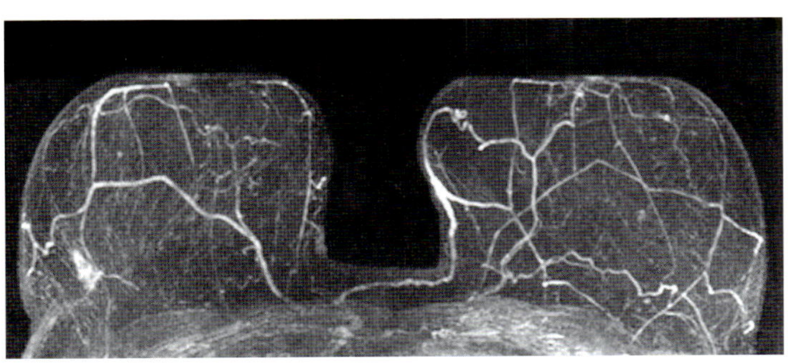

Fig. 67.**6** Contrast-enhanced MR mammography. Maximum intensity projection.

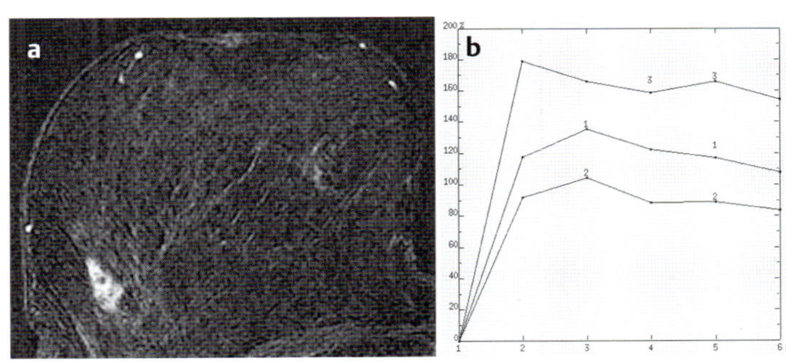


Fig. 67.**7 a, b** Signal-to-time curves.

Please characterize ultrasound, mammography, and MRI findings.
What is your preliminary diagnosis?
What are your next steps?

This case investigates increased tumor marker levels discovered during monitoring of the patient following lumpectomy and radiation therapy for an invasive ductal carcinoma (stage pT1c) 3 years previously.

### Ultrasound

There was an ill-defined, hypoechoic lesion in the upper outer quadrant of the right breast. The surrounding ligamental structures were not displaced. The margins were not hyperechoic and there was no distal echo shadowing. US BI-RADS 3.

### Mammography

The parenchyma was bilaterally symmetric and fibroglandular in texture, ACR type 2. Slight postoperative architectural distortion was seen in the upper outer quadrant of the right breast. There were no suspicious masses or densities and no microcalcifications. BI-RADS right 3/left 1.PGMI: CC view I (lateral superimposition of the shoulder, imaging not repeated); MLO view M (inframammary angle, pronounced abdominal skin fold, pectoralis).

### MR Mammography

MRI demonstrated a segmental, ill-defined inhomogeneously enhancing mass measuring 2 cm between the outer quadrants of the right breast. This lesion showed marked initial signal increase, postinitial washout, and decreased signal in T2-weighted imaging. *Note:* Because of the ptosis of the large breasts and the prone position of the examination, the areola is depicted at the level of the lumpectomy scar in the upper outer quadrant of the left breast.

**MRI Artifact Category:** 1
**MRI Density Type:** 1

| MRM score | Finding | Points |
|---|---|---|
| **Shape** | irregular/segmental | 1 |
| **Border** | ill-defined | 1 |
| **CM Distribution** | inhomogeneous | 1 |
| **Initial Signal Intensity Increase** | strong | 2 |
| **Post-initial Signal Intensity Character** | wash-out | 2 |
| **MRI score (points)** | | **7** |
| **MRI BI-RADS** | | **5** |

### → Differential Diagnosis

Local tumor relapse, focal (e.g., granulomatous) mastitis, focal adenosis.

| BI-RADS Categorization | | |
|---|---|---|
| Clinical Findings | right 1 | left 1 |
| Ultrasound | right 3 | left 1 |
| Mammography | right 3 | left 1 |
| MR Mammography | right 5 | left 1 |
| **BI-RADS Total** | **right 5** | **left 1** |

### Procedure

MR-guided vacuum biopsy of the lesion in the upper outer quadrant of the right breast.

### Histology

Invasive ductal carcinoma.

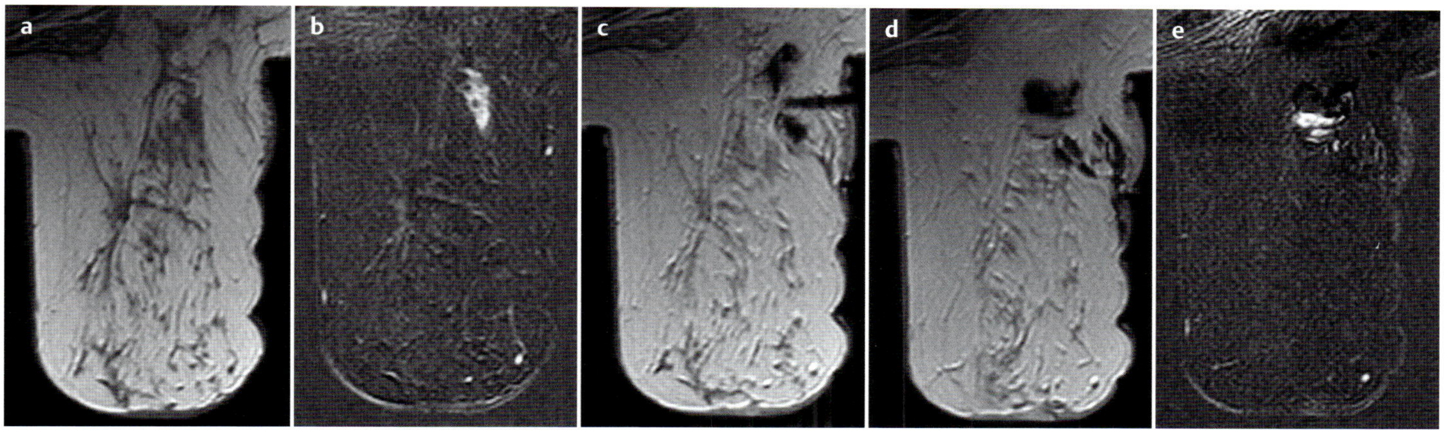


Fig. 67.**8** a–e MR-guided vacuum biopsy of the right breast.
**a** Precontrast T1-weighted image.
**b** Reproducibility of the segmental enhancement in subtraction image.
**c** Coaxial needle after local anesthesia.
**d** Findings after biopsy in precontrast T1-weighted image.
**e** Subtraction image after further contrast administration with enhancement due to bleeding. No residual enhancing tumor component.

### Diagnosis

Local tumor relapse after breast conservation therapy.

### Treatment

Palliative lumpectomy, since liver metastases were discovered in renewed staging.

Enhancements in the operated area after breast conservation therapy are always suspicious for local tumor relapse. Such enhancements can, however, also be caused by focal inflammation (giving false-positive MRI findings).

**Indication:** Sonographically suspicious lesion in the left breast discovered in screening performed elsewhere.
**History:** Unremarkable.
**Risk profile:** No increased risk.
**Age:** 76 years.

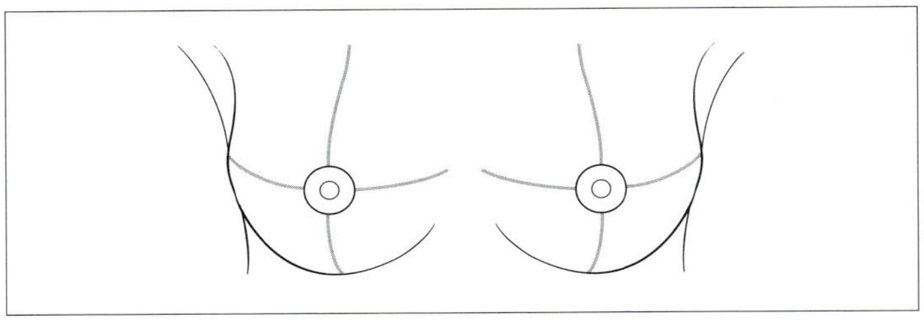

## Clinical Findings

No findings.

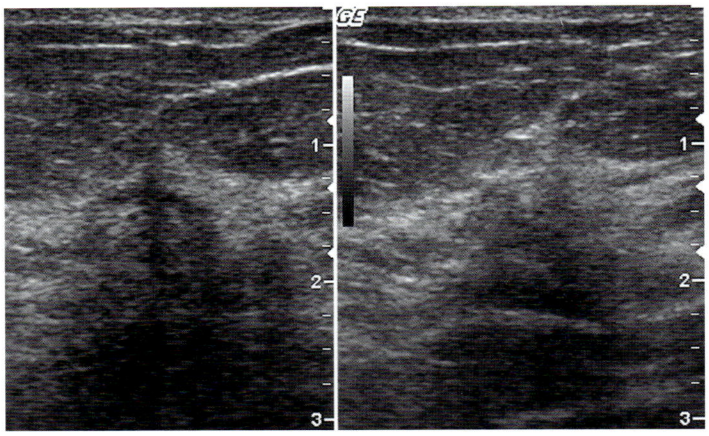

Fig. 68.**1** Ultrasound between the outer quadrants of the left breast.

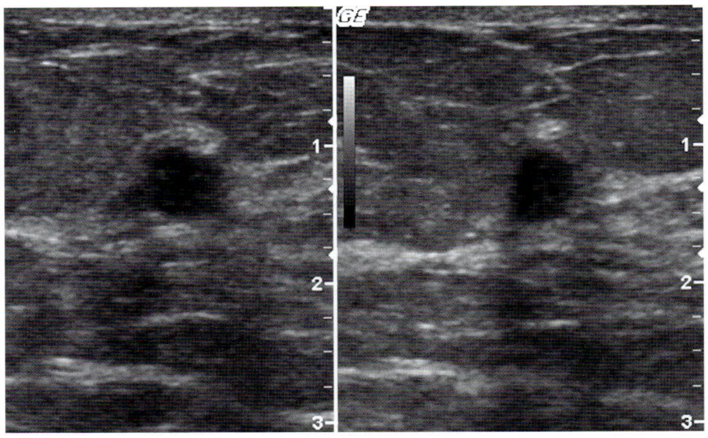

Fig. 68.**2** Ultrasound between the inner quadrants of the left breast.

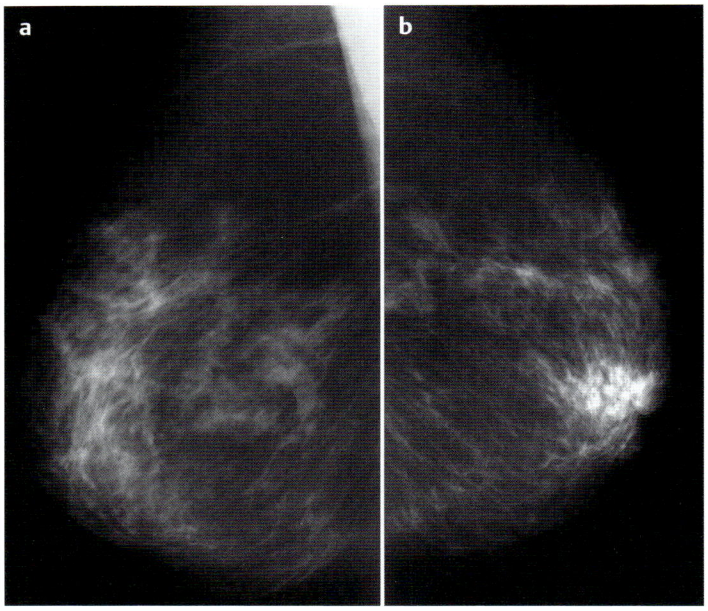


Fig. 68.**3 a, b** Conventional mammography, ML view [imaging not performed by authors].

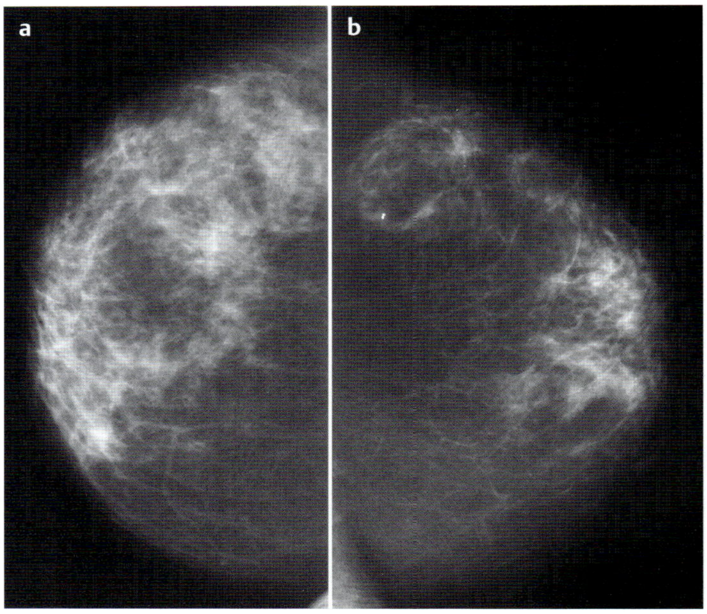


Fig. 68.**4 a, b** Conventional mammography, CC view [imaging not performed by authors].

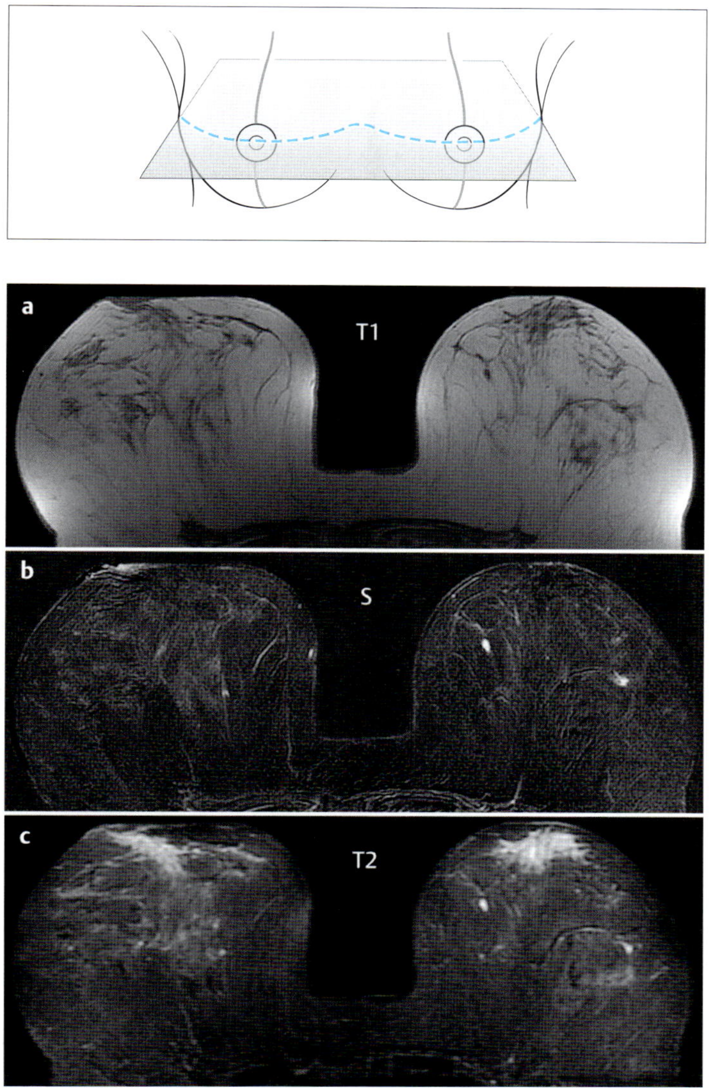


Fig. 68.**5 a – c** Contrast-enhanced MRI of the breasts.

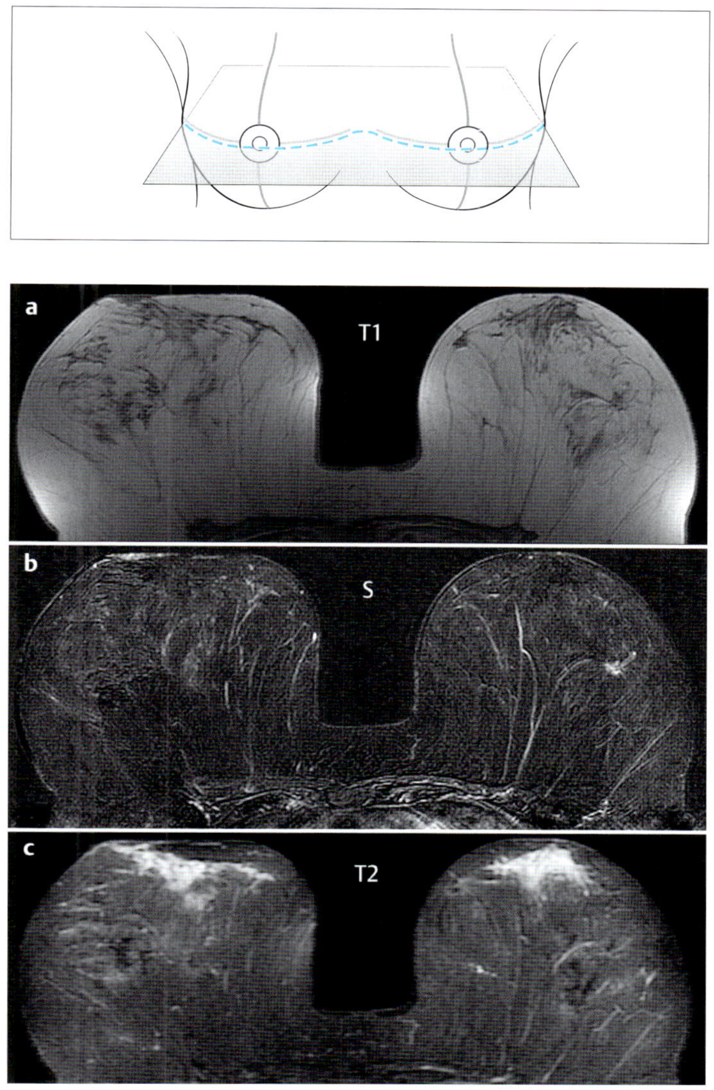


Fig. 68.**6 a – c** Contrast-enhanced MRI of the breasts.

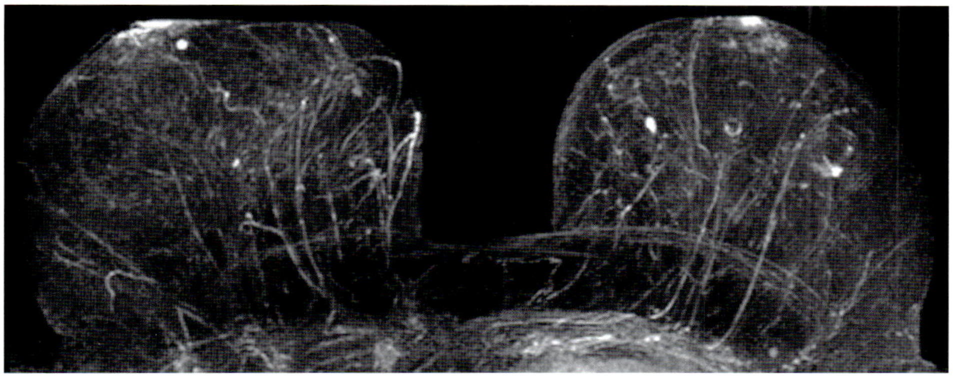

Fig. 68.**7** Contrast-enhanced MR mammography. Maximum intensity projection.

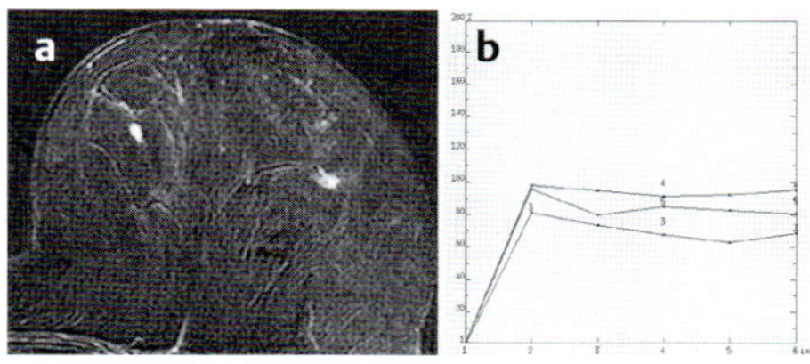


Fig. 68.**8 a, b** Signal-to-time curves, finding between outer quadrants.

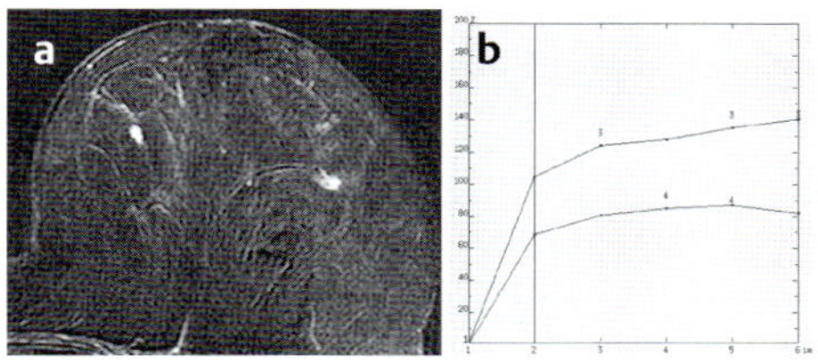


Fig. 68.**9 a, b** Signal-to-time curves, finding between inner quadrants.

Please characterize ultrasound, mammography, and MRI findings.
What is your preliminary diagnosis?
What are your next steps?

This case investigates a suspicious finding in an ultrasound examination performed for screening purposes in another clinic.

### Ultrasound

Between the outer quadrants of the left breast a hypoechoic, lobulated lesion (diameter 4 mm) with lateral echo shadowing and indeterminate distal echo pattern was visible. There was no echogenic margin and no architectural distortion. Between the lower quadrants of the left breast a cyst measuring 1 cm was detected. US BI-RADS left 3.

### Mammography

Mammograms showed an inhomogeneously dense parenchyma, ACR type 3. Particularly between the outer quadrants of the left breast, there were no signs of a lesion. BI-RADS right 1, left 1. PGMI: CC view G (difference in exposure); not defined for ML view.

### MR Mammography

An irregular, well-defined, homogeneously enhancing lesion 5 mm in diameter was demonstrated in MRI between the outer quadrants of the left breast. This lesion had initial signal increase of 95% and a postinitial plateau as well as reduced signal in T2-weighted imaging. Another well-defined homogeneously enhancing lesion 5 mm in diameter was depicted between the inner quadrants of the left breast. This had an initial signal increase of 120% and continuing signal increase as well as an increased signal in T2-weighted imaging. MIP showed a ring enhancement with unsuspicious signal curve and high signal in T2-weighted imaging, corresponding to a complicated cyst.

**MRI Artifact Category:** 1
**MRI Density Type:** 2

| MRM score | Left breast, between outer quadrants | Points | Left breast, between inner quadrants | Points |
|---|---|---|---|---|
| **Shape** | irregular | 1 | oval | 0 |
| **Border** | well-defined | 0 | well-defined | 0 |
| **CM Distribution** | homogeneous | 0 | homogeneous | 0 |
| **Initial Signal Intensity Increase** | moderate | 1 | strong | 2 |
| **Post-initial Signal Intensity Character** | plateau | 1 | continuous | 0 |
| **MRI score (points)** | | **3** | | **2** |
| **MRI BI-RADS** | | **3** | | **2** |

### → Differential Diagnosis

Left breast, between outer quadrants: Adenosis, radial scar, carcinoma (tubular?).
Left breast, between inner quadrants: Fibroadenoma, adenoma, papilloma, carcinoma.

| BI-RADS Categorization | | |
|---|---|---|
| Clinical Findings | right 1 | left 1 |
| Ultrasound | right 1 | left 3 |
| Mammography | right 1 | left 1 |
| MR Mammography | right 1 | left 3 |
| **BI-RADS Total** | **right 1** | **left 3** |

### Procedure

Follow-up examination after 6 months was indicated with regard to the findings in MRI and ultrasound (both categorized BI-RADS 3).

### Diagnosis (without histopathological confirmation)

Left lateral: Adenosis
Left medial: Fibroadenoma

### Treatment

Follow-up after 6 months (US and MRI), perhaps also x-ray mammography because of the nonstandard view of the images available (ML) and the imperfect quality of the CC view images.

There is a second part to this case. You might be curious.
But first: What do you make of the hypervascularized lesion seen in the right breast in MRI (see maximum intensity projection, Fig. 68.**7**)?

**Indication:** Follow-up of findings categorized BI-RADS 3 in the left breast.
**History:** Unremarkable.
**Risk profile:** No increased risk.
**Age:** 77 years.

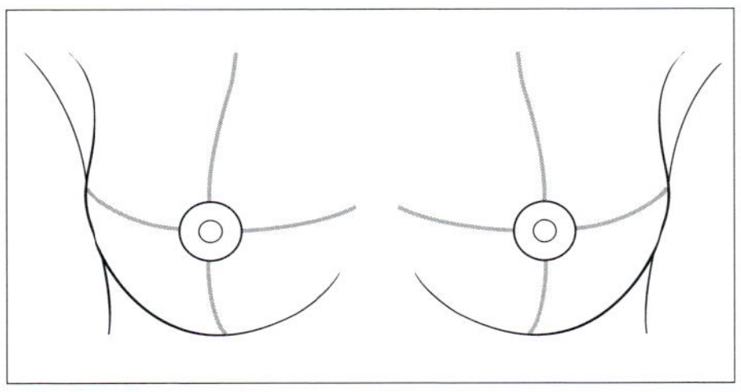

### Clinical Findings

Normal.

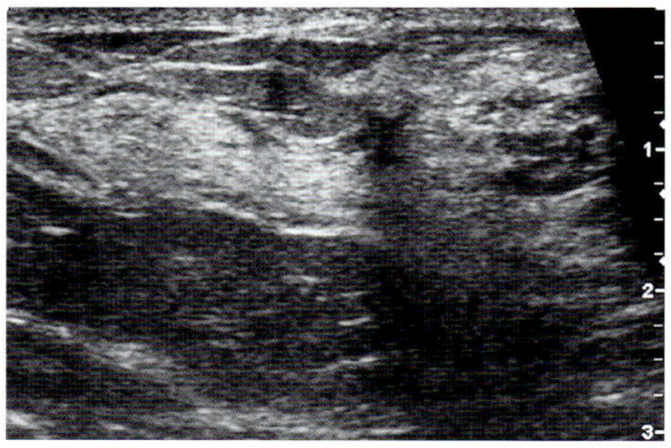

Fig. 69.1 **a, b** Ultrasound between the outer quadrants of the left breast.

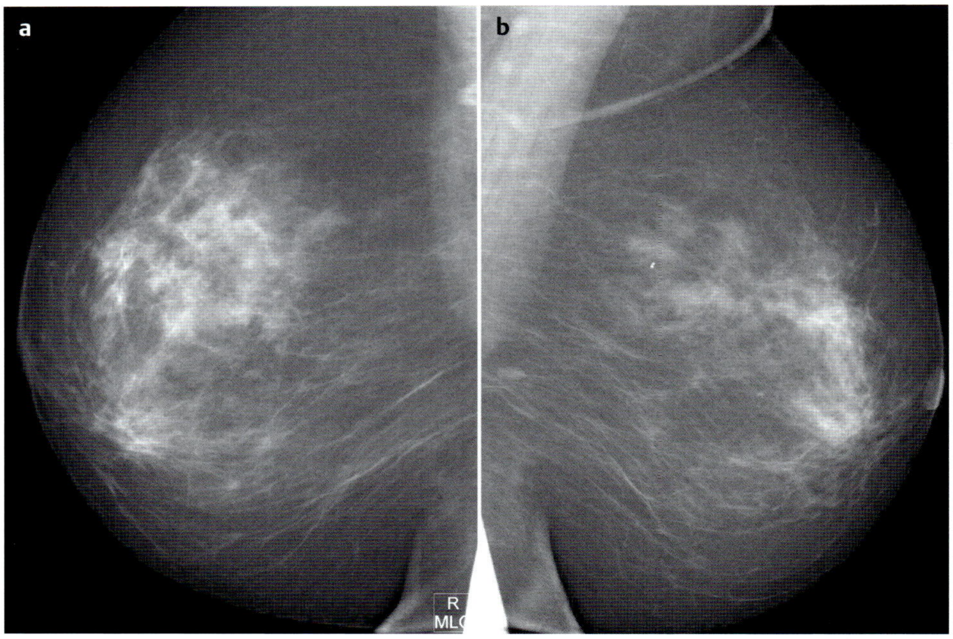


Fig. 69.2 **a, b** Digital mammography, MLO view.

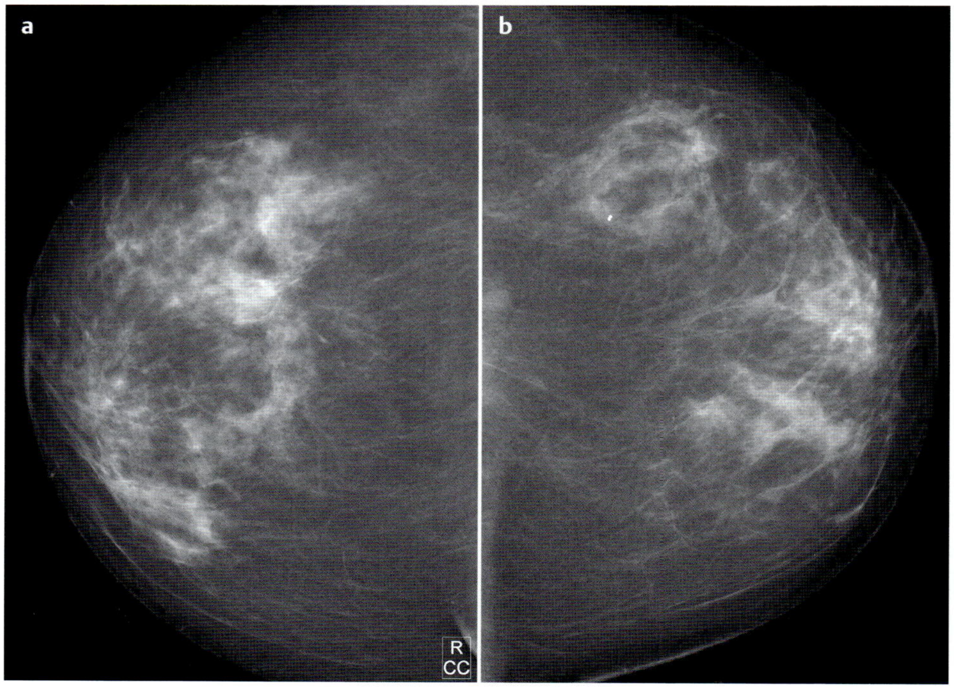


Fig. 69.3 **a, b** Digital mammography, CC view.

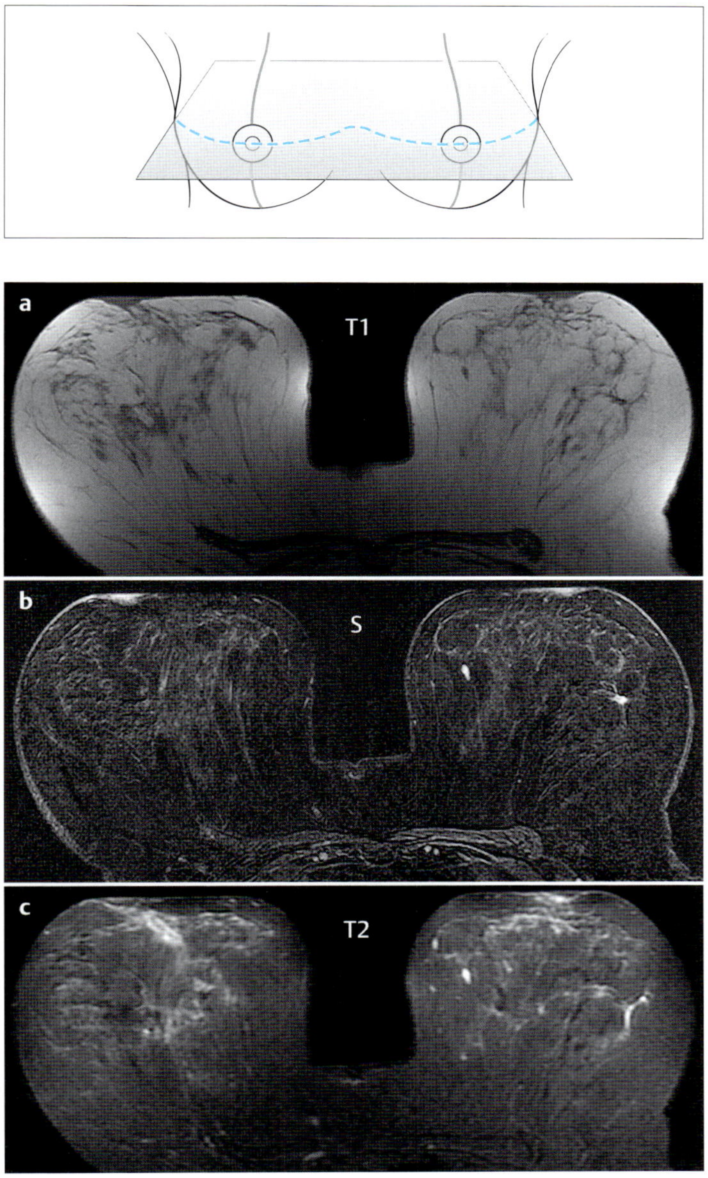


Fig. 69.**4 a – c** Contrast-enhanced MRI of the breasts.

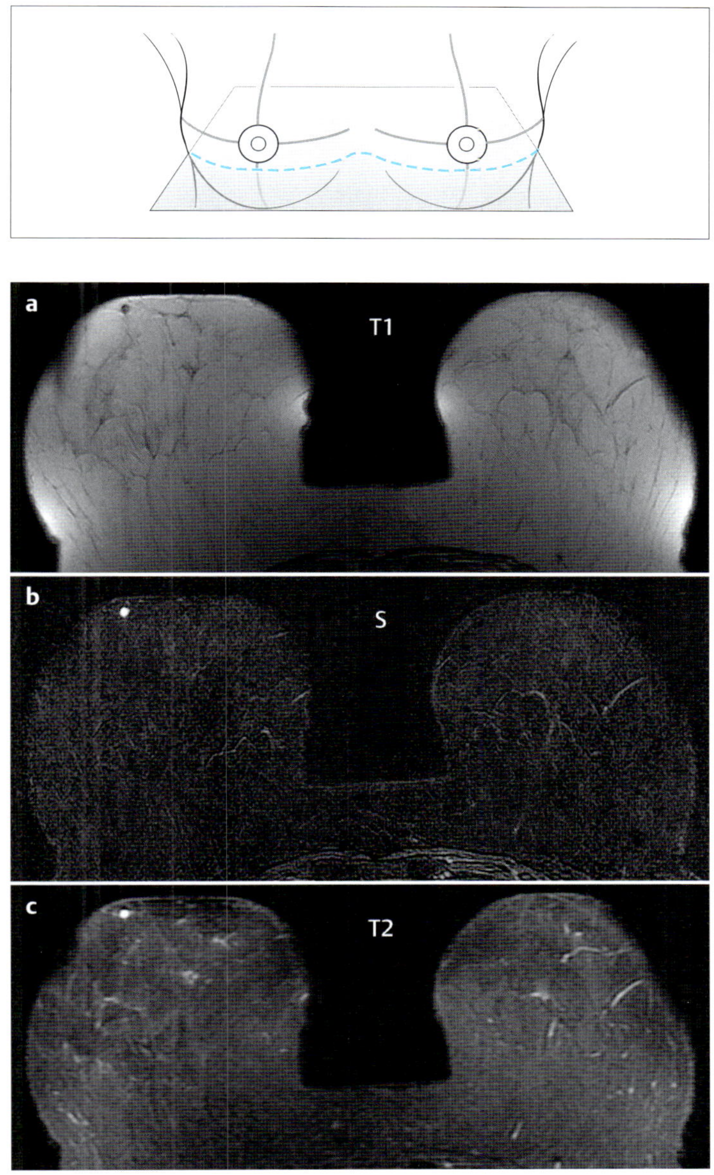


Fig. 69.**5 a – c** Contrast-enhanced MRI of the breasts.

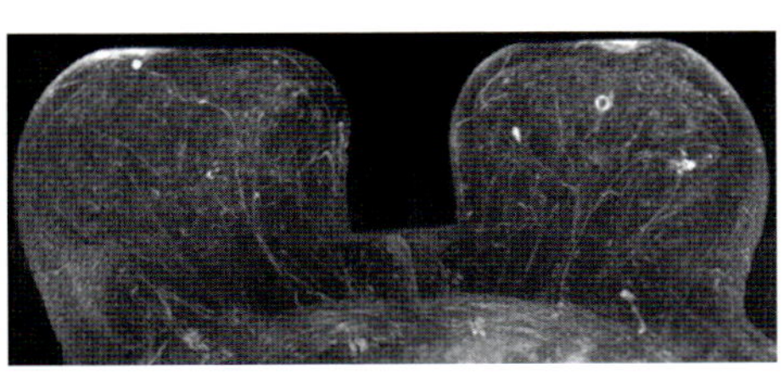

Fig. 69.**6** Contrast-enhanced MR mammography. Maximum intensity projection.

Please characterize ultrasound, mammography, and MRI findings.
What is your preliminary diagnosis?
What are your next steps?

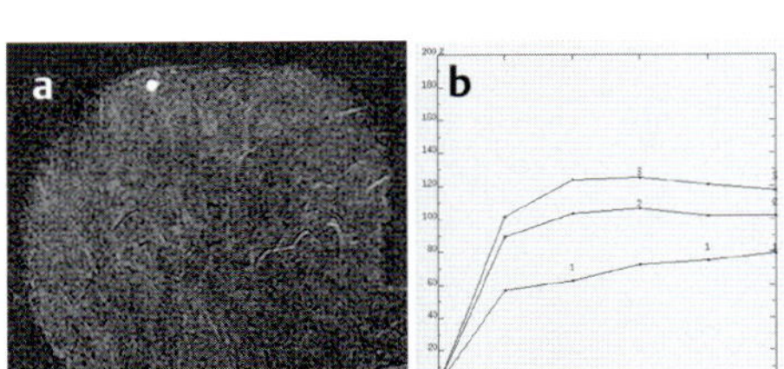


Fig. 89.**7 a, b** Signal-to-time curves, right breast.

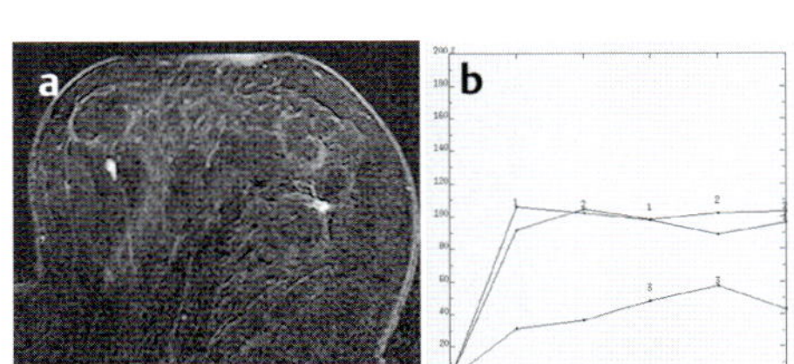


Fig. 69.**8 a, b** Signal-to-time curves, left outer quadrants.

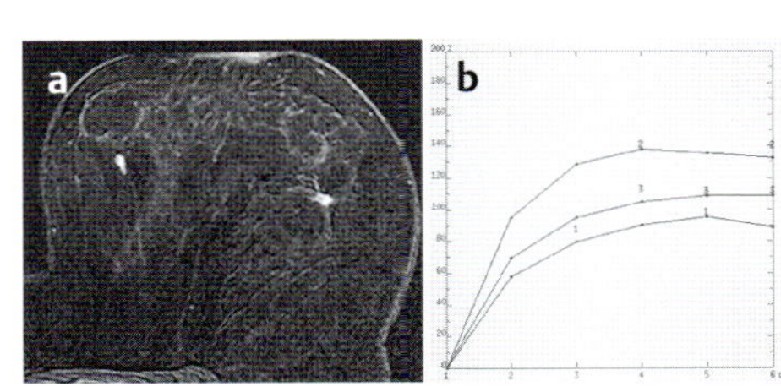


Fig. 69.**9 a, b** Signal-to-time curves, left inner quadrants.

This case shows the follow-up after 6 months of a lesion depicted in sonography and MRI between the outer quadrants of the left breast (Case 68).

### Ultrasound

Again, a hypoechoic, irregular lesion (diameter 4 mm) was seen between the outer quadrants of the left breast. Sonography depicted this lesion only in one plane. A slight increase in possible spiculations was seen. There was also distal shadowing. There were no echogenic margins and there was no architectural distortion. A hypoechoic lesion between the inner quadrants of the left breast (diameter 5 mm) and a cyst (diameter 1 cm) between the lower quadrants of the left breast were visible (these findings were unchanged since the previous examination). US BI-RADS left 4.

### Mammography

Inhomogeneously dense parenchyma, ACR type 3. Particularly between the outer quadrants of the left breast, there were still no signs of suspicious lesions. BI-RADS right 1/left 1. PGMI: CC view G (medial skin fold); MLO view M (angle of right pectoralis muscle, left nipple, inframammary fold).

### MR Mammography

There was an irregular, well-defined lesion between the outer quadrants of the left breast (diameter 5 mm) with homogeneous contrast uptake, an initial signal increase of 110%, and a postinitial plateau as well as reduced signal in T2-weighted imaging. There was also a well-defined lesion measuring 5 mm between the inner quadrants of the left breast with homogeneous enhancement, an initial signal increase of 130%, and a postinitial continuing signal increase as well as increased signal in T2-weighted imaging. Also, unchanged since the previous examination, MRI depicted a well-defined lesion (diameter 4 mm) in the lower outer quadrant of the right breast with an initial signal increase of 130% and a post-initial plateau as well as increased signal in T2-weighted imaging. In maximum intensity projection there was a ring enhancement behind the left nipple with unremarkable signal curve and increased signal in T2-weighted imaging (no quantification, complicated cyst).

**MRI Artifact Category:** 1
**MRI Density Type:** 2

| MRM score | Right | Points | Left breast, between outer quadrants | Points | Left breast, between inner quadrants | Points |
|---|---|---|---|---|---|---|
| **Shape** | round | 0 | irregular | 1 | oval | 0 |
| **Border** | well-defined | 0 | well-defined | 0 | well-defined | 0 |
| **CM Distribution** | homogeneous | 0 | homogeneous | 0 | homogeneous | 0 |
| **Initial Signal Intensity Increase** | strong | 2 | strong | 2 | strong | 2 |
| **Post-initial Signal Intensity Character** | plateau | 1 | plateau | 1 | continuous | 0 |
| **MRI score (points)** | | **3** | | **4** | | **2** |
| **MRI BI-RADS** | | **3** | | **4** | | **2** |

### → Differential Diagnosis

Left lateral: Adenosis, carcinoma.
Left medial: Fibroadenoma, adenoma, papilloma.
Left behind nipple: Complicated cyst.
Right: Fibroadenoma, adenoma, papilloma.

| BI-RADS Categorization | | |
|---|---|---|
| Clinical Findings | right 1 | left 1 |
| Ultrasound | right 1 | left 4 |
| Mammography | right 1 | left 1 |
| MR Mammography | right 3 | left 4 |
| **BI-RADS Total** | right 3 | left 4 |

### Procedure

Although there was no increase in size, the findings appear a little more suspicious in ultrasound and MRI (BI-RADS 4) than 6 months previously. For this reason, a histopathological investigation was indicated.

### Method

MR-guided vacuum biopsy of the lesion between the outer quadrants of the left breast. Histology: Tubular carcinoma.

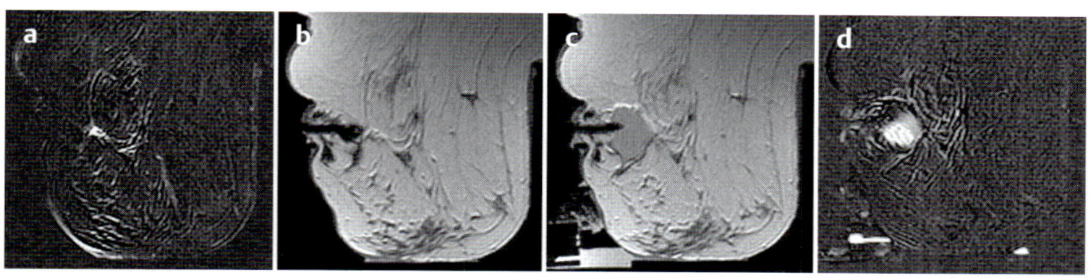

Fig. 69.**10 a – d** MR-guided vacuum core biopsy.
**a** Subtraction image showing lesion.
**b** Coaxial needle.
**c** Biopsy area after removal of tissue specimens.
**d** Final subtraction image after further contrast administration showing enhancement due to bleeding in the resection cavity.

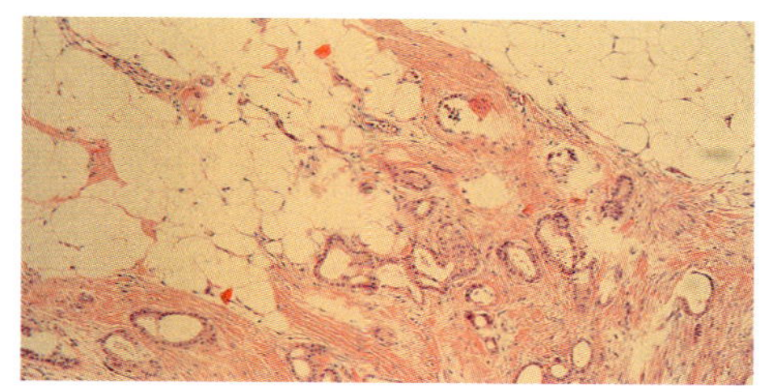

Fig. 69.**11** Histology of the left breast: tubular carcinoma.

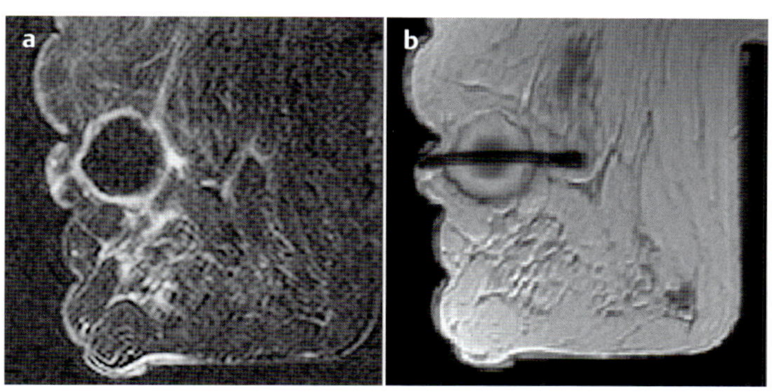

Fig. 69.**12 a, b** Preoperative hook-wire localization of the lesion between the outer quadrants of the left breast after core biopsy.

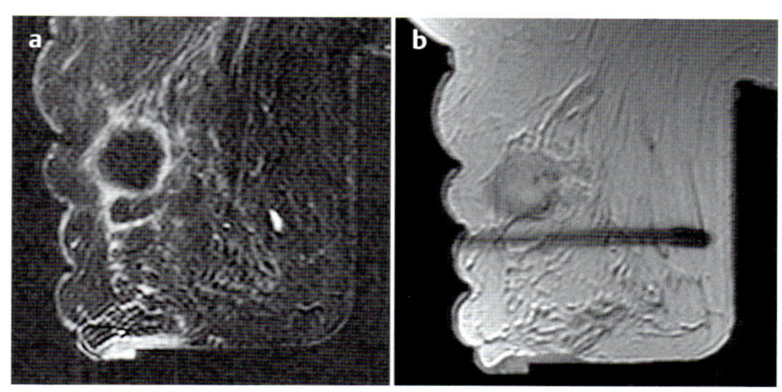

Fig. 69.**13 a – c** Preoperative hook-wire localization of the second lesion between the inner quadrants of the left breast.

### Histology

Tubular carcinoma (diameter 7 mm).

TC pT1b, pN0, G1 left lateral + fibroadenoma left medial.

### Treatment

Breast conservation therapy of the left breast.

A 6-months delay in diagnosis does not negatively affect prognosis. Moreover, G1 graded tumors, such as in the present case, are known to grow very slowly.

**Indication:** Open biopsy of microcalcifications in the right breast was recommended elsewhere.
**History:** Unremarkable.
**Risk profile:** No increased risk.
**Age:** 49 years.

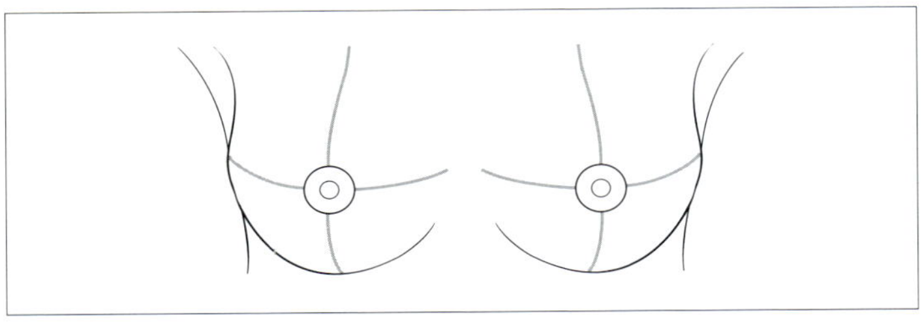

### Clinical Findings

No findings.

### Ultrasound (not shown)

Normal.

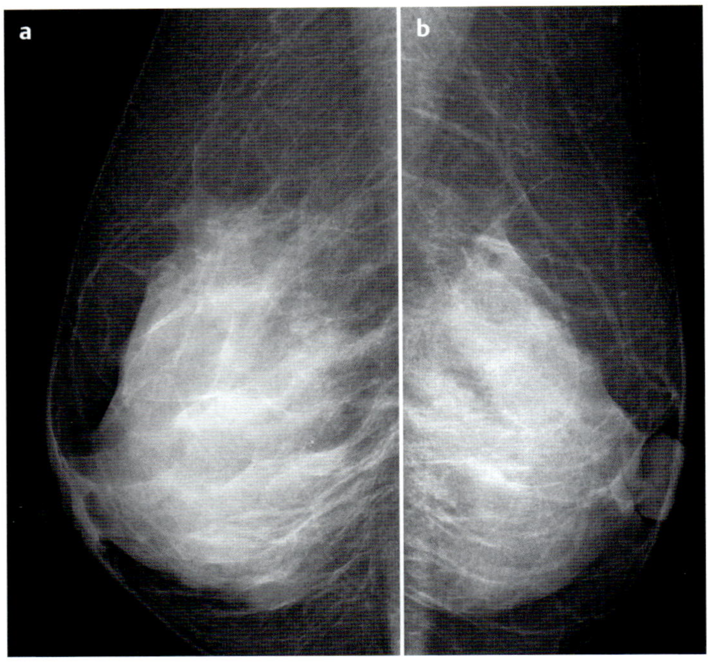


Fig. 70.**1 a, b** Digital mammography, MLO view [imaging not performed by authors].

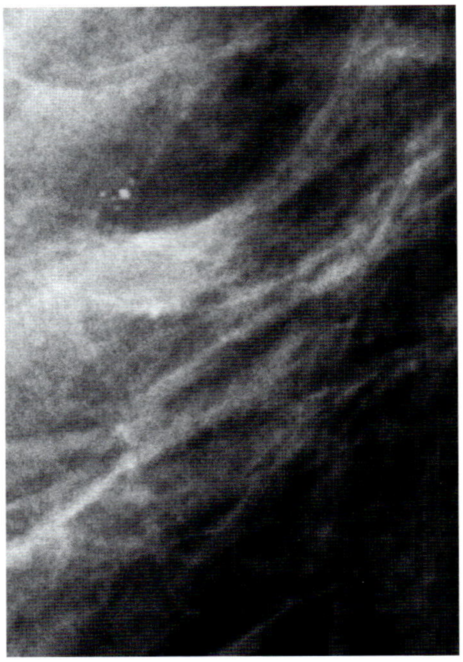

Fig. 70.**2** Digital mammography (MLO), magnification view of the right breast.

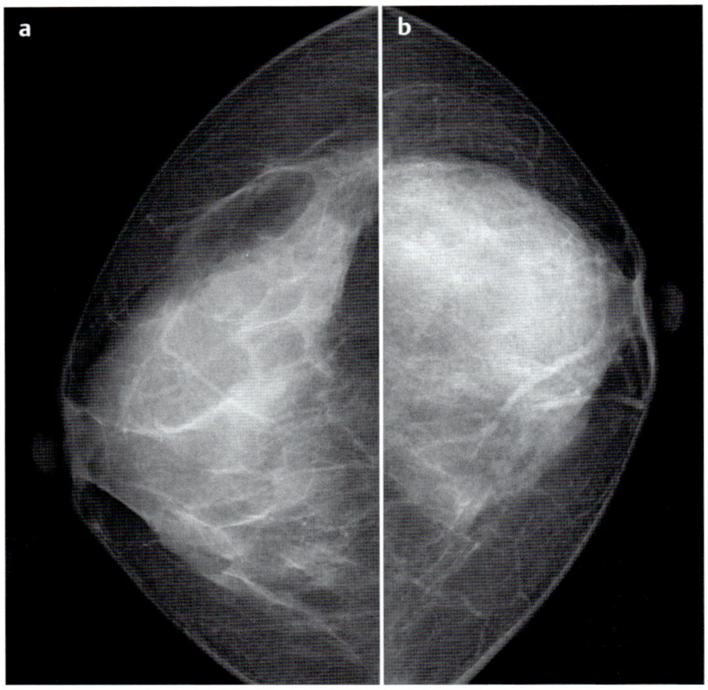


Fig. 70.**3 a, b** Digital mammography, CC view [imaging not performed by authors].

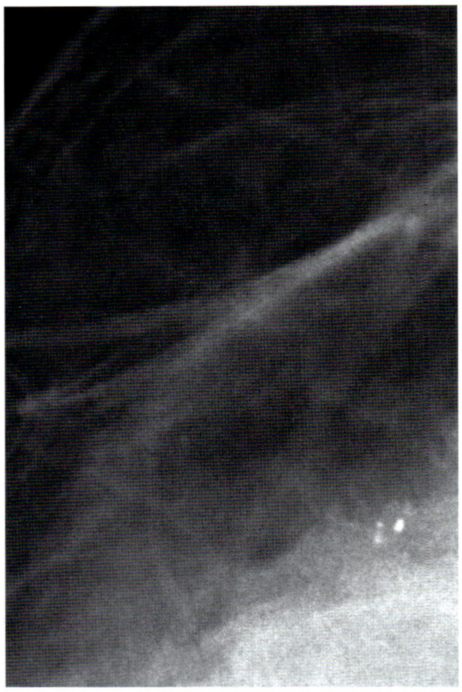

Fig. 70.**4** Digital mammography (CC), magnification view of the right breast.

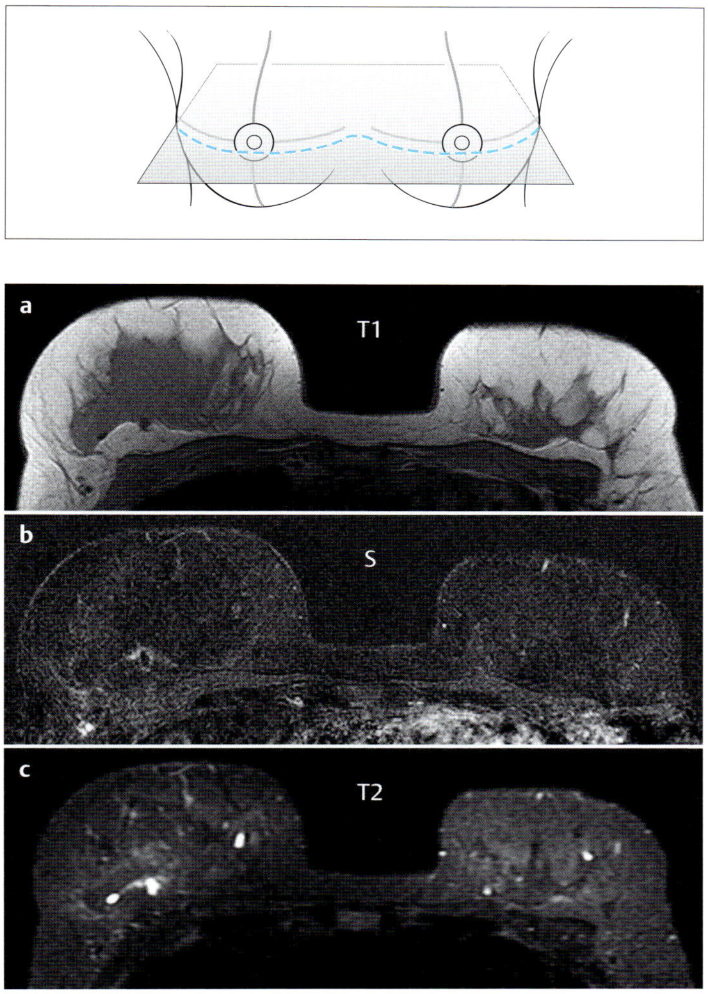


Fig. 70.**5 a – c** Contrast-enhanced MRI of the breasts.

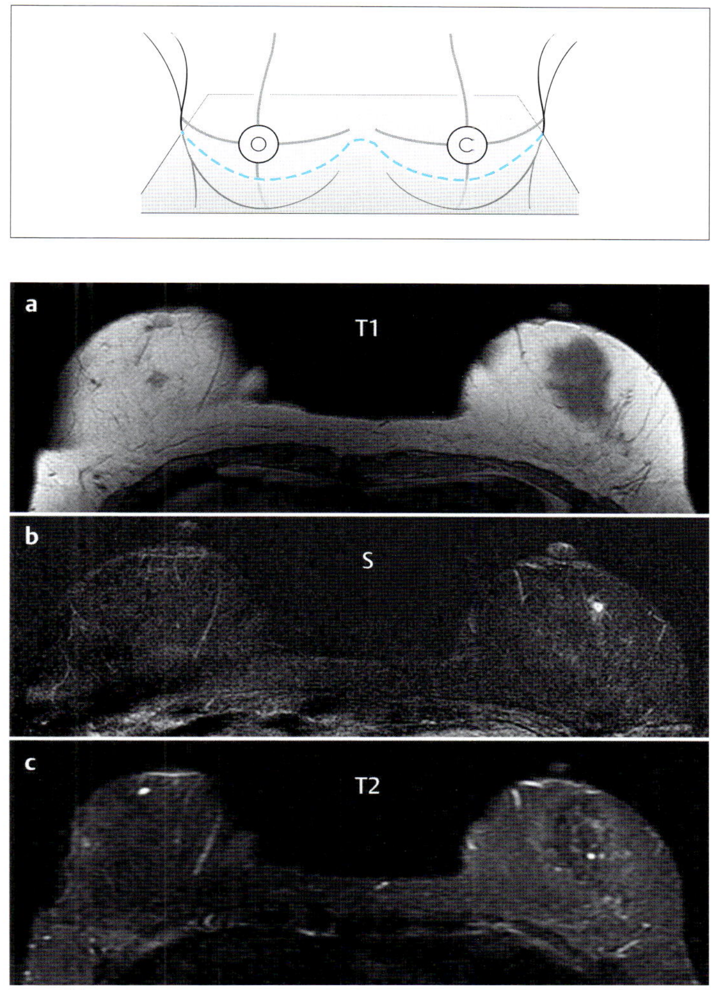


Fig. 70.**6 a – c** Contrast-enhanced MRI of the breasts.

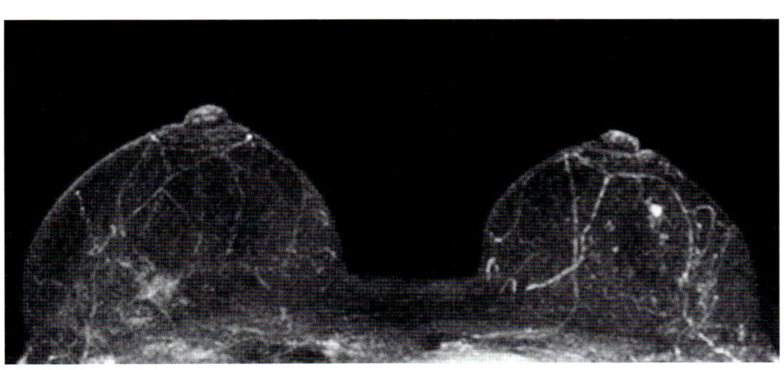

Fig. 70.**7** Contrast-enhanced MR mammography. Maximum intensity projection.

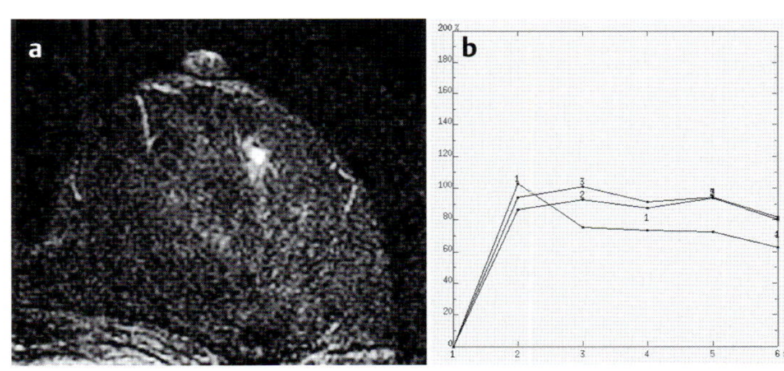


Fig. 70.**8 a, b** Signal-to-time curves.

Please characterize the mammography and MRI findings.
What is your preliminary diagnosis?
What are your next steps?

This case examines a patient with a single cluster of microcalcifications in the right breast. The patient had been referred to a local hospital for open biopsy. However, the surgeon recommended initial investigation by stereotactic vacuum biopsy.

### Ultrasound

No unusual findings bilaterally. US BI-RADS 1.

### Mammography

Mammograms showed bilaterally symmetric extremely dense parenchyma, ACR type 4. In the lower outer quadrant of the right breast, a group of monomorphous microcalcifications was seen. There were no suspicious masses or densities and no architectural distortions. BI-RADS right 3/left 1.PGMI: CC view I (nipple projection); MLO view M (pectoralis muscle, inframammary fold, nipple not in profile).

### MR Mammography*

MRI documented a round, ill-defined lesion measuring 6 mm in the left breast behind the nipple, presenting with a ring enhancement, a strong initial signal increase, and postinitial plateau as well as reduced signal in T2-weighted imaging.

* *Note:* The MRI was performed following stereotactic vacuum biopsy on the right breast for the purpose of preoperative local staging. The biopsy region is visible in MRI, in the area of the parenchyma toward the chest wall, as a slight ring enhancement with increased signal in T2-weighted imaging.

**MRI Artifact Category:** 1
**MRI Density Type:** 1

| MRM score | Finding left | Points |
|---|---|---|
| **Shape** | round | 0 |
| **Border** | ill-defined | 1 |
| **CM Distribution** | ring | 2 |
| **Initial Signal Intensity Increase** | strong | 2 |
| **Post-initial Signal Intensity Character** | wash-out | 2 |
| **MRI score (points)** | | **7** |
| **MRI BI-RADS** | | **5** |

### → Differential Diagnosis

Right: DCIS, invasive carcinoma, adenosis, regressive fibroadenoma.
Left: Carcinoma, complicated cyst, fibroadenoma, papilloma, focal adenosis.

| BI-RADS Categorization | | |
|---|---|---|
| Clinical Findings | right 1 | left 1 |
| Ultrasound | right 1 | left 1 |
| Mammography | right 3 | left 1 |
| MR Mammography | right 3 | left 5 |
| **BI-RADS Total** | **right 3** | **left 5** |

### Procedure

Stereotactic vacuum biopsy of the calcifications in the right breast (Figs. 70.**9** and 70.**10**).

### Histopathology of the right breast

Low grade DCIS.

### Further procedure

Bilateral simultaneous MR-guided localization of the region to be excised in the right breast (Fig. 70.**11**) and the suspicious lesion in the left breast (Fig. 70.**12**).

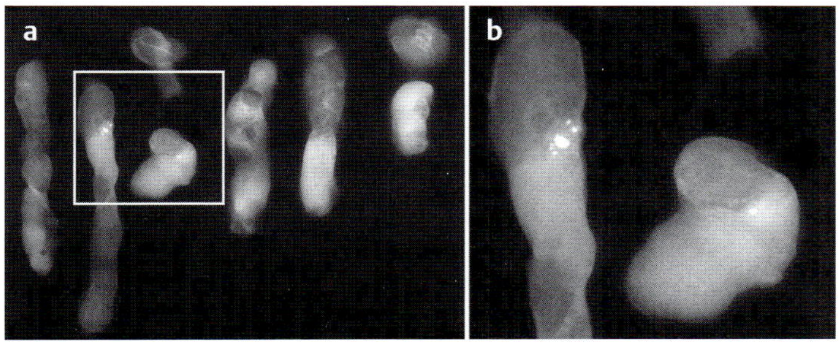

Fig. 70.**9 a, b** Specimen radiography.

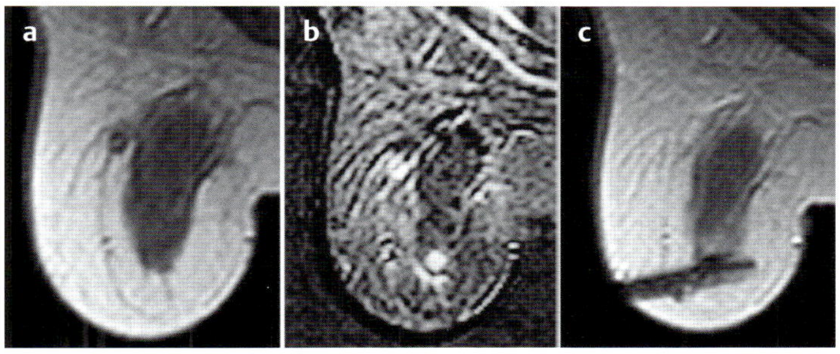

Fig. 70.**12 a – c** MR-guided localization, left breast.

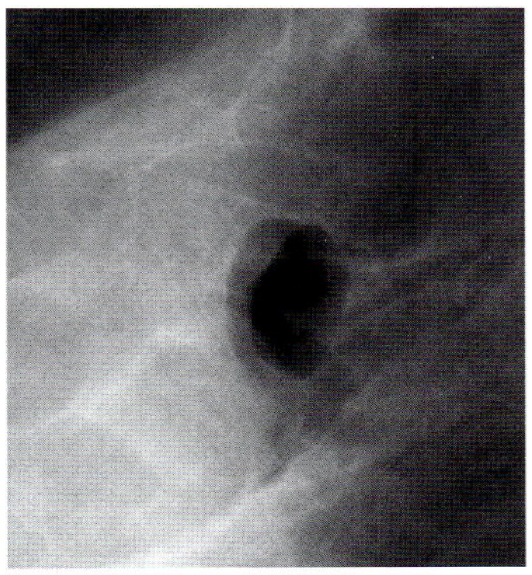

Fig. 70.**10** Air-filled cavity at site of biopsy showing complete removal of calcifications.

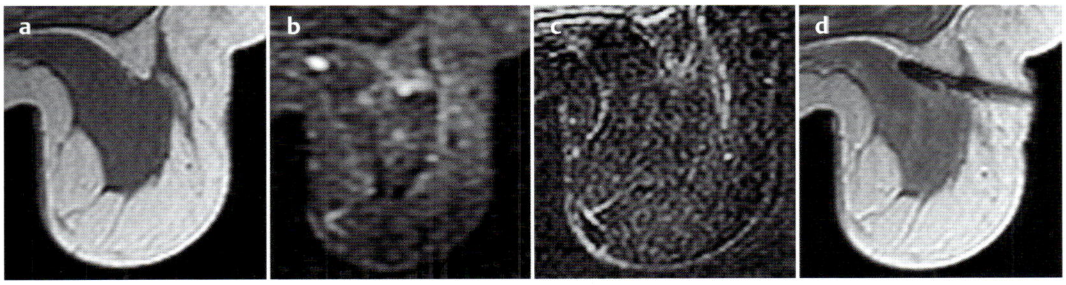

Fig. 70.**11 a – d** MR-guided localization of the biopsy region in the right breast.

## Diagnosis

Right: DCIS (low grade).
Left: Adenosis.

## Treatment

Breast conservation therapy (right breast); open biopsy (left breast).

If no hematoma is visible in mammography after complete removal of a calcification cluster by core biopsy, preoperative hook-wire localization can be either US- or MR-guided.

**Indication:** Screening. Mastodynia of the left breast.
**History:** Unremarkable.
**Risk profile:** No increased risk.
**Age:** 67 years.

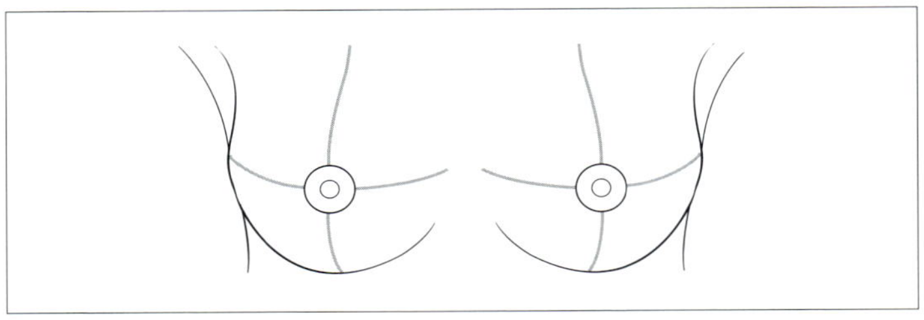

## Clinical Findings

Normal.

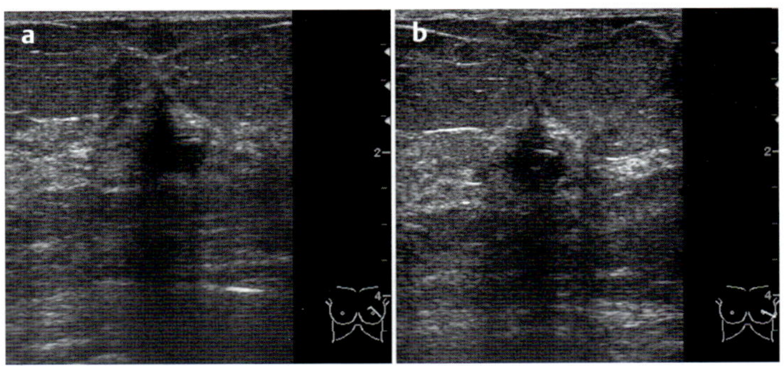


Fig. 71.**1 a, b** Sonography.

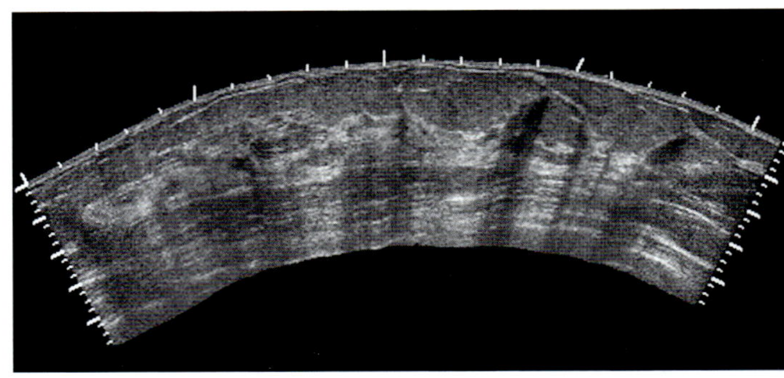

Fig. 71.**2** Sonography. Panoramic view of the left breast.

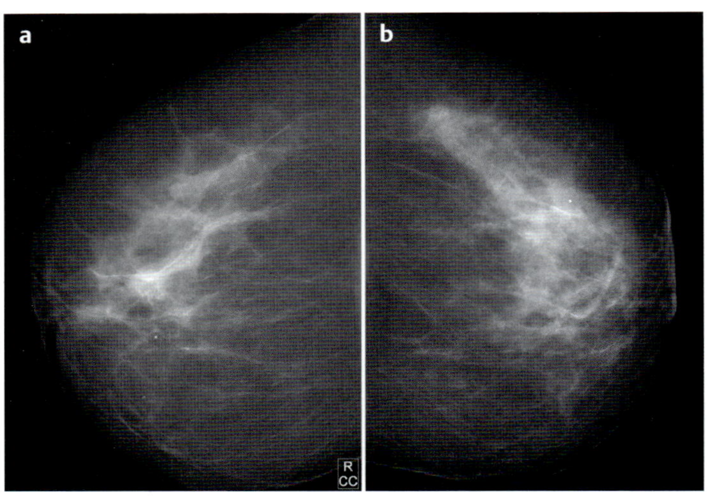


Fig. 71.**3 a, b** Digital mammography, CC view.

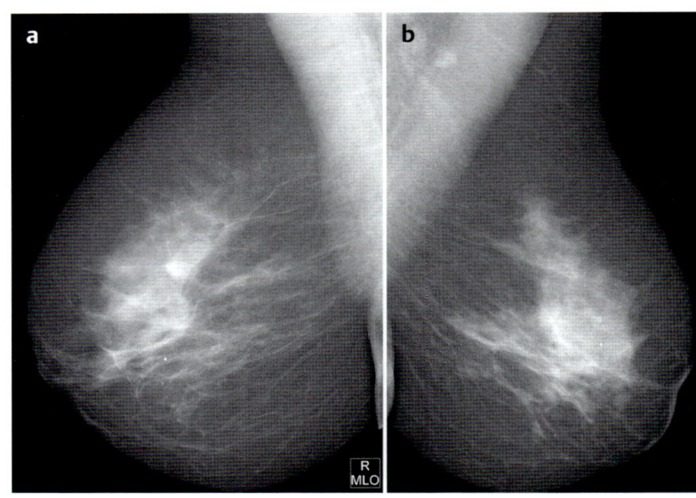


Fig. 71.**4 a, b** Digital mammography, MLO view.

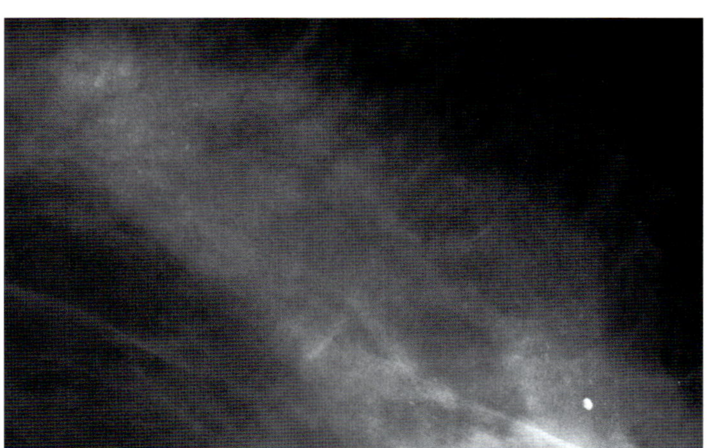

Fig. 71.**5** Magnification view of the outer quadrants of the left breast (CC).

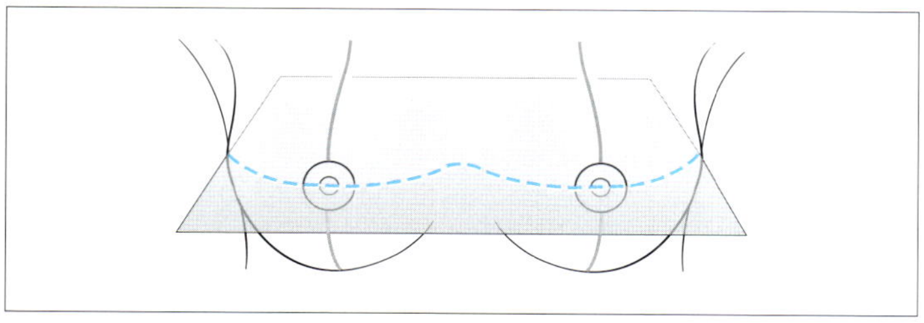

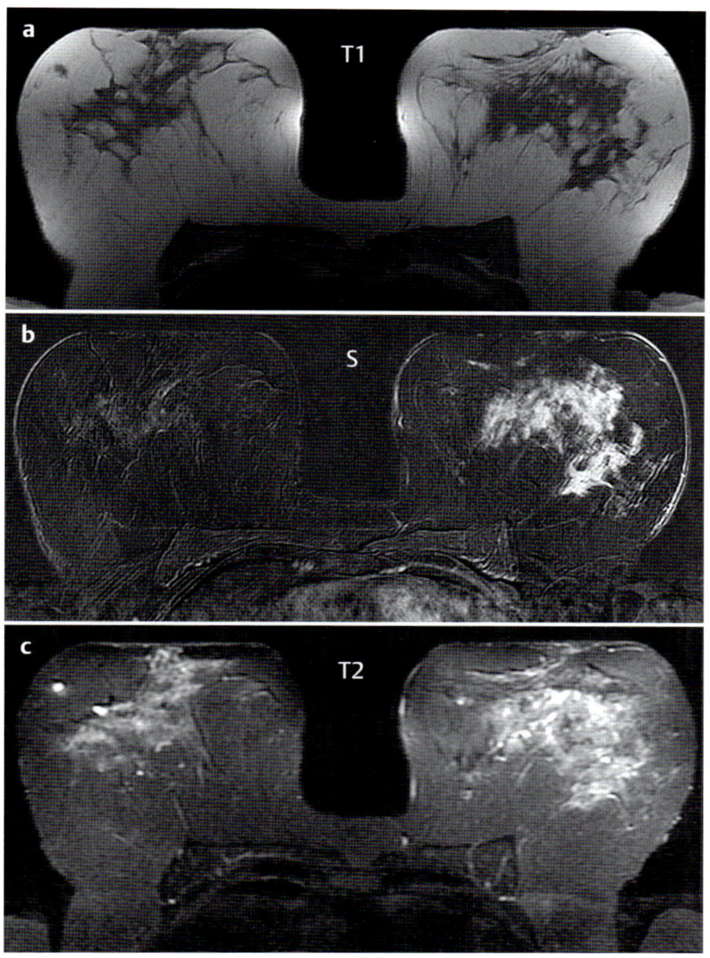


Fig. 71.**6 a – c** Contrast-enhanced MRI of the breasts.

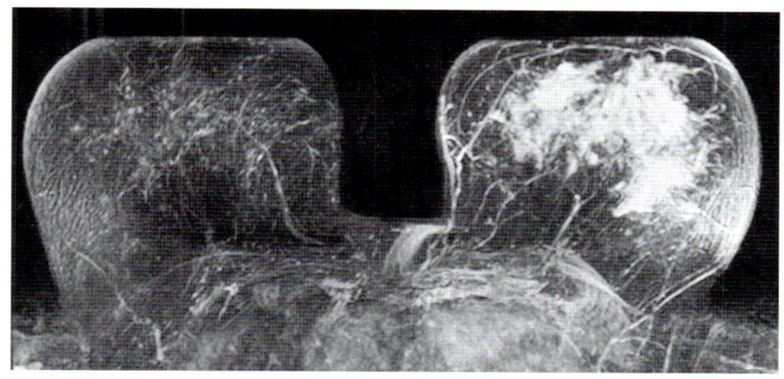

Fig. 71.**7** Contrast-enhanced MR mammography. Maximum intensity projection.

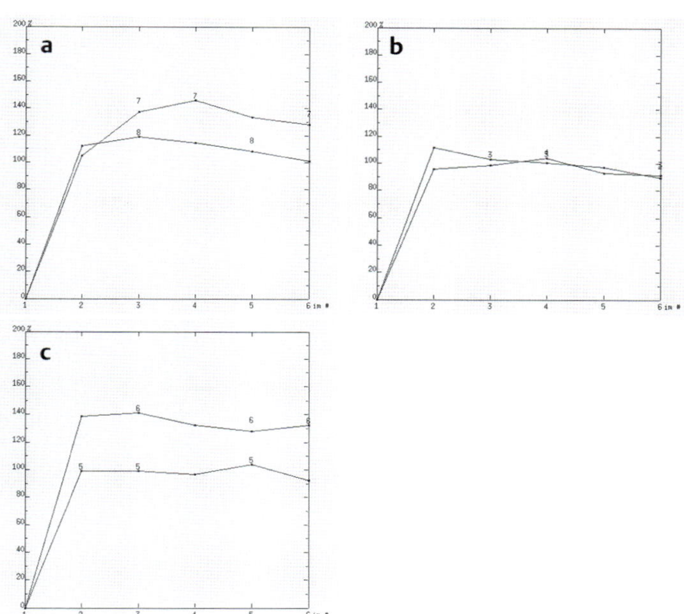


Fig. 71.**8 a – c** Signal-to-time curves of representative regions of the left breast.

Please characterize ultrasound, mammography, and MRI findings.
What is your preliminary diagnosis?
What are your next steps?

These imaging studies were done in a screening situation. However, the criterion of unilateral mastodynia, particularly in postmenopausal women, raises the possibility of malignancy.

### Ultrasound

There was a highly suspicious irregular lesion in the left breast with the long axis perpendicular to the skin and with hyperechoic margin, distortion of ligamental structures, and pathological distal echo shadowing. Panoramic view of the left breast demonstrated multiple linear distal shadows that, taken together with the primary lesion, also point to malignancy. There was a small cyst in the right breast. US BI-RADS right 2/left 5.

### Mammography

The parenchymal texture was inhomogeneously dense, ACR type 3, and asymmetric (right > left). In the upper outer quadrant of the left breast, magnification view depicted multiple predominantly amorphous microcalcifications (Fig. 71.**5**). There were no circumscribed lesions in the left breast. A small round lesion was visible in the right breast (consistent with the cyst seen in ultrasound). BI-RADS right 2/left 5. PGMI CC view P; MLO view G (inframammary fold).

### MR Mammography

Precontrast images of both breasts were unremarkable. However, postcontrast imaging demonstrated unilateral diffuse enhancement of the entire nonlipomatous tissue of the left breast. Signal–time curves were characteristic of malignancy.

**MRI Artifact Category:** 1
**MRI Density Type:** 1

| MRM score | Finding | Points |
|---|---|---|
| **Shape** | irregular | 1 |
| **Border** | ill-defined | 1 |
| **CM Distribution** | homogeneous | 0 |
| **Initial Signal Intensity Increase** | strong | 2 |
| **Post-initial Signal Intensity Character** | wash-out | 2 |
| **MRI score (points)** | | **6** |
| **MRI BI-RADS** | | **5** |

### → Preliminary Diagnosis

Carcinoma of the left breast (most likely diffuse invasive lobular carcinoma, although the calcifications are not typical for this). Non-mass lesion seen in MRI.

### → Differential Diagnosis

Mastitis (very low probability).

| BI-RADS Categorization | | |
|---|---|---|
| Clinical Findings | right 1 | left 1 |
| Ultrasound | right 2 | left 5 |
| Mammography | right 2 | left 5 |
| MR Mammography | right 1 | left 5 |
| **BI-RADS Total** | **right 2** | **left 5** |

**Procedure**

Histological analysis of the suspicious finding in the left breast with US-guided core biopsy.

**Histology of the left breast**

Ductal carcinoma in situ (DCIS) accompanied by atypical ductal hyperplasia (ADH).

## Histology

Extensive malignant tumor with multifocal micropapillary, low-grade ductal carcinoma in situ. Transformation into invasive ductal carcinoma in the upper outer quadrant of the left breast.

IDC pT1c + DCIS (multifocal), pN2a (4/12), G2.

## Treatment

Mastectomy of the left breast.

MRI is the imaging method of choice in preoperative staging of malignant tumors.

**Indication:** Screening.
**History:** Unremarkable.
**Risk profile:** No increased risk.
**Age:** 57 years.

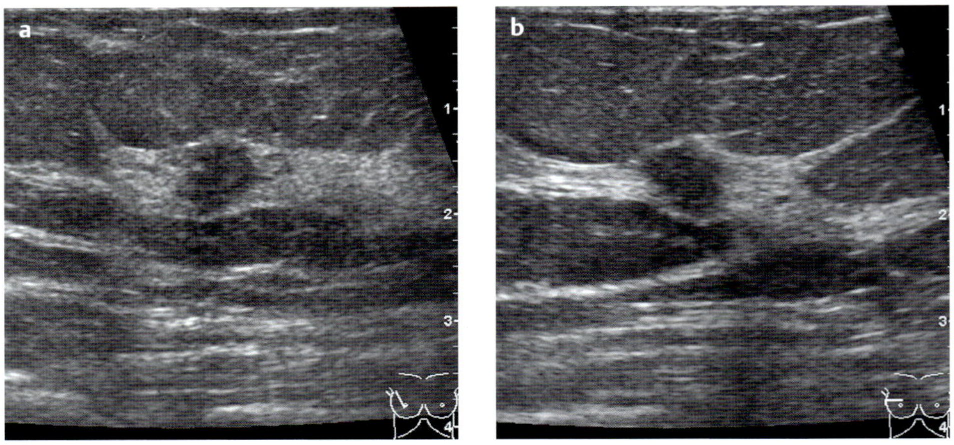


Fig. 72.**1 a, b** Ultrasound.

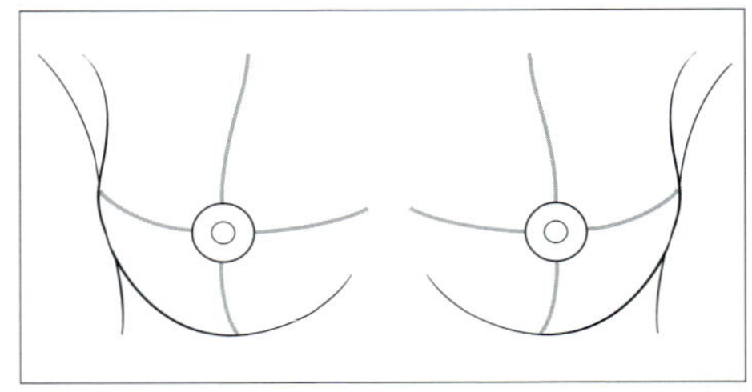

## Clinical Findings

Normal.

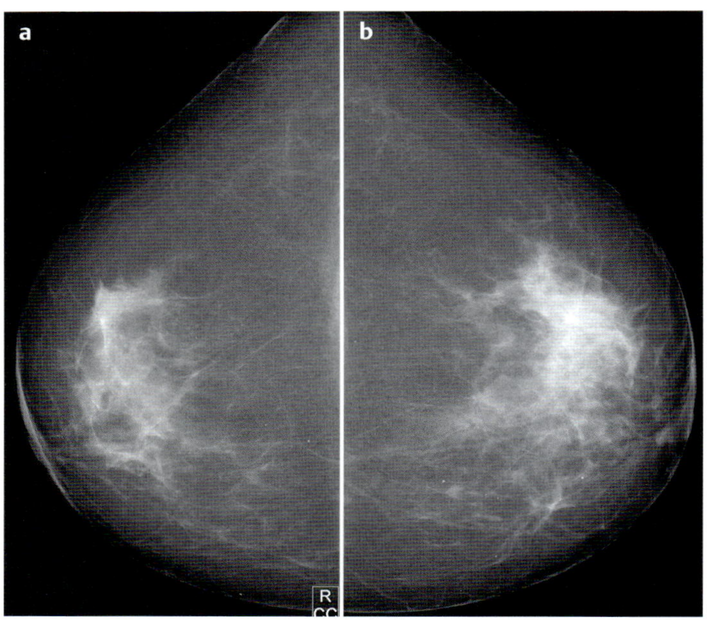


Fig. 72.**2 a, b** Digital mammography, CC view.

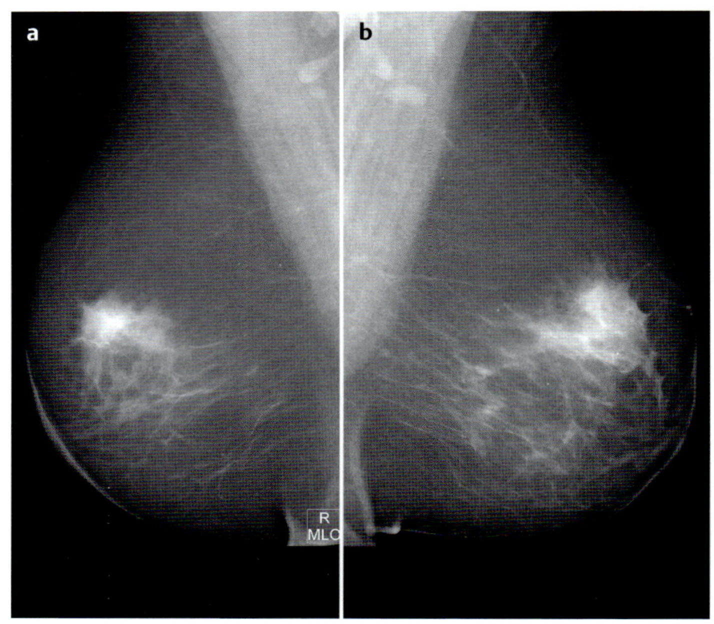


Fig. 72.**3 a, b** Digital mammography, MLO view.

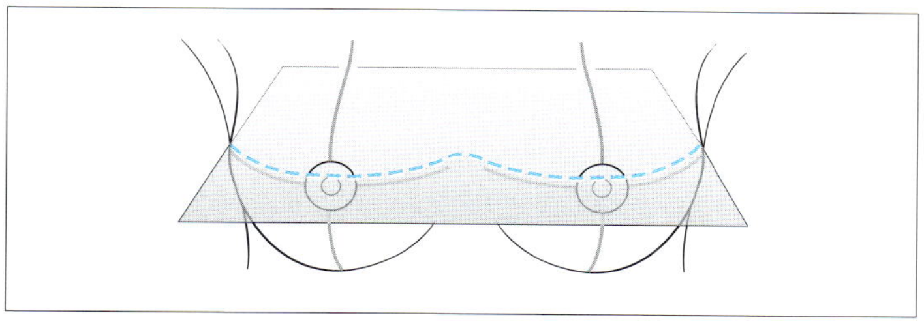

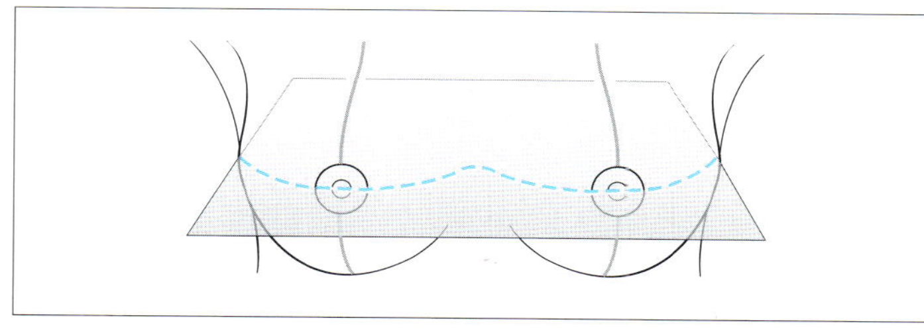

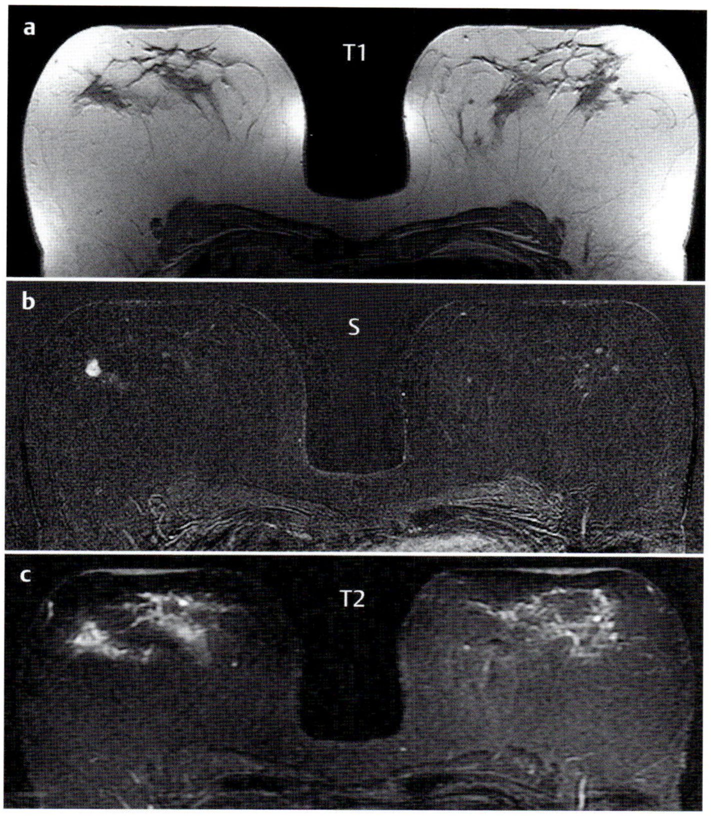


Fig. 72.**4 a–c** Contrast-enhanced MRI of the breasts.

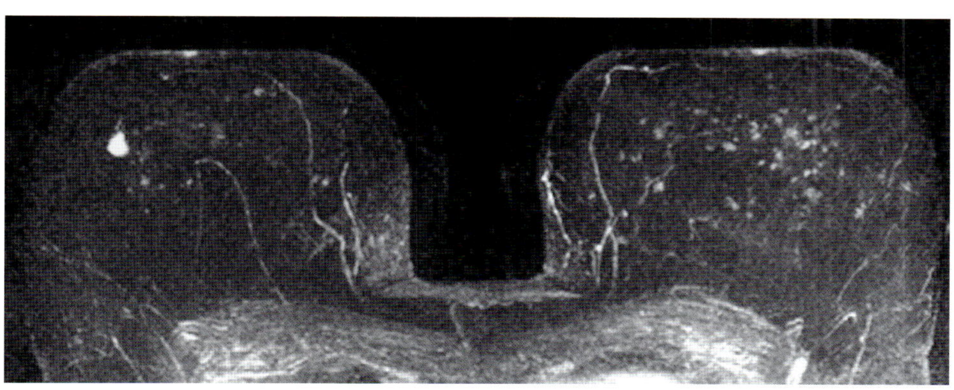

Fig. 72.**5** Contrast-enhanced MR mammography. Maximum intensity projection.

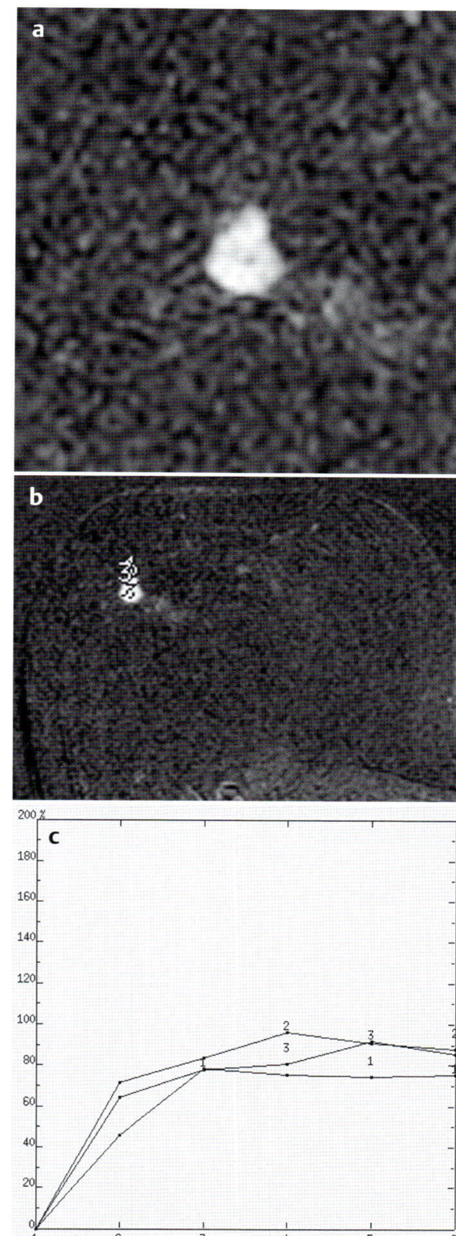


Fig. 72.**6 a–c** Enlarged view of lesion; signal-to-time curves.

Please characterize ultrasound, mammography, and MRI findings.
What is your preliminary diagnosis?
What are your next steps?

This case demonstrates the imaging studies of an asymptomatic woman presenting for screening.

### Ultrasound

In the upper outer quadrant of the right breast, there was an ill-defined, lobulated, hypoechoic area within the glandular tissue with inhomogeneous internal texture. There was no echo alteration of the surrounding structures, but ligamental structures were clearly displaced by this region. US BI-RADS right 3.

### Mammography

Mammograms showed inhomogeneously dense glandular tissue of ACR type 3 with a mild asymmetry of the upper outer quadrants. In the right breast there was a slight shrinking with some peripheral spiculation in the upper outer quadrant. There were no densities or definite lesions. No architectural distortions, and no microcalcifications. BI-RADS right 3/left 1. PGMI CC view P; MLO view G (inframammary fold).

### MR Mammography

MRI demonstrated a single hypervascularized, ill-defined lesion with a ring enhancement between the outer quadrants of the right breast. There were no suspicious signal changes in the analysis of enhancement dynamics. The left breast showed a patchy enhancement, probably attributable to adenosis.

**MRI Artifact Category:** 1
**MRI Density Type:** 2

| MRM score | Finding | Points |
|---|---|---|
| **Shape** | round | 0 |
| **Border** | ill-defined | 1 |
| **CM Distribution** | rim sign | 2 |
| **Initial Signal Intensity Increase** | moderate | 1 |
| **Post-initial Signal Intensity Character** | plateau | 1 |
| **MRI score (points)** | | **5** |
| **MRI BI-RADS** | | **4** |

### → Differential Diagnosis

Right: Carcinoma, adenosis.

| BI-RADS Categorization | | |
|---|---|---|
| Clinical Findings | right 1 | left 1 |
| Ultrasound | right 3 | left 1 |
| Mammography | right 3 | left 1 |
| MR Mammography | right 4 | left 1 |
| **BI-RADS Total** | **right 4** | **left 1** |

### Procedure

Histopathological analysis of the lesion in the right breast by US-guided percutaneous core biopsy.

### Histopathological analysis of the specimen (right breast)

Chronic fibrocystic mastopathy. No malignancy.

### Further procedure

With regard to the discrepancy between the imaging findings in the right breast (in particular MRI) and the histological results, a further percutaneous core biopsy was necessary for increased accuracy. An MR-guided vacuum biopsy was recommended. Instead, in the present case, an excisional biopsy was performed on the lesion in the right breast at the patient's request.

### Histology

Invasive ductal carcinoma measuring 15 mm. Axillary lymph node status normal.

IDC pT1c, pN0 (0/17), G2.

### Treatment

Breast conservation therapy of the right breast.

It is important that the plausibility of imaging and histology results is carefully considered in order to avoid false-negative findings.

**Indication:** Screening.
**History:** Unremarkable.
**Risk profile:** No increased risk.
**Age:** 44 years.

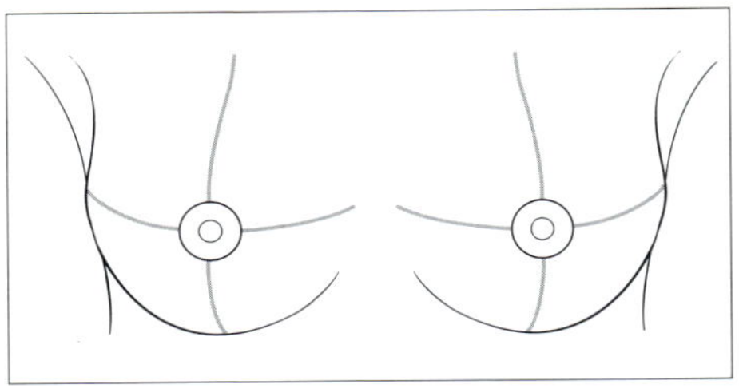

### Clinical Findings

Normal.

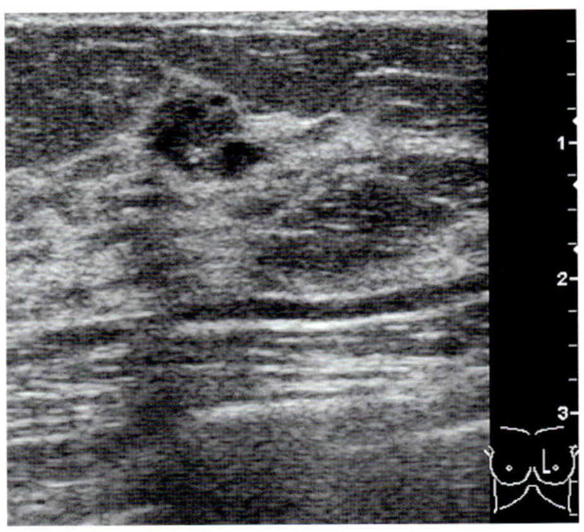

Fig. 73.**1** Ultrasound.

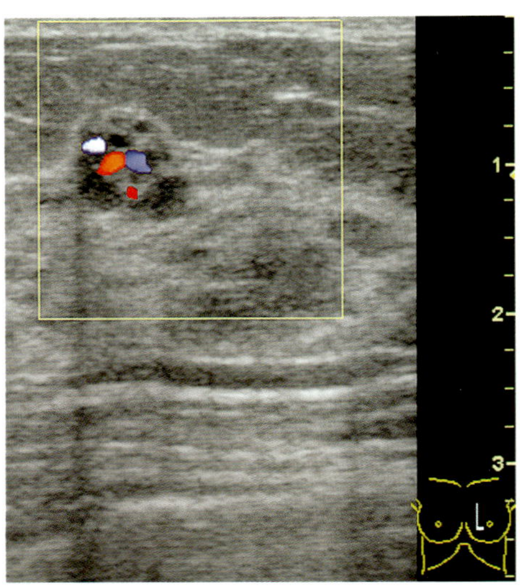

Fig. 73.**2** Color-coded Doppler sonography.

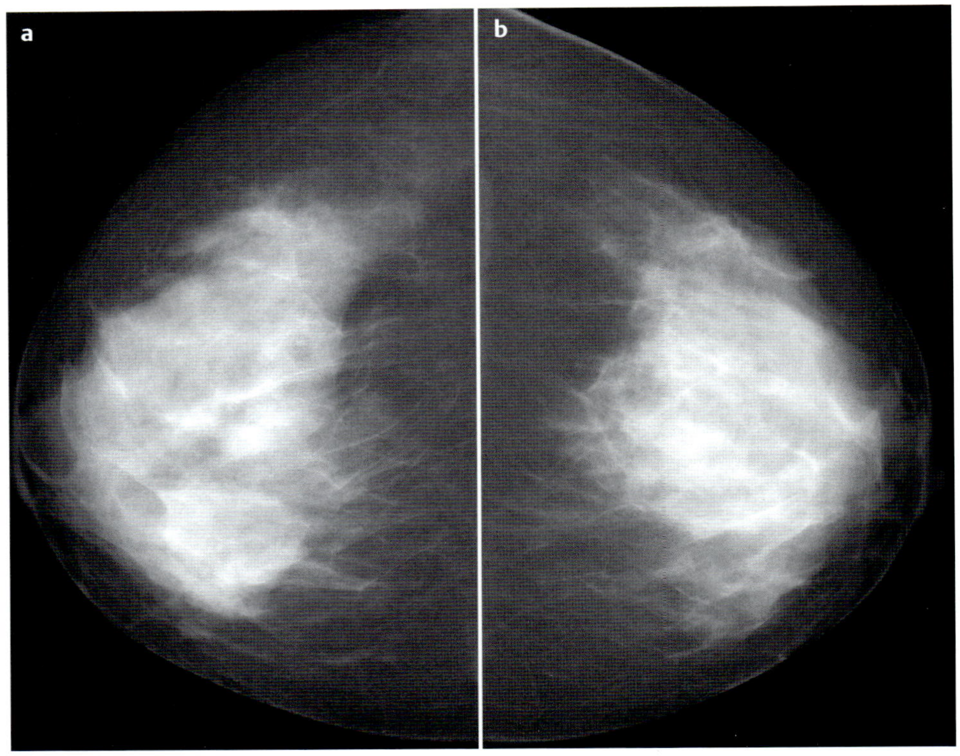

Fig. 73.**3 a, b** Digital mammography, CC view.

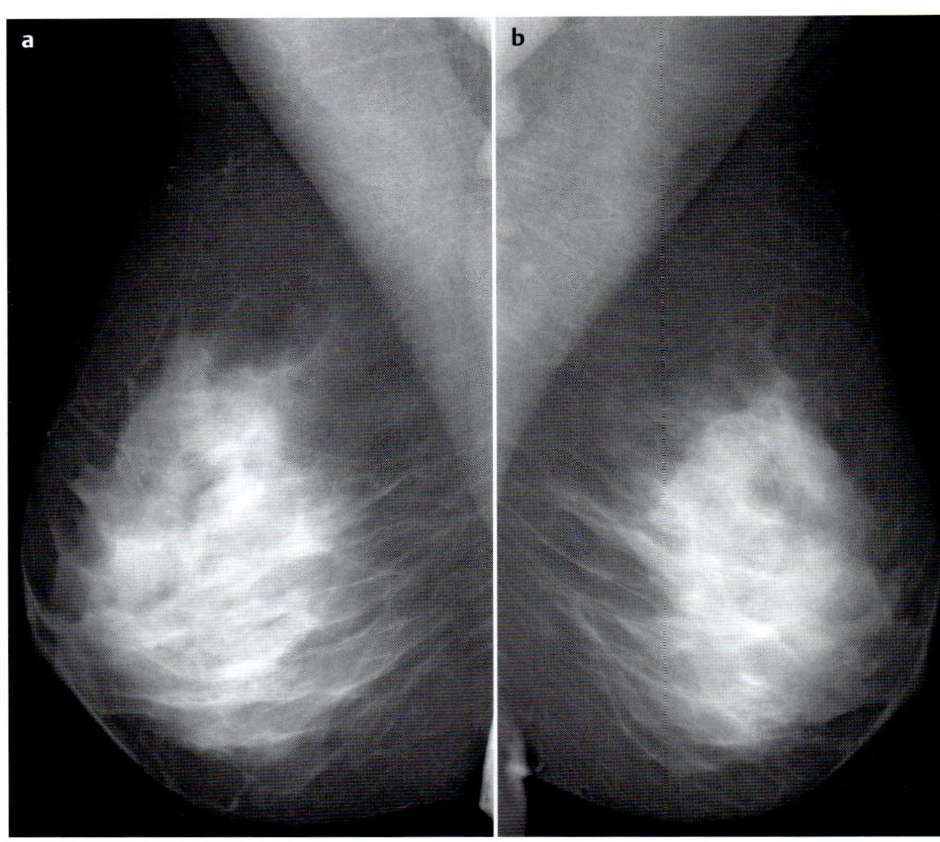

Fig. 73.**4 a, b** Digital mammography, MLO view.

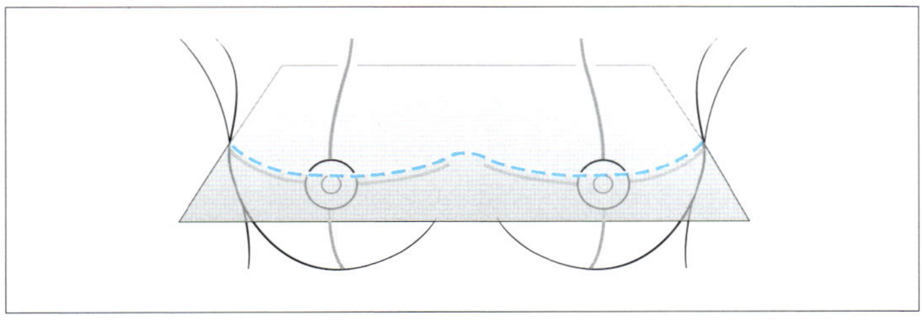

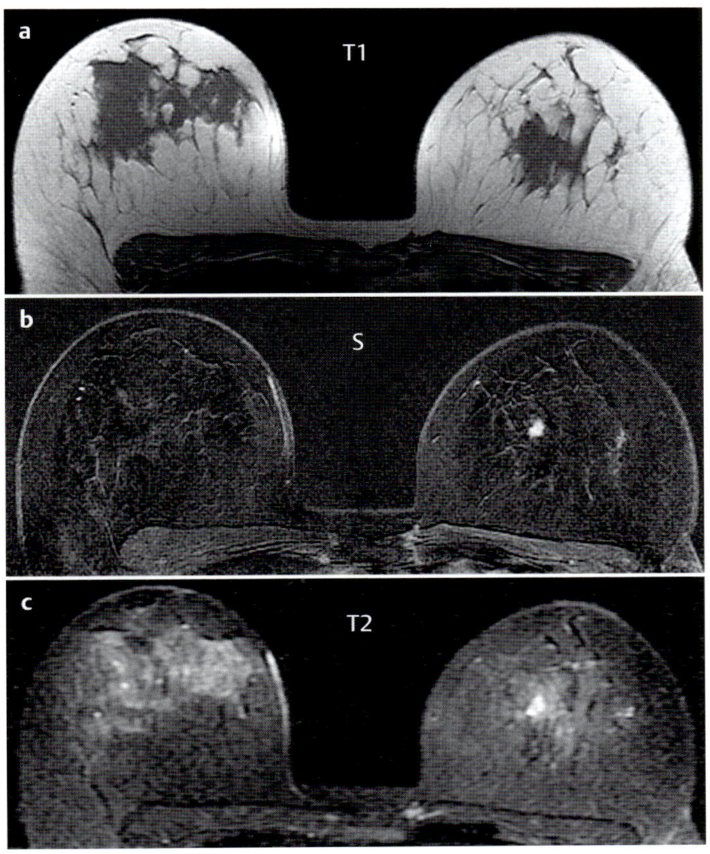

Fig. 73.5 a–c Contrast-enhanced MRI of the breasts.

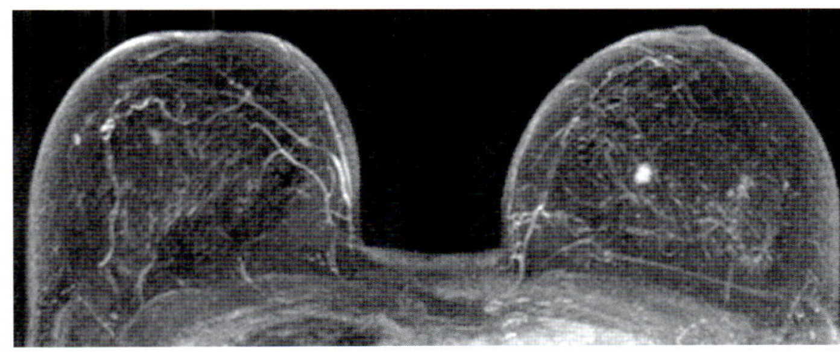
Fig. 73.6 Contrast-enhanced MR mammography. Maximum intensity projection.

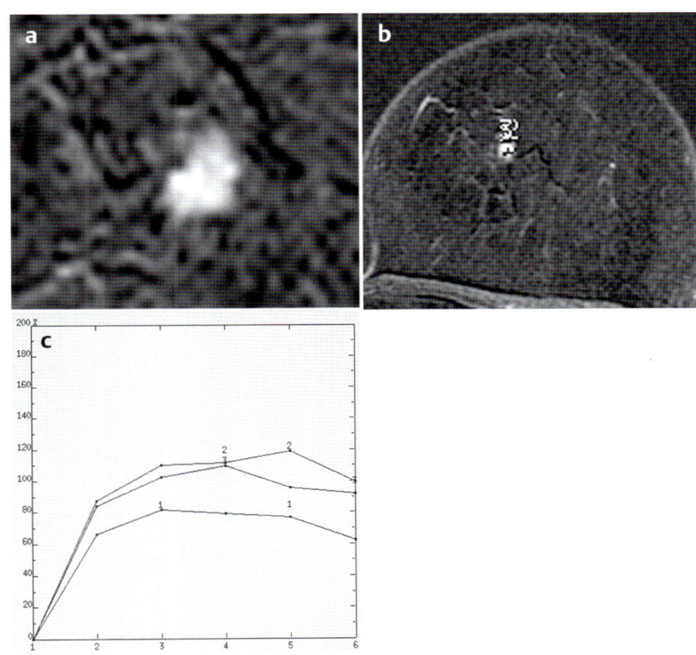

Fig. 73.7 a–c Enlarged view of lesion; signal-to-time curves.

Please characterize ultrasound, mammography, and MRI findings.
What is your preliminary diagnosis?
What are your next steps?

This case demonstrates the imaging in a screening situation of a young asymptomatic woman without increased risk profile.

### Ultrasound

Within the upper inner quadrant of the left breast between the ventral edge of the parenchyma and the subcutaneous fatty tissue, ultrasound showed an irregular, hypoechoic lesion measuring 8 mm with inhomogeneous echo texture. There were signs of a slight distortion of ligamental structures. Moreover, the lesion showed marked internal signal increase in color-coded duplex sonography. US BI-RADS 4.

### Mammography

Mammography showed bilaterally symmetric, extremely dense parenchyma, ACR type 4. Under these limiting conditions, there were no unusual findings, particularly in the inner quadrants of the left breast (the area of the sonographic findings). No densities, no lesions, no architectural distortions, and no microcalcifications were detected. BI-RADS right 1/left 1. PGMI: CC view P; MLO view G (inframammary fold).

### MR Mammography

MRI depicted a single, ill-defined hypervascularized lesion in the upper inner quadrant of the left breast, consistent with the sonographic findings. There was a slight central reduction of signal and overall inhomogeneous enhancement (ring enhancement? septations?). The signal–time curves were non-specific.

**MRI Artifact Category:** 1
**MRI Density Type:** 1

| MRM score | Finding | Points |
|---|---|---|
| **Shape** | irregular | 1 |
| **Border** | ill-defined | 1 |
| **CM Distribution** | inhomogeneous | 1 |
| **Initial Signal Intensity Increase** | strong | 2 |
| **Post-initial Signal Intensity Character** | plateau | 1 |
| **MRI score (points)** | | **6** |
| **MRI BI-RADS** | | **5** |

### → Differential Diagnosis

Carcinoma, focal adenosis, papilloma, adenoma.

| BI-RADS Categorization | | |
|---|---|---|
| Clinical Findings | right 1 | left 1 |
| Ultrasound | right 1 | left 4 |
| Mammography | right 1 | left 1 |
| MR Mammography | right 1 | left 5 |
| **BI-RADS Total** | **right 1** | **left 5** |

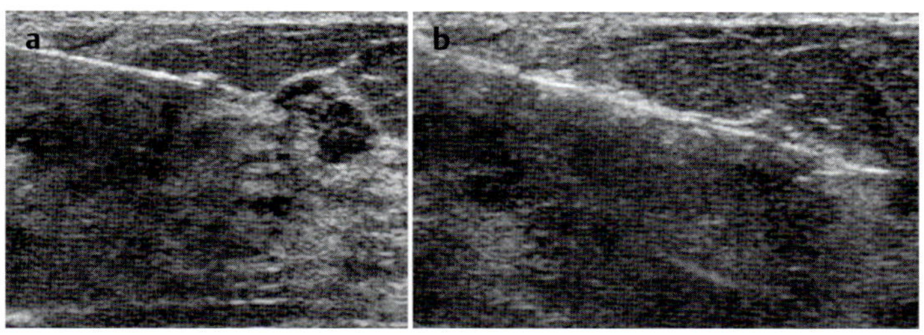


Fig. 73.**8 a, b** US-guided core biopsy (pre-fire, post-fire).

### Procedure

Histopathological investigation with US-guided core biopsy (Fig. 73.**8**).

### Histopathology

Fibrocystic mastopathy. Ductal hyperplasia. Focal apocrine metaplasia. No malignancy.

### Procedure

With regard to the possibility of an inaccurate biopsy (sampling error), an additional biopsy was performed, this time an MR-guided vacuum biopsy, for further histological analysis (Fig. 73.**9**).

### Histopathology

Fibrocystic mastopathy. Sclerosing adenosis with ductal and lobular hyperplasia. No malignancy. (Histopathological double reading.)

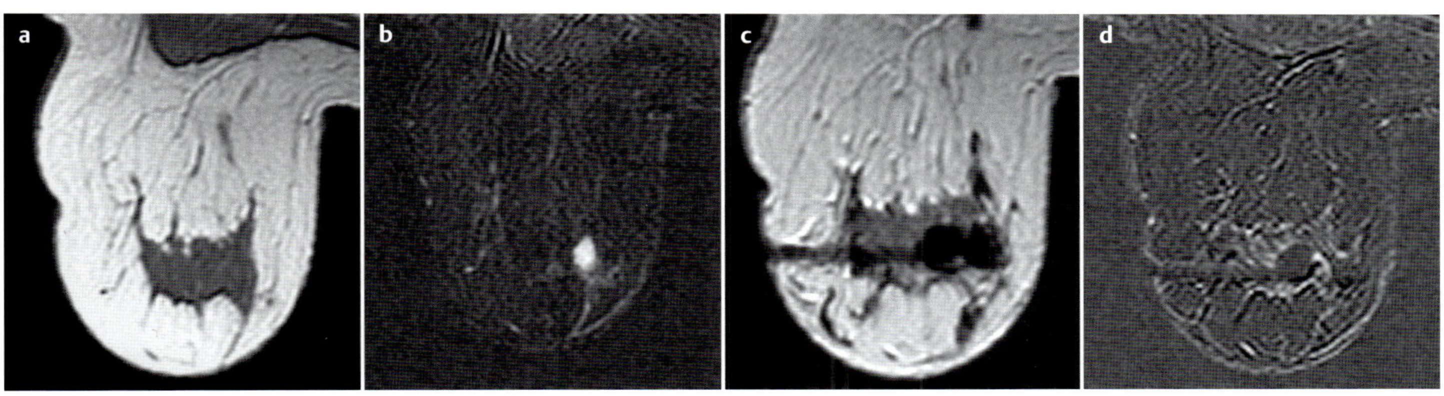


Fig. 73.**9 a – d** MR-guided vacuum biopsy (precontrast, subtraction after contrast administration, T1-weighted image after biopsy, and documentation of complete removal of the lesion after further contrast administration.

### Histology

Tumorous sclerosing adenosis.

### Treatment

None. Follow-up after 6 months. (The lesion was no longer visible in this follow-up examination.)

In this case, an unusual finding in ultrasound triggered a whole range of further diagnostic measures, only to reach a benign diagnosis. All that for “nothing”?
But would ***you*** have acted differently in this case?

**Indication:** Palpable lump in right breast discovered 3 weeks previously.
**History:** Unremarkable.
**Risk profile:** No increased risk.
**Age:** 54 years.

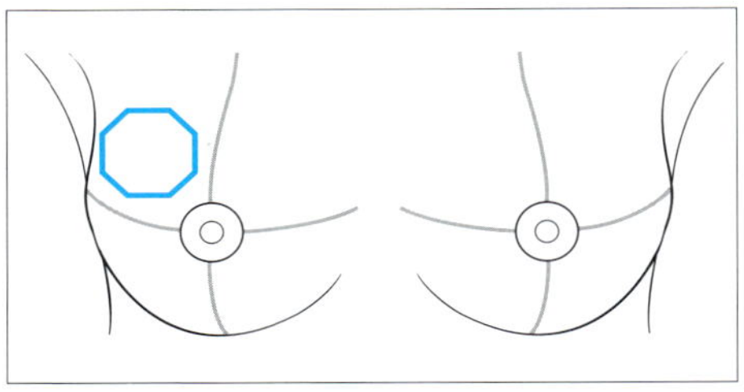

### Clinical Findings

Large, mobile lump in the upper outer quadrant of the right breast. No axillary lymph nodes palpable.

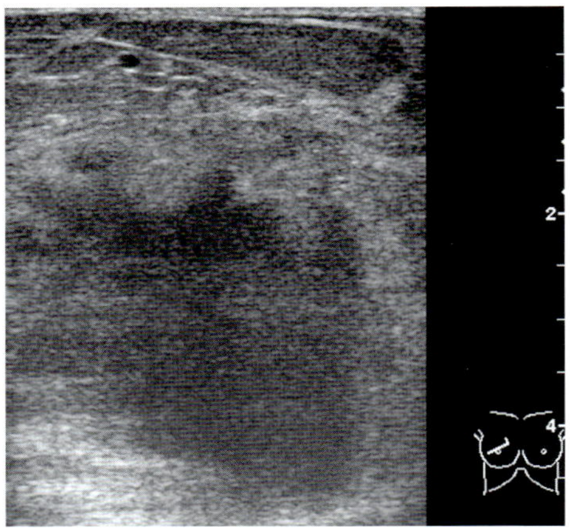

Fig. 74.**1** Ultrasound.

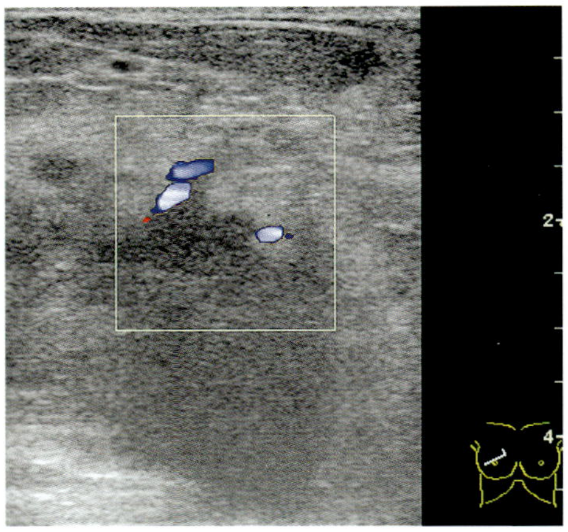

Fig. 74.**2** Color-coded Doppler sonography.

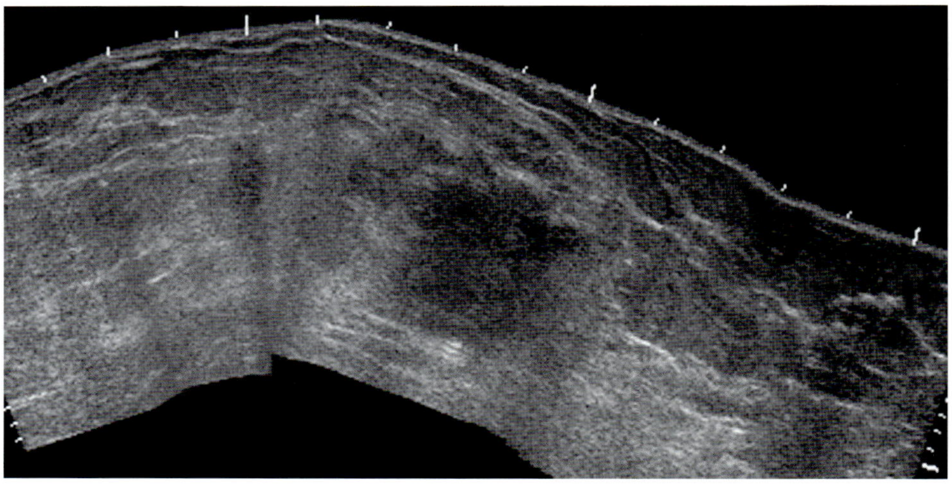

Fig. 74.**3** Ultrasound. Panoramic view of the right breast.

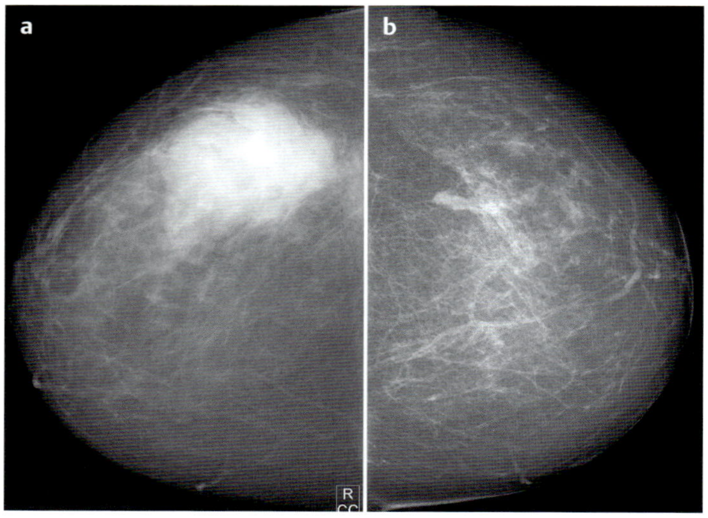

Fig. 74.**4 a, b** Digital mammography, CC view.

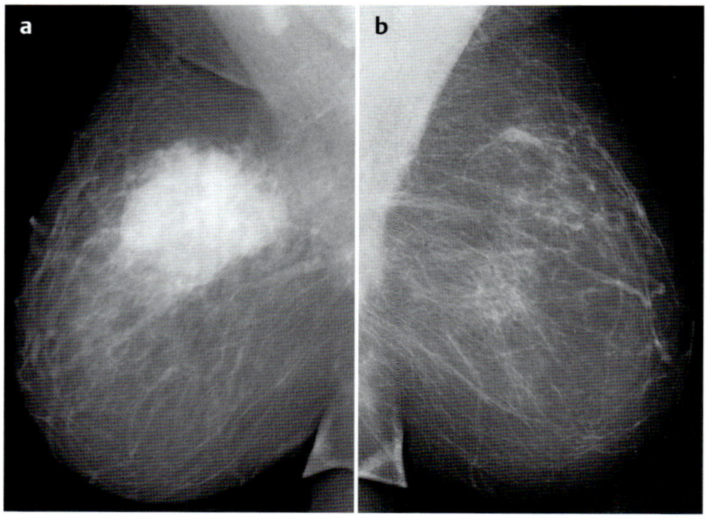

Fig. 74.**5 a, b** Digital mammography, MLO view.

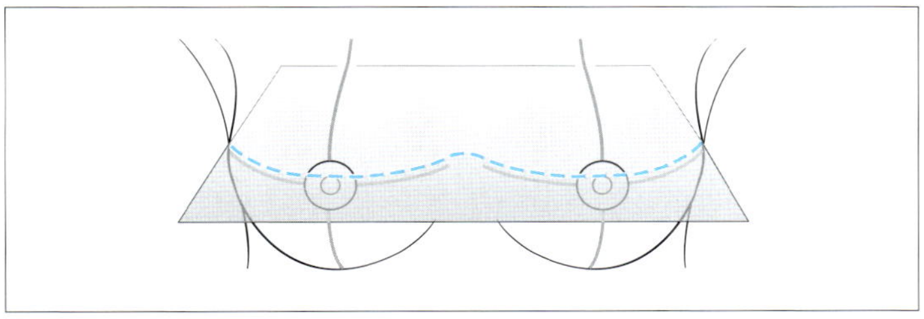

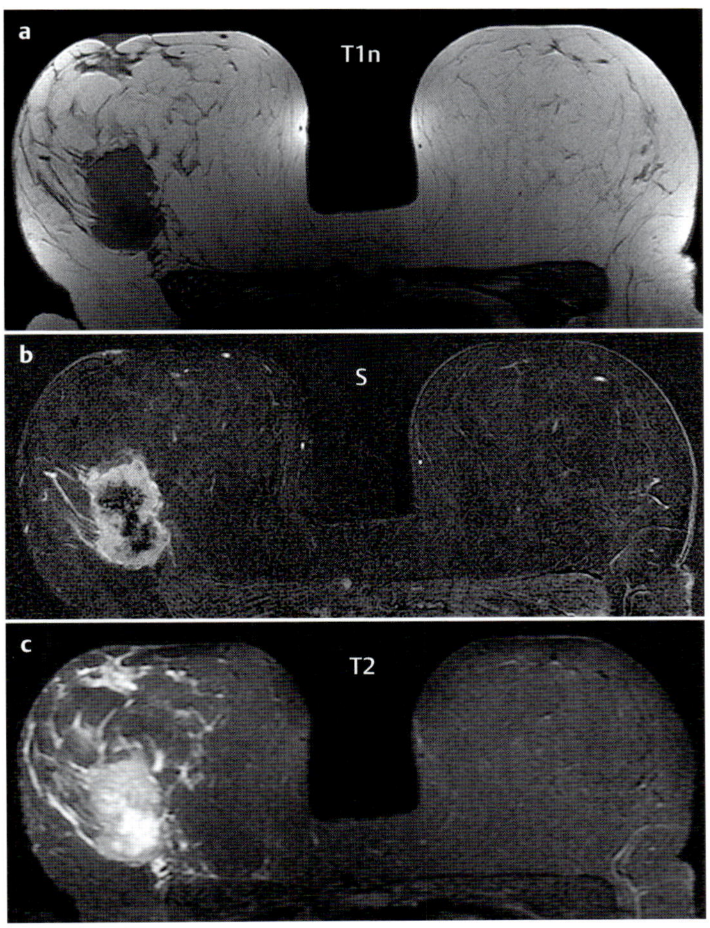


Fig. 74.**6 a–c** Contrast-enhanced MRI of the breasts.

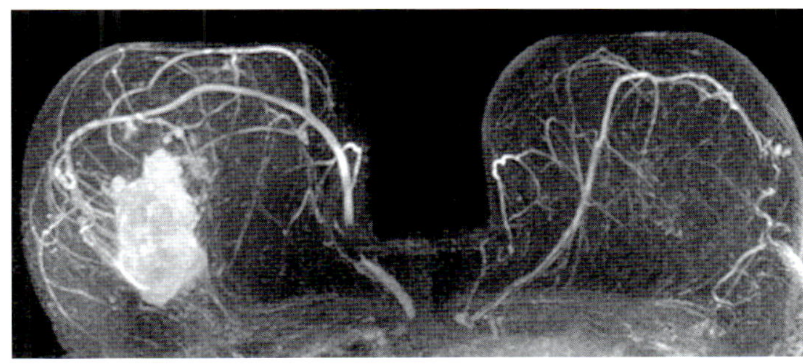

Fig. 74.**7** Contrast-enhanced MR mammograp ıy. Maximum intensity projection.

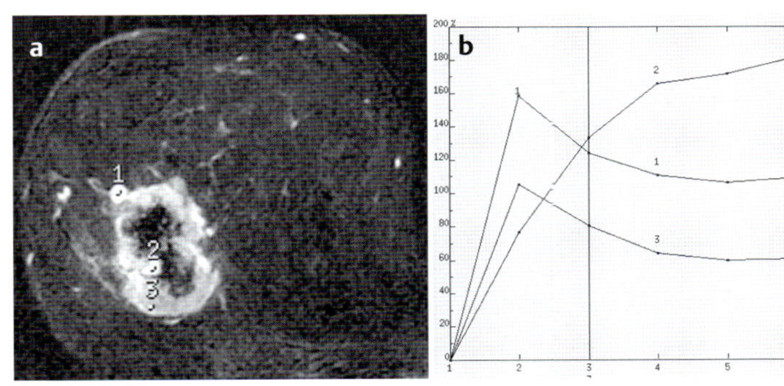


Fig. 74.**8 a, b** Signal-to-time curves.

?

Please characterize ultrasound, mammography, and MRI findings.
What is your preliminary diagnosis?
What are your next steps?

Clinical evidence already pointed to a definitive diagnosis of breast cancer even before the imaging shown here was carried out. The patient's statement that the lump was discovered only 3 weeks before the examination was very surprising, since lumps of this size are known to develop over a period of years. However, see for yourself ...

### Ultrasound

In the area of the palpable mass, ultrasound demonstrated an extensive tumor with multiple criteria of malignancy as well as increased peripheral vascularization in Doppler sonography. The best depiction of the lesion was in panoramic view because of its size. US BI-RADS right 5.

### Mammography

The parenchyma was bilaterally predominantly lipomatous, ACR type 1. A massive, ill-defined, hyperdense mass was seen in the right breast. There were no accompanying microcalcifications and no other suspicious findings. BI-RADS right 5/left 1.

### MR Mammography (in this case unnecessary)

MRI showed a lobulated, ill-defined tumor in the upper outer quadrant of the right breast, with marked central necrosis. Signal–time curves in the region of interest were typical for malignancy (N.B: The most significant curves in terms of malignancy are always used for the MRM score, even if some individual curves appear normal). Interestingly, in the region of the central necrosis, small hypervascularized nodules were depicted, their development evidently metachronous to the primary tumor growth.

**MRI Artifact Category:** 1
**MRI Density Type:** 1

| MRM score | Finding | Points |
|---|---|---|
| **Shape** | lobulated | 0 |
| **Border** | ill-defined | 1 |
| **CM Distribution** | rim sign | 2 |
| **Initial Signal Intensity Increase** | strong | 2 |
| **Post-initial Signal Intensity Character** | wash-out | 2 |
| **MRI score (points)** | | **7** |
| **MRI BI-RADS** | | **5** |

### → Preliminary Diagnosis

Extensive carcinoma. No differential diagnosis.

| BI-RADS Categorization | | |
|---|---|---|
| Clinical Findings | right 5 | left 1 |
| Ultrasound | right 5 | left 1 |
| Mammography | right 5 | left 1 |
| MR Mammography | right 5 | left 1 |
| **BI-RADS Total** | **right 5** | **left 1** |

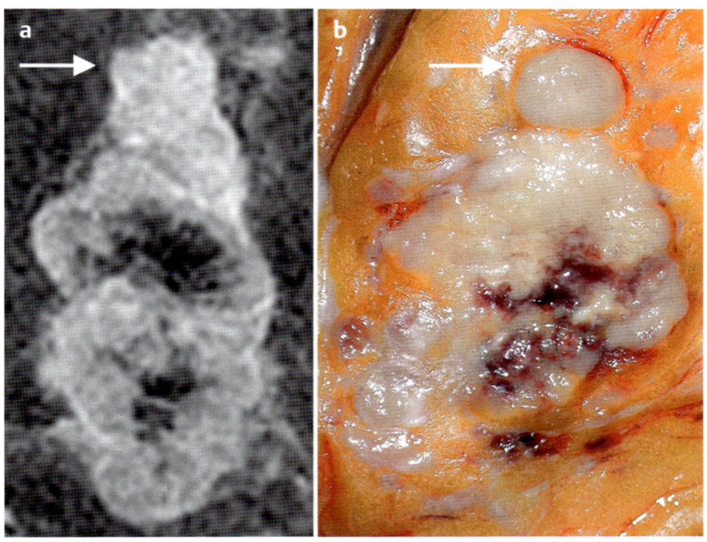


Fig. 74.**9 a, b** The correlation between the MRI findings and the macroscopic sarcoma specimen with respect to the very active peripheral regions, nodular masses (arrows) and central necrosis.

**Procedure**

Histopathological analysis of the palpable lump by US-guided percutaneous core biopsy. In this case, even freehand technique would be feasible.

**Histology**

Carcinosarcoma cells, G4.

### Histology

Carcinosarcoma of the right breast (diameter 4 cm). No involvement of axillary lymph nodes.

Sarcoma of the breast pT3, pN0, G4.

### Treatment

Mastectomy of the right breast, appropriate adjuvant therapy.

Taking the very high grading of the sarcoma into account, the patient's report of discovering the lump only 3 weeks previously can be seen as more plausible than it initially sounded.

**Indication:** Yearly screening examination.
**History:** Unremarkable.
**Risk profile:** No increased risk.
**Age:** 54 years.

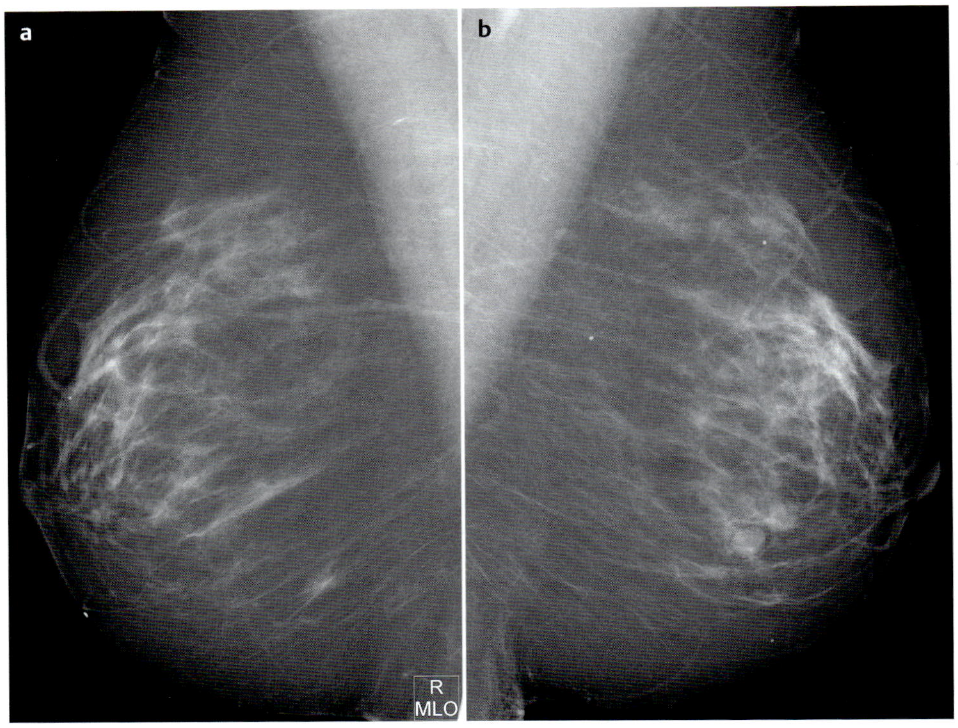


Fig. 75.**2 a, b** Digital mammography, MLO view.

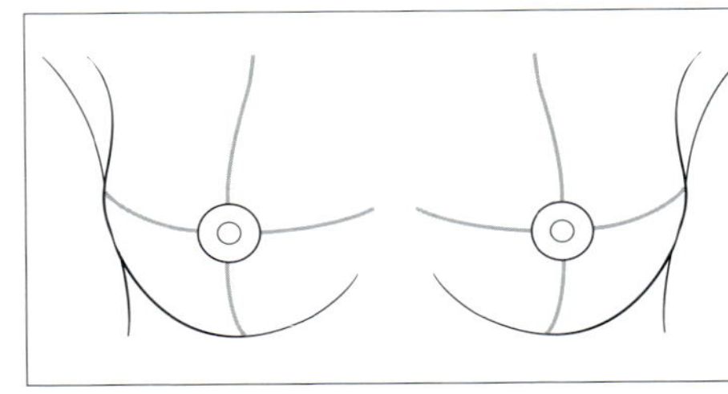

## Clinical Findings

Normal.

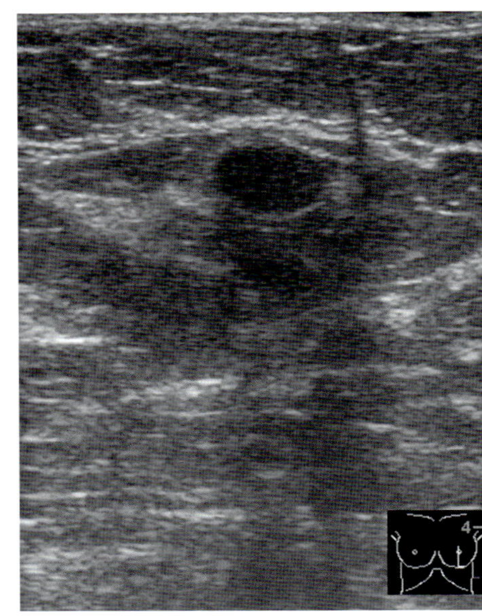

Fig. 75.**1** Sonography.

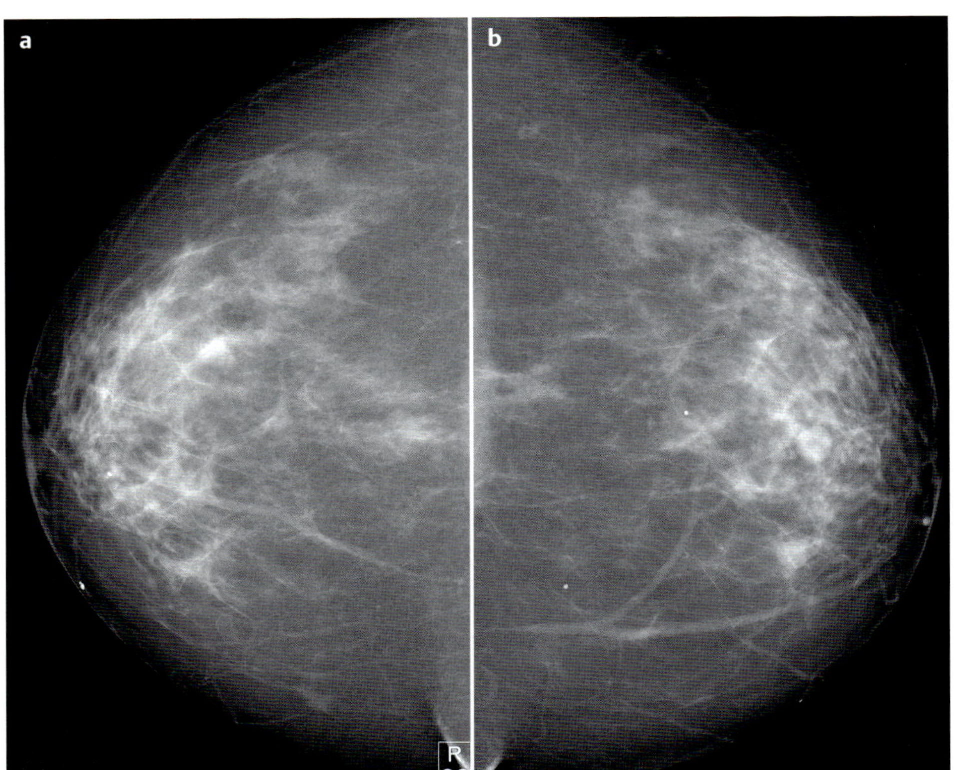


Fig. 75.**3 a, b** Digital mammogaphy, CC view.

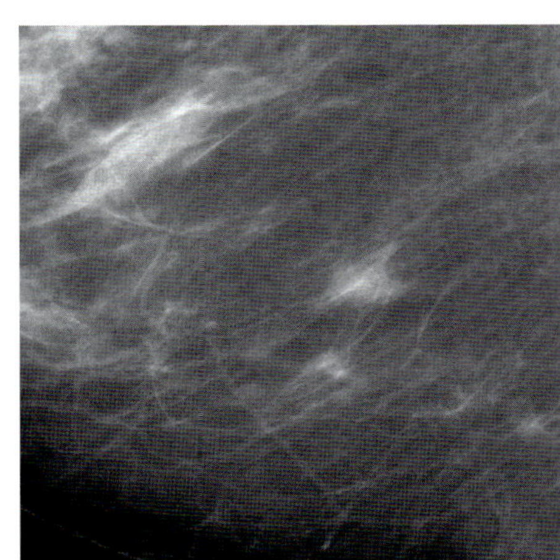

Fig. 75.**4** Spct compression of the right breast, lower quadrants (MLO).

?

Please characterize ultrasound and mammography findings.
What is your preliminary diagnosis?
What are your next steps?

| BI-RADS Categorization | | |
|---|---|---|
| Clinical Findings | right 1 | left 1 |
| Ultrasound | right 1 | left 3 |
| Mammography | right 1 | left 3 |
| **BI-RADS Total** | **right 1** | **left 3** |

This case demonstrates screening imaging studies of an asymptomatic woman.

### Ultrasound

Between the lower quadrants of the left breast there was a round, well-defined lesion with hypoechoic, homogeneous internal texture and unremarkable distal echo pattern. US BI-RADS left (lower quadrants) 3.

### Mammography

Mammograms showed focally asymmetric, inhomogeneously dense parenchyma, ACR type 3. Between the lower quadrants of the left breast, consistent with the finding in ultrasound, there was a round, well-defined, isodense lesion of 1 cm diameter. In the lower quadrants of the right breast there was a circumscribed density, which in spot compression changed shape and appeared equivalent to glandular tissue. There were no architectural distortions and no suspicious microcalcifications BI-RADS right 3/left 3; after spot compression right 1/left 3. PGMI: CC view P; MLO view P.

### → Differential Diagnosis

Left breast: Fibroadenoma, adenoma, papilloma (DD: phyllodes tumor).
Right breast lower quadrants: Isolated parenchymal tissue.

### Procedure

A follow-up ultrasound examination of the lesion between the lower quadrants of the left breast was recommended. Screening examinations at intervals of one year should continue.

### Diagnosis (without histological confirmation)

Left breast: Fibroadenoma.

### Treatment

None.

Are you satisfied with the solution presented? We hope not! Can you suggest an alternative diagnosis?
To have a look at some older mammograms, see part 2 of this case on page 302 (Case 77).
You will see how useful older images can be.

**Indication:** Calcifications detected in a mammogram performed in another clinic.
**History:** Open biopsy of the right breast more than 10 years ago.
**Risk profile:** No increased risk.
**Age:** 72 years.

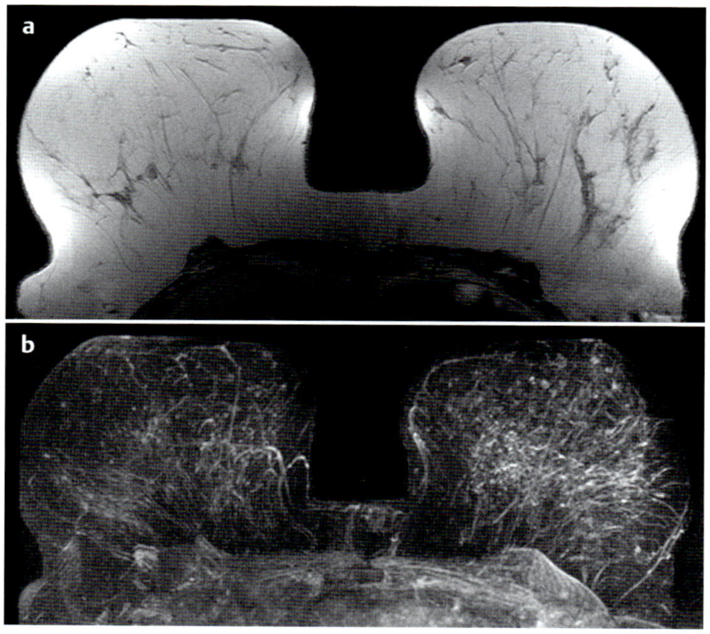


Fig. 76.**1 a, b** Contrast-enhanced MR mammography. Precontrast image and maximum intensity projection.

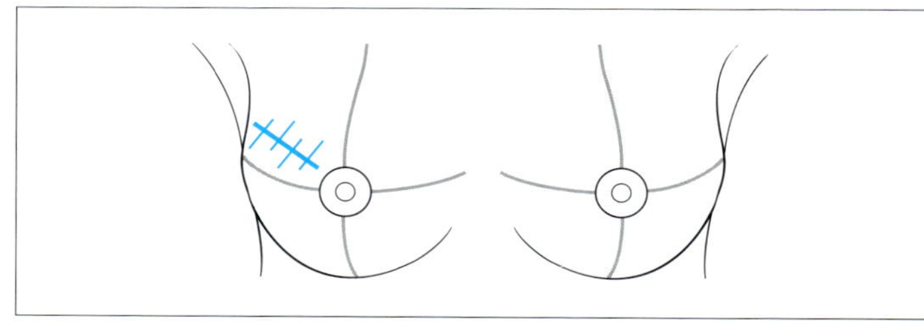

## Clinical Findings

Normal.

## Ultrasound

No unusual findings. (Not shown.)

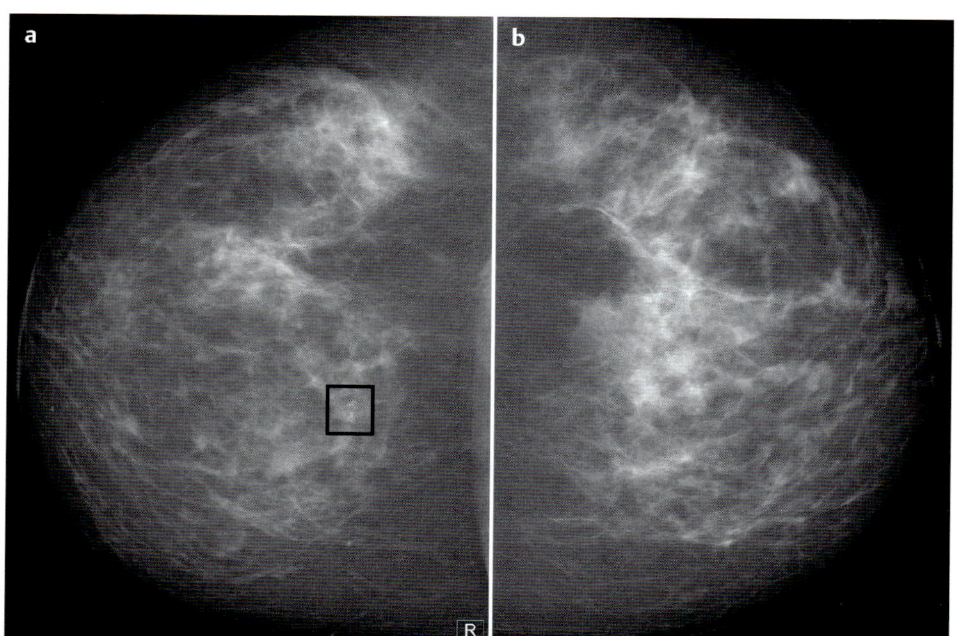


Fig. 76.**2 a, b** Digital mammography, CC view.

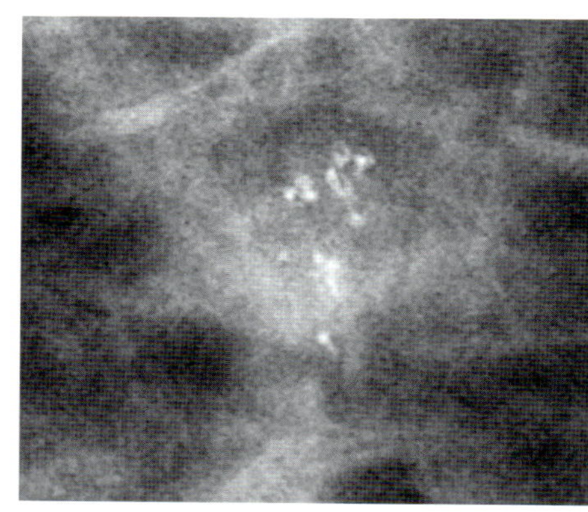

Fig. 76.**3** Magnification view (CC) of the central region of the right breast.

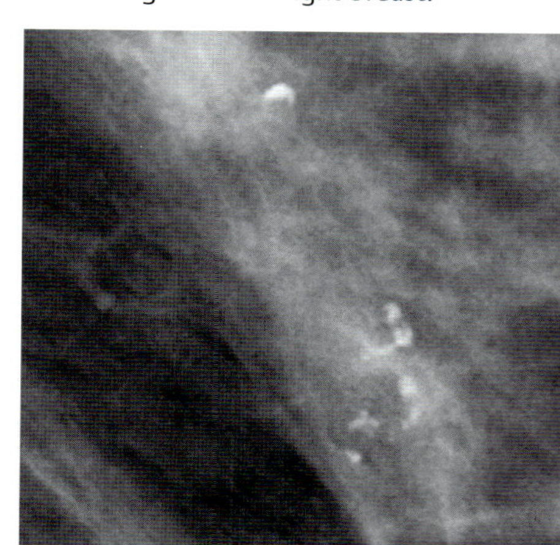

Fig. 76.**4** Magnification view (MLO) of the central region of the right breast.

Please characterize mammography and MRI findings.
What is your preliminary diagnosis?
What are your next steps?

| BI-RADS Categorization | | |
|---|---|---|
| Clinical Findings | right 1 | left 1 |
| Ultrasound | right 1 | left 1 |
| Mammography | right 4 | left 1 |
| MR Mammography | right 1 | left 1 |
| **BI-RADS Total** | **right 4** | **left 1** |

During screening, a cluster of microcalcifications between the inner quadrants of the right breast was detected on a mammogram performed elsewhere.

### Ultrasound (not shown)

Unremarkable.

### Mammography

Bilaterally symmetric, partially inhomogeneously dense parenchyma ACR type 3. A cluster of pleomorphic microcalcifications (some V-shaped, some dumb-bell shaped) was depicted between the inner quadrants of the right breast. No other abnormalities. No densities or lesions. No architectural distortion. BI-RADS right 4/ left 1. PGMI: CC view P.

### MR Mammography

Precontrast imaging at the level of the microcalcifications showed an oval mass within the lipomatous tissue. After administration of contrast there was no pathological enhancement.

### Procedure

Stereotactic vacuum biopsy (Fig. 76.**5**).

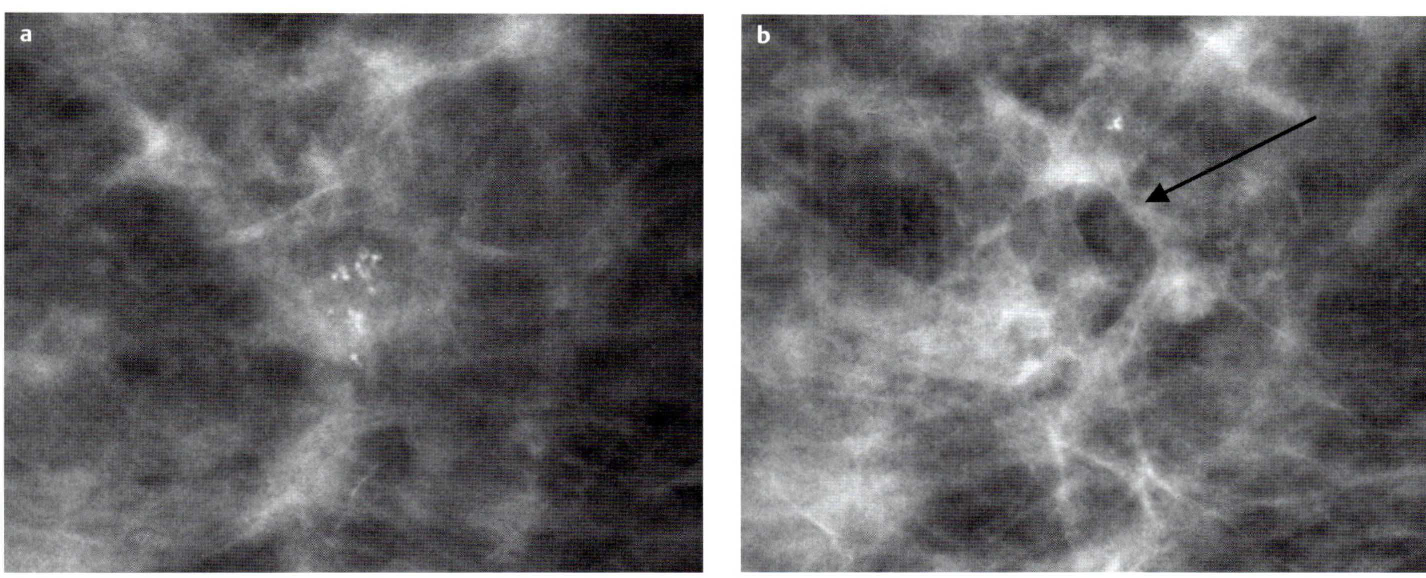


Fig. 76.**5 a, b** Mammography before (**a**) and after (**b**) vacuum biopsy. Documentation of the incomplete removal of the calcifications and tissue damage (arrow).

### Histology

Fibroadenoma (with regressive calcifications).

### Treatment

None.

Stereotactic vacuum biopsy is an ideal method for nonoperative evaluation of microcalcifications categorized BI-RADS 4. The number of unnecessary open biopsies can thus be greatly reduced.

Ah-ha, here are the earlier mammograms from Case 75, just arrived by bike courier!

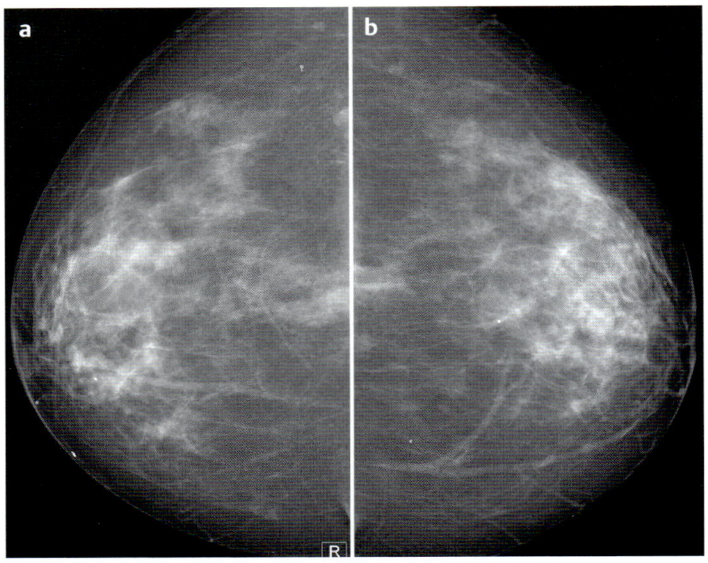

Fig. 77.1 a, b Digital mammography performed 1 year previously, CC view.

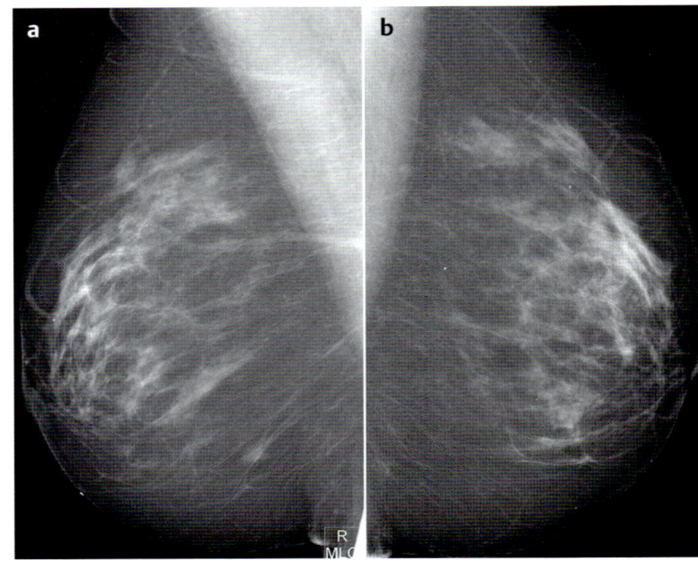

Fig. 77.2 a, b Digital mammography performed 1 year previously, MLO view.

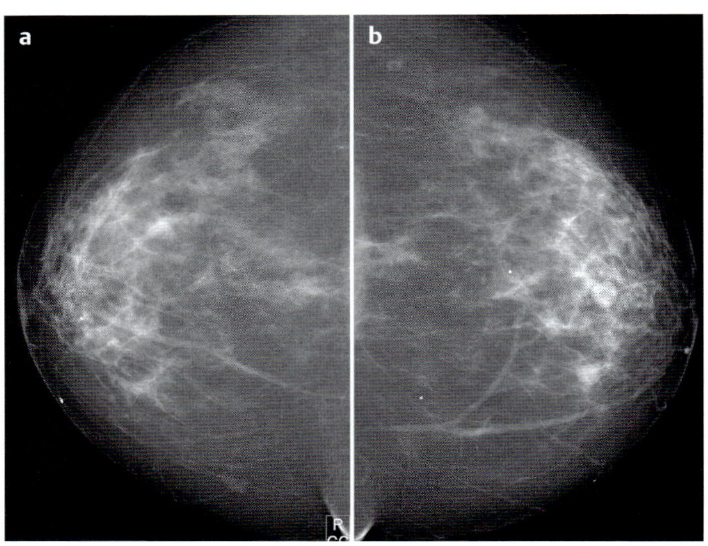

Fig. 77.3 a, b Current mammography, CC view.

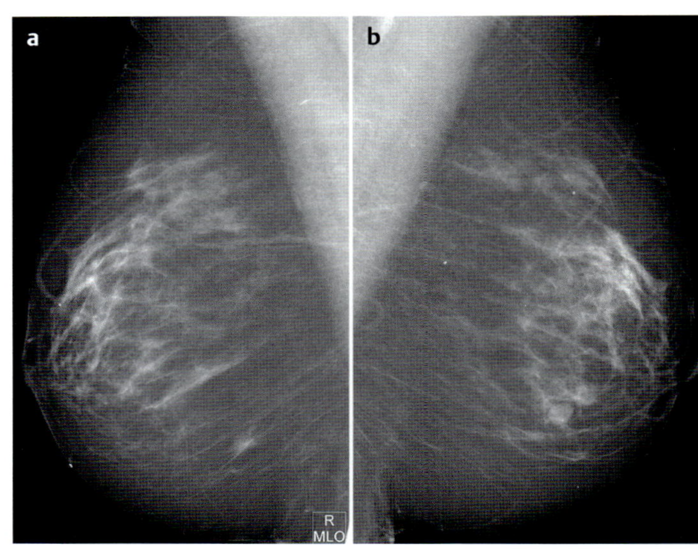

Fig. 77.4 a, b Current mammography, MLO view.

?

Do the earlier mammograms change your interpretation of the recent findings?

Of course you changed your mind: close to the fibroadenoma already identified there is a newly developed mass, which indicates that further investigation is urgently required.

### Ultrasound

Between the inner quadrants of the left breast there was a microlobulated mass measuring 6 mm and disturbing a Cooper's ligament (Fig. 77.**5**). This mass also showed increased peripheral vascularization (Fig. 77.**6**).

### MR Mammography

Solitary hypervascularized lesion in the lower inner quadrant of the left breast (Fig. 77.**7**) with adjoining intraductal tumor component within a milk duct (Fig. 77.**8**).

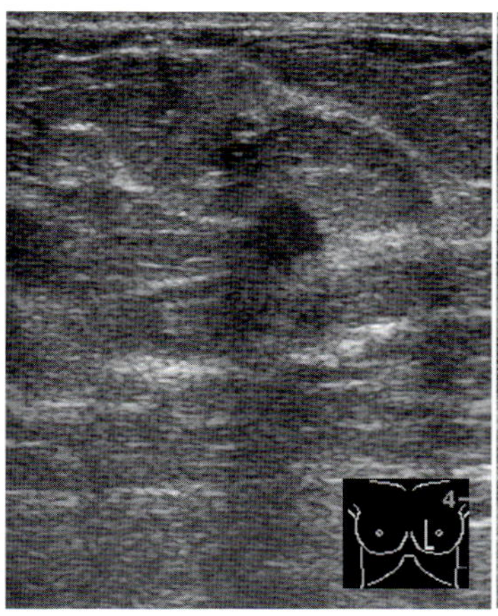

Fig. 77.**5** Sonography.

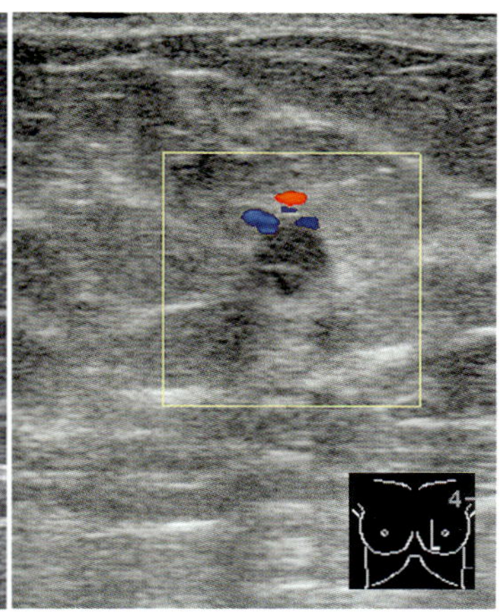

Fig. 77.**6** Color-coded Doppler sonography.

**BI-RADS Categorization**

| | | |
|---|---|---|
| Clinical Findings | right 1 | left 1 |
| Ultrasound | right 1 | left 5 |
| Mammography | right 1 | left 4 |

### Spot compression mammography, left breast (MLO)

Spiculated, highly suspect lesion with internal calcifications (Fig. 77.**9**). Additionally, fibroadenoma with regressive changes. (Note: This lesion showed no enhancement in MRI.)

### Procedure

US-guided core biopsy.

### Histology of the specimen

Invasive ductal carcinoma, G3.

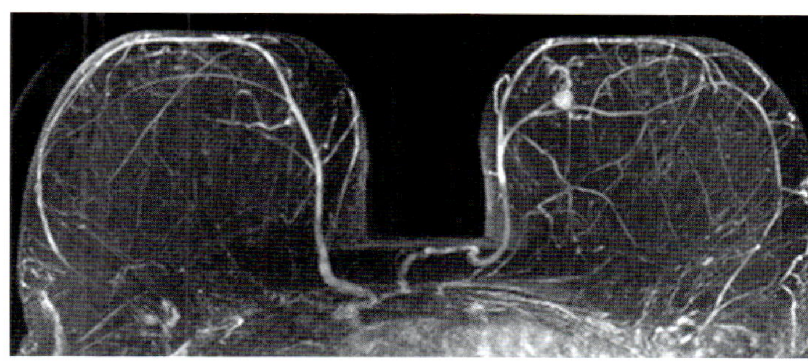

Fig. 77.**7** Contrast-enhanced MR mammography. Maximum intensity projection.

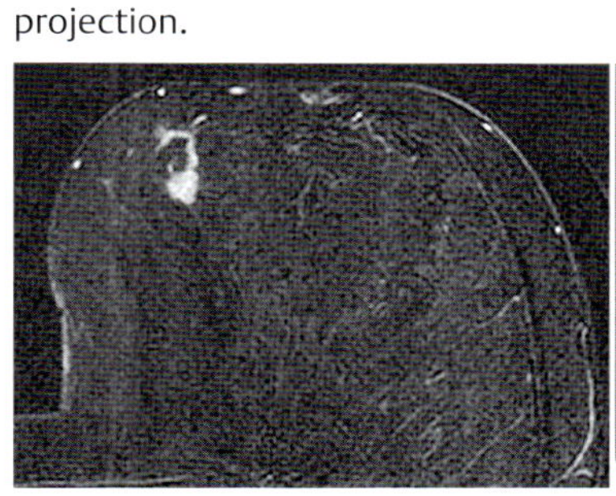

Fig. 77.**8** MR mammography subtraction image. Linear enhancement in tumor region indicates extensive intraductal component.

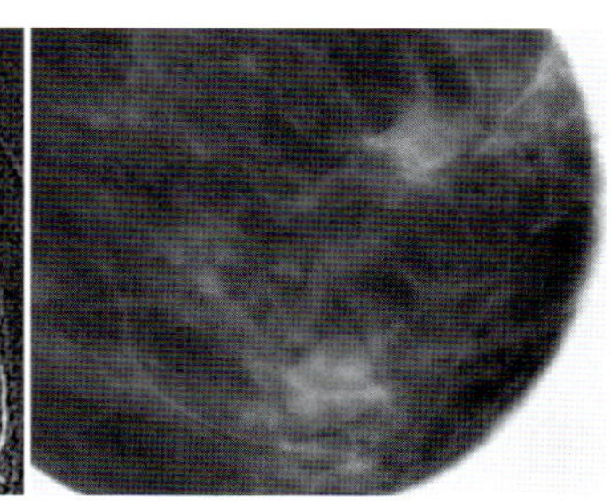

Fig. 77.**9** Spot compression, inner quadrants of left breast.

### Histology

Invasive ductal carcinoma (9 mm) + extensive intraductal component.

IDC pT1b, pN0, G3.

### Treatment

Breast conservation therapy of the left breast.

Older screening images are the radiologist's best friend.

**Indication:** Cutaneous changes of the left nipple.
**History:** Unremarkable.
**Risk profile:** Breast cancer in grandmother at 62 years.
**Age:** 77 years.

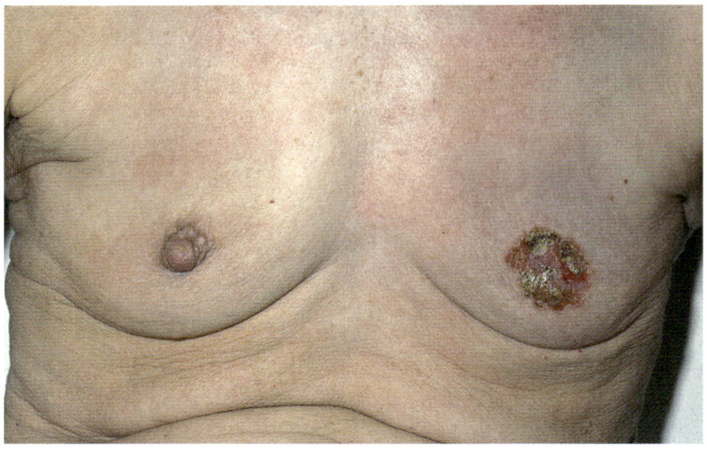

Fig. 78.1 Clinical examination. No findings at palpation.

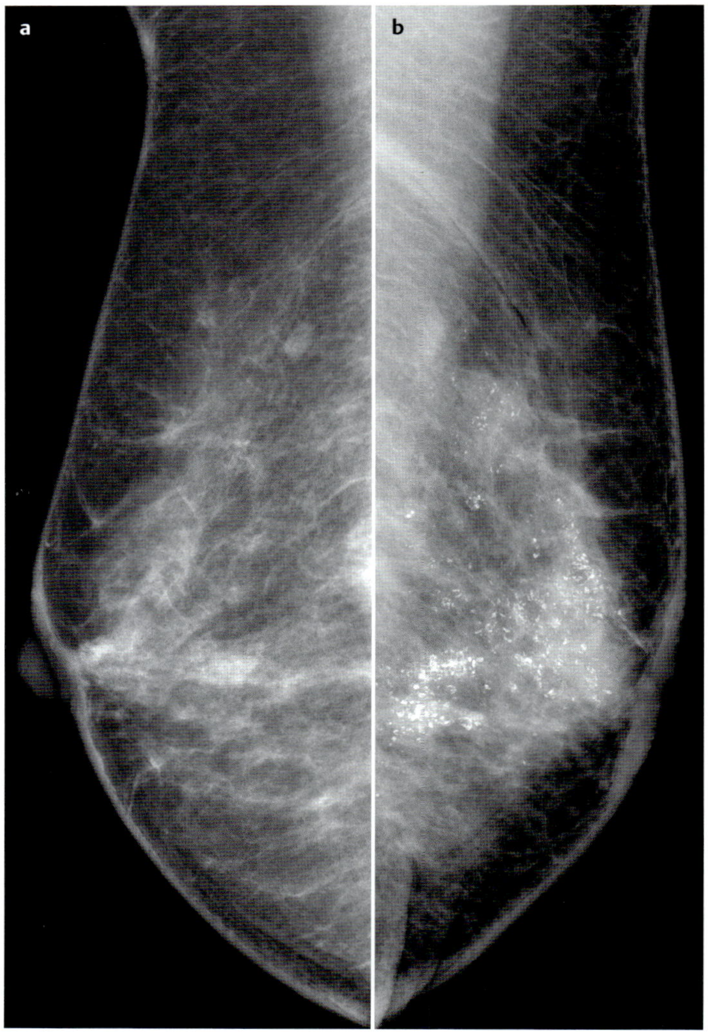


Fig. 78.3 a, b Digital mammography, CC view.

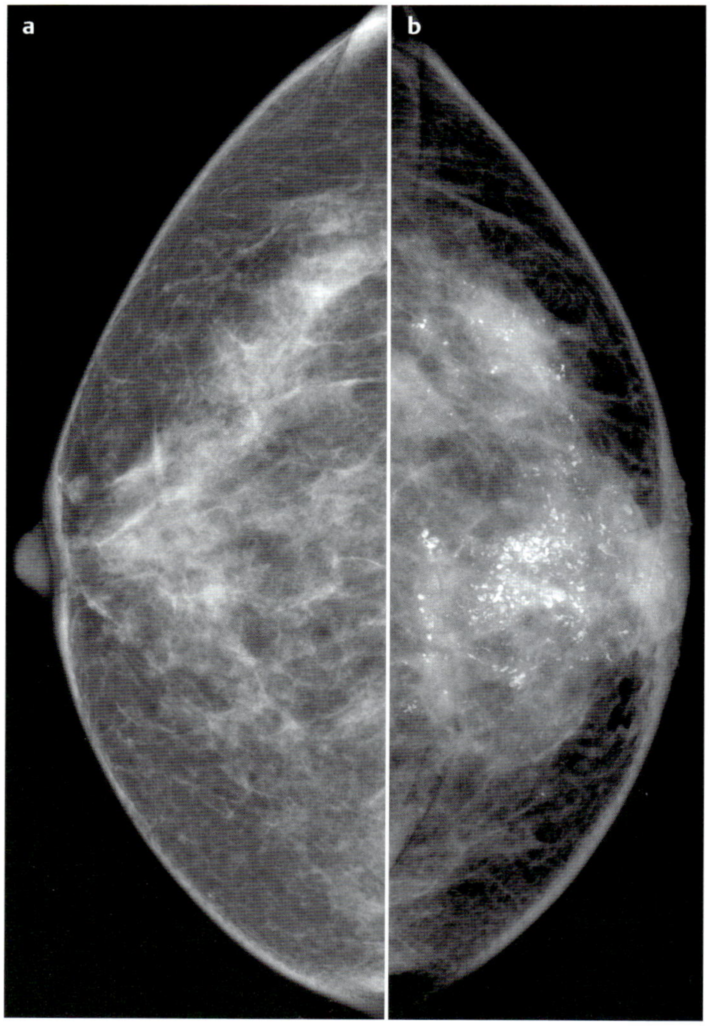


Fig. 78.2 a, b Digital Mammography, MLO view.

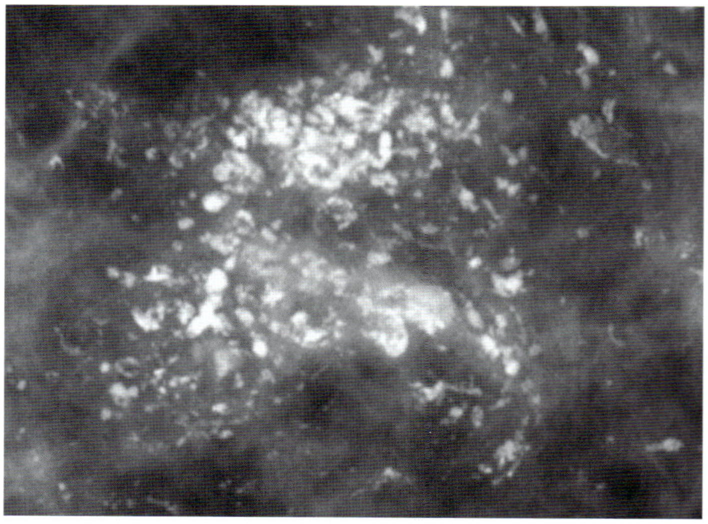

Fig. 78.4 Magnification view (CC), left breast.

?
Please characterize the mammography and clinical findings.
What is your preliminary diagnosis?
What are your next steps?

| BI-RADS Categorization | | |
|---|---|---|
| Clinical Findings | right 1 | left 5 |
| Mammography | right 1 | left 5 |
| **BI-RADS Total** | **right 1** | **left 3** |

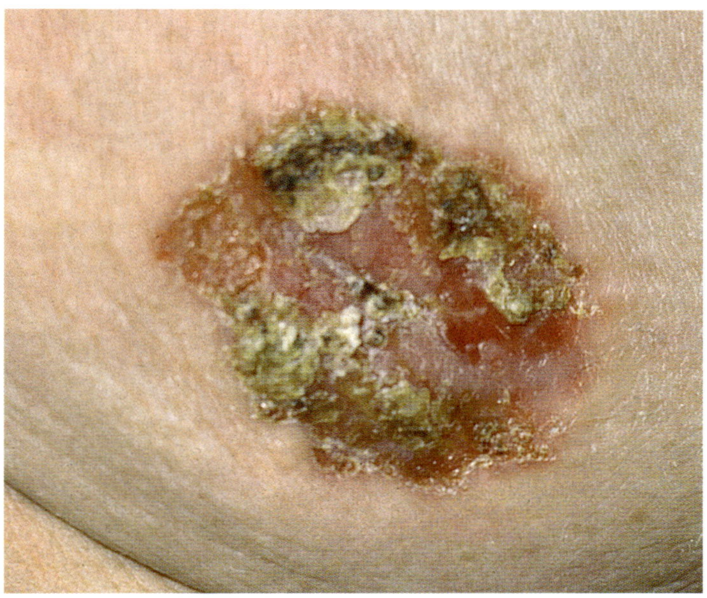

Fig. 78.**5** Enlarged image of the left nipple.

This is the imaging study of a symptomatic patient with eczematous changes of the left nipple (Fig. 78.**5**), and ptosis of both breasts.

### Ultrasound (not shown)

No abnormal findings.

### Mammography

Bilaterally symmetric, inhomogeneously dense parenchyma, ACR type 3. In the upper outer quadrant and central area of the left breast, extensive diffuse pleomorphous micro- and macrocalcifications were depicted. Flattening and thickening of the nipple region of the left breast. No unusual findings in the right breast. BI-RADS right 1/left 5. PGMI CC view G (skin folds); MLO view M (pectoralis muscle).

### → Differential Diagnosis

Paget disease; benign eczema of the nipple (unlikely).

### Procedure

Skin biopsy of the eczematous tissue of the areola.

### Histology

Paget disease.

### Histology

Paget disease with extensive intramammary DCIS.

### Treatment

Mastectomy of the left breast.

Eczematous changes of the nipple or areola region are always suggestive for Paget disease.

**Indication:** Lump in the left breast.
**History:** Unremarkable.
**Risk profile:** No increased risk.
**Age:** 75 years.

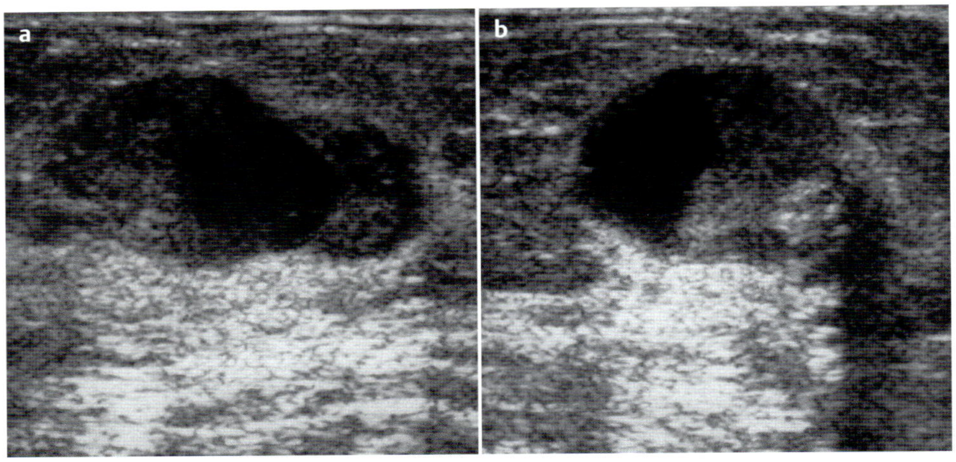

Fig. 79.**1 a, b** Sonography.

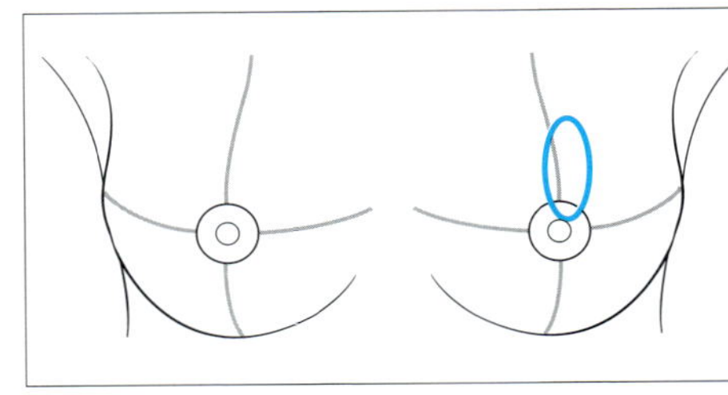

### Clinical Findings

Smooth, oval lump measuring 2 cm in the central part of the left breast.

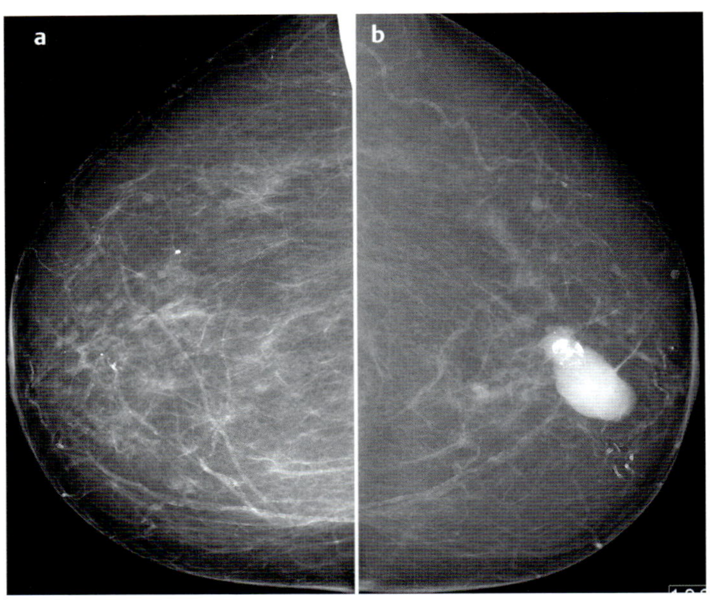

Fig. 79.**2 a, b** Digital mammography, CC view.

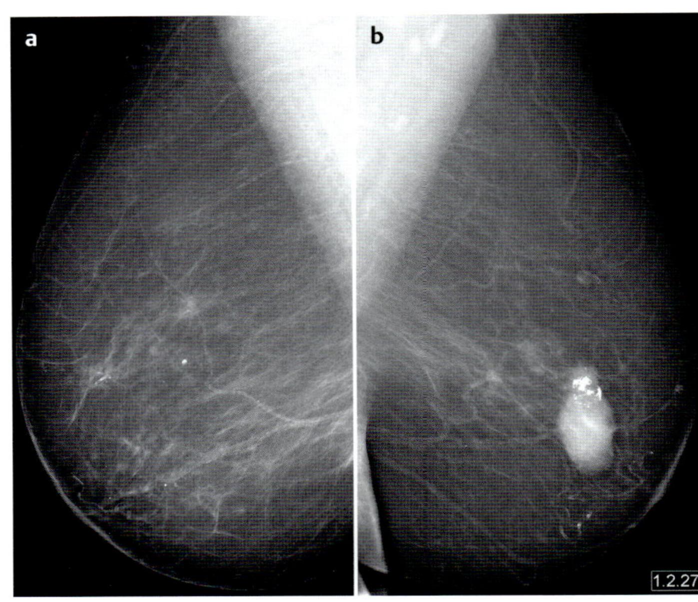

Fig. 79.**3 a, b** Digital mammography, MLO view.

Please characterize the ultrasound and mammography findings.
What is your preliminary diagnosis?
What are your next steps?

| BI-RADS Categorization | | |
|---|---|---|
| Clinical Findings | right 1 | left 2 |
| Ultrasound | right 1 | left 4 |
| Mammography | right 1 | left 4 |
| **BI-RADS Total** | **right 1** | **left 3** |

This is the imaging study of a symptomatic woman with a palpable mass discovered a couple of weeks earlier in the center of the left breast. Clinically this lump seemed benign.

### Ultrasound

Consistent with the clinical findings, sonography showed a well-defined, mainly solid but partially cystic oval mass in the left breast. Due to the possibility of a malign phyllodes tumor, this was categorized US BI-RADS left 4.

### Mammography

Bilaterally predominantly lipomatous glandular tissue, ACR type 1. Consistent with the palpable finding, there was a well-defined, oval, hyperdense lesion measuring 2 cm with internal popcorn-like macrocalcifications in the center of the left breast (Fig. 79.**4**). Arteriosclerosis. Possibility of a malignant phyllodes tumor adjoining a fibroadenoma with regressive changes; hence categorization as BI-RADS right 1/left 4. PGMI CC view M (superimposition of tissue in the right breast laterally, image not repeated); MLO view G (inframammary fold).

## → Differential Diagnosis

Phyllodes tumor, hamartoma, fibroadenoma, papilloma.

### Procedure

Although the lesion was categorized BI-RADS 4, an open biopsy of the lesion was performed without preoperative core biopsy at the request of the patient as well as of her son.

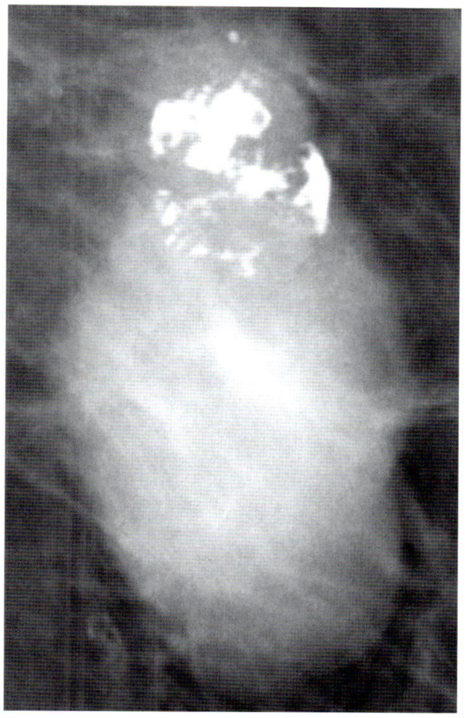

Fig. 79.**4** Magnification view of the left breast.

## Histology

Partially hemorrhagic, partially calcified tumor 17 mm in diameter.

Tumorlike sclerosing adenosis.

## Treatment

Excisional biopsy. No further therapy.

***Macro***calcifications within a tumor are nearly always a sign of benign processes.

**Indication:** Screening.
**History:** Unremarkable.
**Risk profile:** No increased risk.
**Age:** 66 years.

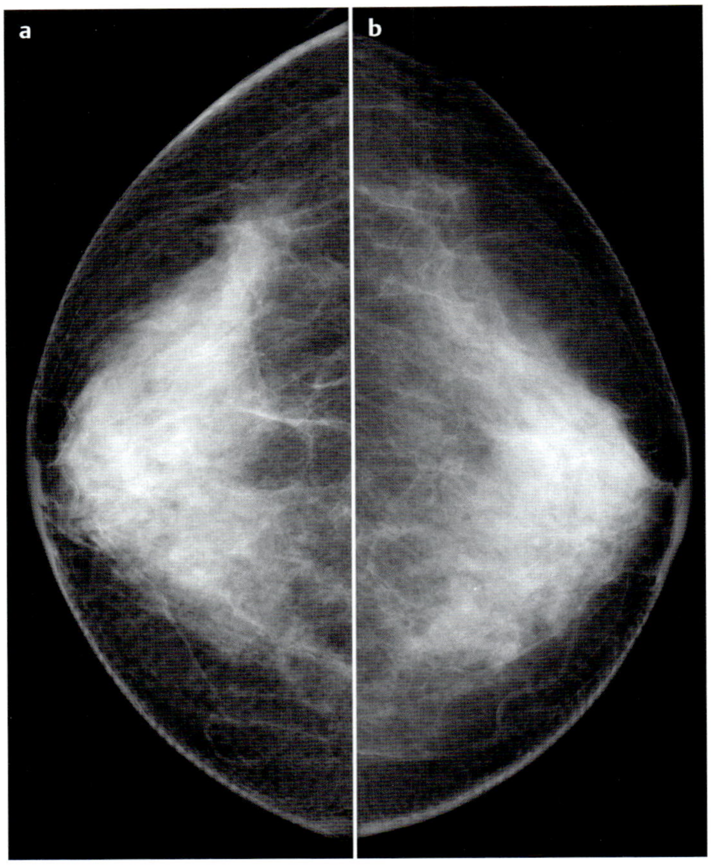

Fig. 80.**1 a, b** Digital mammography, MLO view.

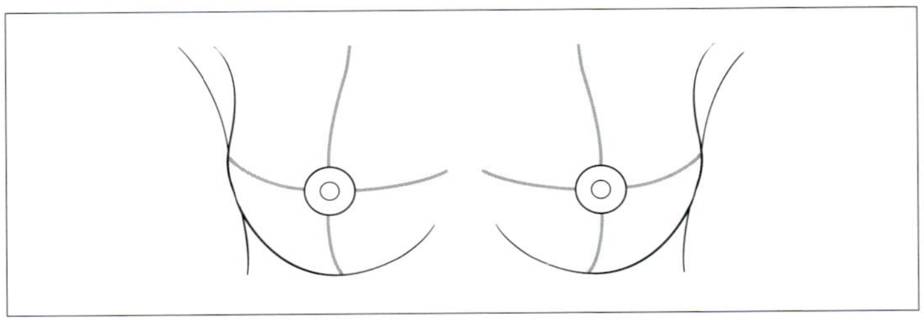

**Clinical Findings**

Normal.

**Ultrasound (not shown)**

No unusual findings.

Please characterize the mammography findings.
What is your preliminary diagnosis?
What are your next steps?

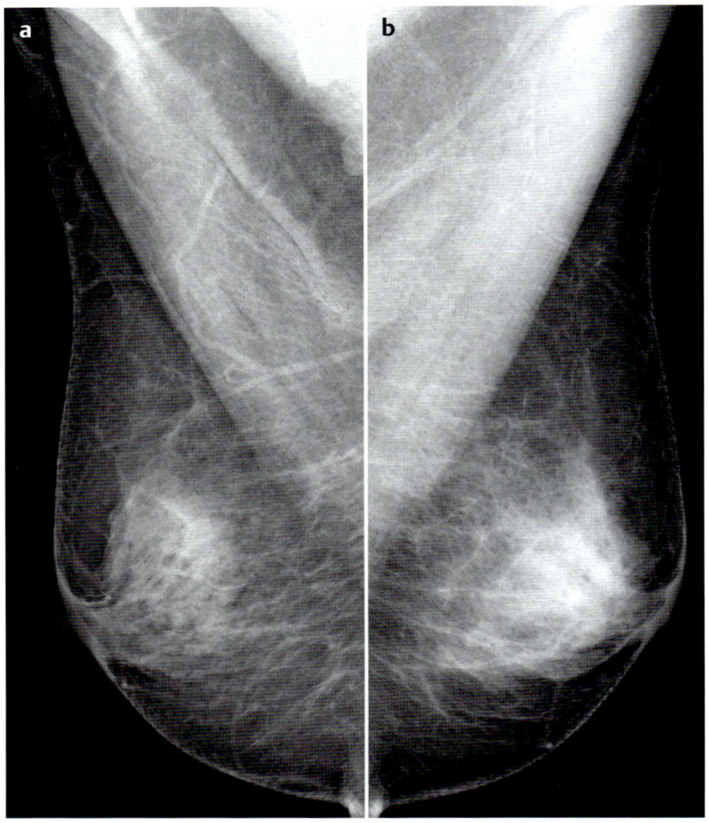

Fig. 80.**2 a, b** Digital mammography, CC view.

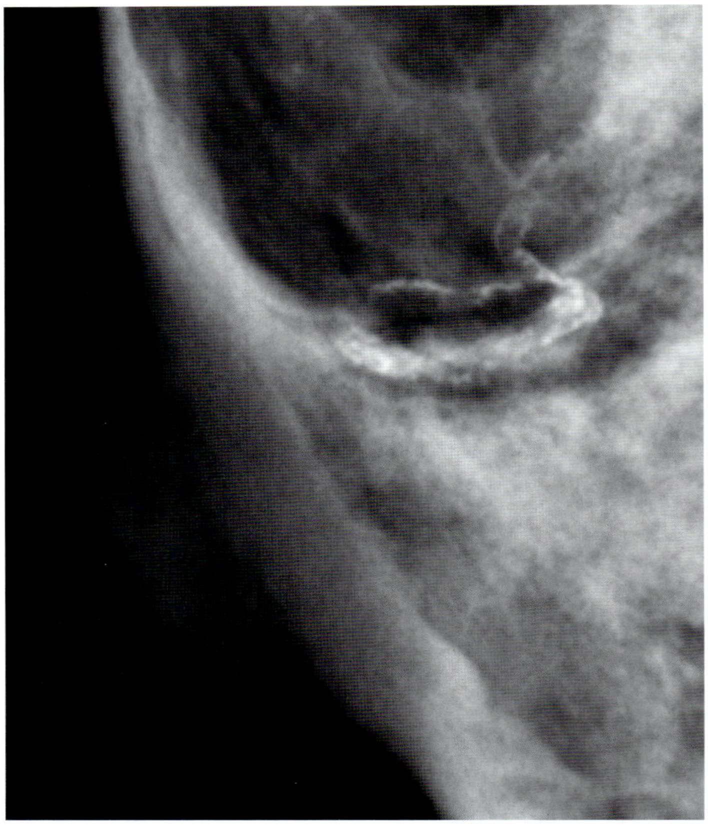

Fig. 80.**3** Zoomed view of the region behind the right nipple, MLO view.

| BI-RADS Categorization | | |
|---|---|---|
| Clinical Findings | right 1 | left 1 |
| Ultrasound | right 1 | left 1 |
| Mammography | right 1 | left 1 |
| **BI-RADS Total** | **right 1** | **left 1** |

This case presents images from screening mammography.

### Ultrasound (not shown)

Normal echogenicity of the parenchyma bilaterally. No unusual findings in the right breast behind the nipple or elsewhere. US BI-RADS right 1/left 1.

### Mammography

Symmetric, inhomogeneously dense parenchyma, ACR type 3. No circumscribed masses or densities. In the area behind the nipple of the right breast there was a lobulated, centrally transparent macrocalcification visible in MLO view. CC view here showed pronounced tramline-like arterial calcifications. No suspicious microcalcifications. BI-RADS right 1/left 1. PGMI: CC view P; MLO view P.

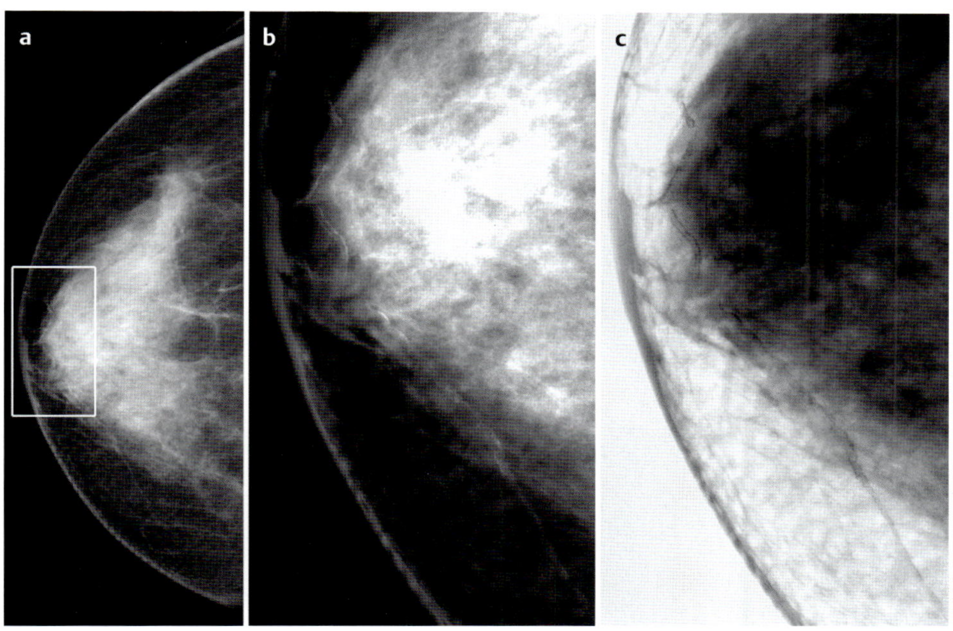


Fig. 80.**4 a–c** Mammography of the right breast in CC view. Enlarged and inverted images.

### Diagnosis (no histological confirmation)

Intramammary arteriosclerosis.

### Treatment

None. In the case of extensive arteriosclerotic changes, the presence of an underlying condition should be investigated.

The MLO view here suggested the presence of fat necrosis.
As in this case, summation artifacts arising coincidentally in mammographic projection can mimic certain tumor entities.

**Indication:** Screening.
**History:** Unremarkable.
**Risk profile:** No increased risk.
**Age:** 46 years.

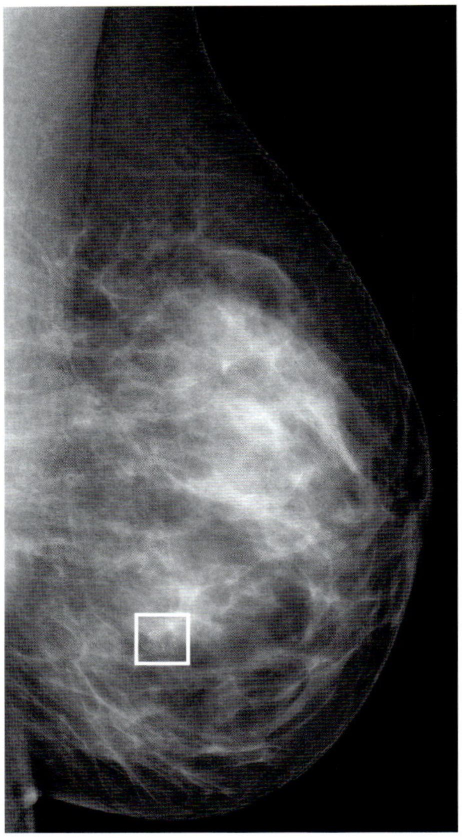

Fig. 81.**1** Digital mammography of the left breast, CC view.

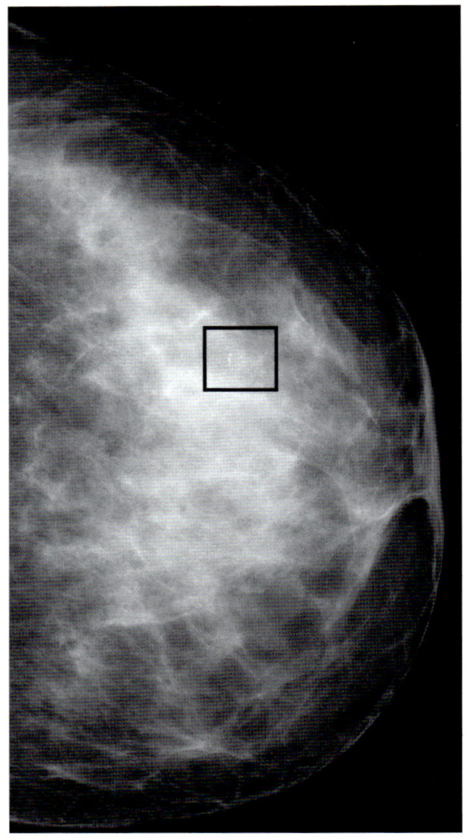

Fig. 81.**2** Digital mammography of the left breast, MLO view.

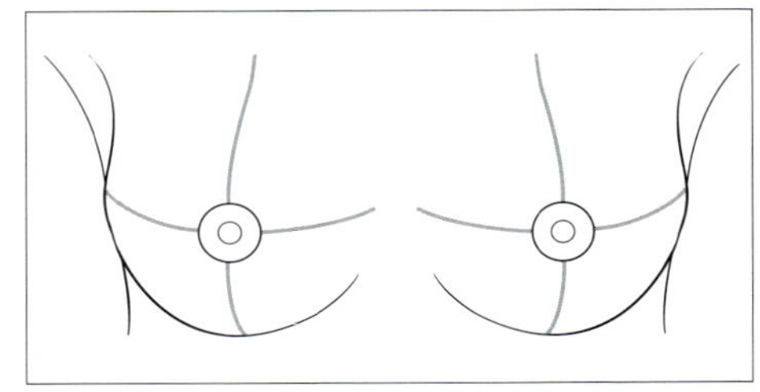

## Clinical Findings

Normal.

## Ultrasound

No unusual findings.

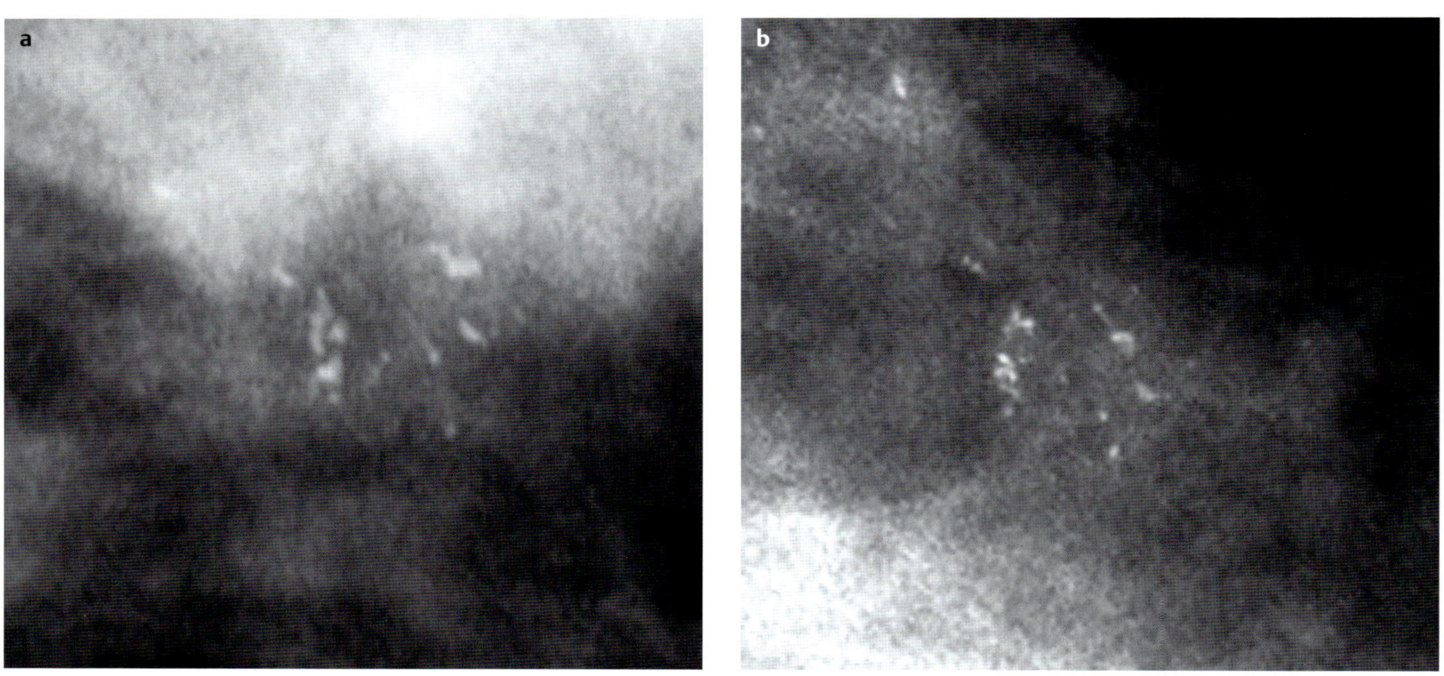


Fig. 81.**3 a, b** Magnification views of the left breast.

?

Please characterize the mammography findings.
What is your preliminary diagnosis?
What are your next steps?

| BI-RADS Categorization | | |
|---|---|---|
| Clinical Findings | right 1 | left 1 |
| Ultrasound | right 1 | left 1 |
| Mammography | right 1 | left 4 |
| **BI-RADS Total** | **right 1** | **left 4** |

This is a typical screening mammography.

### Mammography

ACR type 4 glandular tissue density. In the lower outer quadrant of the left breast at the 4-o'clock position, a cluster of polymorphous microcalcifications could be seen. BI-RADS 4. PGMI is not defined for unilateral mammograms.

### Procedure

Histopathological analysis of the microcalcifications with stereotactic vacuum biopsy.

### Specimen radiography

Characteristic documentation of calcifications in multiple specimens (Fig. 81.**4**).

### Histopathology of the specimen

Ductal carcinoma in situ (DCIS) (Fig. 81.**5**).

### Procedure

Open biopsy after preoperative localization.

### Radiography of the macroscopic specimen

Two residual microcalcifications were depicted near the end of the hook-wire (Fig. 81.**6**).

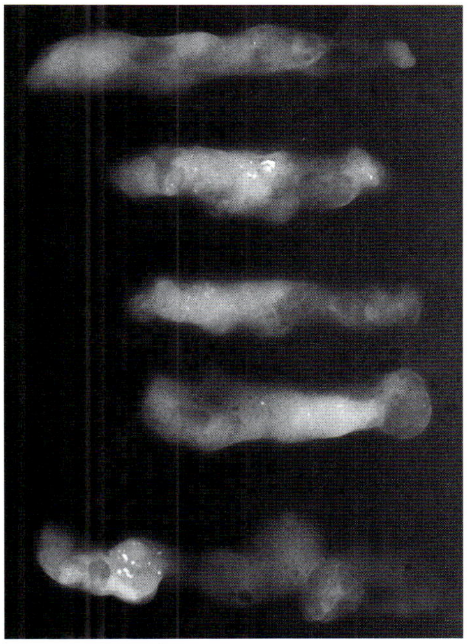

Fig. 81.**4** Specimen radiography.

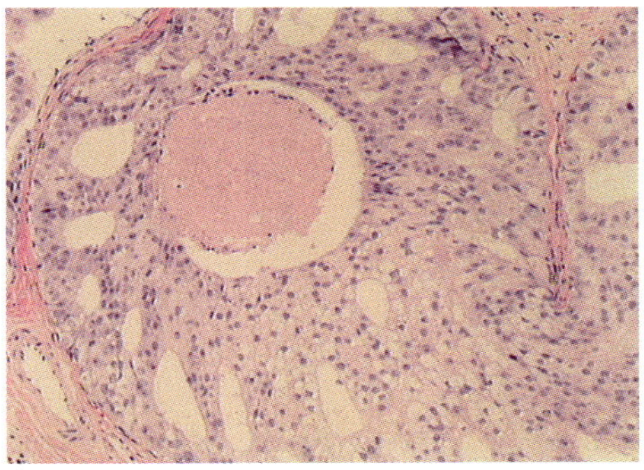

Fig. 81.**5** Histology of the specimens.

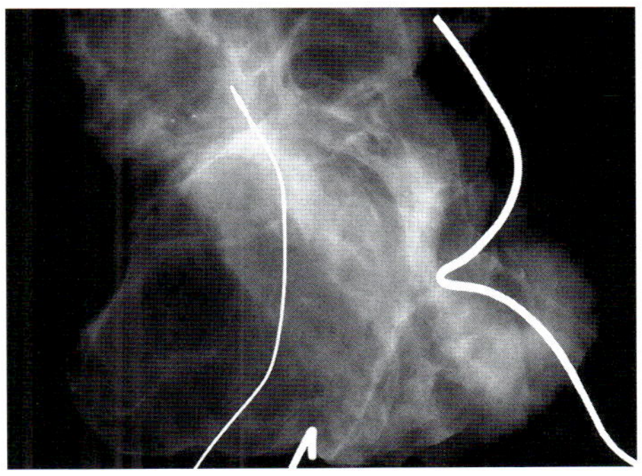

Fig. 81.**6** Radiography of the macroscopic specimen.

### Histology

DCIS pTis, pN0, M0, R0.

### Treatment

No further measures. Follow-up monitoring.

This case shows a classic screening carcinoma that is detectable only by mammography.

**Indication:** Monitoring following carcinoma of the right breast.
**History:** Mastectomy and reconstruction surgery 5 years previously.
**Risk profile:** Increased by previous instance of breast cancer.
**Age:** 44 years.

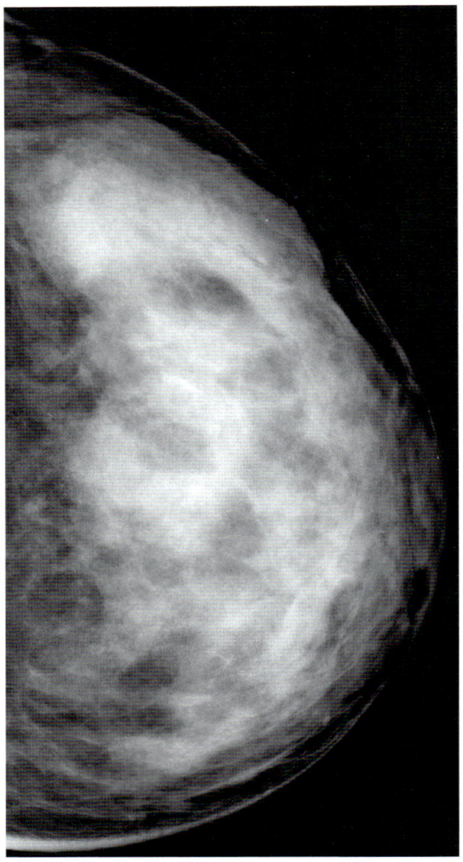

Fig. 82.**1** Digital mammography of the left breast, CC view.

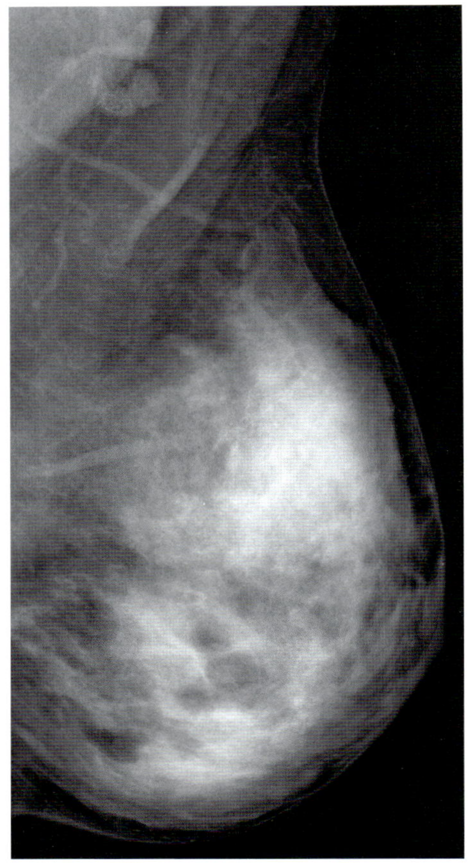

Fig. 82.**2** Digital mammography of the left breast, MLO view.

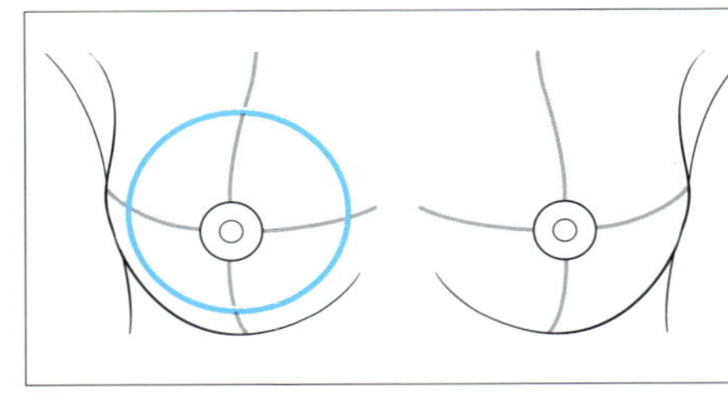

### Clinical Findings

Normal mastectomy scar and implant in the right breast. No other unusual findings at inspection and palpation.

### Ultrasound

Unremarkable (not shown).

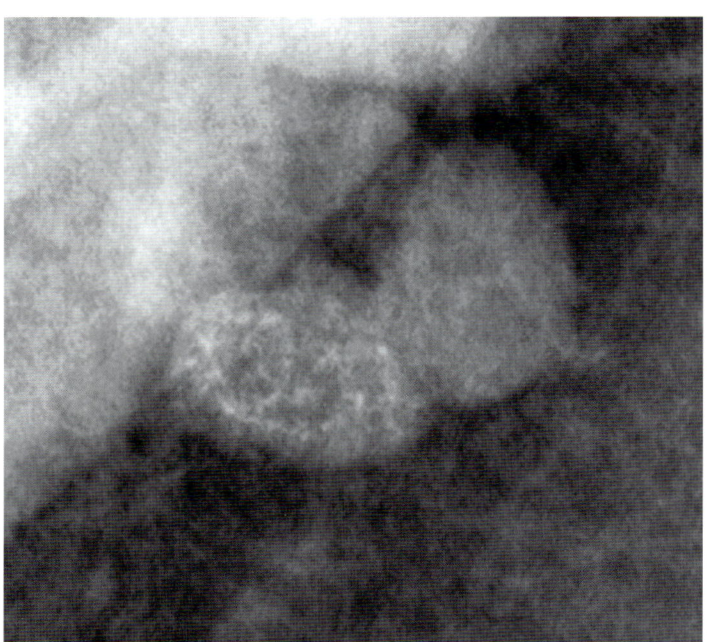

Fig. 82.**3** Digital mammography (magnification view) of the left axilla.

?

Please characterize the mammography findings.
What is your preliminary diagnosis?
What are your next steps?

| BI-RADS Categorization | | |
|---|---|---|
| Clinical Findings | right 1 | left 1 |
| Ultrasound | right 1 | left 1 |
| Mammography | right 1 | left 4 |
| **BI-RADS Total** | **right 1** | **left 4** |

This case demonstrates the imaging from a follow-up examination after mastectomy and reconstruction surgery 5 years earlier.

### Ultrasound

There were no unusual findings. In particular, the left axillary region showed no signs of malignancy. US BI-RADS right 1.

### Mammography

The patient had a normal prosthesis of the right breast (not shown). Mammography of the left breast showed extremely dense parenchyma, ACR type 4, with some benign microcalcifications. No masses or densities were detected. Two axillary lymph nodes were visible, which were not enlarged. One of these included multiple hyperdense flecks. BI-RADS right 1/left 4. PGMI is not defined for unilateral imaging.

### → Preliminary Diagnosis

Microcalcifications within an axillary lymph node, probable metastases of an unknown primary tumor in a woman with increased risk of breast cancer (earlier contralateral carcinoma). Differential diagnosis: foreign bodies within the lymph node.

### Procedure

Excisional biopsy of the lymph node after preoperative hook-wire localization.

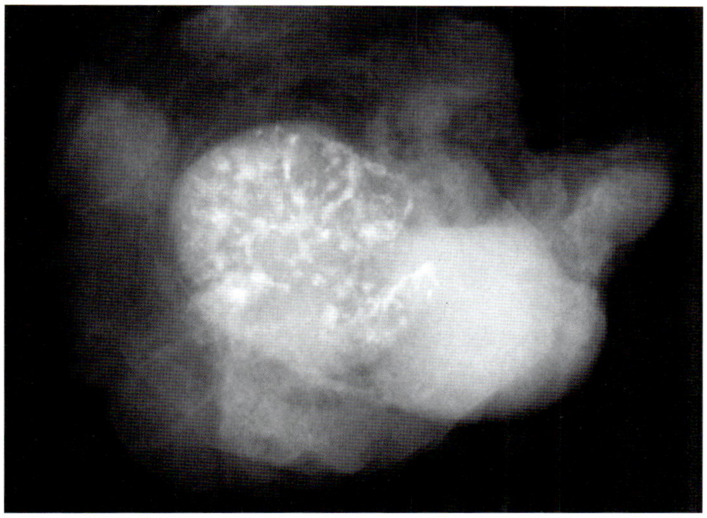

Fig. 82.**4** Specimen radiography.

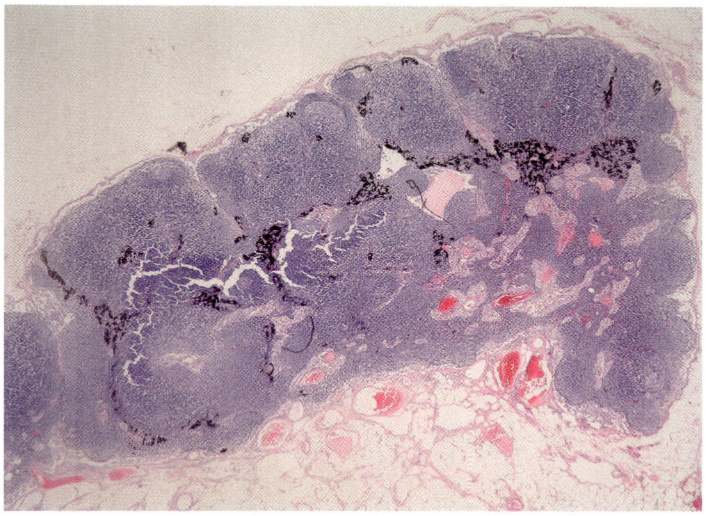

Fig. 82.**5** Histological specimen.

### Histology

Colored particles within an axillary lymph node.

After extensive questioning, it emerged that the patient painted as a hobby. It is possible that paint particles were introduced into the body through tiny hand injuries, and accumulated in the lymph nodes.

**Indication:** Swelling and reddening.
**History:** Possible recent insect bite.
**Risk profile:** No increased risk.
**Age and sex:** 34 years, *male.*

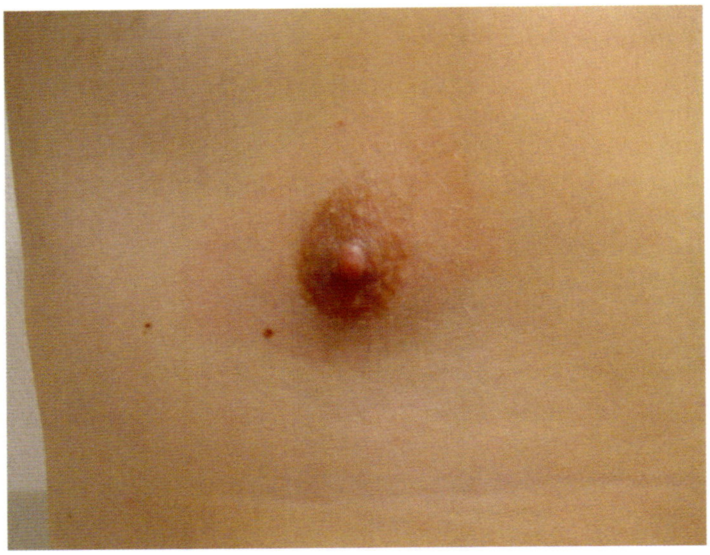

Fig. 83.**1** Clinical examination.

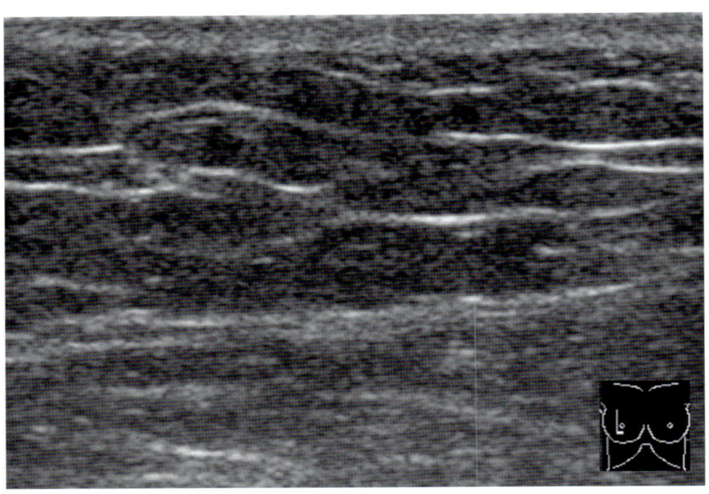

Fig. 83.**2** Ultrasound.

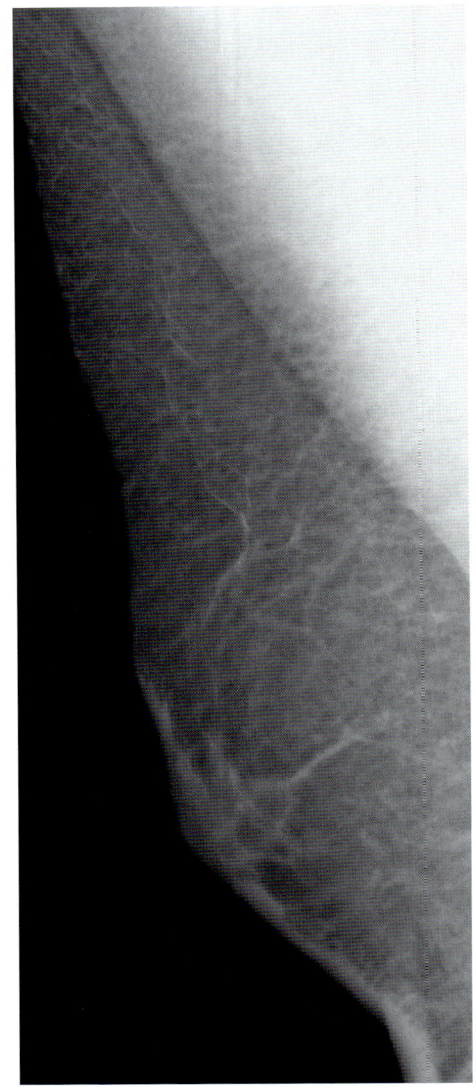

Fig. 83.**3** Digital mammography of the left breast, MLO view.

Please characterize ultrasound, mammography, and clinical findings.
What is your preliminary diagnosis?
What are your next steps?

Diagnostic imaging was carried out to investigate an inflammation in the area around the nipple in a male patient.

### Inspection

The inflamed region around the right nipple was well defined. Two nevi. The location of the insect bite was visible above the nipple at the cranial limit of the inflammation (Fig. 82.**4**).

### Ultrasound

The appearance of the skin and subcutaneous structures was normal. No displacing formations. US BI-RADS right 1.

### Mammography

The MLO view was unremarkable. Cutaneous and subcutaneous structures were normal. There were no tissue-displacing formations and no microcalcifications. BI-RADS right 1. PGMI is not defined for unilateral mammography.

### → Preliminary Diagnosis

Infection, allergic dermatological reaction, mastitis, carcinoma.

### Procedure

Empirical antibiotic treatment; local cooling.
Determination of infection markers and *Borrelia* antibodies.

### Laboratory results

Moderately elevated infection markers. *Bcrrelia* antibody titer highly positive.

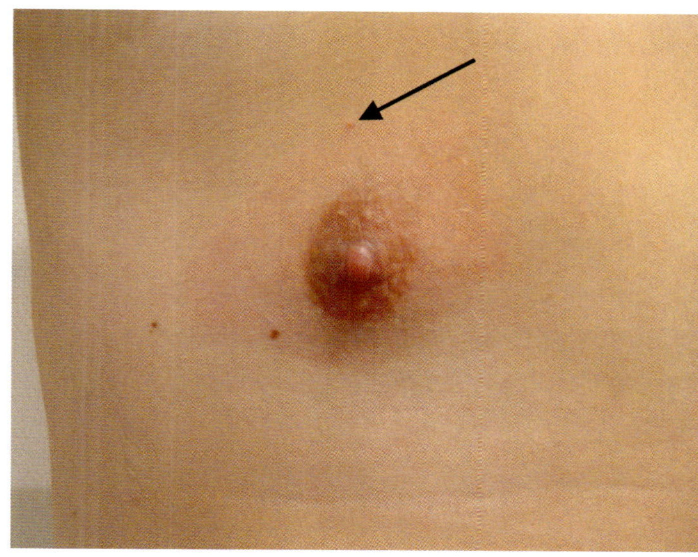

Fig. 83.**4** Location of the mosquito bite (arrow).

### Diagnosis

Erythema cronicum migrans due to Borreliosis (following insect bite).

### Treatment

Antibiotic therapy for 4 weeks. After 2 weeks the inflammation had completely disappeared.

Inflammatory changes of the breast may be treated with antibiotics for a limited period of 10 – 14 days. However, if antibiotic therapy has no effect, a differential diagnosis of inflammatory breast cancer must be considered and histological investigation is essential.

**Indication:** Small lump in the right breast.
**History:** Unremarkable.
**Risk profile:** No increased risk.
**Age:** 39 years.

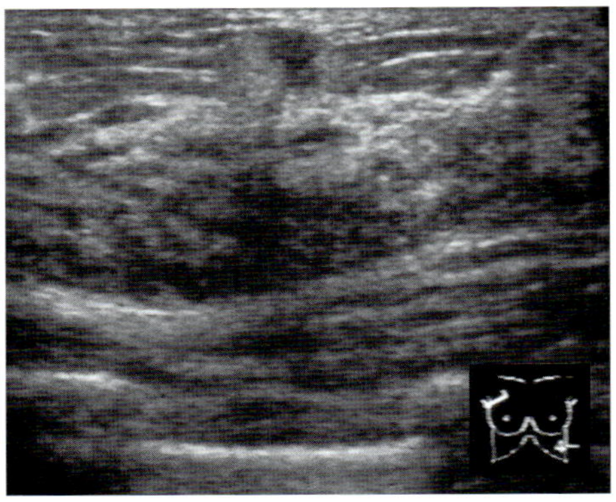

Fig. 84.**1** Sonography.

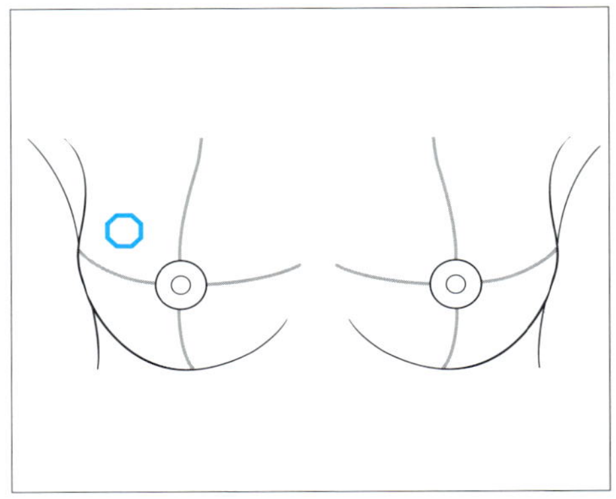

## Clinical Findings

A small resistance with characteristics of a gland measuring 5 mm in the upper outer quadrant of the right breast. Generally nodular parenchymal texture.

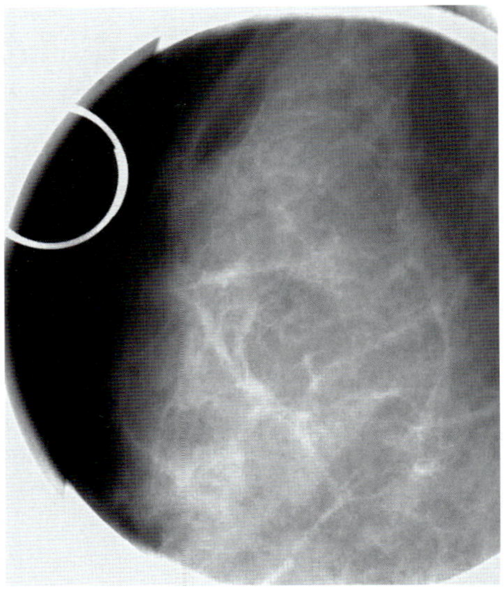

Fig. 84.**4** Spot compression of the upper outer quadrant of the right breast with marker at the site of the palpable mass.

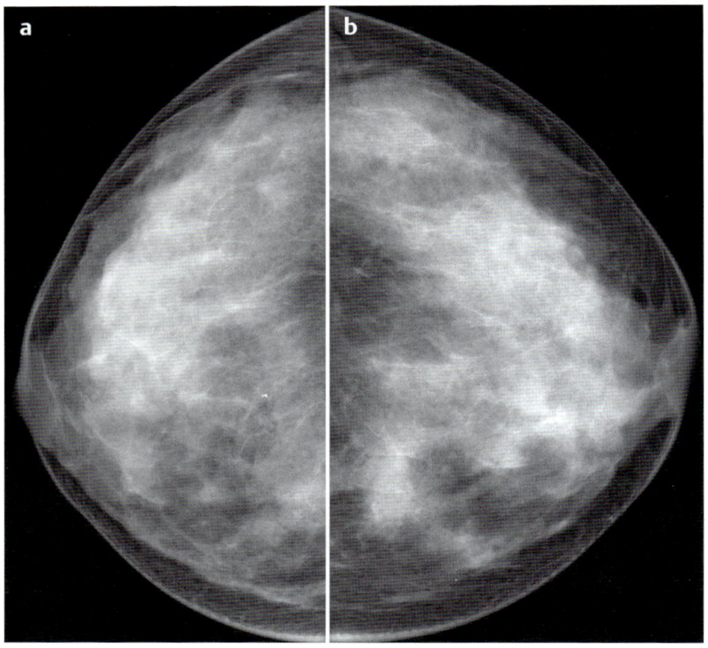


Fig. 84.**2 a, b** Digital mammography, CC view.

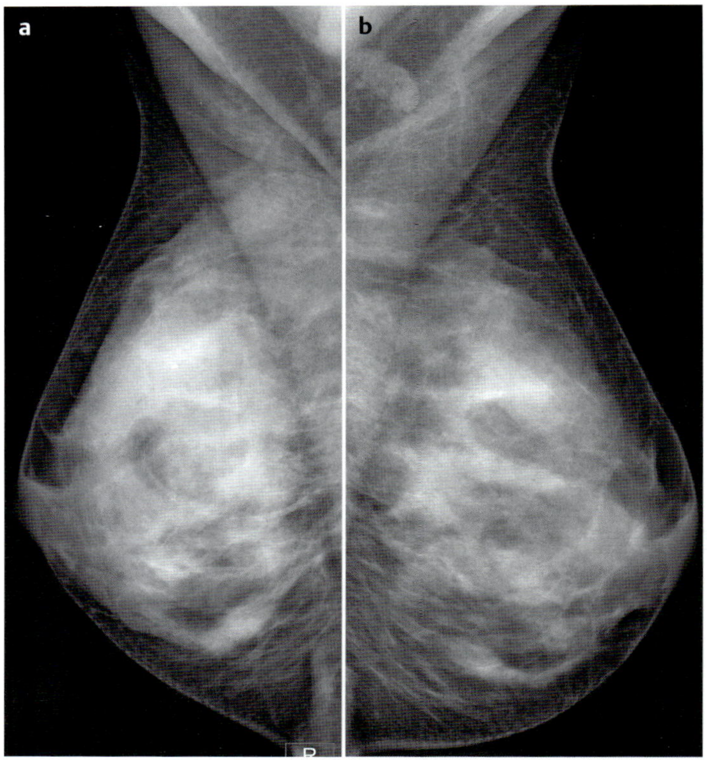


Fig. 84.**3 a, b** Digital mammography, MLO view.

?

Please characterize ultrasound and mammography findings.
What is your preliminary diagnosis?
What are your next steps?

| BI-RADS Categorization | | |
|---|---|---|
| Clinical Findings | right 3 | left 1 |
| Ultrasound | right 5 | left 1 |
| Mammography | right 1 | left 1 |
| **BI-RADS Total** | **right 5** | **left 1** |

This case presents the imaging of a symptomatic woman. The palpable lump had characteristics of a harmless sclerotic gland; nevertheless, this was the reason for the examination.

### Ultrasound

In the area of the palpable lump, ultrasound showed a round, well-defined lesion with markedly hyperechoic margins. This lesion had caused distortion of the surrounding echogenic tissue (Fig. 84.**5**). There was no distal shadowing to indicate a tumor. US BI-RADS right 5.

### Mammography

Bilaterally symmetric, extremely dense parenchyma, ACR type 4. Under these limiting conditions, mammography showed no remarkable findings. Spot compression also showed no circumscribed findings. BI-RADS right 1/left 1. PGMI: CC view P; MLO view P.

### Procedure

Histological analysis of the palpable resistance with US-guided percutaneous core biopsy.

### Histology of the right breast

Invasive ductal carcinoma.

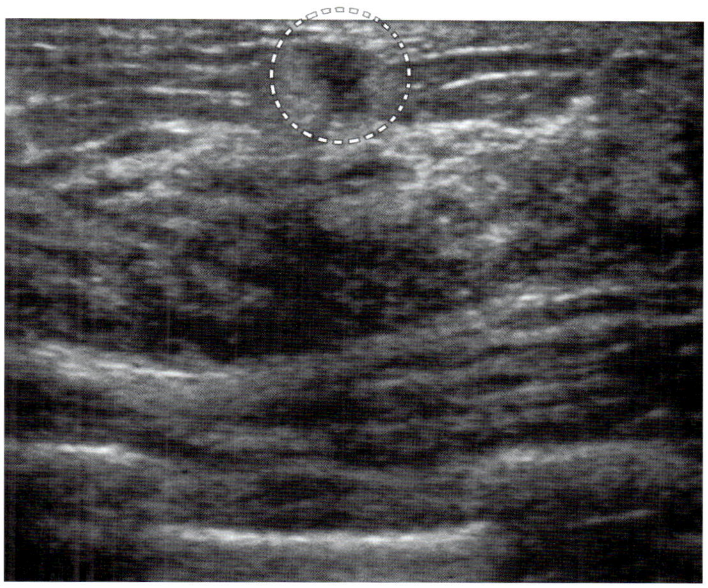

Fig. 84.**5** Sonography findings.

### Diagnosis

After open biopsy, no carcinoma was histologically identified in the specimen. However, there were signs of micrometastasis in one of the excised axillary lymph nodes. Taking into account the original percutaneous biopsy results, the diagnosis is:

IDC pT1b, pN1a, G2.

### Treatment

Breast conservation therapy; later quadrantectomy and mastectomy since the tumor was not found in the excised specimens.

Hyperechoic margins are a very important criterion of malignancy in ultrasound.

**Indication:** Screening.
**History:** Unremarkable.
**Risk profile:** No increased risk.
**Age:** 59 years.

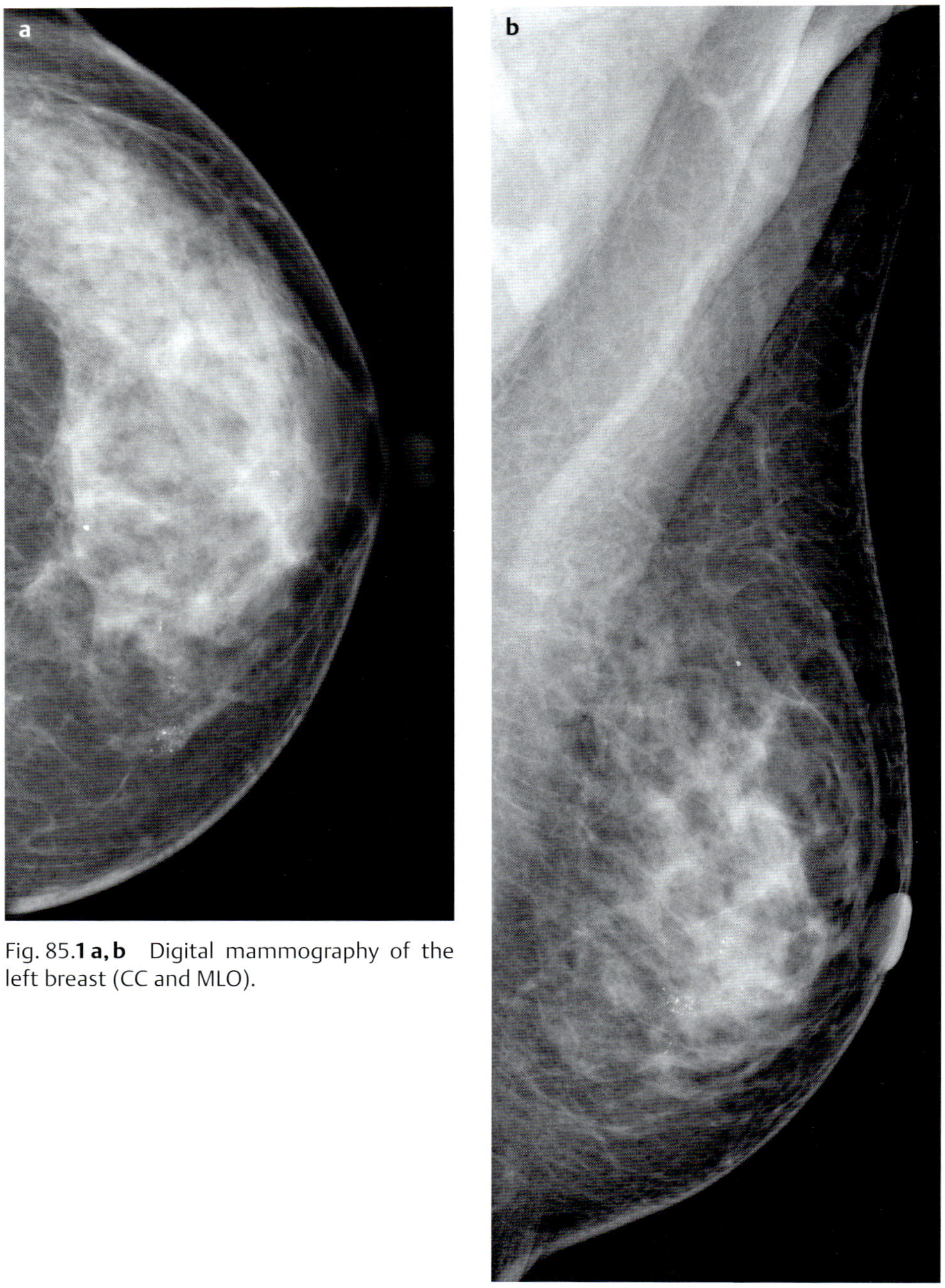


Fig. 85.**1 a, b** Digital mammography of the left breast (CC and MLO).

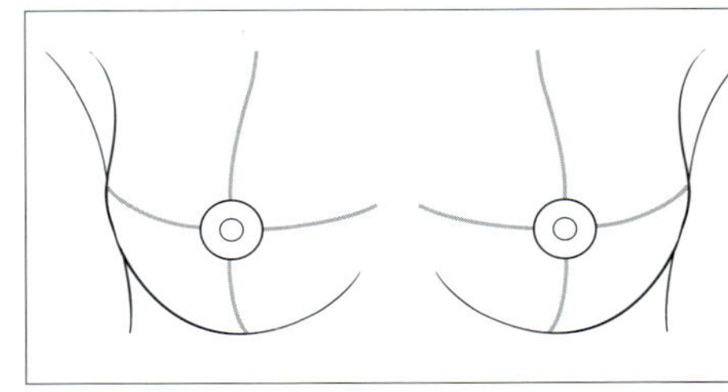

## Clinical Findings

Normal.

## Ultrasound

Unremarkable (not shown).

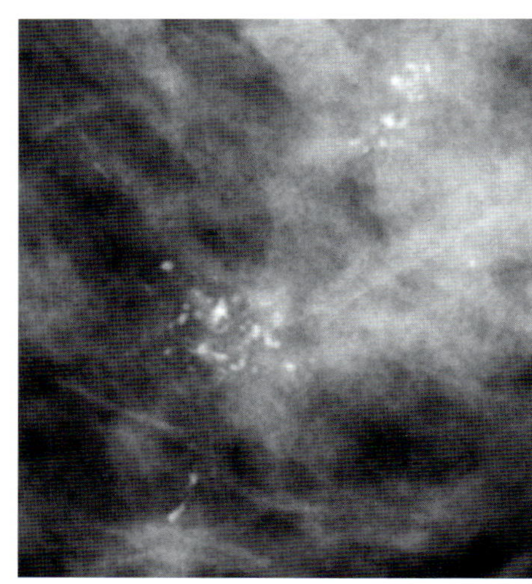

Fig. 85.**2** Digital mammography, magnification view of the left breast.

Please characterize the mammography findings.
What is your preliminary diagnosis?
What are your next steps?

| BI-RADS Categorization | | |
|---|---|---|
| Clinical Findings | right 1 | left 1 |
| Ultrasound | right 1 | left 1 |
| Mammography | right 1 | left 5 |
| **BI-RADS Total** | **right 1** | **left 5** |

This case demonstrates the relevant images of a woman within a screening situation.

### Ultrasound

As expected in the present case, ultrasound showed no unusual findings, including in targeted examination of the area behind the nipple and in the inner quadrants of the left breast.

### Mammography

Markedly dense parenchyma, ACR type 4. Under these limiting conditions, no density or circumscribed lesion was visible. There was no architectural distortion. Mammograms depicted several clustered distributions of polymorphous calcifications in the lower inner quadrant of the left breast. In combination, the distribution of these calcification clusters was segmental. BI-RADS left 5. PGMI is not defined for unilateral mammography.

### Procedure

Histological analysis of the microcalcifications with stereotactic vacuum biopsy. Calcifications were found in 9 of the 12 specimens (Fig. 85.**3**).

### Histology

Extensive ductal carcinoma in situ (high-grade with necroses) with signs of microinvasion of the breast.

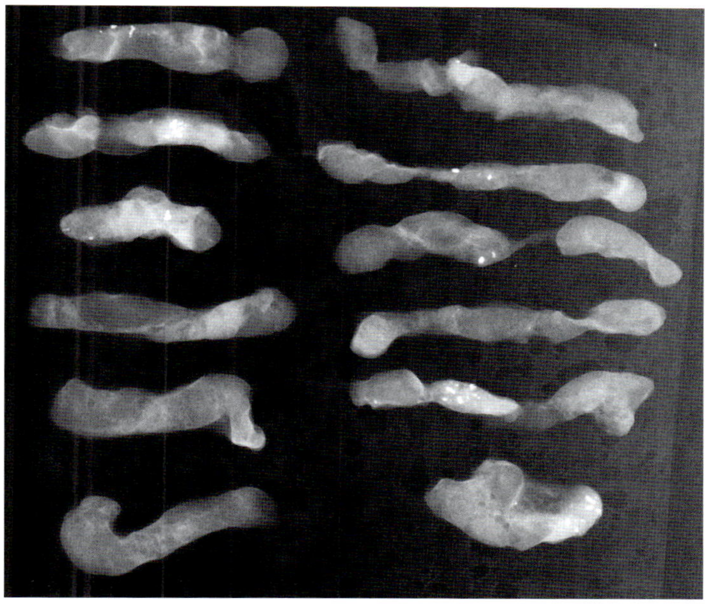

Fig. 85.**3** Specimen radiography.

### Histology

Minimally invasive ductal carcinoma. Axillary lymph node status normal.

DC pT1mic, pN0 (0/4)sn, VNPI 7 – 8 points.

### Treatment

Segmental resection, secondary mastectomy and reconstruction surgery.

When a ductal carcinoma in situ extends over an area greater than 4 cm, mastectomy is usually recommended.

**Indication:** Screening.
**History:** Unremarkable. No previous operations.
**Risk profile:** No increased risk.
**Age:** 43 years.

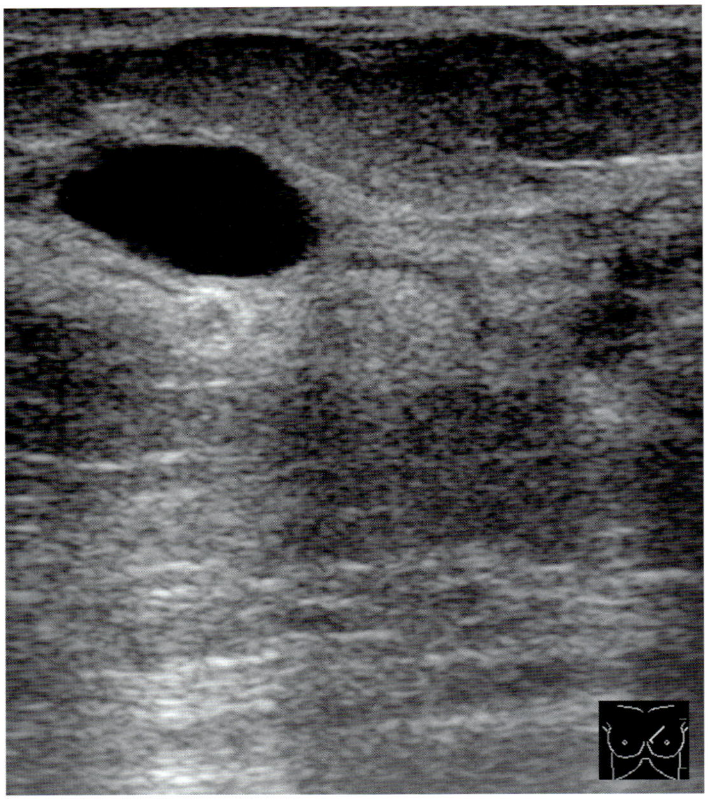

Fig. 86.**1** Sonography.

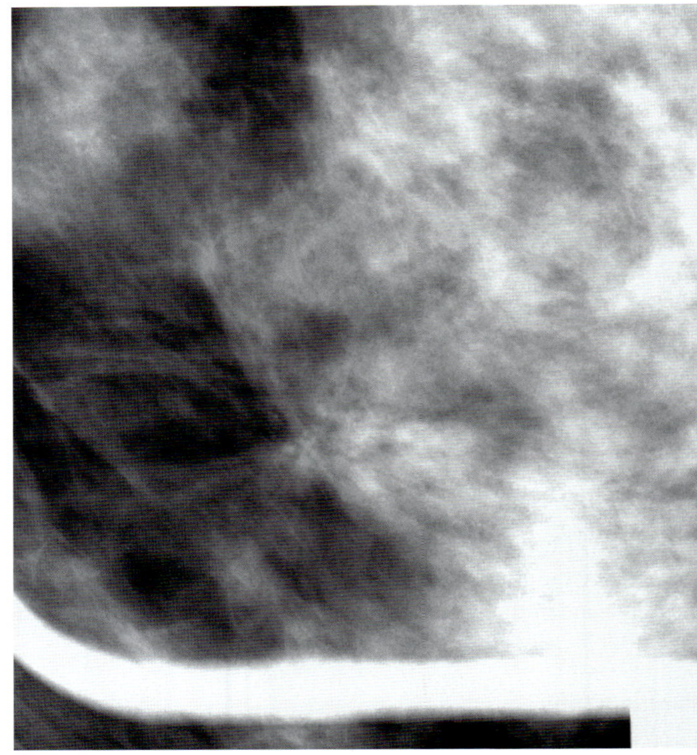

Fig. 86.**4** Spot compression of the central region of the left breast (CC).

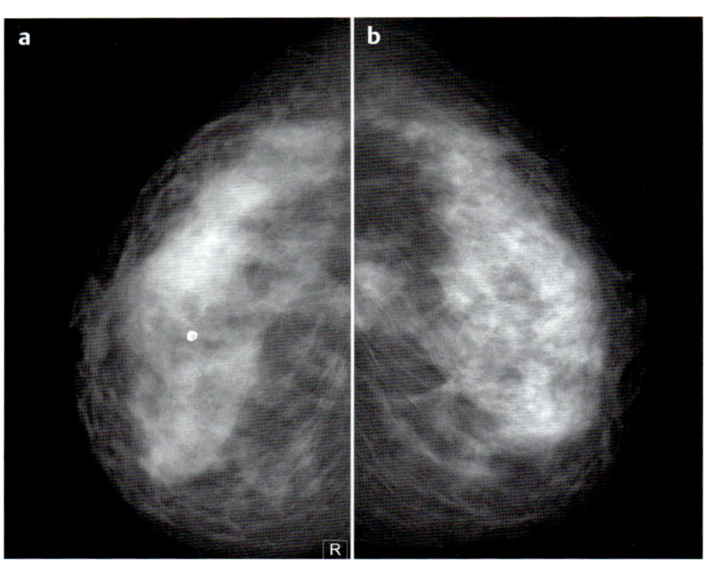


Fig. 86.**2 a, b** Digital mammography, CC view.

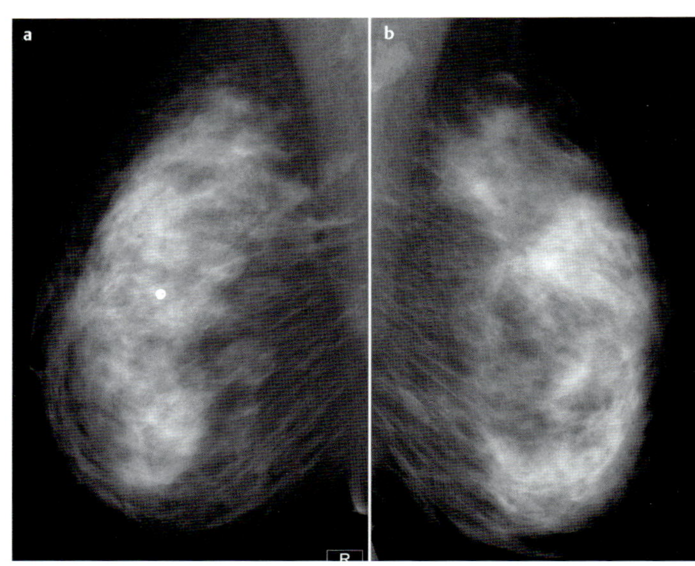


Fig. 86.**3 a, b** Digital mammography, MLO view.

Please characterize ultrasound and mammography findings.
What is your preliminary diagnosis?
What are your next steps?

| BI-RADS Categorization | | |
|---|---|---|
| Clinical Findings | right 1 | left 1 |
| Ultrasound | right 1 | left 2 |
| Mammography | right 1 | left 4 |
| **BI-RADS Total** | **right 1** | **left 4** |

This is a typical screening mammography case.

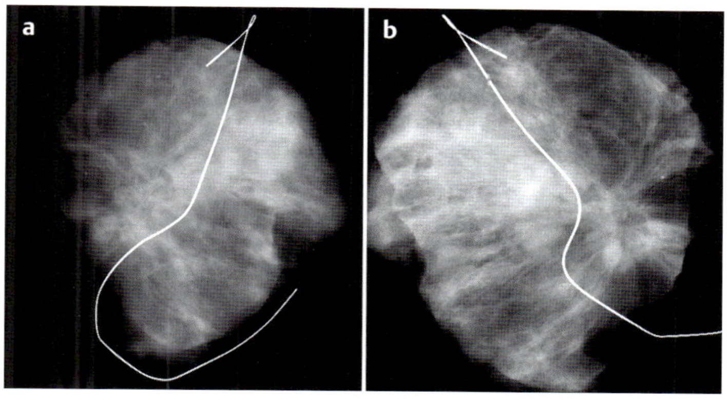


Fig. 86.**5 a, b** Specimen radiograms of the architectural distortion.

### Ultrasound

Ultrasound showed a macrocyst in the central part of the left breast. The acoustic texture was otherwise normal. US BI-RADS left central 2.

### Mammography

Bilaterally symmetric, markedly dense parenchyma, ACR type 4. Architectural distortion in the center of the left breast, visible in both views. Spot compression showed this distortion more clearly. No microcalcifications. BI-RADS right 1/left 4. PGMI: CC view P; MLO view G (angle of pectoralis muscle < 20° both sides).

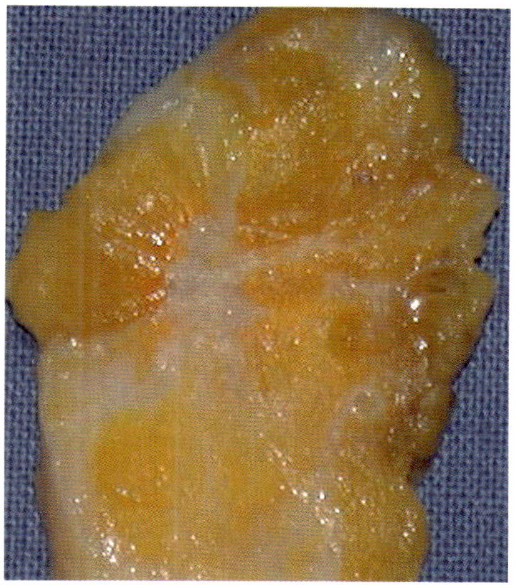

Fig. 86.**6** Macroscopic histological specimen.

### → Differential Diagnosis

Left breast: Radial scar or tubular carcinoma.

### Procedure

Open biopsy of the architectural distortion in the left breast after hook-wire localization (Fig. 86.**5**).

### Diagnosis

Radial scar.

### Treatment

Open biopsy; no further measures.

Open biopsy is recommended in all cases of mammographic findings that suggest a radial scar, since the coincidence of radial scars and breast cancer is 20–30%.

**Indication:** Monitoring following treatment for breast cancer.
**History:** Breast cancer 5 years previously. Breast conservation therapy.
**Risk profile:** Increased by earlier instance of breast cancer.
**Age:** 47 years.

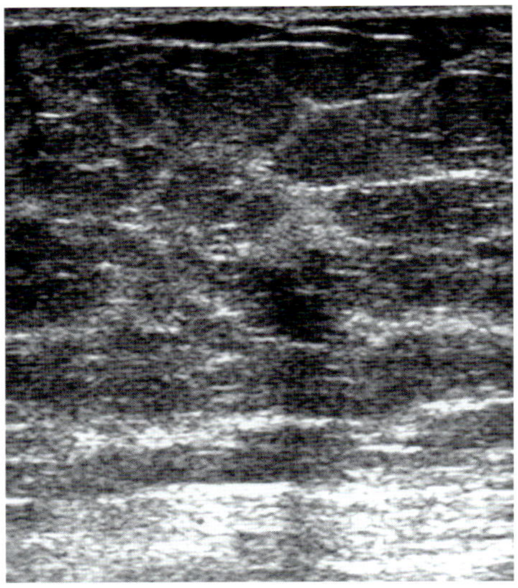

Fig. 87.**1** Sonography.

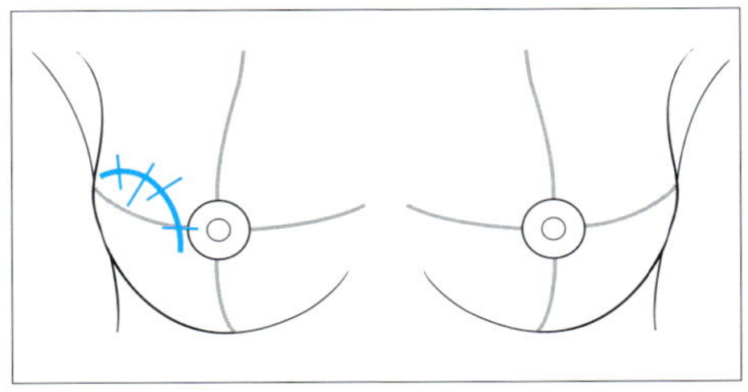

### Clinical Findings

Normal scar after breast conservation therapy (BCT). No palpable mass.

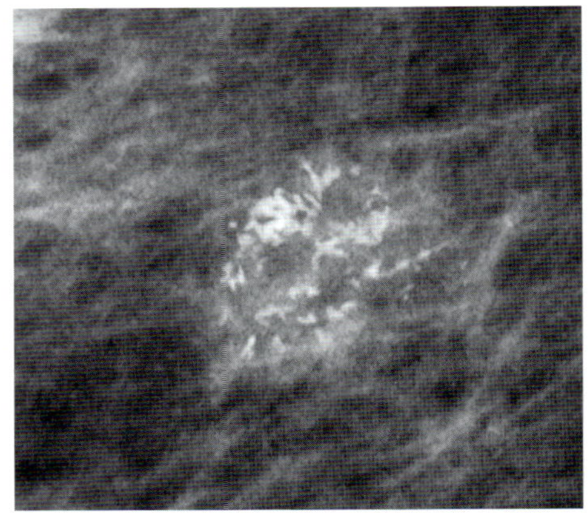

Fig. 87.**4** Magnification view of the right breast close to the chest wall.

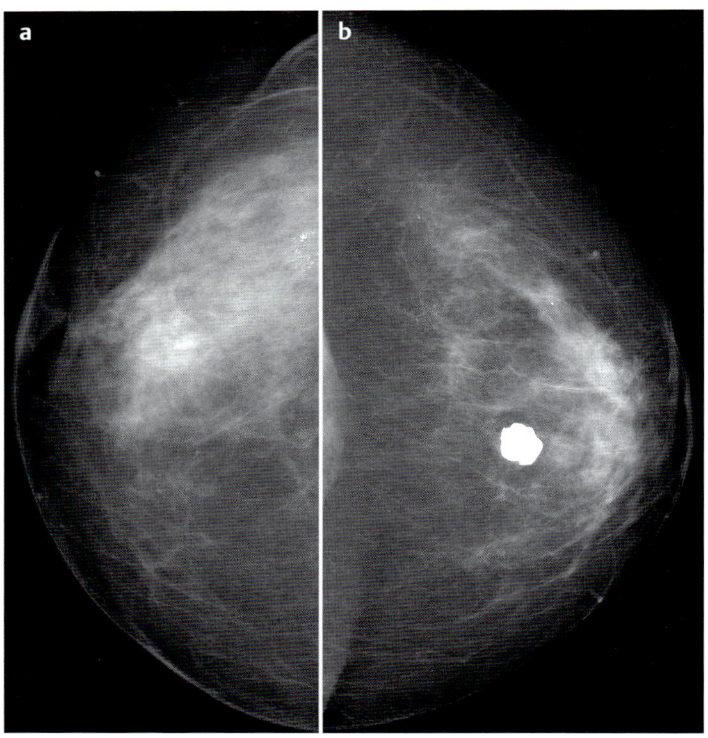


Fig. 87.**2 a, b** Digital mammography, CC view.

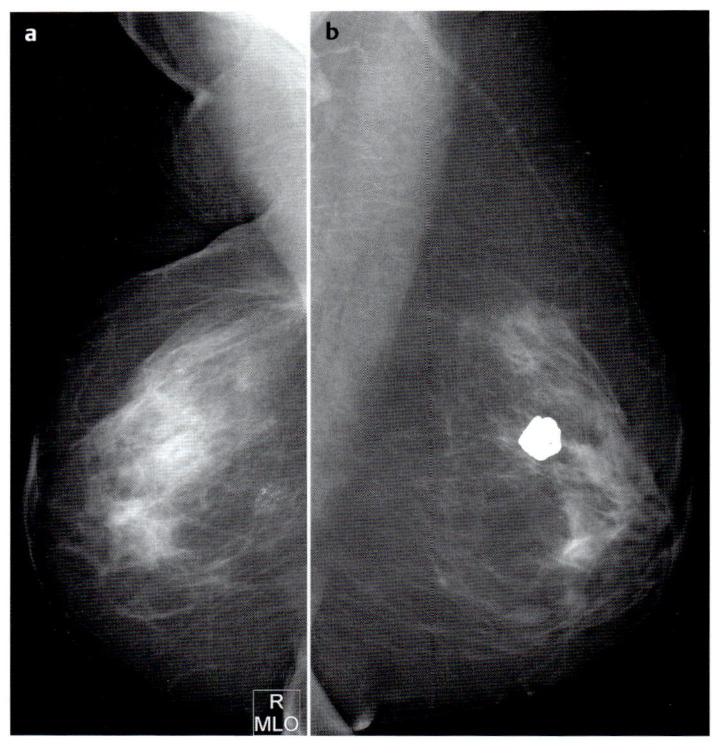


Fig. 87.**3 a, b** Digital Mammography, MLO view.

?

Please characterize ultrasound and mammography findings.
What is your preliminary diagnosis?
What are your next steps?

| BI-RADS Categorization | | |
|---|---|---|
| Clinical Findings | right 1 | left 1 |
| Ultrasound | right 3 | left 2 (no figure) |
| Mammography | right 4 | left 2 |
| **BI-RADS Total** | **right 4** | **left 2** |

A suspicious group of microcalcifications was found in the right breast near the chest wall in mammograms performed elsewhere during follow-up after breast conservation therapy. The present examination was done to investigate these findings further.

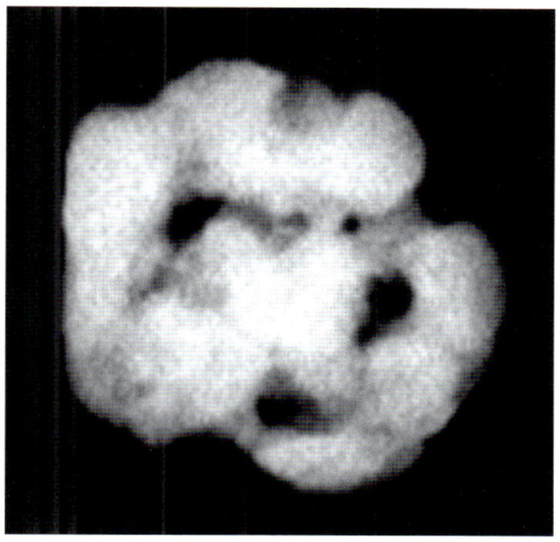

Fig. 87.**5** Calcification in the right breast. Postprocessing of digital image.

### Ultrasound

In the outer quadrants of the right breast there was a nonspecific finding, possibly correlating to the microcalcifications seen in mammography. US BI-RADS 3.

### Mammography

Parenchymal asymmetry after breast conservation therapy (right > left). Mammography positioning was suboptimal with the BCT scar visible in the upper outer quadrant of the right breast. Near the chest wall there was a cluster of polymorphous microcalcifications (round, linear, Y-shaped and V-shaped). There was slight density in this area but no circumscribed lesion. No architectural distortion. Macrocalcification in the left breast (see digital post-processing in Fig. 87.**5**). BI-RADS right 4/left 2.

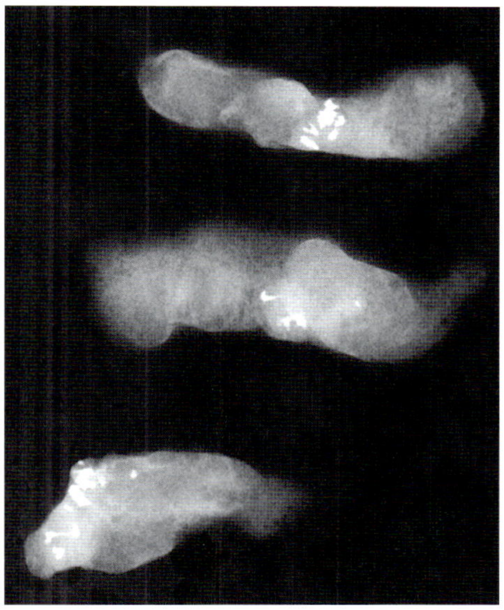

Fig. 87.**6** Specimen radiography.

### Procedure

Histological analysis of the calcifications in the right breast with stereotactic vacuum biopsy.

### Histology of the calcifications (right breast)

Fibroadenoma with regressive changes. No malignancy.

### Diagnosis (left side without histological verification)

Right: Fibroadenoma with regressive calcifications
Left: Fibroadenoma with regressive calcifications

### Treatment

None.

Vacuum biopsy is currently the method of choice for minimally invasive investigation of calcifications categorized BI-RADS 4. This avoids open biopsy in the case of benign histology.

**Indication:** Screening.
**History:** Unremarkable.
**Risk profile:** Postmenopausal breast cancer in a sister.
**Age:** 66 years.

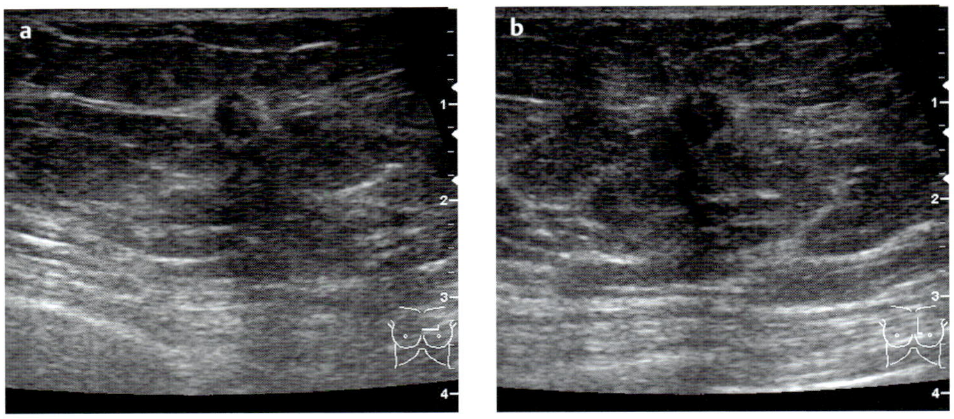

Fig. 88.1 **a, b** Ultrasound.

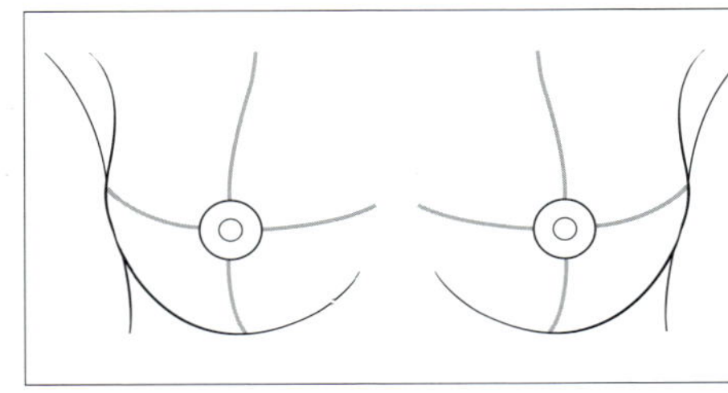

### Clinical Findings

Normal.

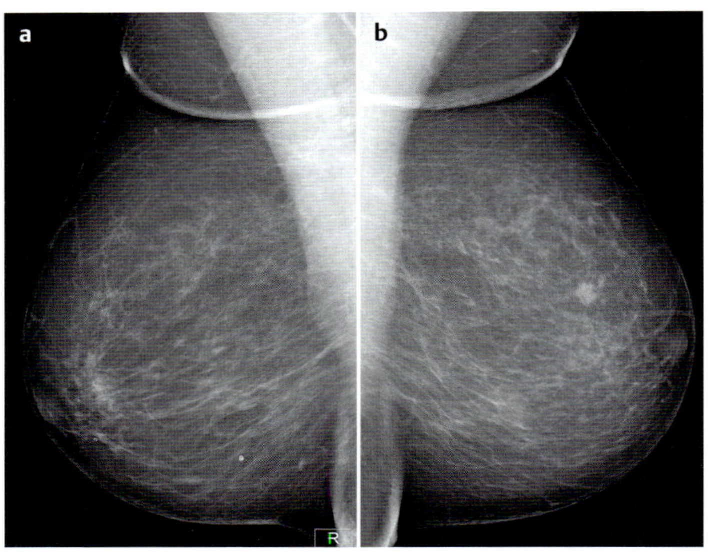

Fig. 88.2 **a, b** Digital mammography, MLO view.

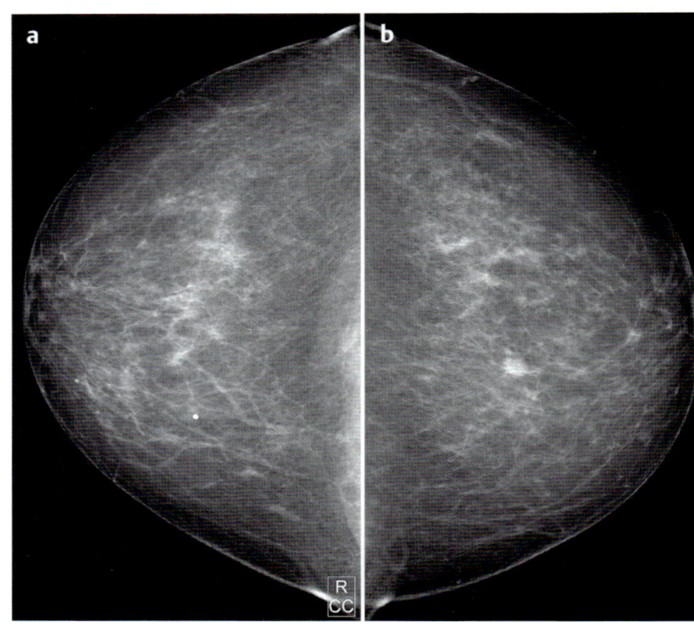

Fig. 88.3 **a, b** Digital mammography, CC view.

?

Please characterize ultrasound and mammography findings.
What is your preliminary diagnosis?
What are your next steps?

| BI-RADS Categorization | | |
|---|---|---|
| Clinical Findings | right 1 | left 1 |
| Ultrasound | right 1 | left 5 |
| Mammography | right 1 | left 5 |
| **BI-RADS Total** | **right 1** | **left 5** |

This case demonstrates a screening mammography and ultrasound in an asymptomatic woman.

### Ultrasound

Ultrasound showed an irregular, hypoechoic lesion (diameter 9 mm) with echogenic borders and distal shadowing in the upper inner quadrant of the left breast. There was distortion of the local ligamental structures by this lesion. US BI-RADS left 5.

### Mammography

Lipomatous parenchyma, ACR type 1. Round, spiculated, hyperdense mass measuring 1 cm between the upper quadrants of the left breast. No density. No suspicious calcifications. No architectural distortions. BI-RADS right 1/left 5. PGMI: CC view P; MLO view G (angle of pectoral muscle, left).

### Procedure

Ultrasound-guided core biopsy (Fig. 88.**4**).

### Histology of the core specimen (left breast)

Invasive tubular-ductal carcinoma.

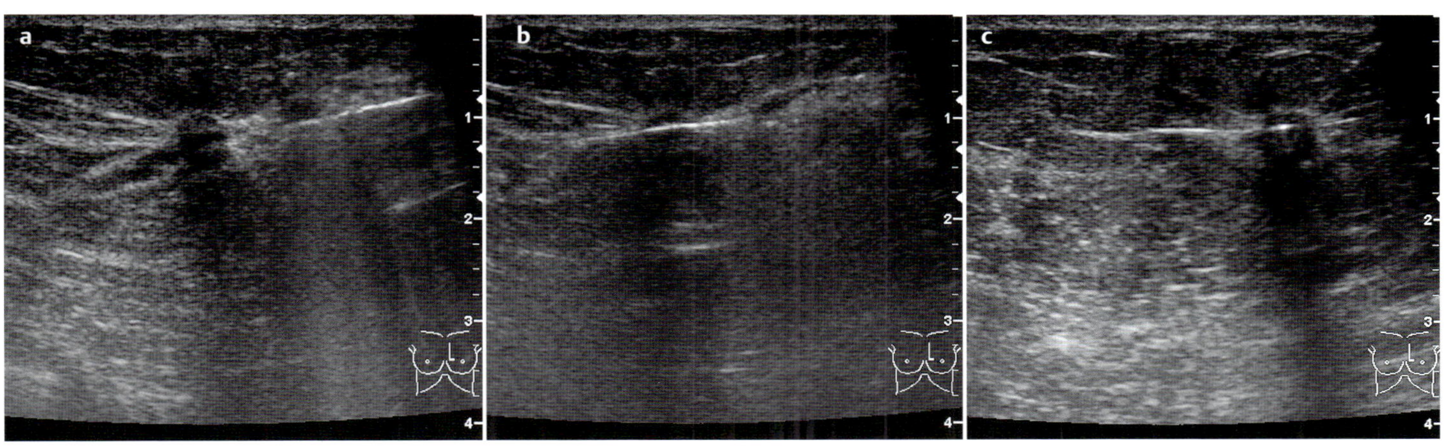


Fig. 88.**4 a–c** US-guided core biopsy.

### Diagnosis

Invasive ductal carcinoma (diameter: 12 mm).

IDC pT1c, pN0 (sn), G2, M0.

### Treatment

Breast conservation therapy.

In cases of lipomatous glandular texture (ACR type 1), the sensitivity of x-ray mammography even for small carcinomas is high.

**Indication:** Screening.
**History:** Unremarkable.
**Risk profile:** No increased risk.
**Age:** 40 years.

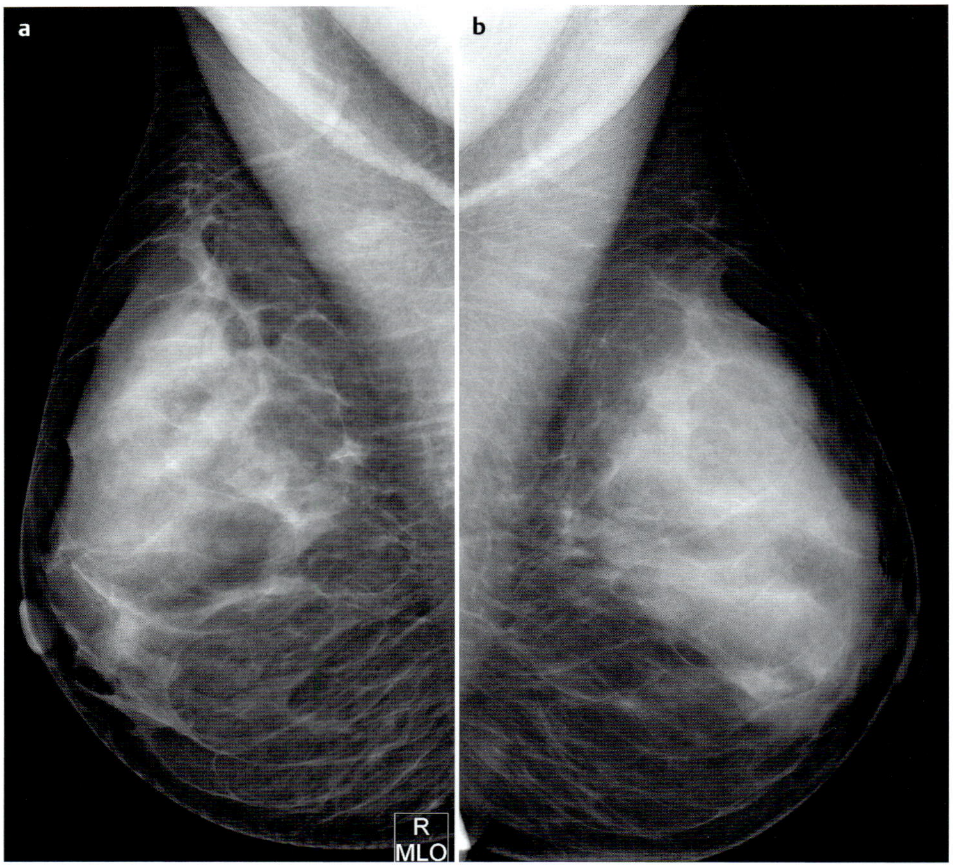


Fig. 89.**1 a, b** Digital mammography, MLO view.

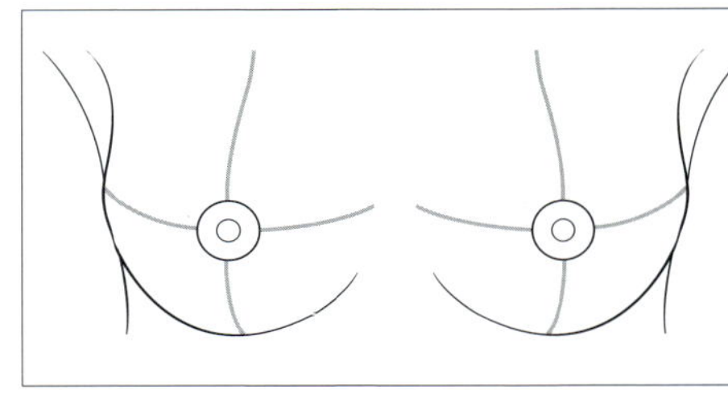

## Clinical Findings

No findings.

## Sonography

Unremarkable.

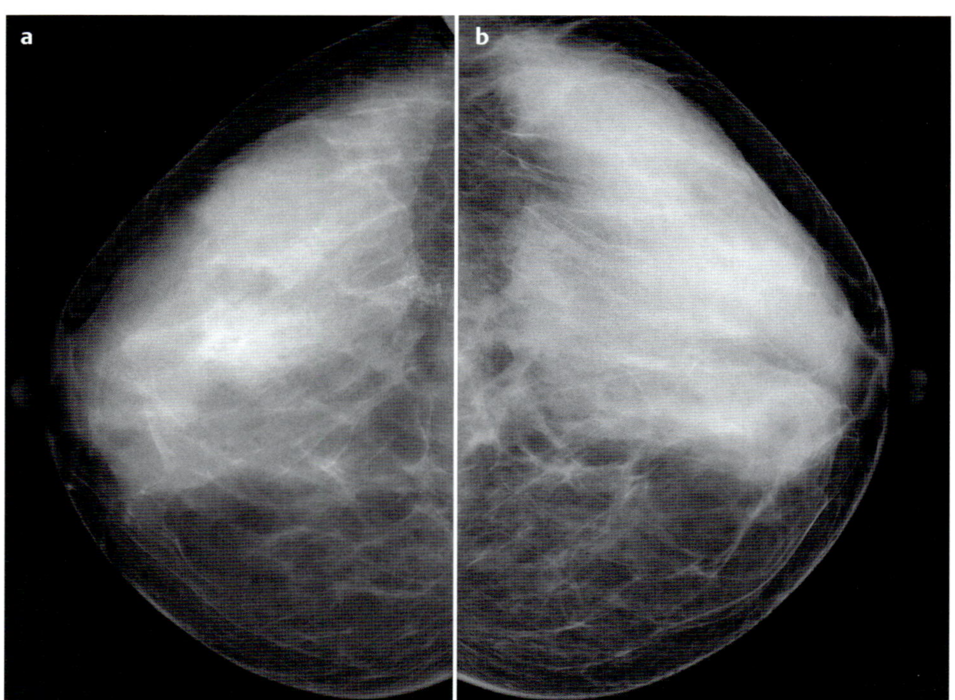


Fig. 89.**2 a, b** Digital mammography, CC view.

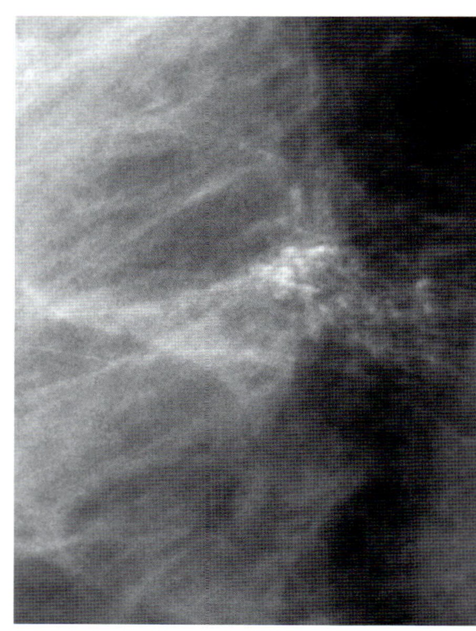

Fig. 89.**3** Magnification view (CC) of the left breast.

?

Please characterize the mammography findings.
What is your preliminary diagnosis?
What are your next steps?

| BI-RADS Categorization | | |
|---|---|---|
| Clinical Findings | right 1 | left 1 |
| Ultrasound | right 1 | left 1 |
| Mammography | right 4 | left 1 |
| **BI-RADS Total** | **right 4** | **left 1** |

This is the screening mammography of a young asymptomatic woman.

### Ultrasound

Bilaterally unremarkable acoustic texture (not shown). US BI-RADS right 1/left 1.

### Mammography

Partially extremely dense glandular tissue, ACR type 4. Polymorphous microcalcifications, somewhat ill-defined, were depicted in a segmental distribution in the prepectoral region of the right breast in CC view. No architectural distortion. BI-RADS right 4/left 1. PGMI: CC view P; MLO view G (inframammary fold incorrectly positioned).

### Reflection

Why were the prepectoral calcifications not visible in MLO view, when this view normally provides excellent documentation of prepectoral findings?

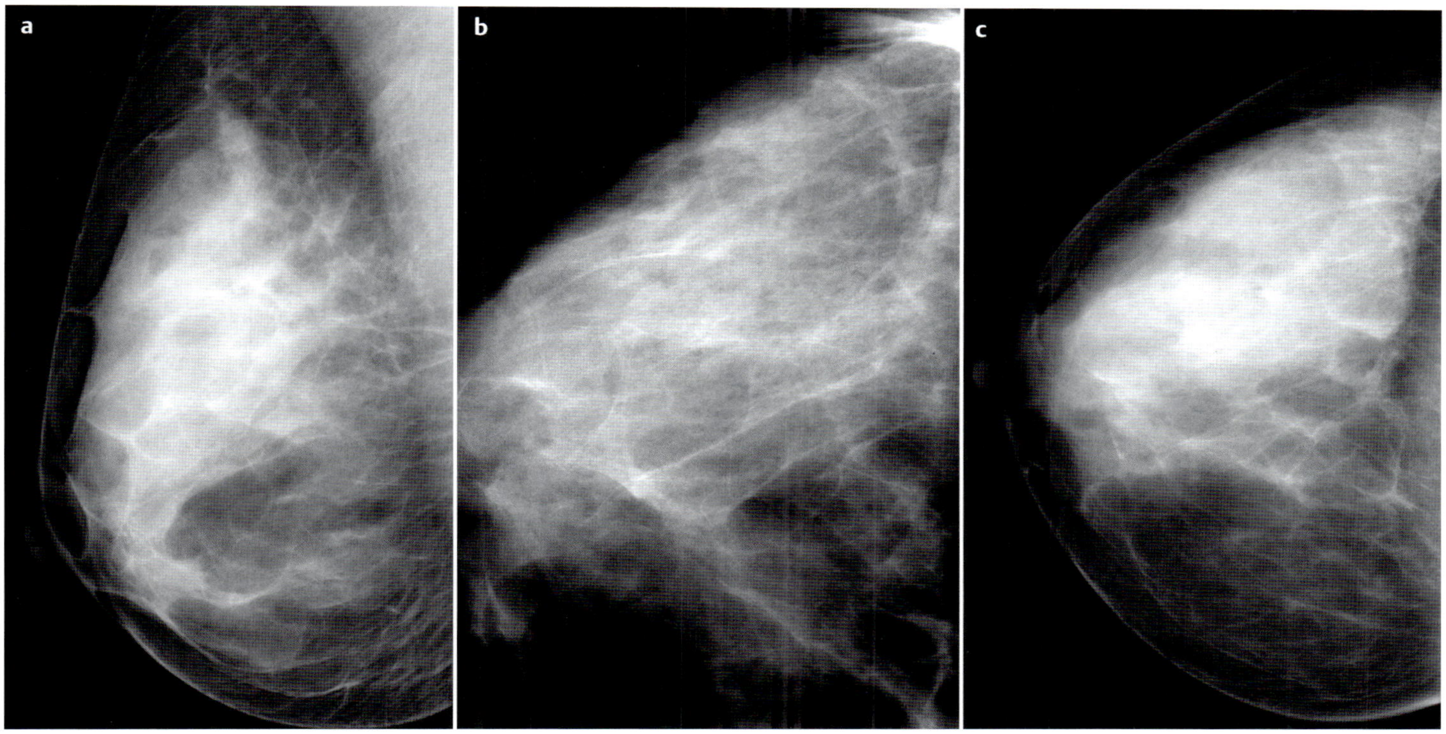


Fig. 89.**4 a – c** Supplementary imaging in lateromedial and magnification views did not reproduce the microcalcifications. Repeated CC imaging also failed to reproduce the earlier findings.

## Diagnosis

Artifact caused by superimposition of hair on image.

## Explanation

The patient's shoulder-length curly hair was treated with hairspray. A strand of hair fell into the path of the x-ray beam between the tube and the compression paddle, and was therefore projected onto the image.

Artifacts can sometimes appear worryingly real.

**Indication:** Screening.
**History:** Unremarkable.
**Risk profile:** No increased risk.
**Age:** 68 years.

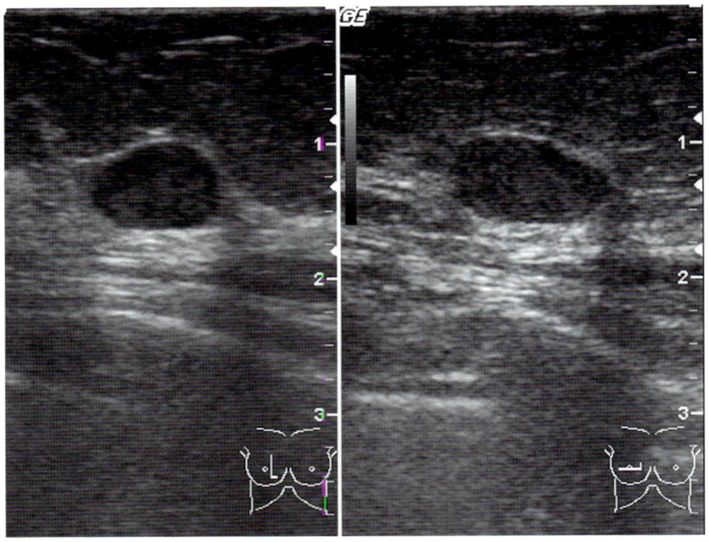

Fig. 90.**1** Ultrasound.

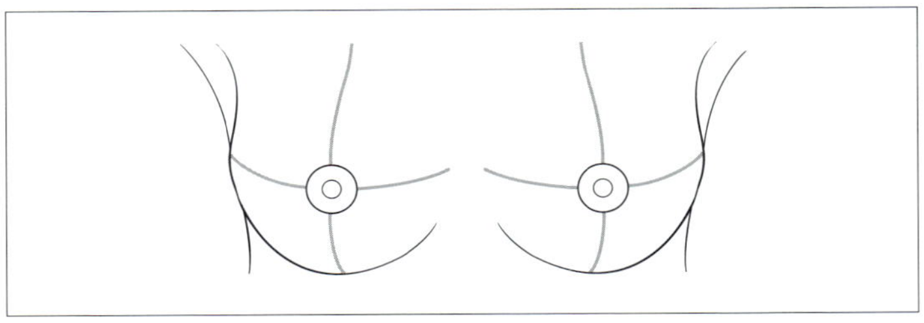

### Clinical Findings

No abnormal findings. Bilateral retracted nipples since puberty.

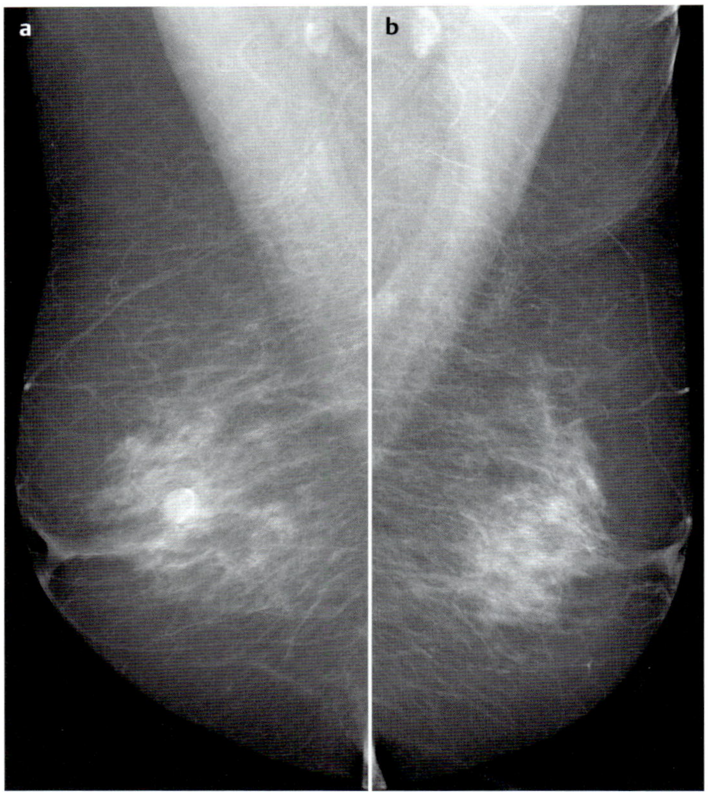


Fig. 90.**2 a, b** Digital mammography, MLO view.

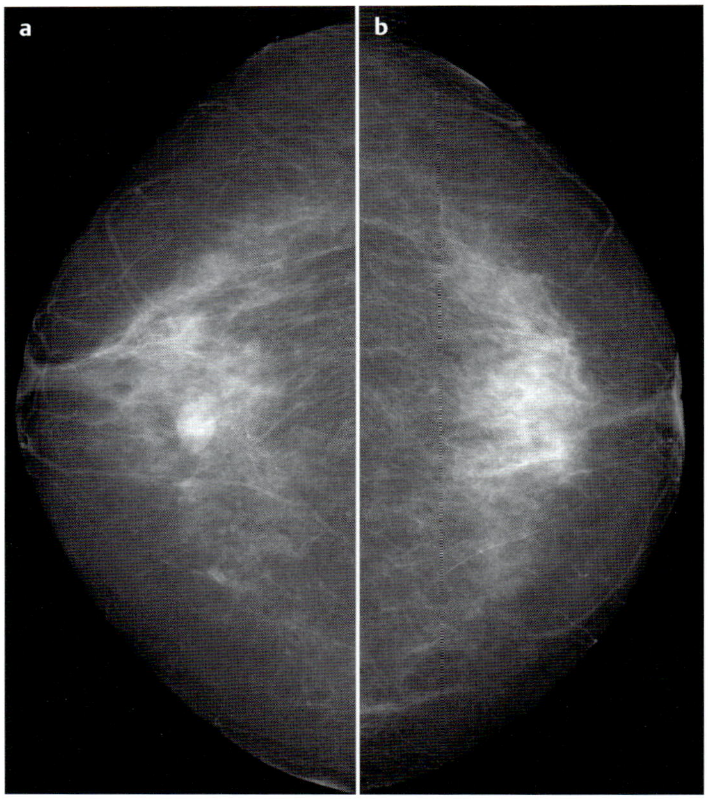


Fig. 90.**3 a, b** Digital mammography, CC view.

?

Please characterize ultrasound and mammography findings.
What is your preliminary diagnosis?
What are your next steps?

| BI-RADS Categorization | | |
|---|---|---|
| Clinical Findings | right 1 | left 1 |
| Ultrasound | right 3 | left 1 |
| Mammography | right 3 | left 1 |
| **BI-RADS Total** | **right 3** | **left 1** |

This is the imaging study of an asymptomatic woman.

### Ultrasound

Ultrasound showed a well-defined lesion measuring 9 mm in the center of the right breast, with increased distal acoustic signal. US BI-RADS right 3/left 1.

### Mammography

Fibroglandular parenchyma, ACR type 2. Compared to the mammograms from 2.5 years previously, a well-defined, oval, isodense lesion had increased from 0.4 cm to 1 cm in diameter. No architectural distortion. BI-RADS right 3/left 1. PGMI: CC view P; MLO view G (inframammary fold incorrectly positioned).

### Procedure

A lesion increasing in size is grounds for further investigation in a 68-year-old patient, even when morphological appearance is benign. For this reason, US-guided core biopsy was performed here.

### Histology

The initial diagnosis was tubular adenoma. However, after immunohistochemical work-up a diagnosis of intraductal papilloma was reached.

### Further procedure

Because of the risk of malignant transformation associated with intraductal papillomas, resection of the benign lesion was recommended.

### Final Histopathology

Intraductal papilloma.

### Treatment

Excisional biopsy.

Papilloma and radial scars are two entities of the breast that should always be resected despite their benign histology. This is because they are associated with increased risk of malignant transformation and coincidence with breast cancers.

**Indication:** Screening.
**History:** Unremarkable.
**Risk profile:** No increased risk.
**Age:** 53 years.

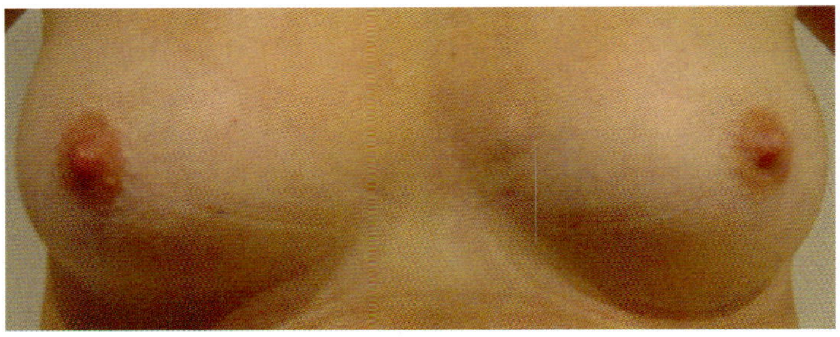

Fig. 91.**1** Inspection.

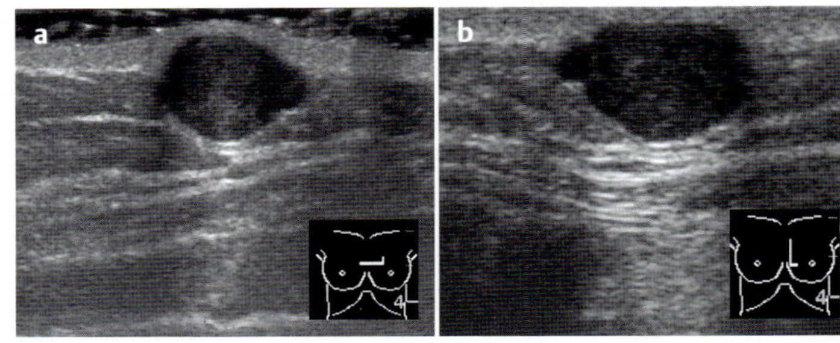


Fig. 91.**2 a, b** Sonography.

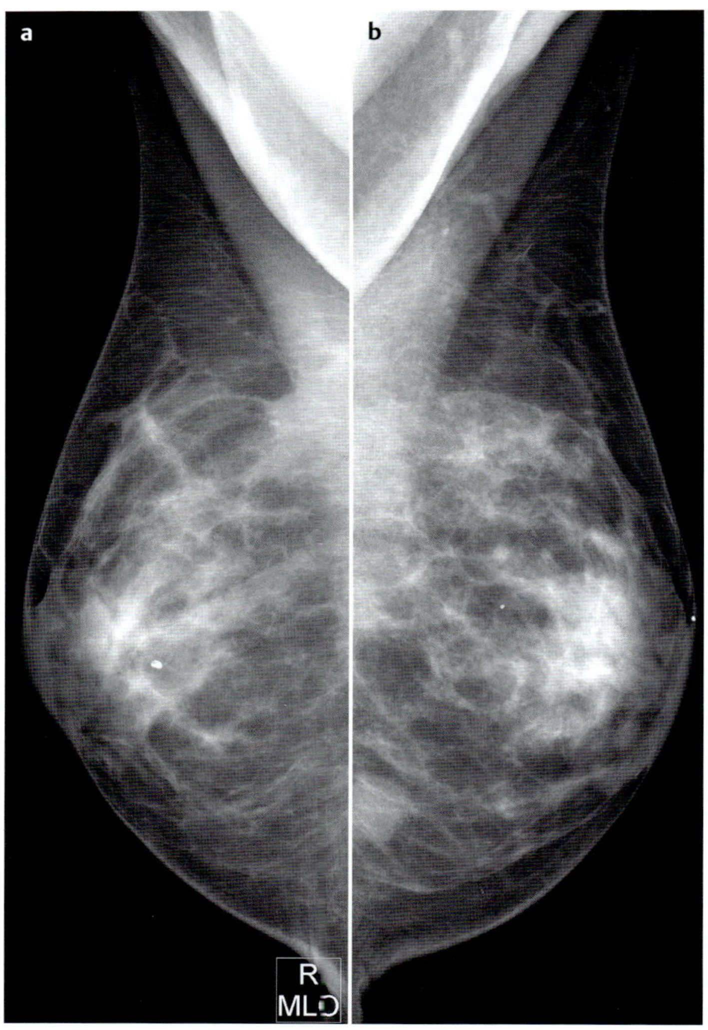


Fig. 91.**3 a, b** Digital mammography, MLO view.

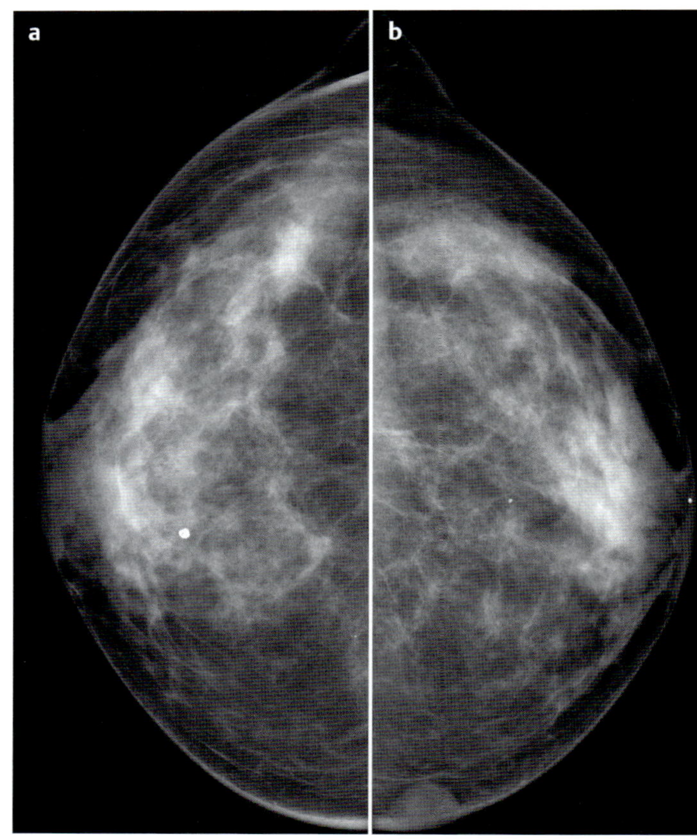


Fig. 91.**4 a, b** Digital mammography, CC view.

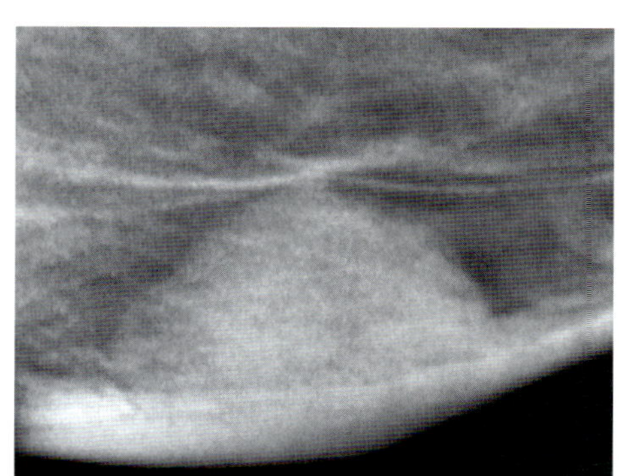

Fig. 91.**5** Magnification view of the inner region of the left breast.

?

Please characterize ultrasound, mammography, and clinical findings.
What is your preliminary diagnosis?
What are your next steps?

| BI-RADS Categorization | | |
|---|---|---|
| Clinical Findings | right 1 | left 3 |
| Ultrasound | right 1 | left 3 |
| Mammography | right 1 | left 3 |
| **BI-RADS Total** | **right 1** | **left 2** |

This imaging study was performed in a screening examination. A raised area of skin in the upper inner quadrant of the left breast was observed clinically. This abnormality was known to the patient but had recently increased in size.

### Ultrasound

In the area of the clinical finding, ultrasound showed a round, well-defined lesion with homogeneous internal echo texture and slight distal signal increase. The location was within the cutaneous and subcutaneous tissue, with slight thinning of the cutis. No signs of malignancy. US BI-RADS left 3.

### Mammography

Bilaterally symmetric, partially very dense parenchyma, ACR type 4. Some benign macrocalcifications. In the inner region of the left breast in the cutaneous/subcutaneous tissue, there was a well-defined, half-moon-shaped isodense lesion of 1 cm diameter. No signs of malignancy. No architectural distortion. No suspicious calcifications. BI-RADS right 1/left 3. PGMI: CC view P; MLO view P.

### Procedure

Due to the increase in size of the lesion in the upper inner quadrant of the left breast, and at the patient's request, the finding was excised without preoperative core biopsy analysis.

### Diagnosis

Atheroma.

### Treatment

Open biopsy.

The topographic location of the lesion suggested a tumorous entity of a sweat gland. A malignant breast process was very unlikely.

**Indication:** Screening.
**History:** Burn trauma in childhood.
**Risk profile:** No increased risk.
**Age:** 55 years.

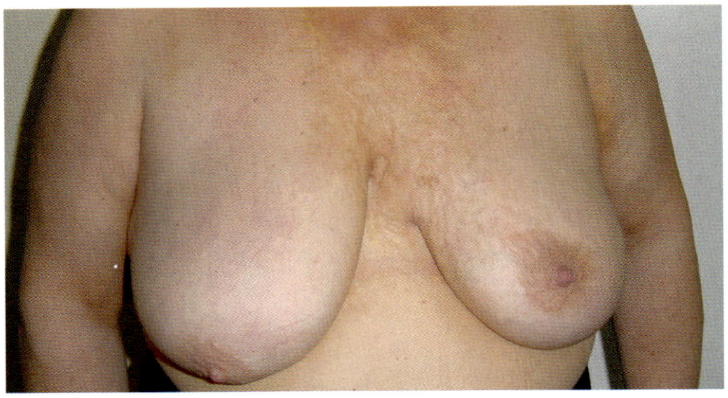

Fig. 92.1 Clinical findings.

## Palpation

Normal. See photograph for findings by inspection (Fig. 92.1).

## Ultrasound

Normal (not shown).

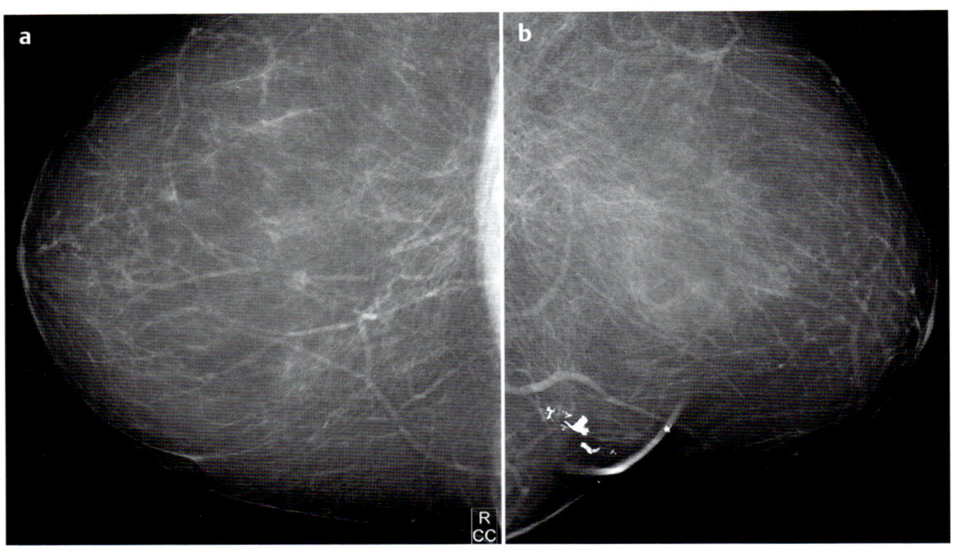


Fig. 92.2 a, b Digital mammography, CC view.

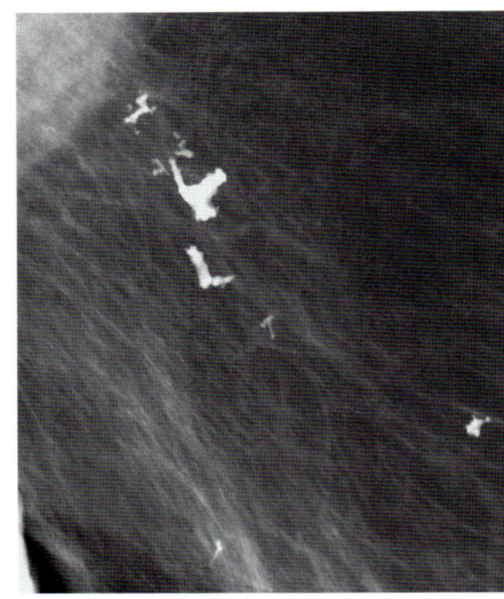

Fig. 92.4 Magnification view.

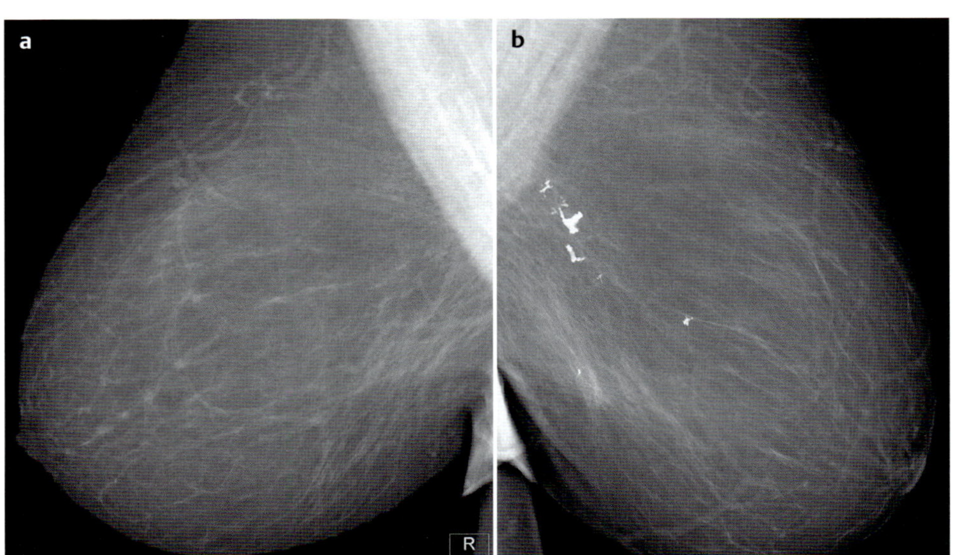


Fig. 92.3 a, b Digital mammography, MLO view.

?

Please characterize the mammography, and clinical findings.
What is your preliminary diagnosis?
What are your next steps?

| BI-RADS Categorization | | |
|---|---|---|
| Clinical Findings | right 1 | left 2 |
| Ultrasound | right 1 | left 1 |
| Mammography | right 1 | left 2 |
| **BI-RADS Total** | **right 1** | **left 2** |

This is the imaging study of a asymptomatic woman.

### Ultrasound

No pathological findings (not shown).

### Mammography

Lipomatous glandular tissue, ACR type 1. Medial skin shrinking in the left breast without evidence of a mass. Segmentally distributed macrocalcifications, predominantly in coarse clumps. No suspicious microcalcifications. BI-RADS right 1/left 2. PGMI: CC view G (lateral part of the breast incompletely documented); MLO view G (inframammary fold).

### Procedure

Clinical examination to establish correlation between skin changes (burn scarring) and the coarse calcifications.

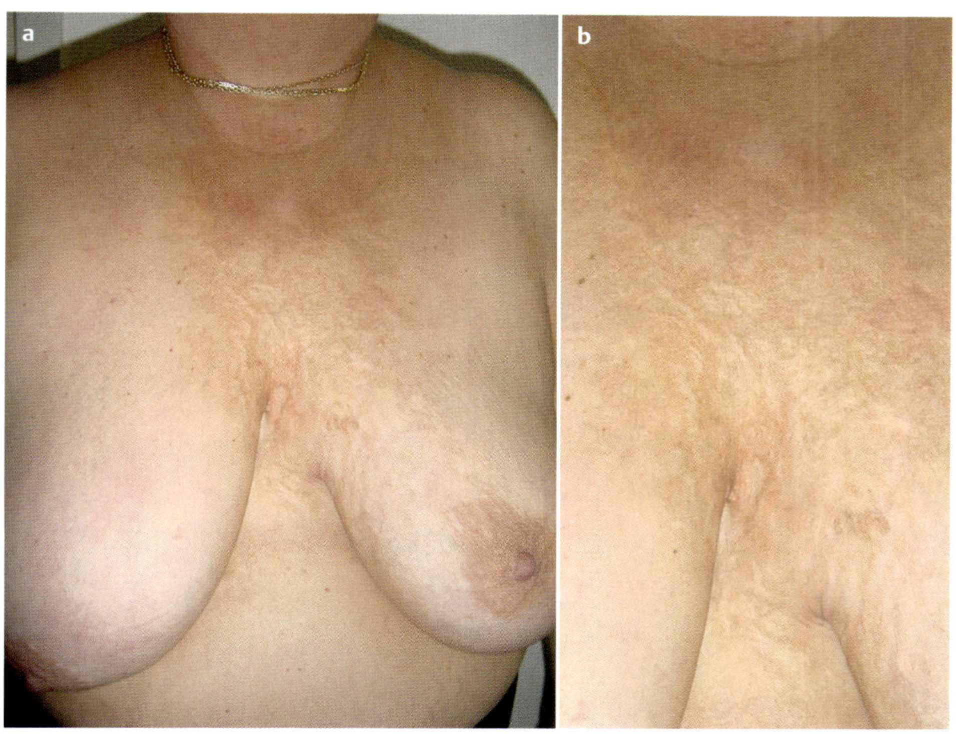


Fig. 92.**5 a, b** Clinical findings in detail.

### Diagnosis (no histological verification)

Macrocalcifications in burn scarring region.

### Treatment

None.

The clinical examination is an essential element of breast diagnostics.

**Indication:** Newly detected microcalcifications in the left breast.
**History:** Unremarkable.
**Risk profile:** Breast cancer in mother at the age of 60 years.
**Age:** 56 years.

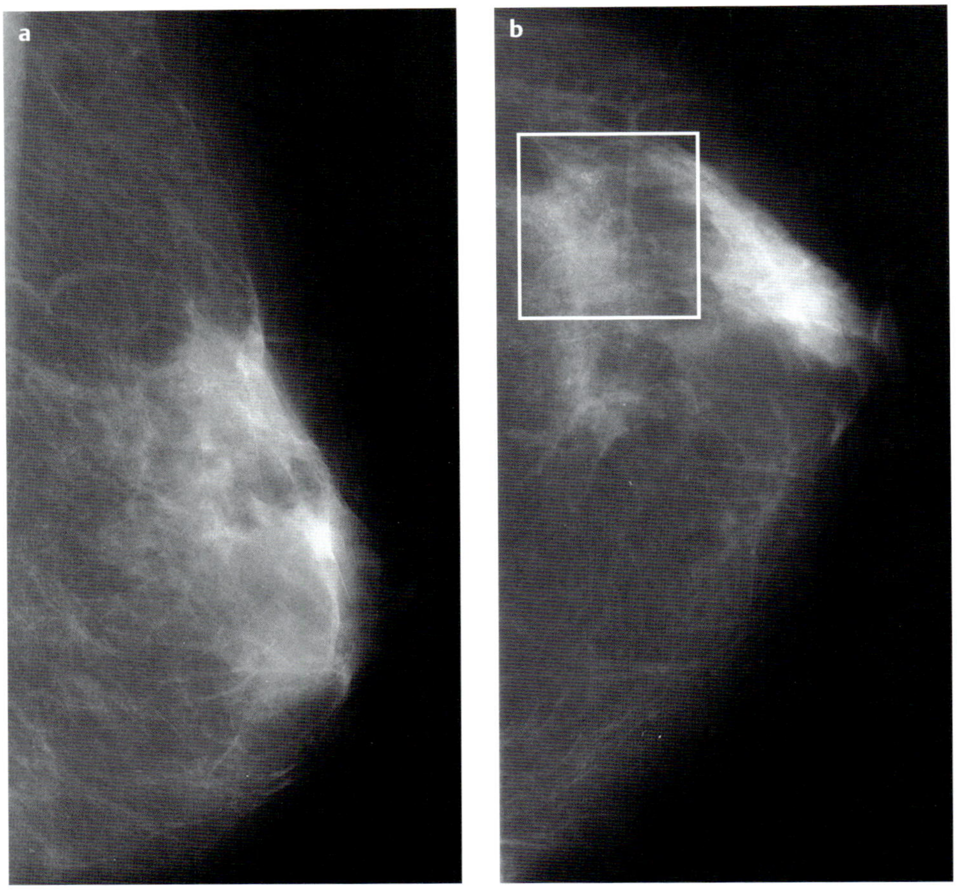


Fig. 93.**1 a, b** Conventional mammography of the left breast, MLO and CC views [imaging not performed by authors].

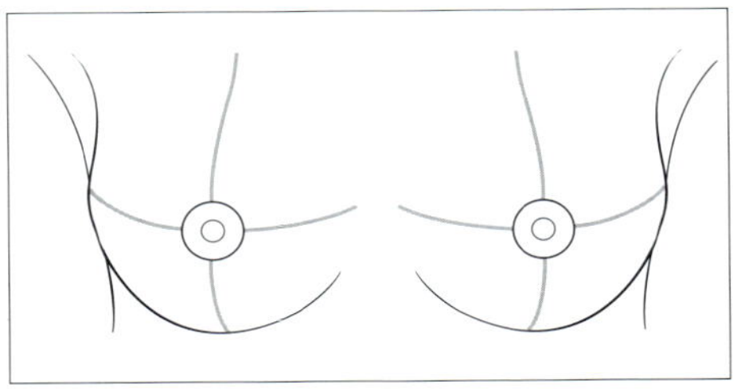

**Clinical Findings**

No findings.

**Ultrasound (not shown)**

Unremarkable.

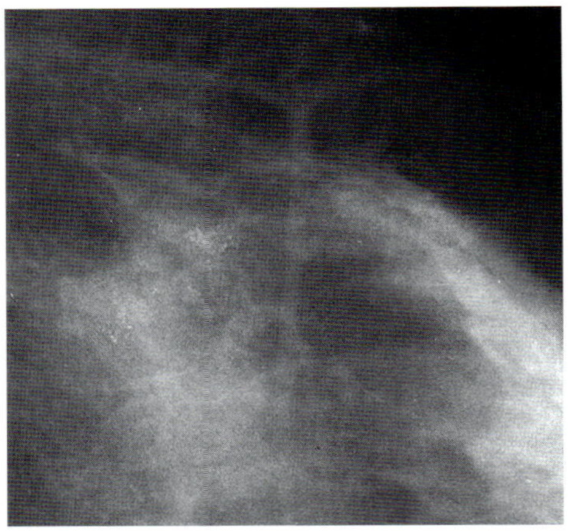

Fig. 93.**2** Magnification view of the outer quadrants of the left breast (CC).

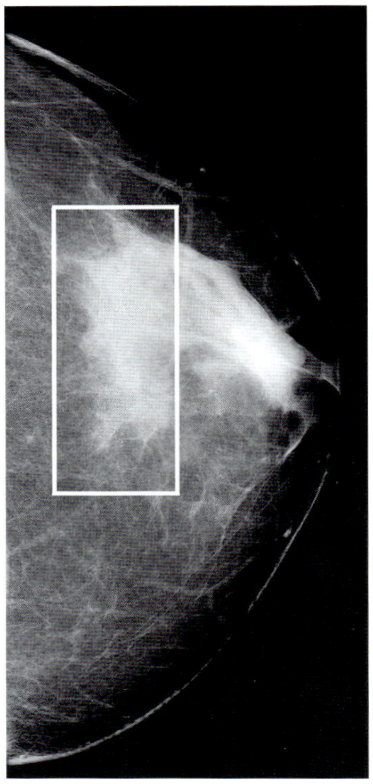

Fig. 93.**3** Digital mammography of the left breast, CC view, in preparation for intervention 5 weeks later.

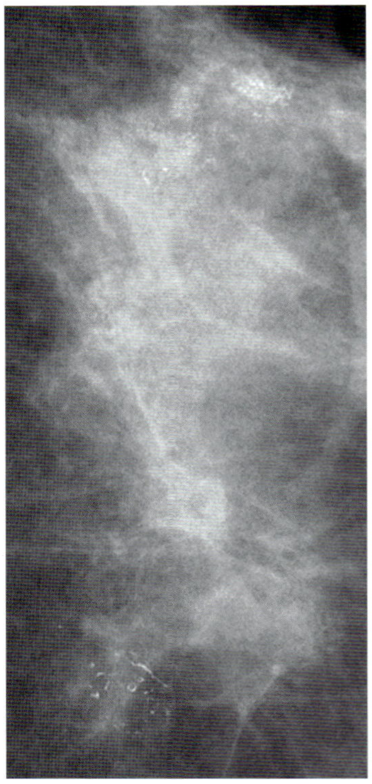

Fig. 93.**4** Magnification view (CC) of the left breast (see section marked in 93.**3**).

?

Please characterize the mammography from 5 weeks earlier and the current images.
What is your preliminary diagnosis?
What are your next steps?

This case demonstrates the imaging studies of an asymptomatic woman. In a recent examination in another clinic, microcalcifications in an apparent segmental distribution were detected in the upper outer quadrant of the left breast, which were not present in earlier mammograms from 2 years previously.

### Ultrasound

There were no unusual sonographic findings in either breast.

Which of the two calcification groups would you biopsy? Or do you have an alternative suggestion?

### Mammography

Inhomogeneously dense parenchyma, ACR type 3. Monomorphous, segmentally distributed microcalcifications were seen in the outer quadrants of the left breast. No suspect masses or densities. Digital mammography was performed on the left breast in preparation for a stereotactic core biopsy (see Figs. 93.**3** and 93.**4**). This showed another polymorphous cluster of calcifications in the central part of the left breast, newly developed since the examination 5 weeks previously. The newly developed cluster was more suspect than the calcifications seen earlier. BI-RADS right 1/ left 5. PGMI is not defined for unilateral mammography.

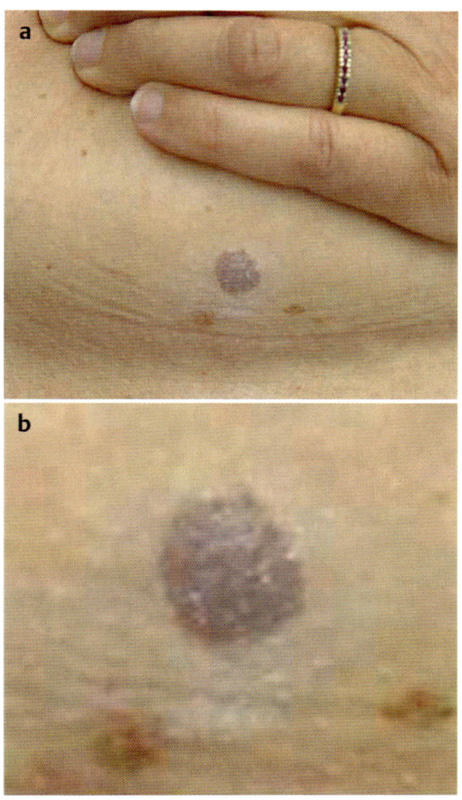

Fig. 93.**5 a, b** Clinical finding!

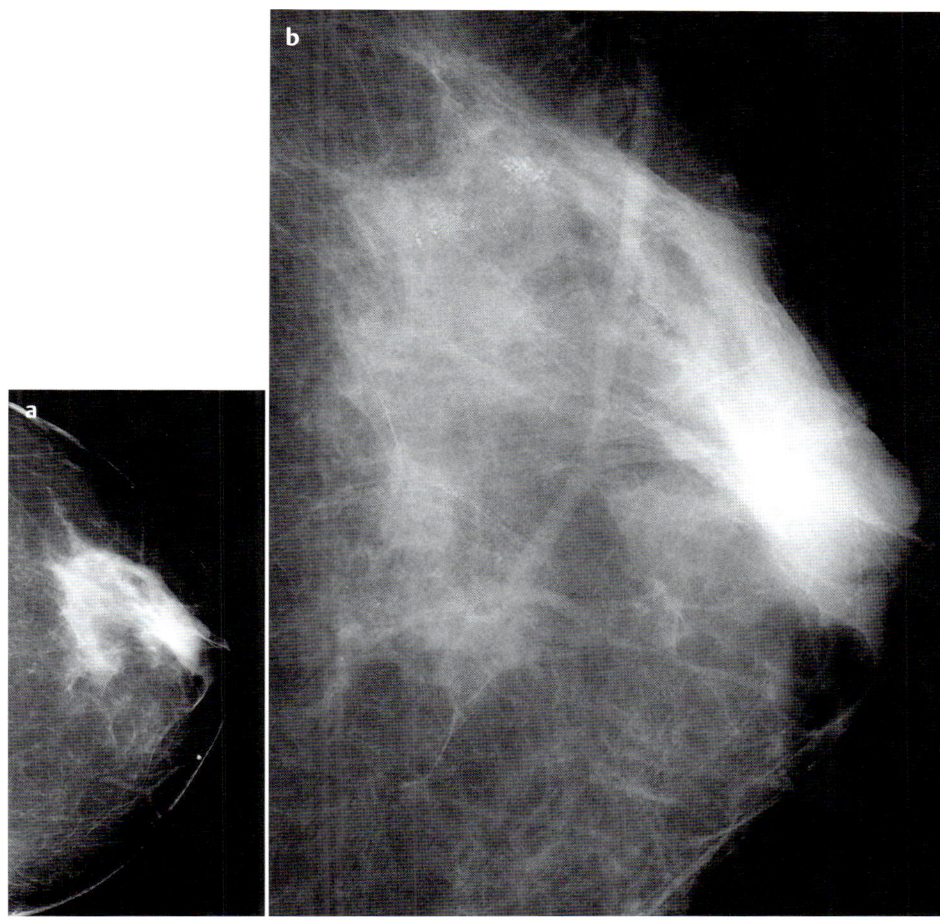

Fig. 93.**6 a, b** Digital mammography and magnification view of the left breast after removal of the cream from the mole.

### Diagnosis (without histopathological confirmation)

The apparent calcifications were in fact a manifestation of zinc-containing cream on a mole on the underside of the left breast (findings left central). Outer quadrants of the left breast: sclerosing adenosis (histology of vacuum biopsy).

### Treatment

None.

Microcalcifications associated with tumors do not develop to the extent seen here in only 5 weeks!

**Indication:** Acute increase in size of the left breast.
**History:** Unremarkable.
**Risk profile:** No increased risk.
**Age:** 18 years.

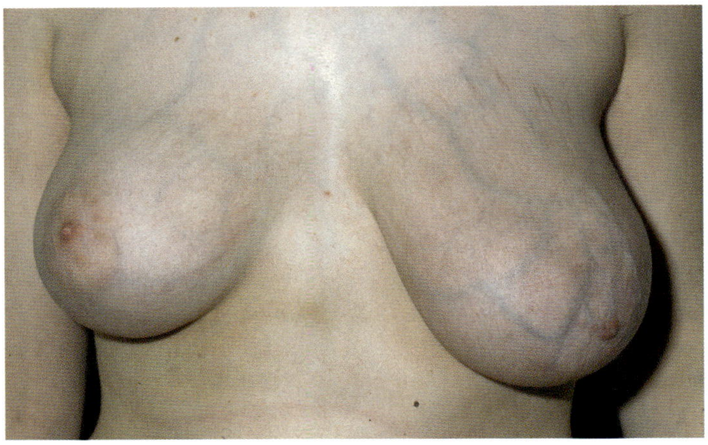

Fig. 94.**1** Clinical examination. The entire left breast had a dense texture at palpation.

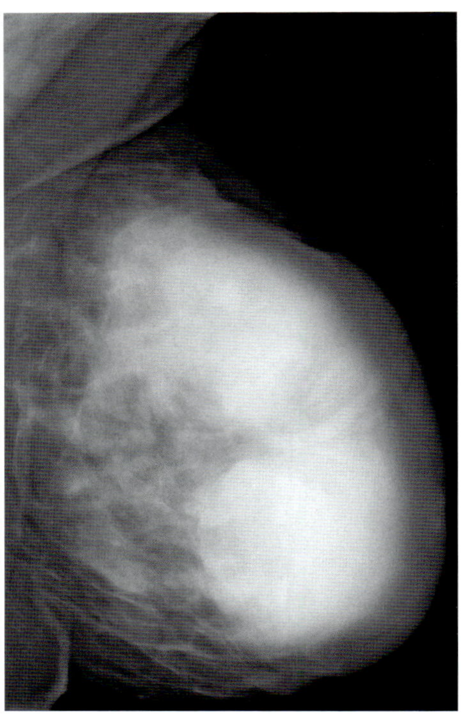

Fig. 94.**2** Digital mammography of the left breast, MLO view.

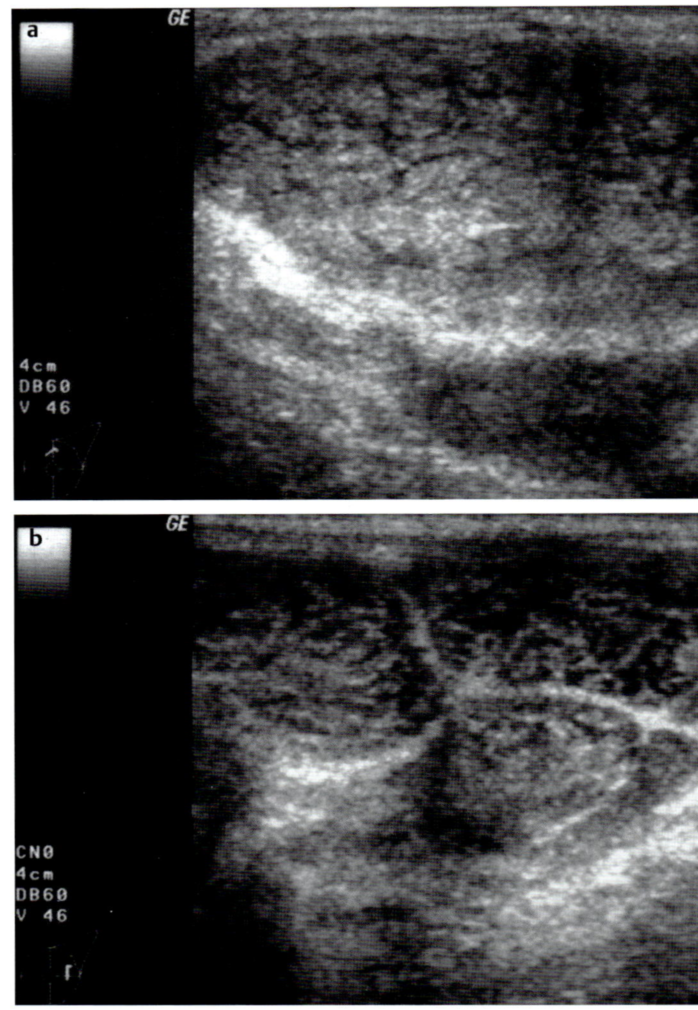


Fig. 94.**3 a, b** Sonography.

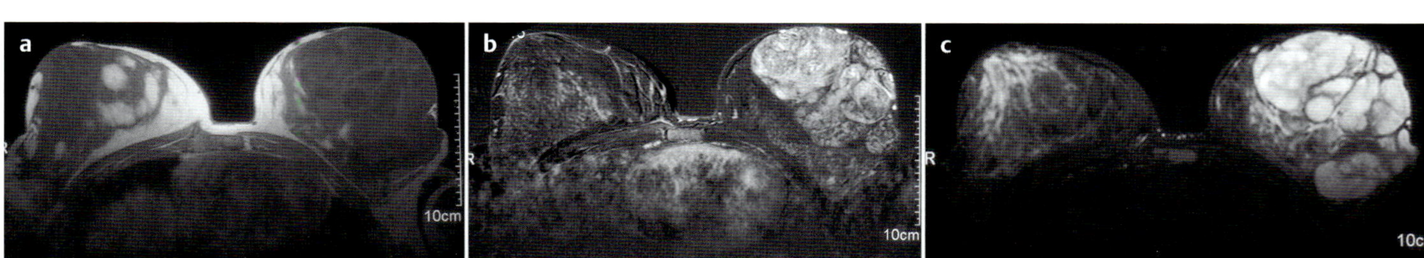


Fig. 94.**4 a – c** Contrast-enhanced MR mammography. Precontrast and postcontrast subtraction images and water-sensitive inversion recovery sequence.

?

Please characterize the clinical, ultrasound, mammography, and MRI findings.
What is your preliminary diagnosis?
What are your next steps?

| BI-RADS Categorization | | |
|---|---|---|
| Clinical Findings | right 1 | left 3 |
| Ultrasound | right 1 | left 3 |
| Mammography | right 1 | left 3 |
| MR Mammography | right 1 | left 3 |
| **BI-RADS Total** | **right 1** | **left 3** |

This young woman presented for further investigation of marked and escalating asymmetry, the left breast having increased considerably in size over the previous months.

### Ultrasound

Documentation of the entire lesion was impossible in sonography. Individual sections showed a conglomerate of multiple round, well-defined nodules with inhomogeneous, reticular internal structure. No cystic areas within the tumor. No unusual distal echo pattern. US BI-RADS left 3.

### Mammography

Taking the extreme growth of the left breast into account, a digital MLO view was performed despite the youth of the patient. It was still considered necessary to exclude any signs of malignancy such as microcalcifications. As expected, mammography depicted a conglomerate of multiple homogeneous, well-defined, hyperdense lesions. No calcifications. BI-RADS left 3. PGMI is not defined for unilateral imaging.

### MR Mammography

MRI was performed as part of preoperative preparation. A massive hypervascularized conglomerate tumor was seen in the left breast. No signs of malignancy. The glandular tissue was displaced toward the chest wall by the tumor. BI-RADS left 3.

### → Differential Diagnosis

Juvenile giant fibroadenoma (high probability); phyllodes tumor, sarcoma, lymphoma (low probability).

### Procedure

The high probability of the tumor being benign was comprehensively explained to the young woman. On aesthetic and psychosocial grounds, resection of the tumor was recommended.

### Histology

Giant fibroadenoma.

### Treatment

Tumor resection. No further therapy.

Performing at least one mammogram (e.g., reduced-dose digital mammography) is justified for diagnostic purposes even in young patients when signs of possible malignancy are present.

**Indication:** Screening.
**History:** Unremarkable.
**Risk profile:** No increased risk.
**Age:** 59 years.

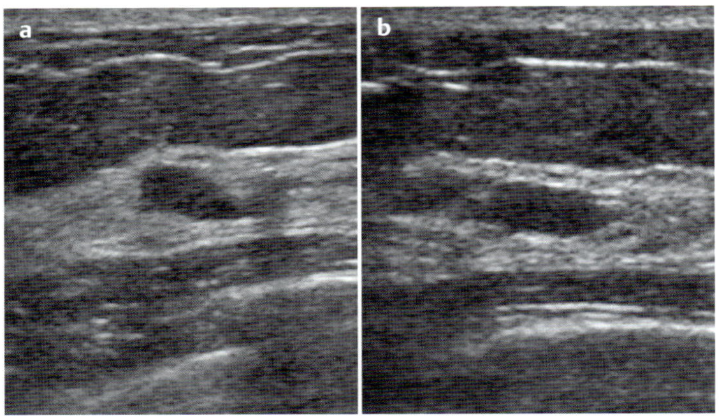


Fig. 95.**1 a, b** Ultrasound of the central region of the left breast.

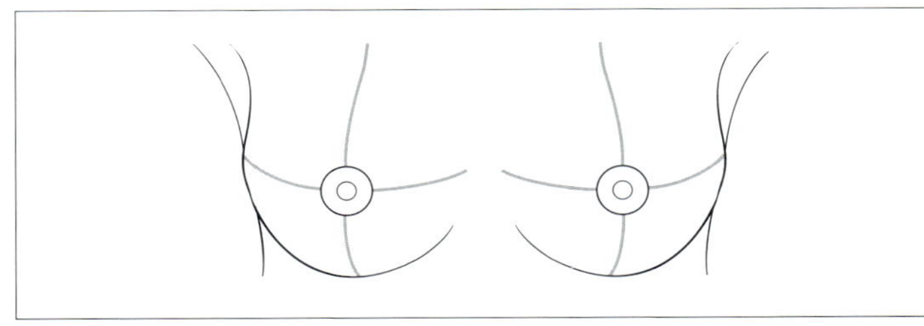

**Clinical Findings**

Normal.

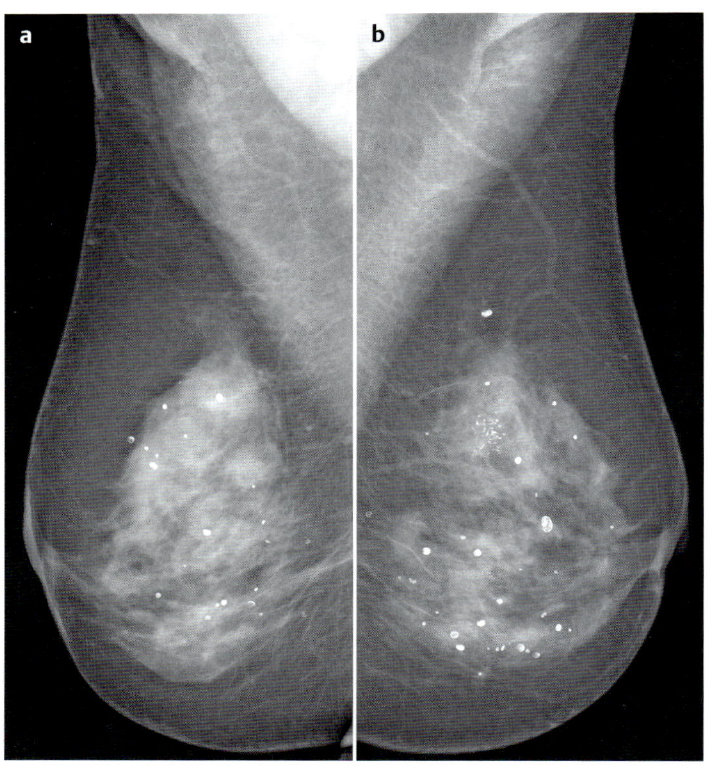


Fig. 95.**2 a, b** Digital mammography, MLO view.

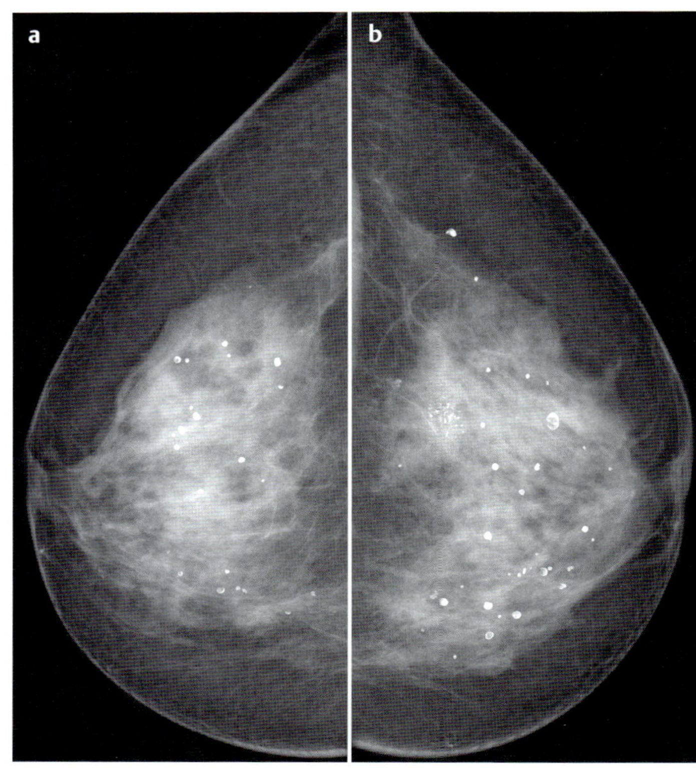


Fig. 95.**3 a, b** Digital mammography, CC view.

Please characterize ultrasound and mammography findings.
What is your preliminary diagnosis?
What are your next steps?

| BI-RADS Categorization | | |
|---|---|---|
| Clinical Findings | right 1 | left 1 |
| Ultrasound | right 1 | left 3 |
| Mammography | right 1 | left 5 |
| **BI-RADS Total** | **right 1** | **left 5** |

This case presents screening mammography images of an asymptomatic woman.

### Ultrasound

Possibly corresponding to the finding in mammography, ultrasound depicted a hypoechoic, lobulated lesion (diameter 7 mm) with indeterminate distal echo pattern. US BI-RADS left 3.

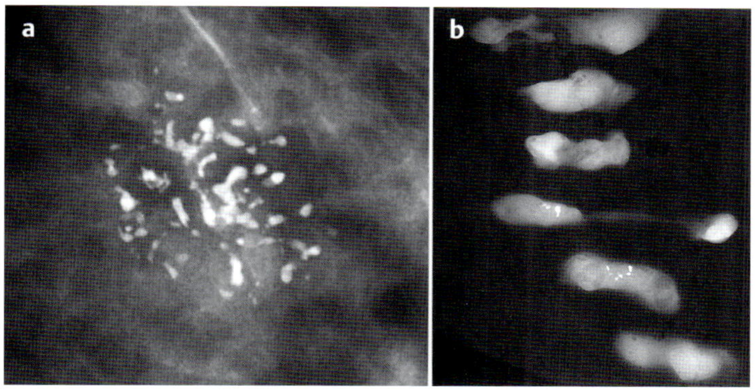


Fig. 95.**4 a, b** Magnification view mammogram and specimen radiogram.

### Mammography

Partially very dense parenchyma, ACR type 4. No suspicious masses or densities. No architectural distortions. Diffuse, monomorphous macrocalcifications. Additionally, there was a cluster of polymorphous microcalcifications in the central part of the left breast, with no accompanying density. BI-RADS right 1/left 5. PGMI: CC view P; MLO view G (inframammary fold).

### Procedure

Stereotactic vacuum biopsy.

### Histology of the specimen

Ductal carcinoma in situ.

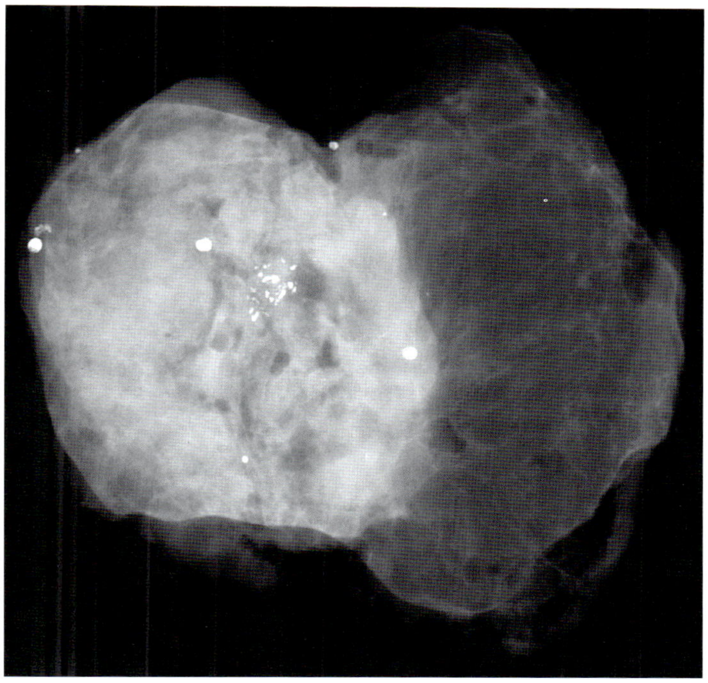

Fig. 95.**5** Specimen radiography after tumor excision.

### Diagnosis

Microinvasive ductal carcinoma in situ.

IDC pT1mic, pN0 (sn), G2, M0.

### Treatment

Breast conservation therapy of the left breast.

Microcalcifications are often the first sign of breast cancer seen in mammography.

**Indication:** Monitoring following earlier breast cancer.
**History:** Carcinoma and mastectomy of the right breast. Reduction surgery on the left breast. Dermatomyositis.
**Risk profile:** Increased by earlier incidence of breast cancer.
**Age:** 68 years.

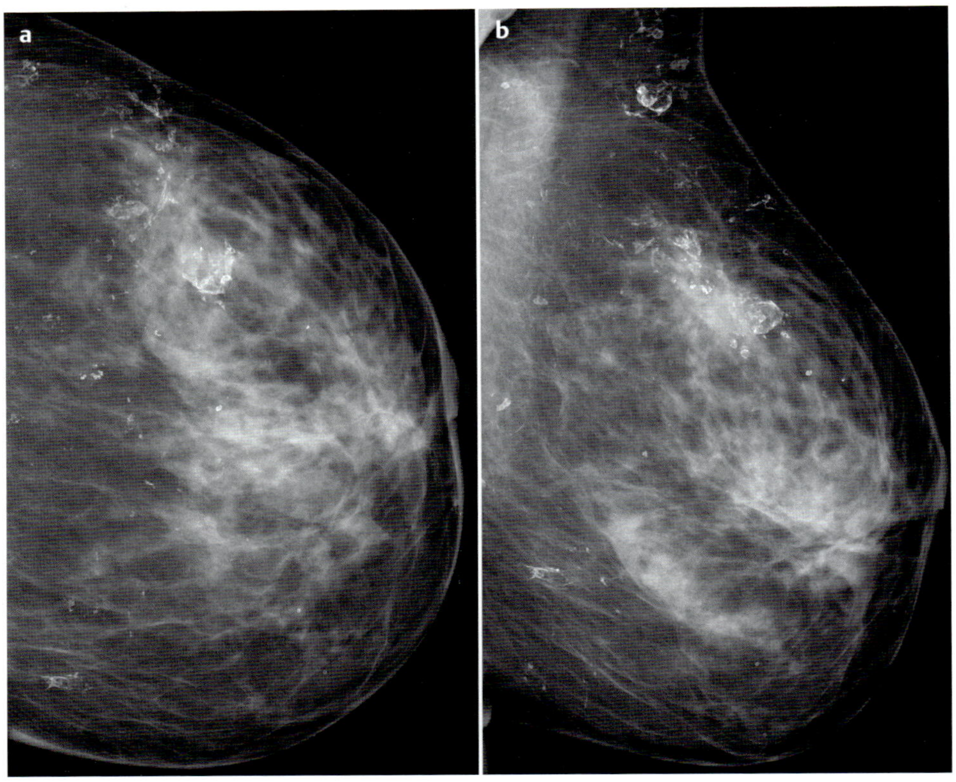


Fig. 96.**1 a, b** Digital mammography of the left breast, CC and MLO views.

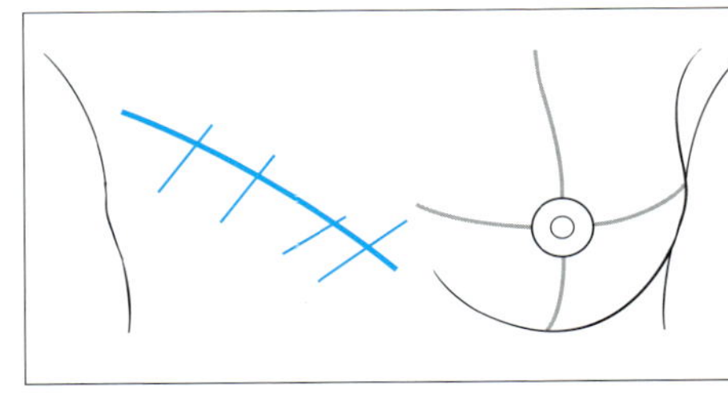

### Clinical Findings

Normal scar on the right side. No unusual findings in the left breast.

### Ultrasound (not shown)

Unremarkable.

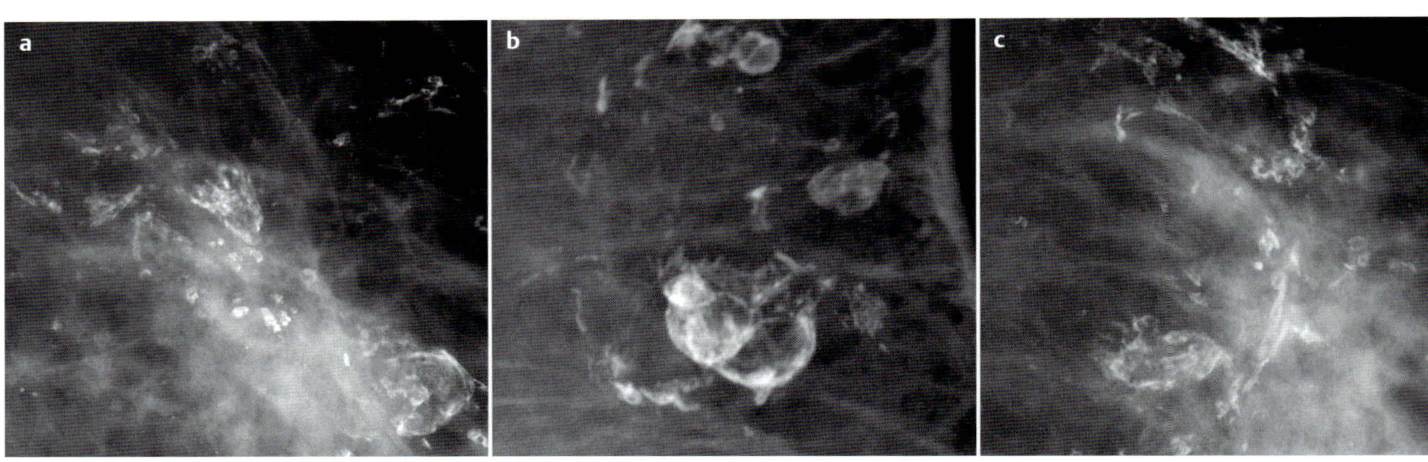


Fig. 96.**2 a, b** Magnification views of the calcifications in three locations within the left breast.

?

Please characterize the mammography findings.
What is your preliminary diagnosis?
What are your next steps?

| BI-RADS Categorization | | |
|---|---|---|
| Clinical Findings | right – | left 1 |
| Ultrasound | right – | left 1 |
| Mammography | right – | left 2 |
| **BI-RADS Total** | **right –** | **left 2** |

The imaging was performed in the context of monitoring following carcinoma and mastectomy of the right breast.

### Ultrasound

Unremarkable (not shown).

### Mammography

Inhomogeneously dense parenchyma, ACR type 3. Particularly in the upper quadrants, mammography depicted bizarre macrocalcifications. No masses or densities. No suspicious microcalcifications. BI-RADS right –/left 2.

### Procedure

No further investigation. It is recommended that mammographic examinations continue at the usual intervals for monitoring purposes.

## Diagnosis (without histological confirmation)

Postoperative fat necroses and oil cysts with macrocalcifications.*

* Findings subsequently remained unchanged over several years.

## Treatment

None.

Macrocalcifications within fat necrosis provide an immediate diagnosis. There is usually no differential diagnosis.

**Indication:** Screening.
**History:** Unremarkable.
**Risk profile:** Breast cancer in an aunt at the age of 30 years.
**Age:** 47 years.

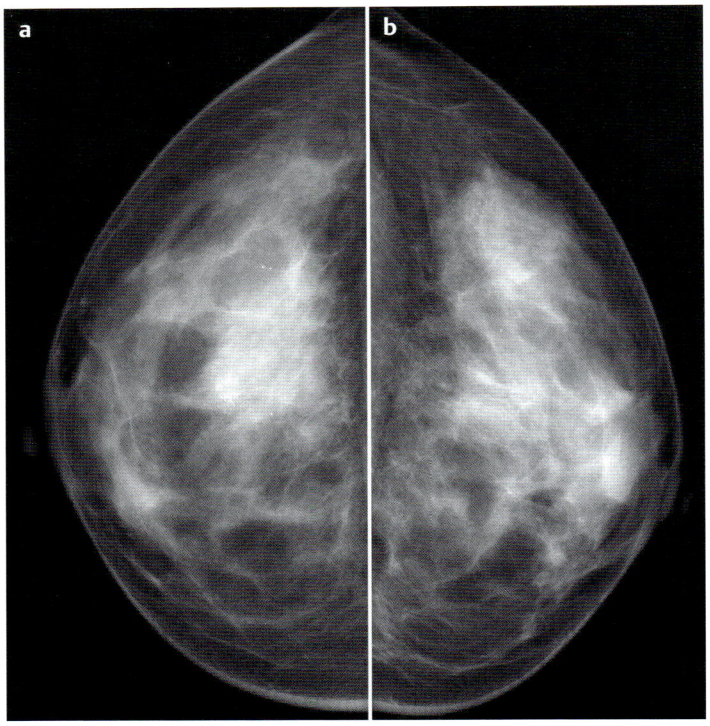

Fig. 97.1 **a, b** Digital mammography, CC view.

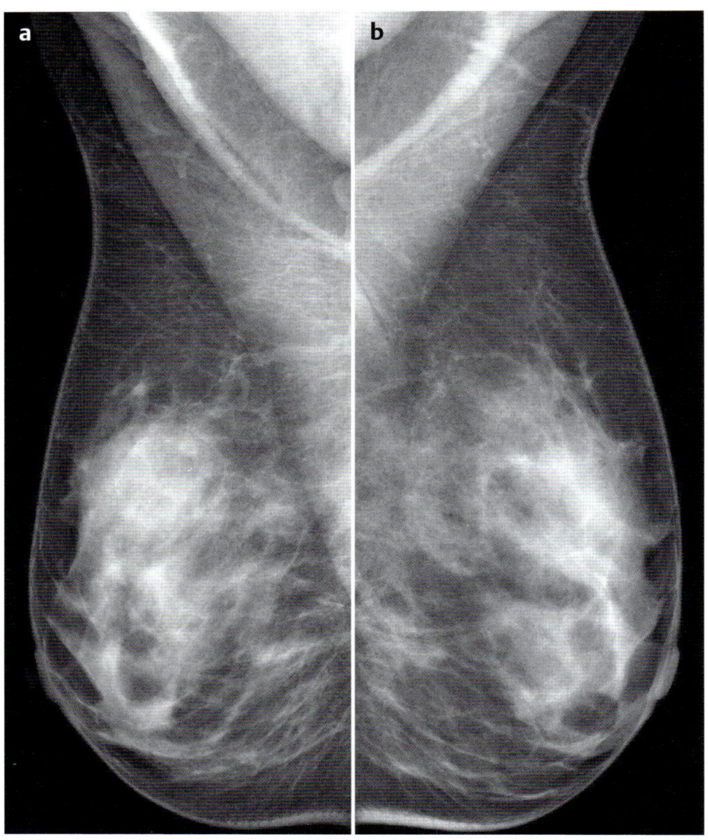

Fig. 97.2 **a, b** Digital mammography, MLO view.

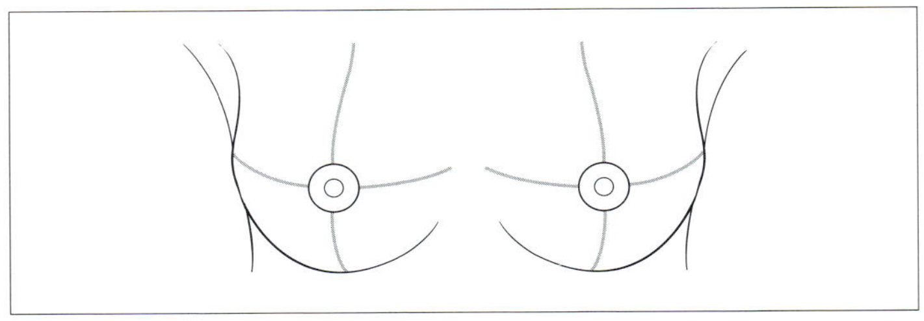

## Clinical Findings

Normal.

## Ultrasound (not shown)

No findings.

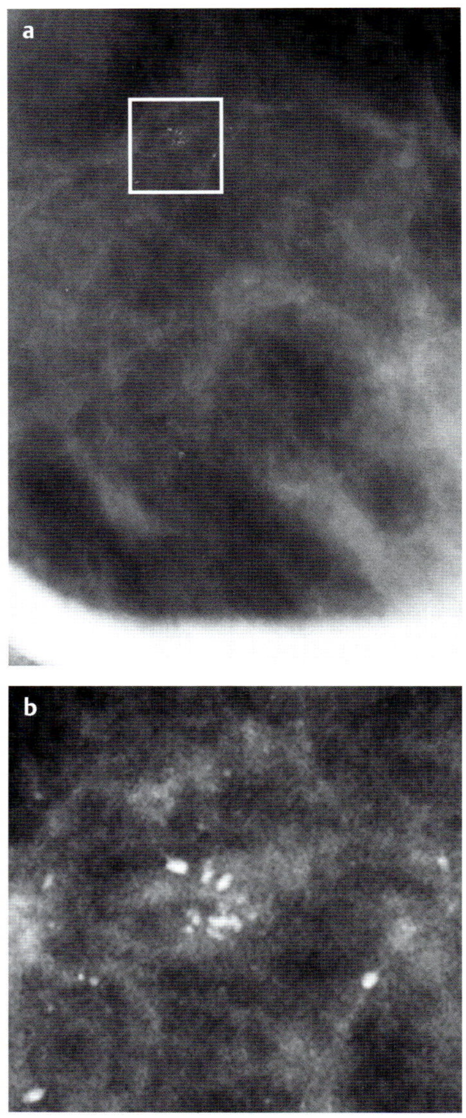

Fig. 97.3 **a, b** Magnification view of the left breast (MLO) and enlarged image.

Please characterize the mammography findings.
What is your preliminary diagnosis?
What are your next steps?

| BI-RADS Categorization | | |
|---|---|---|
| Clinical Findings | right 1 | left 1 |
| Ultrasound | right 1 | left 1 |
| Mammography | right 1 | left 4 |
| **BI-RADS Total** | **right 1** | **left 4** |

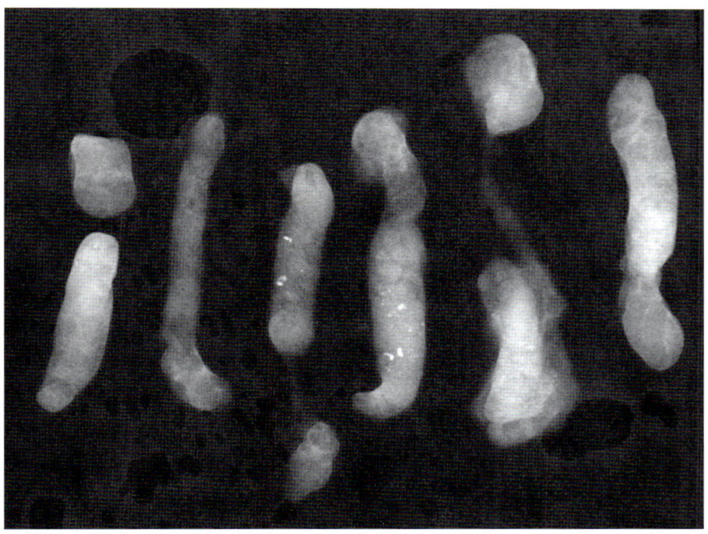

Fig. 97.**4** Specimen radiography.

This is the imaging study of an asymptomatic woman.

### Mammography

Partially extremely dense parenchyma, ACR type 4. Under these limiting conditions, no suspicious masses or densities. No architectural distortions. In the upper outer quadrant of the left breast, there was a cluster of polymorphous microcalcifications with a radial distribution pattern. BI-RADS right 1/left 4. PGMI: CC view P; MLO view G (inframammary fold).

### Procedure

Stereotactic vacuum biopsy.

### Diagnosis

Sclerosing adenosis.

### Treatment

None, but a single follow-up examination after 6 months is recommended.

Microcalcifications caused by sclerosing adenosis sometimes have suspicious characteristics. Vacuum core biopsy avoided the need for this woman to undergo an unnecessary open biopsy.

**Indication:** Screening.
**History:** Unremarkable.
**Risk profile:** No increased risk.
**Age:** 51 years.

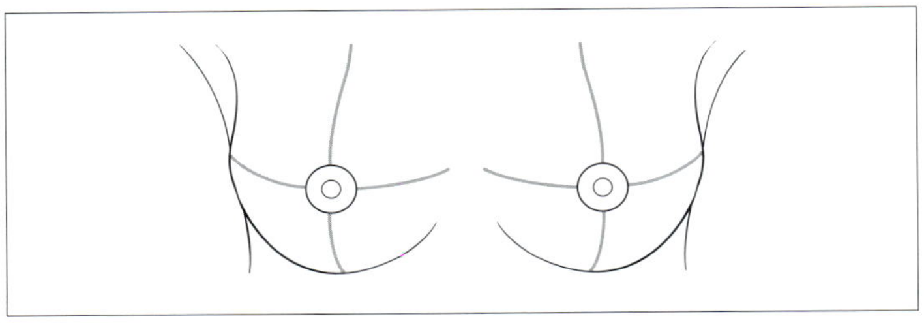

**Clinical Findings**

Normal.

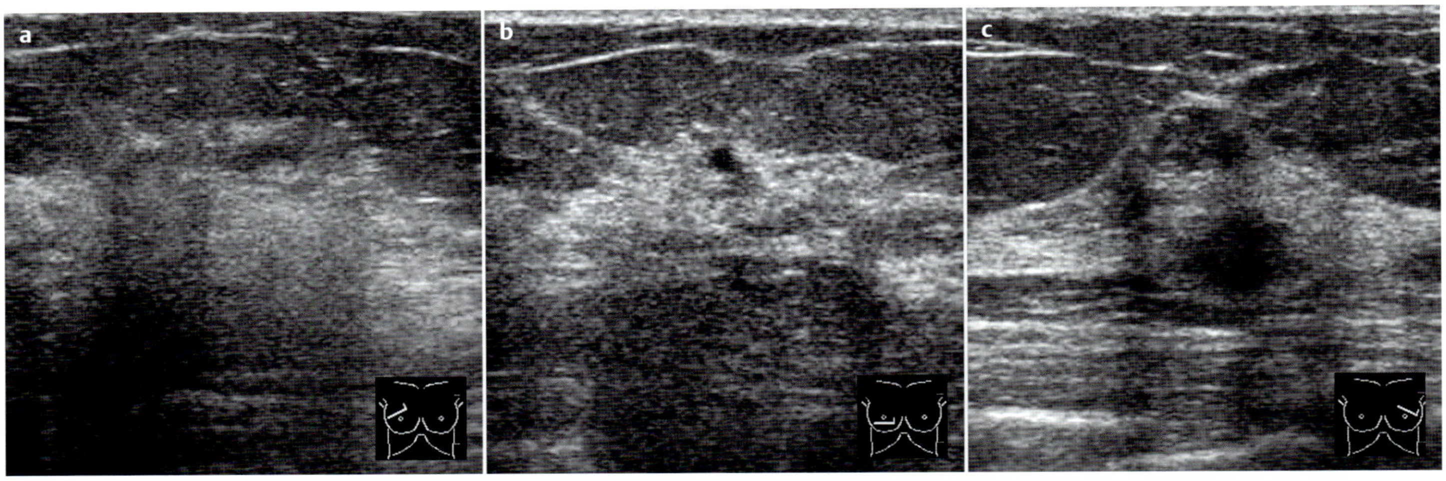

Fig. 98.**1 a – c** Sonography.

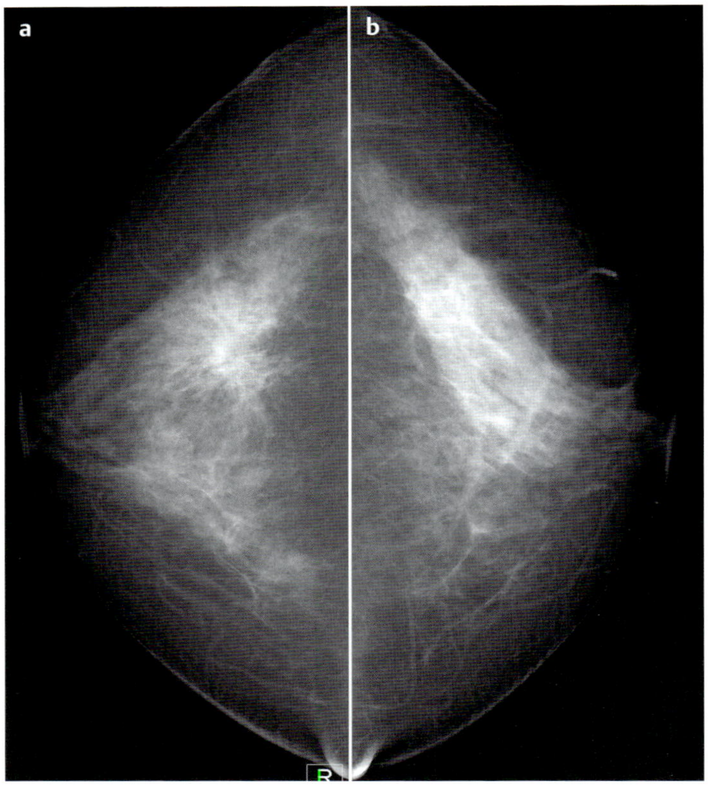

Fig. 98.**2 a, b** Digital mammography, CC view.

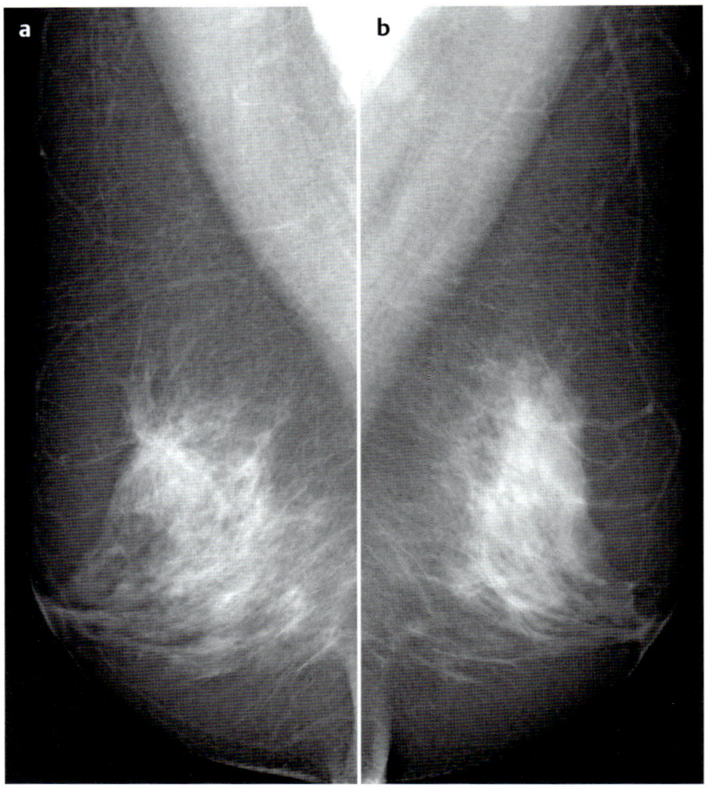

Fig. 98.**3 a, b** Digital mammography, MLC view.

?

Please characterize the ultrasound and mammography findings.
What is your preliminary diagnosis?
What are your next steps?

| BI-RADS Categorization | | |
|---|---|---|
| Clinical Findings | right 1 | left 1 |
| Ultrasound | right 2 | left 2 |
| Mammography | right 4 | left 1 |
| **BI-RADS Total** | **right 4** | **left 2** |

The images presented were obtained in the context of a screening examination.

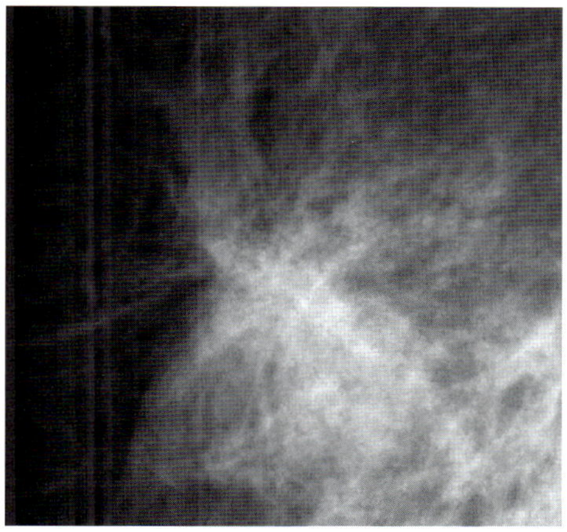

Fig. 98.**4** Magnification view of the cranial region of the right breast.

### Ultrasound

Bilaterally ultrasound showed glandular tissue with macrocysts. No signs of malignancy in the upper outer quadrant of the right breast or elsewhere. US BI-RADS right 2/left 2.

### Mammography

Extremely dense, asymmetric glandular texture (ACR type 4) with signs of tissue retraction in the upper outer quadrant of the right breast (architectural distortion, Fig. 98.**4**). Margins of a tumor could not be distinctly established. No microcalcifications. No further unusual findings. BI-RADS right 4/left 1. PGMI: CC view P; MLO view G (inframammary fold).

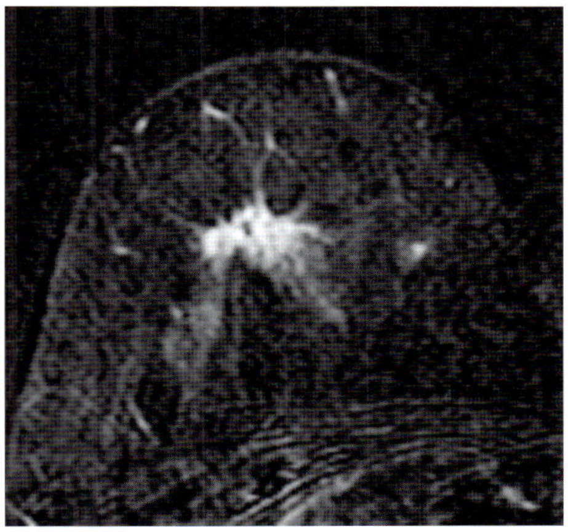

Fig. 98.**5** Contrast-enhanced MR mammography of the right breast.

### Procedure

Histological investigation (here by MR-guided vacuum core biopsy). Diagnostic MR mammography (Fig. 98.**5**).

### Histology of the core biopsy (right breast)

Invasive ductal carcinoma G2 developed from a base of DCIS (high grade, without necrosis).

### Histology

Invasive ductal carcinoma measuring 14 mm with an extensive intraductal component.

IDC pT1c + EIC, pN0 (0/21), G2.

### Treatment

Breast conservation therapy of the right breast.

Architectural distortion seen in mammography can be a sign of malignancy and warrants further investigation in cases where there are no previous operations in the patient's history.

**Indication:** Lump in the right breast.
**History:** Resection of fibroadenoma 16 months previously (right breast).
**Risk profile:** No increased risk.
**Age:** 39 years.

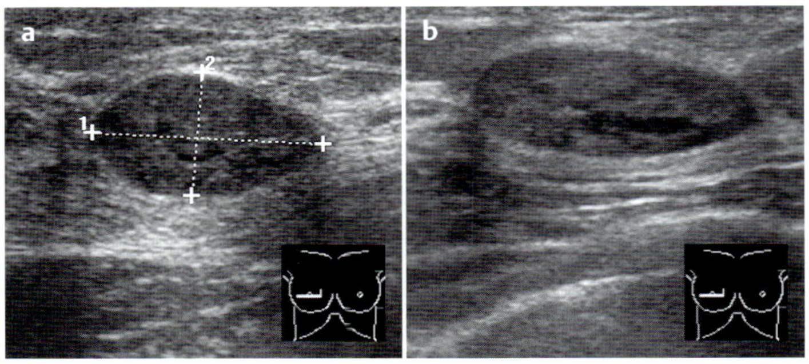

Fig. 99.1 **a, b** Sonography. Conventional (**a**) and with compression (**b**).

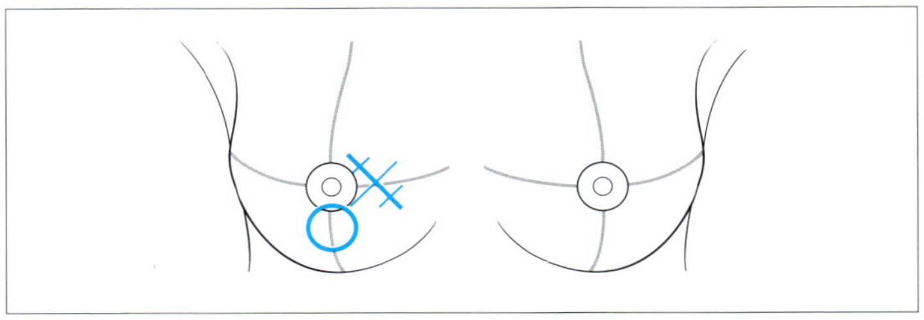

### Clinical Findings

Unremarkable scar on the right breast. Mobile lump between the lower quadrants of the right breast.

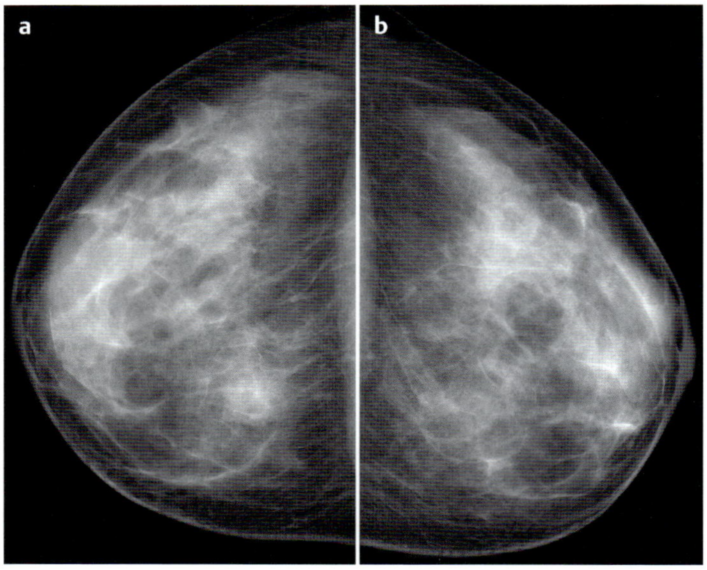

Fig. 99.2 **a, b** Digital mammography, CC view.

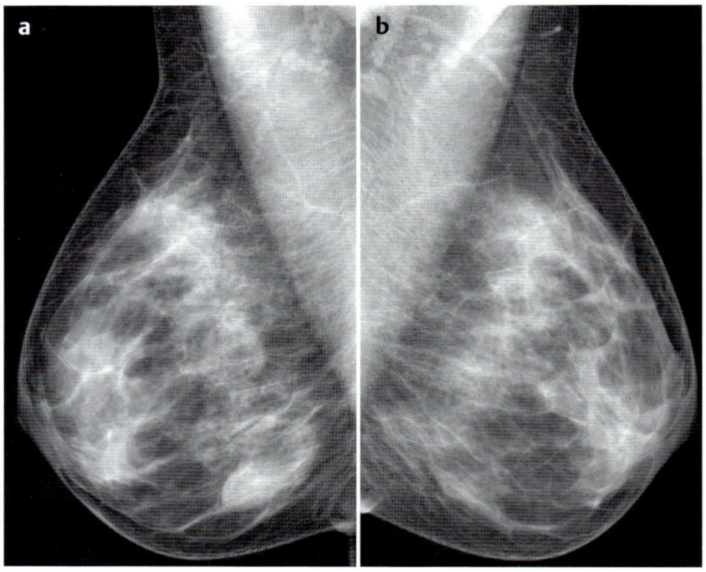

Fig. 99.3 **a, b** Digital mammography, MLO view.

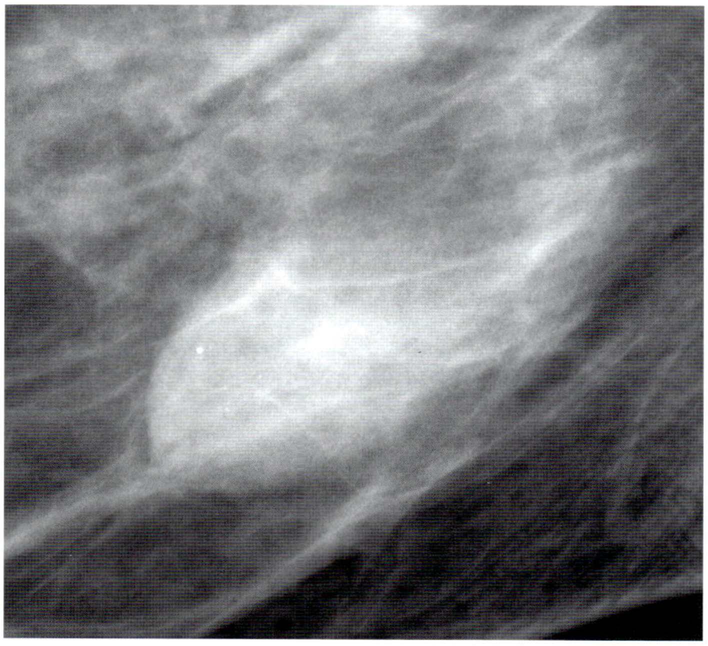

Fig. 99.4 Magnification view of the caudal region of the right breast.

Please characterize ultrasound and mammography findings.
What is your preliminary diagnosis?
What are your next steps?

| BI-RADS Categorization | | |
|---|---|---|
| Clinical Findings | right 3 | left 1 |
| Ultrasound | right 3 | left 1 |
| Mammography | right 3 | left 1 |
| **BI-RADS Total** | **right 3** | **left 1** |

This case presents the diagnostic imaging of a symptomatic young woman with a recently discovered lump in the right breast.

### Ultrasound

Oval lesion with well-defined margins and predominantly homogeneous texture as well as an internal linear anechoic region. Long axis parallel to the skin. Peritumoral no abnormalities. Under compression the lesion's shape clearly altered along the long axis. US BI-RADS right 3.

### Mammography

Bilaterally symmetric, partially markedly dense glandular tissue, ACR type 4. In the lower inner quadrant of the right breast there was a partially superimposed, otherwise well-defined oval and isodense lesion. Both mammography views depicted a solitary calcification within the lesion. No further abnormalities. BI-RADS right 3/left 1. PGMI: CC view P; MLO view G (inframammary fold).

### → Preliminary Diagnosis

Fibroadenoma, adenoma, papilloma, hamartoma (cystic areas within lesion), phyllodes tumor (this gives rise to the categorization as BI-RADS 3), medullary carcinoma (very unlikely).

### Next step according to guidelines

US-guided percutaneous core biopsy.

### Procedure followed here

At the patient's request, the palpable lump was completely resected by open biopsy.

### Histology

Adenomyoepithelioma.

### Treatment

Excisional biopsy, no further therapy.

Adenomyoepithelioma of the breast is a rare benign mixed tumor that forms across both epithelial and myoepithelial tissue structures.

**Indication:** Screening mammography.
**Age:** 52 years.

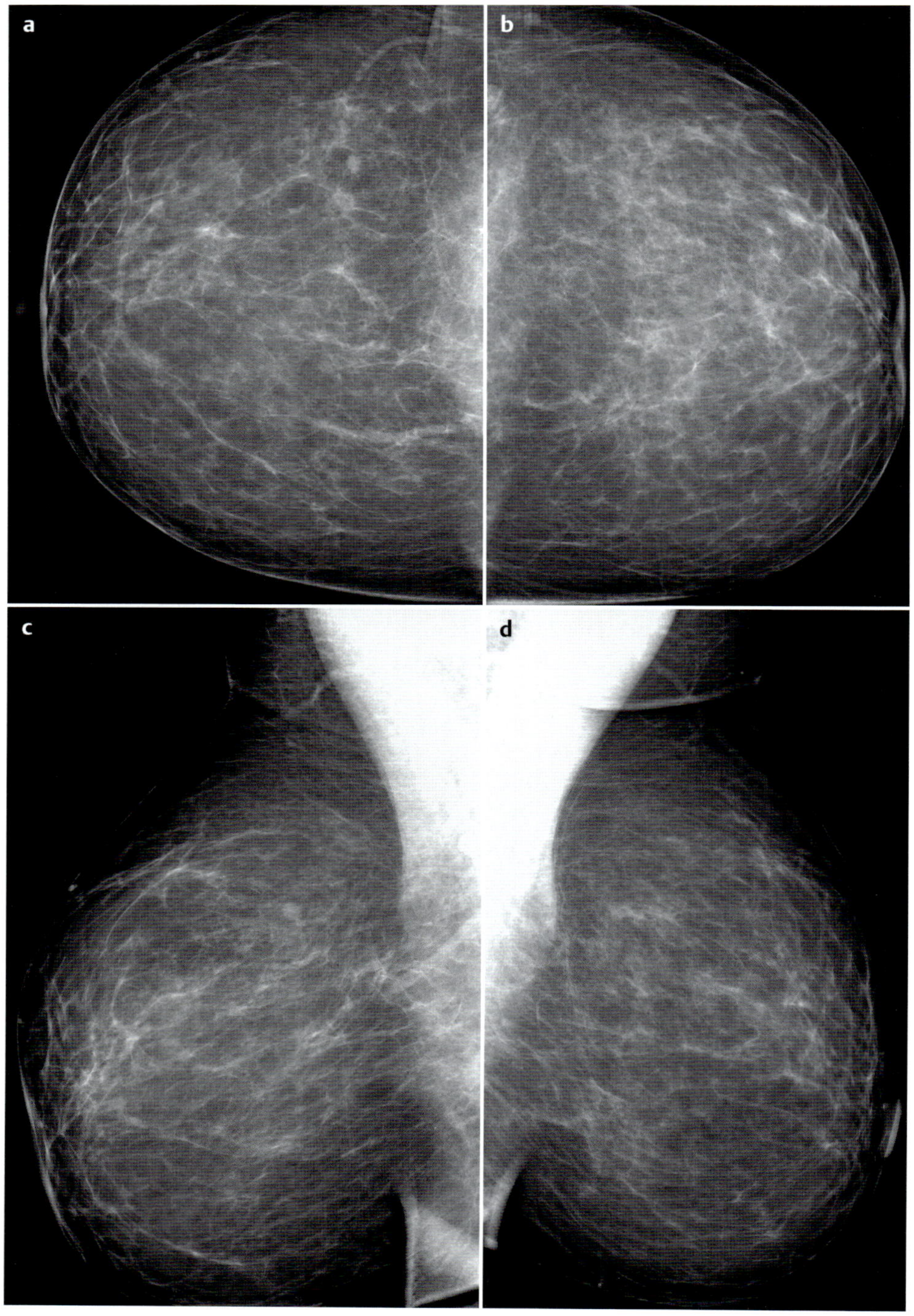


Fig. 100.**1 a – d** Digital mammography of both breasts, CC and MLO views.

?

Would you recall this woman for further investigation?

In conclusion, let's take a look at the future of comprehensive breast diagnostics.

Of course you spotted the spiculated lesion in the right breast at the 11-o'clock position ... didn't you? After the consultation, this woman should be recalled for further investigation, and adjunctive modalities should always be considered.

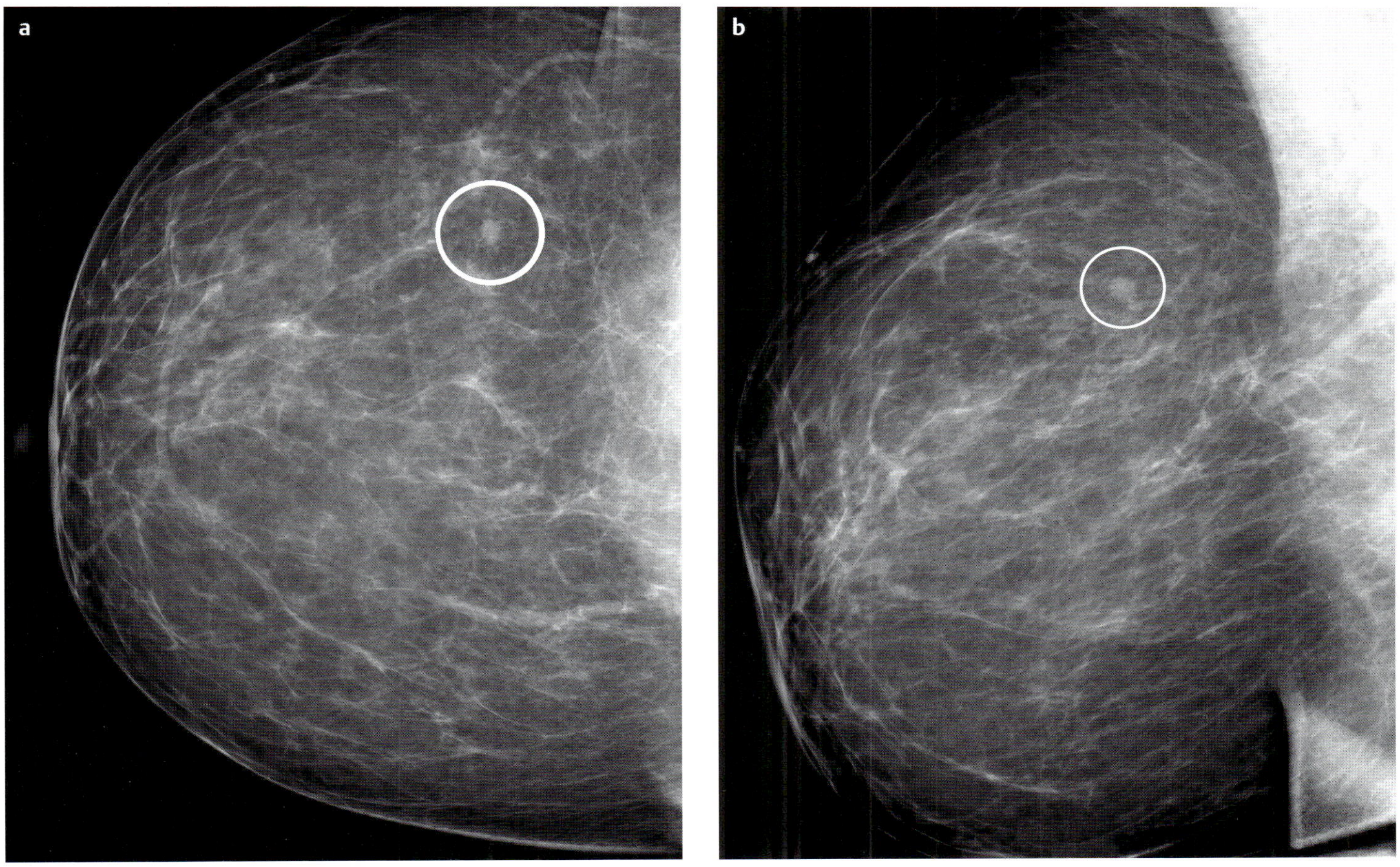


Fig. 100.**2 a, b** Spiculated lesion in the upper outer quadrant of the right breast. Histology: carcinoma.

### Histology

IDC pT1b, pN0, G2.

Take-home point: Only two thirds of all breast carcinomas are detected in classic mammography screening programs. An individually-tailored diagnostic program, including ultrasound and MRI if necessary, could detect a large proportion of the remainder at an equally early stage.

Conclusion: In breast diagnostics we have powerful technology at our disposal–it must now be widely applied.

**With diagnoses**

Numbers in **bold** type refer to case numbers, normal type refers to page numbers.